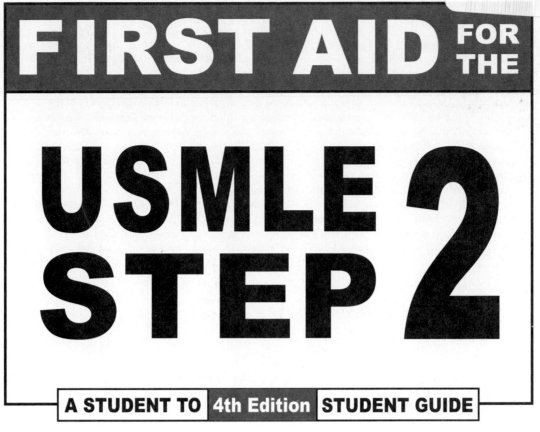

FIRST AID FOR THE

USMLE STEP 2

A STUDENT TO 4th Edition STUDENT GUIDE

FIRST AID FOR THE

USMLE STEP 2

A STUDENT TO 4th Edition **STUDENT GUIDE**

TAO LE, MD
University of California, San Francisco, Class of 1996
Johns Hopkins University, Fellow in Allergy and Immunology

VIKAS BHUSHAN, MD
University of California, San Francisco, Class of 1991
Diagnostic Radiologist

CHIRAG AMIN, MD
University of Miami, Class of 1996
Orthopaedic Surgeon

JENNIFER LaFEMINA, MD
University of California, Los Angeles, Class of 2003
Resident in Surgery, Massachusetts General Hospital

JESSICA NORD, MD
University of California, Los Angeles, Class of 2002
Resident in Psychiatry, UCLA

NADER POURATIAN, MD, PhD
University of California, Los Angeles, Class of 2003
Resident in Neurological Surgery, University of Virginia

McGraw-Hill
Medical Publishing Division

New York Chicago San Francisco Lisbon London Madrid
Mexico City Milan New Delhi San Juan Seoul
Singapore Sydney Toronto

First Aid for the USMLE Step 2, Fourth Edition

1 2 3 4 5 6 7 8 9 0   CUS/CUS   0 9 8 7 6 5 4 3

ISBN 0-07-140930-0

ISSN 1532-320X

This book was set in Goudy by Rainbow Graphics.
The editor was Catherine A. Johnson.
The production supervisor was Phil Galea.
Project management was provided by Rainbow Graphics.
Editorial services was provided by Andrea Fellows.
The interior designer was Elizabeth Sanders.
The index was prepared by Oneida Indexing.

Von Hoffman Graphics was printer and binder.

This book is printed on acid-free paper.

ISBN 0-07-121915-3 (international)
Copyright © 2003. Exclusive rights by The McGraw-Hill Companies, Inc. for manufacture and export. This book cannot be re-exported from the country to which it is consigned by McGraw-Hill. The International Edition is not available in North America.

To our families, friends, and loved ones, who endured
and assisted in the task of assembling this guide.

&

To the contributors to this and future editions, who took
time to share their knowledge, insight, and
humor for the benefit of students.

Contributing Authors

ZACHARY V. EDMONDS
UCLA School of Medicine & Anderson School of
   Management, Class of 2004

ASHKAN LASHKARI, MD
UCLA School of Medicine, Class of 2003

ROBERT A. LEE, MD, PhD
UCLA School of Medicine, Class of 2003

TIMOTHY PLATTS-MILLS, MD
UCLA School of Medicine, 2003

JENNIFER SERRANO, MD
UCLA School of Medicine, Class of 2003

Faculty Reviewers

ANDREW D. WATSON, MD, PhD
Fellow in Cardiology
UCLA Medical Center
Cardiovascular

DANIEL BEHROOZAN, MD
Chief Resident, Dermatology
Los Angeles County/King-Drew Medical Center
Charles R. Drew University of Medicine and Science
Dermatology

IRINA A. URUSOVA, MD
Fellow in Endocrinology
Cedars Sinai Medical Center
Endocrinology

FRANK DAY, MD
Associate Professor of Medicine
UCLA Medical Center
Epidemiology and Public Health

STANLEY G. KORENMAN, MD
Associate Dean, Ethics and Medical Scientist
    Training Program
UCLA School of Medicine
Ethics

WALEED SHINDY, MD
Fellow in Gastroenterology
UCLA School of Medicine
Gastroenterology

GARY SCHILLER, MD
Associate Professor of Medicine
UCLA Medical Center
Hematology/Oncology

GUNTER RIEG, MD
Fellow in Infectious Disease
Harbor-UCLA Medical Center
Infectious Disease

GARY GHISELLI, MD
Chief Resident, Orthopaedic Surgery
UCLA Department of Orthopaedic Surgery
Musculoskeletal

LARA M. SCHRADER, MD
Assistant Professor
UCLA Department of Neurology
Neurology

ASHIM KUMAR, MD
Fellow in Reproductive Endocrinology and Infertility
UCLA Medical Center
Obstetrics and Gynecology

BYRON PATTERSON, MD
Fellow in Pediatric Sports Medicine
UCLA
Pediatrics

SVETLANA ANIC, MD
Fellow in Child and Adolescent Psychiatry
Neuropsychiatric Institute and Hospital
UCLA
Psychiatry

DANI HACKNER, MD
Director, Transitional Critical Care Service
Associate Chair, Medicine
Cedars-Sinai Medical Center
Pulmonary

RUTH WINTZ, MD
Fellow in Nephrology
UCLA Medical Center
Renal

CHRISTIAN DE VIRGILIO, MD
General Surgery Residency Program Director
Harbor-UCLA Medical Center
Associate Professor of Surgery
UCLA
Selected Topics in Emergency Medicine

Contents

Color Illustration Section (16 pages) between pages 520 and 521

Preface

With the fourth edition of *First Aid for the USMLE Step 2*, we continue our commitment to providing students with the most useful and up-to-date preparation guide for the USMLE Step 2. The fourth edition represents a thorough revision in many ways and includes:

- A completely revised and updated exam preparation guide for the new computerized USMLE Step 2. Includes detailed analysis as well as all new study and test-taking strategies for the new computer-based testing (CBT) format.
- Revisions and new material based on student experience with the 2001 and 2002 administrations of the USMLE Step 2.
- Concise summaries of over 300 heavily tested clinical topics.
- A basic science primer for each medical subspecialty, focusing on clinically relevant high-yield basic science facts from the 2003 edition of *First Aid for the USMLE Step 1*.
- A "rapid review" that tests your knowledge of each topic.
- Boards-type clinical vignettes, with explanations, from McGraw-Hill's updated *PreTest®* series for the USMLE Step 2.
- A revised collection of over 120 high-yield glossy photos similar to those appearing on the USMLE Step 2 exam.
- Useful reference links to prototypical clinical cases from the popular *Underground Clinical Vignette* series (Blackwell Science).
- A completely revised, in-depth guide to clinical science review and sample examination books.

The fourth edition would not have been possible without the help of the many students and faculty members who contributed their feedback and suggestions. We invite students and faculty to continue sharing their thoughts and ideas to help us improve *First Aid for the USMLE Step 2*. (See How to Contribute, p. xv, and User Survey, p. xxiii.)

Baltimore   Tao Le
Los Angeles   Vikas Bhushan
Los Angeles   Chirag Amin
Boston   Jennifer LaFemina
Los Angeles   Jessica Nord
Charlottesville   Nader Pouratian

Acknowledgments

This has been a collaborative project from the start. We gratefully acknowledge the thoughtful comments, corrections, and advice of the many medical students, international medical graduates, and faculty who have supported the authors in the continuing development of *First Aid for the USMLE Step 2.*

For significant contributions to the fourth edition, we would like to thank Patricia Moore, Seth Goldbarg, Biren Modi, and Brian Lester. For review of the International Medical Graduate section, a special thank you to Mae Sheikh-Ali and Fadi Abu Shahin. Thanks to Elizabeth Sanders and Ashley Pound for the interior design.

For support and encouragement throughout the process, we are grateful to Thao Pham and Selina Bush.

Thanks to our publisher, McGraw-Hill, for the valuable assistance of their staff. For enthusiasm, support, and commitment for this challenging project, thanks to our editor, Catherine Johnson. For outstanding editorial work, we thank Andrea Fellows. A special thanks to Jimmy and Bennie Sauls (Rainbow Graphics) for remarkable production work.

For contributions, corrections, and surveys we thank Geneen Gin, Jennifer L. Sigsbee-Gonzales, Leslie Huddleston, Kristofer S. Matullo, Sara Best, Jennifer Bang, Constance Lynne, Tracey Mueller, Jennifer B. Higgins, Borislava Burt, L. Andrew Evans, Daniel Bytnar, Anna Flinn, Luc Readinger, Tiffany Heutel, Lauren F.C. Jones, Amy Williams, Hoang T. Vu, Kaman Chong, Leslie Huddleston, Anna Flinn, Ajay V. Raman, Tiffany Heutel, Elizabeth Chung, Tran Hung, Ruben Kalra, Carla Kovacs, Brian Freeman, Derek Rosner, Ernest Lee, J. Douglas Miles, Eric Lee, Bruce Gelb, Debby Rovine, Ashishkumar Shah, and Steven Zeddun.

Our apologies if we accidentally omitted or misspelled your name.

Baltimore	Tao Le
Los Angeles	Vikas Bhushan
Los Angeles	Chirag Amin
Boston	Jennifer LaFemina
Los Angeles	Jessica Nord
Charlottesville	Nader Pouratian

How to Contribute

This version of *First Aid for the USMLE Step 2* incorporates hundreds of contributions and changes suggested by faculty and student reviewers. We invite you to participate in this process. We also offer **paid internships** in medical education and publishing ranging from three months to one year (see next page for details).

Please send us your suggestions for:

- Study and test-taking strategies for the computerized USMLE Step 2
- New facts, mnemonics, diagrams, and illustrations
- High-yield topics that may reappear on future Step 2 exams
- Low-yield topics to remove
- Personal ratings and comments on review books that you have examined

For each entry incorporated into the next edition, you will receive a $10 gift certificate, as well as personal acknowledgment in the next edition. Diagrams, tables, partial entries, updates, corrections, and study hints are also appreciated, and significant contributions will be compensated at the discretion of the authors. Also let us know about material in this edition that you feel is low yield and should be deleted.

The **preferred way** to submit entries, suggestions, or corrections is via **electronic mail.** Please include name, address, school affiliation, phone number, and e-mail address (if different from the address of origin). If there are multiple entries, please consolidate into a single e-mail or file attachment. Please send submissions to:

firstaidteam@yahoo.com

Otherwise, please send entries, neatly written or typed or on disk (Microsoft Word), to: First Aid for the USMLE Step 2, P.O. Box 27, Woodstock, MD 21163-9982, Attention: Contributions. Please use the contribution and survey forms on the following pages. Each form constitutes an entry. Attach additional pages as needed.

Internship Opportunities

The author team is pleased to offer part-time and full-time paid internships in medical education and publishing to motivated medical students and physicians. Internships may range from three months (e.g., a summer) up to a full year. Participants will have an opportunity to author, edit, and earn academic credit on a wide variety of projects, including the popular *First Aid* series. Writing/editing experience, familiarity with Microsoft Word, and Internet access are desired. For more information, e-mail a résumé or a short description of your experience along with a cover letter to the authors at their e-mail address above.

Note to Contributors

All entries become property of the authors and are subject to editing and reviewing. Please verify all data and spellings carefully. In the event that similar or duplicate entries are received, only the first entry received will be used. Include a reference to a standard textbook to facilitate verification of the fact. Please follow the style, punctuation, and format of this edition if possible.

Contribution Form I

Contributor Name: _____

School/Affiliation: _____

Address: _____

_____

Telephone: _____

E-mail: _____

Topic:

Signs and Symptoms:

Diagnosis:

Management:

Notes, Diagrams, Tables, and Mnemonics:

Reference:

You will receive personal acknowledgment and $10 gift certificate for each entry that is used in future editions.

Please seal with tape only.
No staples or paper clips.

-- (fold here) --

FIRST AID FOR THE USMLE STEP 2
P.O. BOX 27
WOODSTOCK, MD 21163

-- (fold here) --

Contribution Form II

Contributor Name: _____

School/Affiliation: _____

Address: _____

_____

Telephone: _____

E-mail: _____

Please place the clinical topic (e.g., ulcerative colitis) on the first line and the high-yield vignette or topic on the following two lines.

1. Subject: _____
    Vignette: _____
    _____

2. Subject: _____
    Vignette: _____
    _____

3. Subject: _____
    Vignette: _____
    _____

4. Subject: _____
    Vignette: _____
    _____

5. Subject: _____
    Vignette: _____
    _____

6. Subject: _____
    Vignette: _____
    _____

7. Subject: _____
    Vignette: _____
    _____

8. Subject: _____
    Vignette: _____
    _____

9. Subject: _____
    Vignette: _____
    _____

10. Subject: _____
    Vignette: _____
    _____

You will receive personal acknowledgment and $10 gift certificate for each entry that is used in future editions.

Please seal with tape only.
No staples or paper clips.

-------------------------------- (fold here) --------------------------------

FIRST AID FOR THE USMLE STEP 2
P.O. BOX 27
WOODSTOCK, MD   21163

-------------------------------- (fold here) --------------------------------

Contribution Form III

Contributor Name: _____

School/Affiliation: _____

Address: _____

_____

Telephone: _____

E-mail: _____

We welcome additional comments on review resources rated in Section III as well as reviews of resources not rated in Section III. Please fill out each review entry as completely as possible. Please do not leave "Comments" blank. Rate texts using the letter grading scale provided on p. 523, taking into consideration current ratings of other books on that subject.

1. **Title/Author:** _____ Days needed to read: _____

   Publisher/Series: _____ ISBN Number: _____

   Rating: _____ **Comments:** _____

   _____

   _____

2. **Title/Author:** _____ Days needed to read: _____

   Publisher/Series: _____ ISBN Number: _____

   Rating: _____ **Comments:** _____

   _____

   _____

3. **Title/Author:** _____ Days needed to read: _____

   Publisher/Series: _____ ISBN Number: _____

   Rating: _____ **Comments:** _____

   _____

   _____

   _____

4. **Title/Author:** _____ Days needed to read: _____

   Publisher/Series: _____ ISBN Number: _____

   Rating: _____ **Comments:** _____

   _____

   _____

5. **Title/Author:** _____ Days needed to read: _____

   Publisher/Series: _____ ISBN Number: _____

   Rating: _____ **Comments:** _____

   _____

   _____

You will receive personal acknowledgment and $10 gift certificate for each entry that is used in future editions.

Please seal with tape only.
No staples or paper clips.

-------------------------------- (fold here) --------------------------------

Place
Stamp
Here

FIRST AID FOR THE USMLE STEP 2
P.O. BOX 27
WOODSTOCK, MD   21163

-------------------------------- (fold here) --------------------------------

User Survey

Contributor Name: _____

School/Affiliation: _____

Address: _____

_____

_____

Telephone: _____

E-mail: _____

What student-to-student advice would you give someone preparing for the computerized USMLE Step 2?

What commercial review courses have you been enrolled in, and what were your overall assessments of the courses?

Please list any high-yield facts, topics, or vignettes that should be added.

Please list any current high-yield facts, topics, or vignettes in Section II that you think were inaccurate, low-yield, or should be deleted.

What review resources for the USMLE Step 2 are not covered in Section III? Would you change the rating of any of the review resources in Section III? If so, which one(s) and why?

What other suggestions do you have for improving *First Aid for the USMLE Step 2*? Any other comments or suggestions? What did you dislike most about the book? What did you like most?

You will receive personal acknowledgment and $10 gift certificate for each entry that is used in future editions.

Please seal with tape only.
No staples or paper clips.

(fold here)

FIRST AID FOR THE USMLE STEP 2
P.O. BOX 27
WOODSTOCK, MD   21163

(fold here)

Guide to Efficient Exam Preparation

The goal of Step 2 is to apply your knowledge of medical facts to actual situations you may encounter as a resident.

INTRODUCTION

For many U.S. medical graduates, the United States Medical Licensing Examination (USMLE) Step 2 is looked upon as an afterthought—an event shoved somewhere in between residency applications, "away" rotations, and matching. Nevertheless, the clinical approach of Step 2 allows you to pull together your clinical experience on the wards with the numerous "factoids" and classical disease presentations that you have memorized over the years. Whereas Step 1 stresses basic mechanisms and principles, Step 2 places more emphasis on clinical diagnosis, disease pathogenesis, and preventive medicine.

USMLE STEP 2—COMPUTER-BASED TESTING BASICS

The USMLE Step 2 is the second of three examinations that you must pass in order to become a licensed physician in the United States. The computerized Step 2 exam is a one-day (nine-hour) multiple-choice exam. Starting in 2002, the number of exam questions on Step 2 was reduced from 400 to 370, although test length remained the same. The exam includes questions in internal medicine, obstetrics and gynecology, pediatrics, preventive medicine, neurology, psychiatry, and surgery.

The computer-based test (CBT) is administered by Prometric, Inc.®, a subsidiary of Thomson Learning. Prometric test centers offer Step 2 testing on a year-round basis, except for the first two weeks in January. The exam is given every day except Sunday at most centers, although the schedule may vary at international test centers. Some schools administer the exam on their own campuses. The National Board of Medical Examiners (NBME) is currently developing new test software, known as FRED™, for the USMLE. FRED™ may replace the Prometric software in 2004. For the most up-to-date information, refer to *www.usmle.org*.

How Will the CBT Be Structured?

- **Test format.** The CBT is a one-day exam with 370 questions divided into eight blocks of 60 minutes each (see Figure 1). During the time allotted for each block, the examinee can answer test questions in any order as well as review responses and change answers. Once the allotted block time has expired, however, further review of test questions or changing of answers within that block is not possible. Expect to spend nine hours at the test center.
- **Test blocks.** The CBT's 60-minute blocks were designed to reduce eyestrain and fatigue during the exam. Once an examinee finishes a particular block, he or she must click on a screen icon to continue to the next block. Examinees cannot go back and change answers from previous blocks.

Testing Conditions: What Will the CBT Be Like?

Given the unique environment of the CBT, it is important that you familiarize yourself ahead of time with your test-day conditions. In particular, getting to know the testing interface before the exam can add to your break time. This is because a 15-minute tutorial, offered on exam day, may be skipped if you are already familiar with the exam procedures and the testing interface

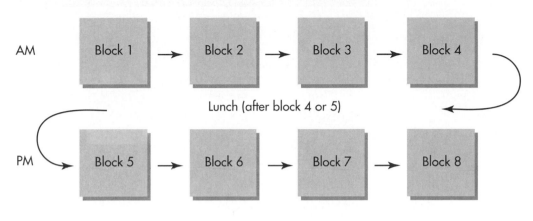

FIGURE 1. Schematic of CBT Exam

(CD-ROM, see below). These 15 minutes are added to your allotted break time of 45 minutes (should you choose to skip the tutorial).

For security reasons, examinees are not allowed to bring any personal electronic equipment into the testing area. This includes digital watches, watches with computer communication and/or memory capability, cellular telephones, and electronic paging devices. Food and beverages are also prohibited. Examinees are given laminated writing surfaces for note taking that must be returned after the examination. The testing centers are monitored by audio and video surveillance equipment.

The following information is based on software previews from the NBME. Check the USMLE Web site (*www.usmle.org*) or with your medical school for updates.

The typical question screen (see Figure 2) has a question followed by a number of answer choices and navigational buttons at the bottom of the screen. A

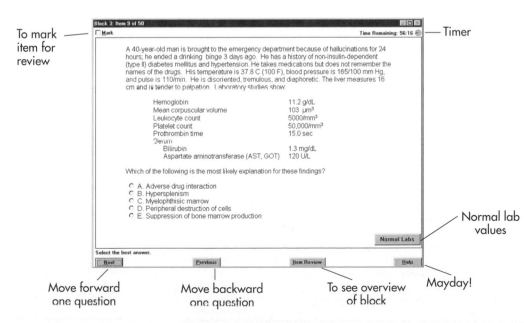

FIGURE 2. Typical Question Screen

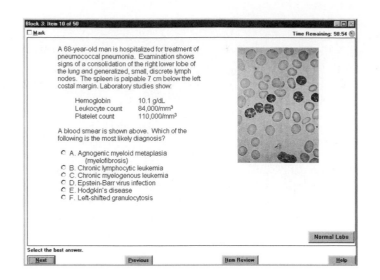

FIGURE 3. Question Screen with Illustration

countdown timer occupies the upper right-hand corner of the screen. If a question happens to be longer than the screen, a scroll bar will appear on the right, allowing the examinee to see the rest of the question. No matter whether the examinee clicks on an answer or leaves it blank, he or she must click the "Next>>" button in order to advance to the next question.

Some questions contain figures or color illustrations (see Figure 3). These are typically situated to the right of the question. Although the contrast and brightness of the screen can be adjusted, there are no other ways to manipulate the picture (e.g., zooming, panning).

The examinee can also call up a window displaying normal lab values (see Figure 4). However, if he or she does not click on "Tile" in the normal-values screen, the normal-values window will often obscure the question. In addition, the examinee will have to scroll down for most laboratory values.

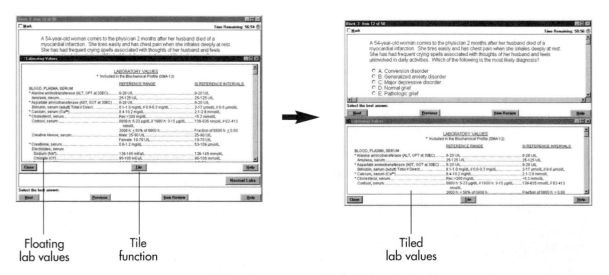

Floating lab values   Tile function   Tiled lab values

FIGURE 4. Lab Values Screen—Floating and Tiled

4

There is a button that allows an examinee to mark a question for review at a later time. Clicking "Item Review" at the bottom of the screen accesses a screen (see Figure 5) that displays an overview of the block, allowing the examinee to pinpoint questions marked for review along with any unanswered questions. This also serves as a quick way for users to navigate to any question in the block—even unmarked, completed questions.

What Does the CBT Format Mean for Me?

For most test takers, the CBT format is nothing new, since it is the same format you saw when you took the USMLE Step 1. However, if you still hate computers and freak out whenever you see one, you might want to confront your fears as soon as possible. Spend some time playing with a Windows-based system and pointing and clicking icons or buttons with a mouse. These are the absolute basics, and you will not want to waste valuable exam time figuring them out on test day. Your test taking will proceed by pointing and clicking, essentially without the use of the keyboard.

For those who feel they would benefit, the USMLE offers an opportunity to take a simulated test, or "Practice Session" at a Prometric center. Students are eligible to take the three-and-one-half-hour practice session after they have received their fluorescent orange scheduling permit (see below).

The same USMLE Step 2 sample test items (150 questions) that are available on the CD-ROM or the USMLE Web site (*www.usmle.org*) are used at CBT practice sessions. *No new items will be presented.* The session is divided into three one-hour blocks of 50 test items each. The cost is about $42 for U.S. and Canadian students but is higher for international students. The student receives a printed percent-correct score after completing the session. No explanations of questions are provided. You may register for a practice session online at *www.usmle.org*.

Keyboard shortcuts:
A–E—Letter choices.
Enter or Alt-N—Move to next question.
Alt-P—Move back one question.
Alt-T—Countdown timers for current session and overall test.

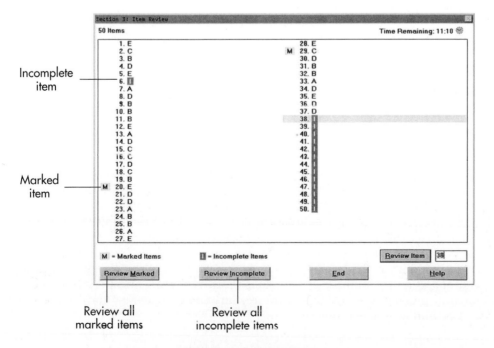

FIGURE 5. Item Review Screen

Ctrl-Alt-Delete are the keys of death during the exam. Don't touch them!

How Do I Register to Take the Exam?

Your medical school should have a supply of the Step 2 CD-ROM, which contains electronic files of all of the printed materials, including the USMLE Bulletin of Information. Step 2 applications, which are not included on the CD-ROM, are available online. To register for the exam in the United States and Canada, apply online at the NBME Web site (*www.nbme.org*). A printable version of the application is also available on this site.

The preliminary registration process for the USMLE Step 2 requires that students complete a registration form and send exam fees to the NBME. The application form allows applicants to select one of 12 overlapping three-month blocks in which to be tested (e.g., June/July/August, July/August/September). The application also includes a photo ID form that must be certified by an official at your medical school to verify your enrollment. After the NBME processes your application, it will send you a fluorescent orange slip of paper called a scheduling permit. It takes four to six weeks to process applications.

The scheduling permit you receive from the NBME will contain your USMLE identification number, the eligibility period in which you may take the exam, and two unique numbers, one of which is known as your "scheduling number." You will need this number to make your exam appointment with Prometric. The other unique number is known as the "Candidate Identification Number," or CIN. Examinees must enter their CIN at the Prometric workstation in order to access their exam. Prometric has no access to the codes and will not be able to supply these numbers. **Do not lose your permit!** You will not be allowed to take the boards unless you present your permit along with an unexpired, government-issued photo identification that contains your signature (such as a driver's license or a passport). Make sure the name on your photo ID exactly matches the name that appears on your scheduling permit.

Because the exam is scheduled on a "first-come, first-served" basis, call Prometric as soon as you receive your scheduling permit!

Once you have received your scheduling permit, you must call Prometric's toll-free number to arrange a time to take the exam. Although requests for taking the exam may be completed more than six months before the test date, examinees will not receive their scheduling permits earlier than six months before the eligibility period. (The eligibility period is the three-month period you have chosen to take the exam.) Because exam scheduling is given on a "first-come, first-served" basis, it is recommended that you telephone Prometric as soon as you have received your permit. Be sure to consult *www.usmle.org* for further details.

When Should I Register for the Exam?

Although there are no deadlines for registering for Step 2, you should plan to register at least nine months ahead of your desired test date to ensure that you get your Prometric center of choice. You should also be able to schedule a date within two weeks of your desired test date. Because of the limited number of computers available, only a certain number of examinees will be able to take the computer exam on any given day. Of course, precisely how difficult it will be to schedule an exam will depend on the location of the Prometric testing center and on the number of test takers (both U.S. students and international medical graduates, or IMGs) in the region. Some areas may have more test takers than available Prometric centers.

What if I Need to Reschedule the Exam?

You can change your date and/or center within your three-month period by contacting Prometric, so choose your eligibility period carefully. If space is available, you may reschedule up to five days before your test date. If you need to reschedule outside your initial three-month period, you can apply for a single three-month extension (e.g., April/May/June can be extended through July/August/September) after your eligibility period has begun. The form is on the NBME Web site and the cost is $50, although Prometric may also impose rescheduling fees. For other rescheduling needs, you must submit a new application along with another $385 application fee.

Where Can I Take the Exam?

Your testing location is arranged with Prometric when you call for your test date (after you receive your scheduling permit). For a list of Prometric locations nearest you, visit *www.prometric.com.*

What Did Other Students Like/Dislike About the CBT Format?

Student feedback about the CBT format has been overwhelmingly positive. Students note that the testing environment was not as stressful as they had imagined and add that they enjoyed the test's point-and-click simplicity. "It's nice to be able to work at your own pace and take breaks whenever you want," commented one student.

Of all the complaints expressed, students were most concerned with image quality, eyestrain, temperature extremes (heat/cold), and background noise at the Prometric center. Students noted that the quality of some images made it difficult to answer certain questions and added that they would like to be able to enlarge images. Eyestrain seemed to affect many other test takers, although taking a short break usually afforded relief. In addition, some students noted that the clicking of mice and keyboard chatter by other students bothered them. Earplugs (provided by the testing center) helped but did not completely block such sounds.

Beware of the awkward lab-values screen, background noise, variable image quality, and eyestrain.

What About Time?

Time is of special interest on the CBT exam. Here is a breakdown of the exam schedule:

Tutorial	15 minutes
60-minute question blocks (46 questions per block)	8 hours
Break time (includes time for lunch)	45 minutes
Total test time	9 hours

The computer will keep track of how much time has elapsed. However, the computer will show you only how much time you have remaining in a given block. Therefore, it is up to you to determine if you are pacing yourself properly (at a rate of approximately one question per 77 to 78 seconds).

The computer will not warn you if you are spending more than your allotted time for a break. Thus, taking long breaks between early question blocks or for lunch may mean that you will not be able to take breaks later in the day. You should budget your time so that you can take a short break when you need one but still have time to eat.

Be especially careful not to waste too much time between blocks (you should keep track of how much time elapses between finishing a block of questions and starting the next block). After you finish one question block, you will need to click the mouse when you are ready to proceed to the next block of questions.

It should be noted that 45 minutes is allowed for break time. However, you can elect not to use all of your break time, or you can gain extra break time (but not time for the question blocks) either by skipping the tutorial or by finishing a block ahead of the allotted time.

Since digital watches are not allowed, get used to keeping track of break time with an analog watch.

For security reasons, digital watches are not allowed at testing centers. This means that only analog watches are permitted. You should therefore get used to timing yourself with an analog watch in your efforts to gauge exactly how much time you have left. Some analog watches come with a bevel that helps keep track of 60-minute periods. This may be useful for keeping track of break time.

If I Leave During the Exam, What Happens to My Score?

Your scheduling permit shows a CIN that you will enter onto the computer screen to start your exam. Entering the CIN is the same as breaking the seal on a test book; thus, you are considered to have started the exam once you have done so. However, no score will be reported if you do not complete the exam. In fact, if you leave at any time from the start of the test to the last block, no score will be reported. However, the fact that you started but failed to complete the exam will appear on your USMLE score transcript.

The exam ends when all blocks have been completed or time has expired. As you leave the testing center, you will receive a written test-completion notice to document your completion of the exam.

In order to receive an official score, you must finish the entire exam. This means that you must start and either finish or run out of time for each block of the exam. Again, if you do not complete all the blocks, your exam will be documented as an incomplete attempt, and no score will be reported.

What Types of Questions Are Asked?

Almost all questions are case based.

- Almost all questions on Step 2 are case based. Some are two to three sentences in length, while others are two to three paragraphs long and contain laboratory data. Very often, a substantial amount of extraneous information is given, making for dense, slow reading. It is also common for a clinical scenario to be given, followed by a question that could be answered without actually reading the case. It is your job to determine which information is superfluous and which is pertinent to the case at hand.
- Questions often describe clinical findings instead of naming eponyms (e.g., they cite "audible hip click" instead of "positive Ortolani's sign"), so it is important to know what each sign or "keyword" actually represents.

■ Subject areas vary randomly from question to question, although groups of matching questions often have a unifying theme.

Most questions have a single best answer, and there have been no negatively phrased questions on recent exams. Some questions are matching sets that call for multiple responses, with the number to select specified at the end of each question. The questions usually describe clinical situations requiring that you identify a diagnosis, the underlying pathophysiology of the disease being described, the next appropriate step in management, interpretation of laboratory findings, potential for prevention, or overall prognosis. The part of the vignette that actually asks the question—the stem—is usually found at the end of the scenario. From student experience, there are a few stems that are consistently addressed throughout the exam:

■ What is the most likely diagnosis? (40%)
■ Which of the following is the most appropriate initial step in management? (20%)
■ Which of the following is the most appropriate next step in management? (20%)
■ Which of the following is the most likely cause of . . . ? (5%)
■ Which of the following is the most likely pathogen . . . ? (3%)
■ Which of the following would most likely prevent . . . ? (2%)
■ Other (10%)

How Long Will I Have to Wait Before I Get My Scores?

The USMLE reports scores three to four weeks after the examinee's test date. However, score reporting may be delayed by an extra one to two weeks owing to recent formatting adjustments to the exam. During peak times, score reports may take up to six weeks. Official information concerning the time required for score reporting is posted on the USMLE Web site, *www.usmle.org*.

How Are the Scores Reported?

Like the Step 1 score report, your Step 2 report includes your pass/fail status, two numeric scores, and a performance profile organized by discipline and disease process (see Figures 6A and 6B). The first score is a three-digit scaled score based on a predefined proficiency standard reviewed in 2000. For recent examinations, the mean for first-time test takers from U.S. and Canadian medical schools was 213 and the standard deviation (SD) was 24. Most scores fell between 160 and 240. In 2002, a score of 174 was required to pass. The second score scale, the two-digit score, defines 75 as the minimum passing score (equivalent to a score of 174 on the first scale). This score is not a percentile. A score of 82 is equivalent to a score of 200 on the first scale.

The overall pass rate for first-time U.S. and Canadian examinees from Liaison Committee for Medical Education (LCME)-accredited medical schools was 95% in 1999–2001. The pass rate for first-time examinees registered by the Educational Commission for Foreign Medical Graduates (ECFMG) rose from 70% in 1999–2000 to 75% in 2000–2001 (see Table 1).

US·MLE
United States
Medical
Licensing
Examination

UNITED STATES MEDICAL LICENSING EXAMINATION™

USMLE Step 2 is administered to students and graduates of U.S. and Canadian medical schools by the
NATIONAL BOARD OF MEDICAL EXAMINERS® (NBME®)
3750 Market Street, Philadelphia, Pennsylvania 19104-3190.
Telephone: (215) 590-9700

STEP 2 SCORE REPORT

Schmoe, Joe T	USMLE ID: 1-234-567-8
Anytown, CA 12345	Test Date: August 1998

The USMLE is a single examination program for all applicants for medical licensure in the United States; it has replaced the Federation Licensing Examination (FLEX) and the certifying examinations of the National Board of Medical Examiners (NBME Parts I, II and III). The program consists of three Steps designed to assess an examinee's understanding of and ability to apply concepts and principles that are important in health and disease and that constitute the basis of safe and effective patient care. **Step 2** is designed to assess whether an examinee possesses the medical knowledge and understanding of clinical science considered essential for the provision of patient care under supervision, including emphasis on health promotion and disease prevention. The inclusion of Step 2 in the USMLE sequence ensures that attention is devoted to principles of clinical science that undergird the safe and competent practice of medicine. Results of the examination are reported to medical licensing authorities in the United States and its territories for use in granting an initial license to practice medicine. The two numeric scores shown below are equivalent; each state or territory may use either score in making licensing decisions. These scores represent your results for the administration of Step 2 on the test date shown above.

PASS	This result is based on the minimum passing score set by USMLE for Step 2. Individual licensing authorities may accept the USMLE-recommended pass/fail result or may establish a different passing score for their own jurisdictions.

200	This score is determined by your overall performance on Step 2. For recent administrations, the mean and standard deviation for first-time examinees from U.S. and Canadian medical schools are approximately 208 and 23, respectively, with most scores falling between 140 and 260. A score of 170 is set by USMLE to pass Step 2. The standard error of measurement (SEM)‡ for this scale is approximately six points.

82	This score is also determined by your overall performance on the examination. A score of 82 on this scale is equivalent to a score of 200 on the scale described above. A score of 75 on this scale, which is equivalent to a score of 170 on the scale described above, is set by USMLE to pass Step 2. The SEM‡ for this scale is one point.

‡Your score is influenced both by your general understanding of clinical science and the specific set of items selected for this Step 2 examination. The standard error of measurement (SEM) provides an estimate of the range within which your scores might be expected to vary by chance if you were tested repeatedly using similar tests.

267PU007

NOTE: Original score report has copy-resistant watermark.

FIGURE 6A. Sample Score Report—Front Page

NBME/USMLE Publications

We strongly encourage students to use the free materials provided by the testing agencies and to study the following NBME publications:

- **USMLE Bulletin of Information.** This publication provides you with nuts-and-bolts details about the exam (included on the Web site *www. usmle.org*; free to all examinees).
- **USMLE Step 2 Computer-Based Content and Sample Test Questions.** This is a hard copy of test questions and test content also found on the CD-ROM.
- **USMLE Web site (*www.usmle.org*).** In addition to allowing you to become familiar with the CBT format, the sample items on the USMLE Web site provide the only questions that are available directly from the test makers. Student feedback varies as to the similarity of these questions to those on the actual exam, but they are nonetheless worthwhile

Consider saving a block of questions from the sample test to take a few days before the exam.

INFORMATION PROVIDED FOR EXAMINEE USE ONLY
The Performance Profile below is provided solely for the benefit of the examinee.
These profiles are developed as assessment tools for examinees only and will not be reported or verified to any third party.

USMLE STEP 2 PERFORMANCE PROFILES

PHYSICIAN TASK PROFILE	Lower Performance	Borderline Performance	Higher Performance
Preventive Medicine & Health Maintenance			xxxxxxxxxxxx*
Understanding Mechanisms of Disease			xxxxx*
Diagnosis			xxxxxx*
Principles of Management			xxxxxxxxxxx*

NORMAL CONDITIONS & DISEASE CATEGORY PROFILE

	Lower Performance	Borderline Performance	Higher Performance
Normal Growth & Development; Principles of Care			xxxxxxxxxxxxxxxxx*
Immunologic Disorders			xxxxxxxxxxxx*
Diseases of Blood & Blood Forming Organs			xxxxxxxxxx*
Mental Disorders			xxxxxxxxxxxx*
Diseases of the Nervous System & Special Senses			xxxxxxxxxxx*
Cardiovascular Disorders		xxxxxxxxxxxxxxxx	
Diseases of the Respiratory System			xxxxxxxxxxxxx*
Nutritional & Digestive Disorders			xxxxxxxxxxx*
Gynecologic Disorders			xxxxxxxxxxxxx*
Renal, Urinary & Male Reproductive Systems			xxxxxxxxxxx*
Disorders of Pregnancy, Childbirth & Puerperium			xxxxxxxxxxxxxxxxxxxx
Musculoskeletal, Skin & Connective Tissue Diseases			xxxxxxxxxx*
Endocrine & Metabolic Disorders			xxxxxxxxxxxxxxx*

DISCIPLINE PROFILE

	Lower Performance	Borderline Performance	Higher Performance
Medicine			xxx*
Obstetrics & Gynecology			xxxxxxxxxxxx*
Pediatrics			xxxxxxxxx*
Psychiatry			xxxxxxxxxxxxx*
Surgery			xxx*

The above Performance Profile is provided to aid in self-assessment. The shaded area defines a borderline level of performance for each content area; borderline performance is comparable to a HIGH FAIL / LOW PASS on the total test.

Performance bands indicate areas of relative strength and weakness. Some performance bands are wider than others. The width of a performance band reflects the precision of measurement: narrower bands indicate greater precision. An asterisk indicates that your performance band extends beyond the displayed portion of the scale. Small differences in the location of bands should not be over interpreted. If two bands overlap, the performance in the associated areas should not be interpreted as significantly different.

This profile should not be compared to those from other Step 2 administrations.

Additional information concerning the topics covered in each content area can be found in the *USMLE Step 2 General Instructions, Content Description, and Sample Items.*

007PU267

FIGURE 6B. Sample Score Report—Back Page

to know. Consider taking one block of questions, allowing yourself a little over one minute per question to approximate the pacing of the "real thing." The extremely detailed Step 2 content outline provided by the USMLE has not proved useful for students preparing for the exam. The USMLE even states that the content outline is not intended to be a study guide. We agree with this assessment.

CLINICAL SKILLS EXAMINATION

The Clinical Skills Examination (CSE) is a one-day interactive exam with "role-playing" standardized patients (SPs). It is currently being pilot tested for incorporation into the licensing requirements of U.S. graduates. The CSE is slated to become an official part of the USMLE in mid-2004 and will most likely be taken in the fourth year of medical school, around the time students

	Number Tested	Passing (%)
TABLE 1. Passing rates for the 2000–2001 USMLE Step 2[a]		
Type of Student	**Number Tested**	**Passing (%)**
U.S./Canadian examinees (NBME registered) overall	17,661	93
Allopathic students	17,361	93
First-time takers	16,205	95
Repeaters	1,156	66
Osteopathic students overall	300	91
First-time takers	288	93
Repeaters	12	42
Non-U.S./Canadian examinees (ECFMG registered) overall	10,354	66
First-time takers	7,131	75
Repeaters	3,223	48

[a]Step 2 data are provided for examinees tested during the period from July 1 to June 30 and reflect the most current data available at the time of publication.

take the USMLE Step 2. A similar test called the Clinical Skills Assessment (CSA) has been required for IMGs since 1998.

The goal of the CSE is to ensure that students from more than 1,600 medical schools worldwide, with varying curricula and educational standards, can collect and interpret a history, perform a physical exam, and communicate with patients at a comparable level. The exam is designed to simulate a typical day in an ambulatory medical clinic. Students examine ten SPs—laypeople who have been trained to simulate various clinical problems—for approximately 15 minutes each. Tasks include establishing rapport, obtaining a relevant history, performing a focused physical exam, formulating diagnostic impressions and treatment plans, and providing appropriate information and counseling. Cases are mixed with respect to age, gender, ethnicity, organ system, and discipline. All, however, are designed to focus on common or important situations that a doctor will likely encounter in an outpatient clinic setting.

Unfortunately, given the requirement for SPs, specialized test centers, and individualized testing, the exam will cost an estimated $950 per student. Many students will incur additional hotel and airline costs to reach the nearest test center.

Test Administration

Before they enter the exam room, examinees are given an opportunity to review preliminary information, including patient characteristics (i.e., age, name, and gender), chief complaint, and vital signs. Once they have entered the room, examinees are given 15 minutes (with a warning bell sounded at ten minutes) to perform the clinical encounter, which includes introducing themselves, obtaining a relevant history, performing a focused physical exam, formulating a differential diagnosis, and planning a diagnostic workup. Examinees are expected to answer any questions the patient might ask, discuss possible diagnoses, and advise the patient regarding follow-up plans. After leaving the room, examinees have ten minutes to write a patient note.

"Do's and Don'ts"

Ground rules for the clinical encounter are:

- Examinees are not allowed to perform rectal, pelvic/genital, or female breast exams. If one of these exams is warranted, it can be suggested as part of the diagnostic workup.
- Examinees are not allowed to reenter the room after they have left, so it is recommended that they obtain all necessary information before ending the encounter.
- Time is not on the examinee's side, so it is advisable to "home in" on relevant problems and conduct a focused clinical exam. For example, if a diabetic patient presents with chest pain, examinees should rule out cardiopulmonary, gastrointestinal, and musculoskeletal etiologies first and focus the examination on these systems. A complete CNS exam would be the last on the examinee's list.

DEFINING YOUR GOAL

Arguably the first and most important thing to do in your Step 2 preparation is define how well you want to do on the Step 2 exam, as the goals you set will ultimately determine the extent of preparation that will be necessary. The amount of time spent in preparation for this exam varies widely among medical students, ranging anywhere from several months to two days (as in the jokingly stated adage "Two weeks for Step 1, two days for Step 2, and a number 2 pencil for Step 3") to no preparation at all. Possible goals include:

- **"Simply passing."** This goal may be sufficient for the majority of U.S. medical students. This may apply to you if you are entering a less competitive specialty.
- **Beating the mean.** Beating the mean (213 for recent exam administrations) signifies an ability to integrate your clinical and factual knowledge to an extent that is superior to that of your peers. Others redefine this goal as achieving a score one SD above the mean (237). This figure is also the so-called "magic number" that many students have aimed for on the USMLE Step 1, as it supposedly represents the score one must receive in order to be strongly considered by the more competitive residency programs (see Figure 7). Highly competitive residency programs may use your Step 1 and Step 2 (if available) scores as a screening tool or as selection criteria (see Figure 8). IMGs should aim to beat the mean, as USMLE scores are likely to be a selection factor even for less competitive U.S. residency programs. For additional discussion of the residency application process and the USMLE Step 2, please refer to *First Aid for the Match*.

Less Competitive	More Competitive	Most Competitive
Pediatrics	Emergency Medicine	Dermatology
Family Practice	OB/GYN	ENT
Internal Medicine	Radiology	Orthopedics
Anesthesiology	General Surgery	Ophthalmology
Psychiatry		

FIGURE 7. Competitive Specialties

- **Acing the exam.** Perhaps you are one of those individuals for whom nothing less than the best will do—and for whom excelling on standardized exams is a source of pride and satisfaction. For you, the USMLE Step 2 represents the culmination of several years of exam taking as well as a final opportunity as a medical student to excel at what you do best. Alternatively, an exceptional score on the USMLE Step 2 might also represent a way to "make up" for a less-than-satisfactory score on Step 1, especially if taken in the fall, so that it can be seen by residency programs and used to strengthen your application.
- **Evaluating your clinical knowledge.** This is a commendable goal that can be considered an addendum to any of the other goals mentioned in this section. Indeed, in many ways this goal should serve as the ultimate

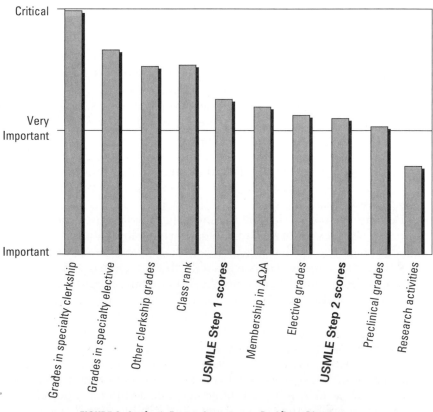

FIGURE 8. Academic Factors Important to Residency Directors

rationale for taking the exam, since it is technically the reason the exam was designed in the first place. Specifically, the case-based nature of the USMLE Step 2 differs significantly from the more fact-based Step 1 exam in that it more thoroughly examines your ability to recognize classic clinical presentations, deal with acute emergent situations, and follow the step-by-step thought processes involved in the treatment of particular diseases. In short, the Step 2 exam allows you to assess your ability to apply your vast collection of medical facts to the situations you are likely to encounter during your residency.

■ **Preparing for internship.** Making the transition to internship can be challenging. Studying for the USMLE Step 2 is an excellent way to review and consolidate all of the information that has slowly but surely been fading from memory during your third year. Use your Step 2 preparation as an opportunity to gear up for internship, especially if you are taking the exam in the spring.

Step 2 is an opportunity to consolidate your clinical knowledge and prepare for internship.

When to Take the Exam

With the CBT, you now have a wide variety of options regarding when to take Step 2. Here are a few factors to consider:

■ **The nature of your objectives,** as defined above.

■ **The specialty to which you are applying.** Some competitive residency programs may request your Step 2 scores. Ask your adviser or the residency director at your school if this applies to you. If you already have a strong application, taking Step 2 in the fall could potentially hurt you if you do poorly. However, if you need to shore up your application for a competitive field, consider taking the exam (and truly preparing for it) in the fall.

■ At many medical schools, passing the USMLE Step 2 is a prerequisite to graduation. This would be another reason to take the exam in the fall or winter. Should you fail, the NBME will allow you to retake the exam 60 days after your last exam date.

■ **Proximity to clerkships.** Many students feel that the core clerkship material is fresher in their minds early in the fourth year, making a good argument for taking Step 2 earlier in the fall. Many students organize their rotation schedules so that they have numerous electives and a relatively "light" clinical load during their fourth year. Such students often discover that much of the clinical information they learned on their core rotations has faded. On the other hand, preparation for the USMLE Step 2 is also an excellent tool for review before internship.

■ **The extent to which you seek a stress-free fourth year.** If you think it is highly likely that you will pass, you may want to take the exam later so that you will not have to worry about the possibility that your score will affect your match possibilities. On the other hand, taking the USMLE Step 2 exam early gets it out of the way, giving you a stress-free fourth year without the specter of an exam looming over you.

■ **The nature of your schedule.** Some students like to plan the test around a clerkship or vacation month in which they have some free time—or at least not when they are on their toughest fourth-year clerkship. It would be counterproductive to take the exam at the same time that you have scheduled a subinternship in your planned specialty, since you will want to concentrate on performing well on the rotation for a good evaluation and, possibly, a letter of recommendation.

Quality and Cost Considerations

Although there is an ever-increasing number of USMLE Step 2 review books and software on the market, the quality of this material is highly variable (see Section III). Some common problems are as follows:

- Some review books are too detailed to be reviewed in a reasonable amount of time or cover subtopics not emphasized on the exam (e.g., a 400-page anesthesiology book).
- Many sample question books were originally written years ago and have not been updated to reflect trends on the revised USMLE Step 2.
- Many sample question books use poorly written questions or contain factual errors in their explanations.
- Explanations for sample questions range from nonexistent to overly detailed.
- Software for boards review is of highly variable quality, may be difficult to install, and may be fraught with bugs.

Clinical Review Books

The best review book for you reflects the way you like to learn.

Most review books are the products of considerable effort on the part of experienced educators. Many such books are available, however, so you must decide which ones to buy on the basis of their relative merits. Although recommendations from other medical students are useful, many students simply recommend whatever books they themselves used without first comparing those books to others on the same subject. In a similar manner, some students blindly advocate one publisher's series without considering the broad range of quality encountered within other series. You should therefore weigh different opinions against each other, read the reviews and ratings in Section III of this guide, and examine the various books closely in the bookstore. You are investing not only money but also your limited study time. Do not worry about finding the "perfect" book, as many subjects simply do not have one.

There are two types of review books: books that are stand-alone titles and books that are part of a series. Books in a series generally have the same style, and you must decide if that style is helpful for you. However, a given style is not optimal for every subject.

If a given review book is not working for you, stop using it no matter how highly rated it may be.

Find out which books are up to date. Some new editions represent major improvements, whereas others contain only cursory changes. You should take into consideration how a book reflects the format of the USMLE Step 2. Some may not have been adequately updated to reflect the changing question style and format of the current USMLE Step 2.

Texts and Notes

Unless you are planning an all-out offensive against Step 2 (and actually have the time), avoid standard texts in preparing for it. Many textbooks are too detailed for high-yield boards review. Even popular handbooks such as the *Washington Manual* can be a chore to read, as they were designed for directed reading and reference rather than for cover-to-cover perusal. When using texts or notes, engage in active learning by making tables, diagrams, new mnemonics, and conceptual associations whenever possible. If you already have your own mnemonics, do not bother trying to memorize someone else's. You should also supplement incomplete or unclear material with reference to other appropriate textbooks. Finally, keep a good medical dictionary on hand to sort out definitions.

Commercial Courses

Commercial preparation courses can be helpful for some students, but they are costly and require a significant time commitment. At the same time, they frequently offer an effective way to organize study material for students who feel overwhelmed by the sheer volume of material involved in preparing for Step 2. Note, however, that multiweek courses may be quite intense and may thus leave limited time for independent study. Note also that some commercial courses are designed for first-time test takers, whereas others focus on students who are repeating the examination. Still other courses focus on IMGs, who must take all three Steps in a limited amount of time.

Practice Tests

Taking practice tests can give you valuable information about strengths and weaknesses in your fund of knowledge and test-taking skills. Some students use practice examinations simply as a means of breaking up the monotony of studying and adding variety to their study schedule. Others study almost entirely from practice tests. Students report that many practice tests have questions that are, on average, shorter and less clinically oriented than those on the current USMLE Step 2. Step 2 questions demand fast reading skills and application of clinical facts in a problem-solving format. Approach sample examinations critically, and do not waste time with low-quality questions until you have exhausted better sources.

After you have taken a practice test, try to identify concepts and areas of weakness, not just the facts that you missed. Use the experience to motivate your study and prioritize what areas need the most work.

Use quality practice examinations to improve your test-taking skills. This is especially important in helping you familiarize yourself with the style of the USMLE Step 2. Analyze your ability to pace yourself so that you have enough time to complete each block comfortably. Practice examinations can also help you train yourself to concentrate for long periods of time under appropriate time pressure. Analyze the pattern of your responses to questions to determine if you have made systematic errors in answering questions. Common mistakes are reading too much into the question, second-guessing your initial impression, and misinterpreting the question.

Use practice tests to identify concepts and areas of weakness, not just facts that you missed.

TEST-TAKING STRATEGIES

By now, you are probably familiar with USMLE exams and most likely have worked out some of your own strategies. However, the clinical vignette style of the USMLE Step 2 may be unfamiliar to you. Listed below are a few strategies that may be helpful, drawn from student experience from recent Step 2 exams.

Planning

If you are unfortunate enough to be on a difficult rotation at the time of the USMLE Step 2, you will need to plan ahead and start studying earlier, as a demanding call schedule may leave you chronically tired. Ask your resident early if you can take a couple of call nights off in order to catch up on some rest just before the exam. Regardless of what rotation you are on, make sure to give your resident and attending advance warning of exam dates. This will allow them to make adjustments in the call schedule and arrange for coverage of your patients if you are on a subinternship.

Things to Bring with You to the Exam

On the morning of the exam, don't forget your scheduling permit and a photo ID that includes your signature. You will not be admitted to the exam if you fail to bring your permit, and Prometric will charge a rescheduling fee. A watch can help you pace yourself, although digital timers are not allowed. It may also be of benefit to have some snacks on hand for a little "sugar rush." However, snacks will need to be stored in a locker until you take a break. In addition, it might be a good idea to bring your lunch given that break time is limited. Also consider bringing fluids, but not too much, as you don't want to waste valuable time running to the bathroom. Should you need earplugs, remember that they will be provided at the Prometric center. Finally, consider layering clothing to accommodate temperature variations at the testing center.

Pacing

Pacing is key with lengthy clinical vignettes.

You have 60 minutes per block in which to complete approximately 46 questions. The test is quite fast-paced. Many scenarios are lengthy and time-consuming to read. Many students report feeling pressed for time before they find a rhythm, so keep close track of time using the clock in the corner of the screen and possibly your analog watch. With the CBT, examinees report that the most efficient use of time is to answer questions in order. You may, however, return to any problematic question within the same block.

Difficult Questions

Do not waste valuable time on difficult or impossible questions.

The cruel reality of the USMLE Step 2 exam is that no matter how much you study, there will still be questions you will not be able to answer. Plan for these. If you recognize that a question is not solvable in a reasonable period of time, do not waste time on it. Move on after making an educated guess; you will not be penalized for wrong answers. Remember, each USMLE exam contains 10–20% experimental questions that will not count toward your score. Don't let tough questions throw you.

Images

Many of the questions can be answered without the picture.

Don't be afraid of questions that include imaging, which may arise with topics such as radiology, dermatology, and ophthalmology. Most questions will be basic and will include common diagnoses. A quick review, however, can be helpful. Use the high-yield glossy section of this book and consider using short glossy segments of other textbooks. Try reading the clinical scenario, question, and answers prior to studying the x-ray or picture. If all else fails, pick the most common diagnosis. It is helpful to know the normal radiographic appearance of the hands, feet, chest, and pelvis in order to recognize gross abnormalities that may be given on the exam.

Guessing

There is no penalty for wrong answers. Thus, no test block should be left with unanswered questions. A hunch is better than a random guess. We suggest that you select an answer you recognize over one that is totally unfamiliar. If you have studied a subject and do not recognize a particular option, it is more likely a distractor than a correct answer.

Finding the "Meat" of the Question

Many of the clinical vignettes in Step 2 are painfully long and contain a significant amount of information. If you think you may be pressed for time, consider reading the stem of the question first and then skimming the answers before reading the vignette. After you have read the stem and answers, you may be able to seek out key pieces of information in the vignette to help you answer the question. A word of caution, however: Do not overlook details in tricky or tough questions. If you have time, it may indeed be worthwhile to read each vignette carefully to avoid making errors. Try the "meat of the question" technique on the sample items. It may not be useful for everyone.

Changing Your Answer

The conventional wisdom regarding "reconsidering" answers is not to change answers that you have already marked unless there is a convincing and logical reason to do so. In other words, when in doubt, go with your first hunch.

Other Tidbits

Other helpful hints include the following:

- Note the age and race of the patient in each clinical scenario. In most questions, ethnicity is not given. When it is given, however, the patient's ethnicity is often relevant. For example, African-American heritage contributes to the epidemiology, pathophysiology, prognosis, outcome, and even treatment of some diseases. Know these well (see high-yield facts), especially for more common diagnoses.
- Some of the questions that many students felt were the most difficult involved choosing the "most important initial step" or the "next step in management" of a disease. It can be difficult to prioritize treatment options, so pay close attention to management strategies as you study. Students who took the Step 2 exam noted that treatment and management issues are often more important than differentials.
- Be able to recognize key factors that distinguish major diagnoses.
- Consider completing an emergency medicine rotation prior to taking Step 2. Questions about acute patient management (e.g., trauma) in an emergency setting are common.

TESTING AGENCIES

National Board of Medical Examiners (NBME)
Department of Licensing Examination Services
3750 Market Street
Philadelphia, PA 19104-3102
215-590-9500
www.nbme.org

Educational Commission for Foreign Medical Graduates (ECFMG)
3624 Market Street, Fourth Floor
Philadelphia, PA 19104-2685
215-386-5900 or 202-293-9320
Fax: 215-386-9196
www.ecfmg.org

Federation of State Medical Boards (FSMB)
P. O. Box 619850
Dallas, TX 75261-9850, 817-868-4000
Fax: 817-868-4099
www.fsmb.org

USMLE Secretariat
3750 Market Street
Philadelphia, PA 19104-3190
215-590-9700
www.usmle.org

Many figures in this chapter are reproduced, with permission, from the NBME.

First Aid for the International Medical Graduate

"International medical graduate" (IMG) is the term now used to describe any student or graduate of a non-U.S., non-Canadian, non-Puerto Rican medical school, regardless of whether he or she is a U.S. citizen. The old term "foreign medical graduate" (FMG) was replaced because it was misleading when applied to U.S. citizens attending medical schools outside the United States.

THE IMG'S STEPS TO LICENSURE IN THE UNITED STATES

If you are an IMG, you must go through the following steps (not necessarily in this order) to become licensed to practice in the United States. You must complete these steps even if you are already a practicing physician and have completed a residency program in your own country.

- Complete the **basic sciences program** of your medical school (equivalent to the first two years of U.S. medical school).
- Take the **USMLE Step 1.** You can do this while still in school or after graduating—but in either case, your medical school must certify that you have completed the basic sciences part of your school's curriculum before you can be allowed to take the USMLE Step 1.
- Complete the **clinical clerkship program** of your medical school (equivalent to the third and fourth years of U.S. medical school).
- Take the **USMLE Step 2.** If you are still in medical school, your school must certify that you are within one year of graduating before you can take Step 2.
- Take the Test of English as a Foreign Language **(TOEFL),** recognized by the ECFMG.
- Take the Clinical Skills Assessment **(CSA).**
- Graduate with your **medical diploma.**
- Then, send the ECFMG a copy of your degree, which they will verify with your medical school.
- Obtain an **ECFMG certificate.** To do this, candidates must accomplish the following:
  - Graduate from a medical school that is listed in the International Medical Education Directory (IMED). The list can be accessed at *www.ecfmg.org.*
  - Pass Step 1 and Step 2 within a seven-year period.
  - Pass the TOEFL.
  - Pass the CSA.
  - Have medical credentials verified by the ECFMG. The standard certificate is usually sent two weeks after all the above requirements have been fulfilled. You must have a valid certificate before entering an accredited residency program, although you may begin the application process before you receive your certification.
- Apply for residency positions in your field of interest, either directly or through the Electronic Residency Application Service **(ERAS)** and the National Residency Matching Program **("the Match").** To be entered into the Match, you need to have passed all the examinations necessary for ECFMG certification (Step 1, Step 2, the CSA, and the TOEFL) by a certain deadline (e.g., January 31, 2003, for the 2003 Match) prior to rank list submission. If you do not pass these exams by the deadline, you will be withdrawn from the Match.
- Obtain a **visa** that will allow you to enter and work in the United States if you are not already a U.S. citizen or a green-card holder (permanent resident).

More detailed information can be found in the ECFMG Information Booklet, available at www.ecfmg.org/pubshome.html.

- If required of IMGs by the state in which your residency is located, obtain an educational/training/limited **medical license.** Your residency program may assist you with this application. Note that medical licensing is the prerogative of each individual state, not of the federal government, and that states vary with respect to their laws about licensing (although all 50 states recognize the USMLE).
- In order to begin your residency program, make sure your TOEFL and CSA scores are valid. A passing TOEFL score is valid for two years, and a passing CSA score is valid for three years. If more time has elapsed, scores must be revalidated by passing a subsequent TOEFL or CSA exam.
- Take the **USMLE Step 3** before or during your residency, and then obtain a full medical license. Once you have a license in any state, you are permitted to practice in federal institutions such as Veterans Administration (VA) hospitals and Indian Health Service facilities in any state. This can open the door to "moonlighting" opportunities and possibilities for an H1B visa application. For details on individual state rules, write to the licensing board in the state in question or contact the FSMB.
- Complete your residency and then take the appropriate specialty **board exams** in order to become board certified (e.g., in internal medicine or surgery). If you already have a specialty certification in your home country (e.g., in surgery or cardiology), some specialty boards may grant you six months' or one year's credit toward your total residency time.
- Currently, the majority of residency programs are accepting applications through ERAS. For more information, see *First Aid for the Match* or contact:

> ECFMG/ERAS Program
> P.O. Box 11746
> Philadelphia, PA 19101-1746
> 215-386-5900
> Fax: 215-222-5641
> *www.ecfmg.org/eras*
> e-mail: eras-support@ecfmg.org

Applicants may apply online for the USMLE Step 1 or Step 2, for the ECFMG CSA, or to request an extension of the USMLE eligibility period at http://iwa.ecfmg.org.

The USMLE and the IMG

The USMLE is a series of standardized exams that gives IMGs a level playing field. It is the same exam series taken by U.S. graduates even though it is administered by the ECFMG rather than by the NBME. This means that passing marks for IMGs for both Step 1 and Step 2 are determined by a statistical process that is based on the scores of U.S. medical students in 1991. For example, to pass Step 1, you will probably have to score higher than the bottom 8–10% of U.S. and Canadian graduates.

Timing of the USMLE

For an IMG, the timing of a complete application is critical. It is extremely important that you send in your application early if you are to garner the maximum number of interview calls. A rough guide would be to complete all exam requirements by August of the year in which you wish to apply. This would translate into sending both your score sheets and your ECFMG certificate in with your application.

In terms of USMLE exam order, arguments can be made for taking the Step 1 or Step 2 exam first. For example, you may consider taking the Step 2 exam first if you have just graduated from medical school and the clinical topics are still fresh in your mind. However, keep in mind that there is a large overlap between Step 1 and Step 2 topics in areas such as pharmacology, pathophysiology, and biostatistics. You might therefore consider taking the Step 1 and Step 2 exams close together to take advantage of this overlap in your test preparation.

USMLE STEP 1 AND THE IMG

What is the USMLE Step 1? It is a computerized test of the basic medical sciences consisting of 350 multiple-choice questions.

Significance of the test. Step 1 is required for the ECFMG certificate as well as for registration for the CSA. Since most U.S. graduates apply to residency with their Step 1 scores only, it may be the only objective tool available with which to compare IMGs with U.S. graduates.

Official Web sites. *www.usmle.org/step1* and *www.ecfmg.org/usmle.*

Eligibility. Both students and graduates from medical schools that are listed in IMED are eligible to take the test. Students must have completed at least two years of medical school by the beginning of the eligibility period selected.

Eligibility period. A three-month period of your choice.

Fees. The fee for Step 1 is $660 plus an international test delivery surcharge (if you choose a testing region other than the United States or Canada).

Retaking the exam. In the event that you failed the test, you can reapply and select an eligibility period that begins at least 60 days after the last attempt. You cannot take the same Step more than three times in any 12-month period. You cannot retake the exam if you passed.

Statistics. In 2001, only 66% of ECFMG candidates passed Step 1 on their first attempt, compared with 91% of U.S. and Canadian medical students and graduates. Of note, 1994–1995 data showed that USFMGs (U.S. citizens attending non-U.S. medical schools) performed 0.4 SD lower than IMGs (non-U.S. citizens attending non-U.S. medical schools). Although their overall scores were lower, USFMGs performed better than IMGs on behavioral sciences. In general, students from non-U.S. medical schools perform worst in behavioral science and biochemistry (1.9 and 1.5 SDs below U.S. students) and comparatively better in gross anatomy and pathology (0.7 and 0.9 SD below U.S. students). Although derived from data collected in 1994–1995, these data may help you focus your studying efforts.

Developing a good test-taking strategy is especially critical for the IMG.

A good Step 1 score is key to a strong IMG application.

Tips. Although few if any students feel totally prepared to take Step 1, IMGs in particular require serious study and preparation to reach their full potential on this exam. It is also imperative that IMGs do their best on Step 1, as a poor score on Step 1 is a distinct disadvantage in applying for most residencies. Remember that if you pass Step 1, you cannot retake it to try to improve your score. Your goal should thus be to beat the mean, because you can then confidently assert that you have done better than average for U.S. students. Good Step 1 scores will lend credibility to your residency application.

Commercial review courses. Do commercial review courses help improve your scores? Reports vary, and such courses can be expensive. Many IMGs decide to try the USMLE on their own and then consider a review course only if they fail. Just keep in mind that many states require that you pass the USMLE within three attempts. (For more information on review courses, see Section III.)

USMLE STEP 2 AND THE IMG

What is the USMLE Step 2? It is a computerized test of the clinical sciences consisting of 370 multiple-choice questions.

Significance of the test. Step 2 is required for the ECFMG certificate. It reflects the level of the clinical knowledge of the applicant.

Official Web sites. *www.usmle.org/step2* and *www.ecfmg.org/usmle*.

Eligibility. Students and graduates from medical schools that are listed in IMED are eligible to take Step 2. Students must be within 12 months of graduation by the beginning of the eligibility period selected.

Eligibility period. A three-month period of your choice.

Fees. The fee for Step 2 is $660 plus an international test delivery surcharge (if you choose a testing region other than the United States or Canada).

Retaking the exam. In the event that you fail Step 2, you can reapply and select an eligibility period that begins at least 60 days after the last attempt. You cannot take the same Step more than three times in any 12-month period. You cannot retake the exam if you passed.

Statistics. In 2000–2001, 75% of ECFMG candidates passed Step 2 on their first attempt, compared with 95% of U.S. and Canadian candidates.

Tips. Because this is a clinical sciences exam, cultural and geographic considerations play a greater role than is the case with Step 1. For example, if your medical education gave you ample exposure to malaria, brucellosis, and malnutrition but little to alcohol withdrawal, child abuse, and cholesterol screening, you must work to familiarize yourself with topics that are more heavily emphasized in U.S. medicine. You must also have a basic understanding of the legal and social aspects of U.S. medicine, because you will be asked questions about communicating with and advising patients.

THE ENGLISH LANGUAGE TEST

Native English-speaking IMGs are also required to take the English language test.

What is the TOEFL? The TOEFL is a computer-based or paper-based test of English language that evaluates grammar, structure, reading, listening, and writing. Topics include proper use of grammar and vocabulary, proper evaluation of sentence structure, comprehension of reading texts, comprehension of audio dialogues, and writing a brief essay.

Significance of the test. The TOEFL is required for the ECFMG certificate and for registration for the CSA.

Official Web sites. *www.toefl.org* and *www.ecfmg.org/elpt/index.html.*

Scoring. The minimum passing score accepted by the ECFMG is 550 with the paper-based test or 213 with the computer-based test. Test results are valid for two years.

CLINICAL SKILLS ASSESSMENT

What is the CSA? The CSA is a test of clinical and communication skills administered as a one-day, eight-hour exam. It includes 10 to 11 encounters with standardized patients (15 minutes each, with 10 minutes to write a note after each encounter). Test results are valid for three years.

There is a big difference between textbook learning of a language and actually being immersed in the culture that goes with it.

Topics covered by this exam. The CSA tests the ability to communicate in English as well as interpersonal skills, data-gathering skills, the ability to perform a physical exam, and the ability to formulate a brief note, a differential diagnosis, and a list of diagnostic tests. The areas that are covered in the exam are:

- Internal medicine
- Surgery
- Obstetrics and gynecology
- Pediatrics
- Psychiatry
- Family medicine

Significance of the test. The CSA is required for the ECFMG certificate.

Official Web site. *www.ecfmg.org/csa.*

Eligibility. Both medical school students and graduates must have passed the USMLE Step 1 and TOEFL exams. Students should be within 12 months of graduation from medical school.

Fee. The fee for the CSA is $1,200.

Scheduling. You must schedule your CSA within **four months** of the date indicated on your notification of registration. You must take the CSA within 12 months of the date indicated on your notification of registration.

By 2004, the CSA will be mandatory for all applicants for licensure (including U.S. graduates).

Retaking the exam. If you fail the CSA, the period of time you must wait before retaking it depends on the total number of times you have failed.

- If you have failed the CSA **one** time, you must wait at least **three months** from the date of your most recent CSA fail before retaking it.
- If you have failed the CSA **two** times, you must wait at least **six months** from the date of your most recent CSA fail before retaking it.
- If you have failed the CSA **three or more** times, you must wait at least **one year** from the date of your most recent CSA fail before retaking it.

Test site locations. The CSA is currently administered at the following locations:

ECFMG CSA Center—Philadelphia
3624 Market Street, Third Floor
Philadelphia, PA 19104-2685

ECFMG CSA Center—Atlanta
Two Crown Center
1745 Phoenix Boulevard, Suite 500
Atlanta, GA 30349-5585

For more information about the CSA, please refer to *First Aid for the CSA*, which will be available in early 2004.

USMLE STEP 3 AND THE IMG

What is the USMLE Step 3? It is a computerized test in clinical medicine consisting of multiple-choice questions and computer-based case simulations (CCS).

Significance of the test. Taking Step 3 before residency is critical if the IMG is seeking an H1B visa and is a bonus that can be added to the application for residency. Step 3 is also required to obtain a full medical license in the United States and can be taken during residency for this purpose.

Official Web site. *www.usmle.org/step3*.

Fee. The fee for Step 3 is $590 (the total application fee can vary among states).

Eligibility. Most states require that applicants have completed one, two, or three years of postgraduate training (residency) prior to applying for Step 3 and permanent state licensure. The exceptions are the 11 states mentioned below, which allow IMGs to take Step 3 at the beginning of or even before residency. So if you don't fulfill the prerequisites to take Step 3 in your state of choice, simply use the name of one of the 11 states in your Step 3 application. You can take the exam in any state you choose regardless of the state that you mentioned on your application. Once you pass Step 3, it will be recognized by all states. Basic eligibility requirements for the USMLE Step 3 are as follows:

- Obtaining an MD or DO degree (or its equivalent) by the application deadline.
- Obtaining an ECFMG certificate if you are a graduate of a foreign medical school or successfully completing a "fifth pathway" program (at a date no later than the application deadline).

- Meeting the requirements imposed by the individual state licensing authority to which you are applying to take Step 3. Please refer to *www.fsmb.org* for more information.

The following states do not have postgraduate training as an eligibility requirement to apply for Step 3:

- Arkansas
- California
- Connecticut
- Florida
- Louisiana
- Maryland
- Nebraska*
- New York
- South Dakota
- Texas
- Utah*
- Washington
- West Virginia

Step 3 applications can be found online at *www.fsmb.org* and must be submitted to the FSMB.

RESIDENCIES AND THE IMG

It is becoming increasingly difficult for IMGs to obtain residencies in the United States given the rising concerns about an oversupply of physicians in the United States. Official bodies such as the Council on Graduate Medical Education (COGME) have recommended that the total number of residency slots be reduced from the current 144% of the number of U.S. graduates to 110%. Furthermore, ongoing changes in immigration laws and regulations influenced by homeland security are likely to make it much harder for noncitizens or legal residents of the United States to remain in the country after completing a residency.

In the residency Match, the number of U.S.-citizen IMG applications has been stable for the last few years, while the percentage accepted has slowly increased. For non-U.S.-citizen IMGs, applications fell from 7,977 in 1999 to 4,556 in 2002, while the percentage accepted significantly increased (see Table 2). This decrease in the total number of IMGs applying for the Match may be attributed to several factors:

- A decrease in the CSA passing rate to 80%.
- Increased difficulty obtaining a U.S. visa.
- Increased expenses associated with the USMLE exams, the CSA, ERAS, and travel to the United States.
- An increase in the number of IMGs who are withdrawing from the Match to sign a separate "pre-Match" contract with programs. This will be eliminated in the 2004 Match through a new policy adopted by the NRMP stating that "beginning with the 2004 Match, all sponsoring institutions participating in the NRMP Main Match must register and at-

---

*A "Valid indefinitely" ECFMG certificate is required (which means that you can be eligible as soon as you start your residency but not before). For complete contact information, refer to *www.fsmb.org/members.htm.*

tempt to fill all their positions in the Match except for those specialties or programs participating in other national matching programs." For more information, refer to *www.nrmp.org*.

VISA OPTIONS FOR THE IMG

If you are living outside the United States, you will need to apply for a visa that will allow you lawful entry into the United States in order to take the CSA and/or do your interviews for residency. A B1 or B2 visitor visa may be issued by the U.S. consulate in your country. Upon entry to the United States, either the B1 or, more commonly, the B2 will be issued on your I-94. Both visas allow you a limited period to stay in the United States (two to six months) in order to take the exam. If the given period is not sufficient, you may apply for an extension before the expiration of your I-94.

Documents that are recommended to facilitate this process include:

- The CSA admission permit and a letter from the ECFMG (which explains why the applicant must enter the United States).
- Your medical diploma.
- Transcripts from your medical school.
- Your USMLE score sheets.
- A sponsor letter or affidavit of support stating that you (if you are sponsoring yourself) or your sponsor will bear the expense of your trip and that you have sufficient funds to meet that expense.
- An alien status affidavit.

Individuals from certain countries may be allowed to enter the United States for up to 90 days without a visa under the Visa Waiver Program. See *www.immigration.gov*.

As an IMG, you need a visa to work or train in the United States unless you are a U.S. citizen or a permanent resident (i.e., hold a green card). Two types of visas enable you to accept a residency appointment in the United States: J1 and H1B. Most sponsoring residency programs (SRPs) prefer a J1 visa. Above all, this is because SRPs are authorized by the Department of Homeland Secu-

TABLE 2. IMGs in the Match

Applicants	2000	2001	2002
U.S.-citizen IMGs	2,169	1,999	2,029
% U.S. citizens accepted	51	52	54
Non-U.S.-citizen IMGs	7,287	5,116	4,556
% non-U.S. citizens accepted	38	45	51
U.S. graduates (non-IMGs)	14,358	14,455	14,336
% U.S. graduates accepted	94	94	94

rity (DHS)—which in 2003 took the place of the U.S. Immigration and Naturalization Service—to issue a Form DS-2019 (which replaced Form IAP-66 as of September 1, 2002) directly to an IMG. By contrast, SRPs must complete considerable paperwork, including an application to the Immigration and Labor Department, to apply to the DHS for an H1B visa on behalf of an IMG.

The J1 Visa

Also known as the Exchange Visitor Program, the J1 visa was introduced to give IMGs in diverse specialties the chance to use their training experience in the United States to improve conditions in their home countries. As mentioned above, the DHS authorizes most SRPs to issue Form DS-2019 in the same manner that I-20s are issued to regular international students in the United States.

To enable an SRP to issue a DS-2019, you must obtain a certificate from the ECFMG indicating that you are eligible to participate in a residency program in the United States. First, however, you must ask the Ministry of Health in your country to issue a statement indicating that your country needs physicians with the skills you propose to acquire from a U.S. residency program. This statement, which must bear the seal of your country's government and must be signed by a duly designated government official, is intended to satisfy the U.S. Secretary of Health and Human Services (HHS) that there is such a need. The Health Ministry in your country should send this statement to the ECFMG (or they may allow you to mail it to the ECFMG).

How can you find out if the government of your country will issue such a statement? In many countries, the Ministry of Health maintains a list of medical specialties in which there is a need for further training abroad. You can also consult seniors in your medical school. A word of caution: If you are applying for a residency in internal medicine and internists are not in short supply in your country, it may help to indicate an intention to pursue a subspecialty after completing your residency training.

The text of your statement of need should read as follows:

> Name of applicant for visa: _____. There currently exists in _____ (your country) a need for qualified medical practitioners in the specialty of _____. (Name of applicant for visa) has filed a written assurance with the government of this country that he/she will return to _____ (your country) upon completion of training in the United States and intends to enter the practice of medicine in the specialty for which training is being sought.
>
> Stamp (or seal and signature) of issuing official of named country.
> Dated _____

To facilitate the issuing of such a statement by the Ministry of Health in your country, you should submit a certified copy of the agreement or a contract from your SRP in the United States. The agreement or contract must be signed by you and the residency program official responsible for the training.

Armed with Form DS-2019, you should then go to the U.S. consulate closest to the residential address indicated in your passport. As for other nonimmigrant visas, you must show that you have a genuine nonimmigrant intent to return to your home country. You must also show that all your expenses will be paid.

When you enter the United States, bring your Form DS-2019 along with your visa. You are usually admitted to the United States for the length of the J1 program, designated as "D/S," or duration of status. The duration of your program is indicated on the DS-2019.

In the wake of the terrorist attacks of September 11, 2001, a number of new regulations have been introduced to improve the monitoring of exchange visitors during their time in the United States. As of January 30, 2003, all SRPs and students are required to register with the Student and Exchange Visitor Program (SEVP) via the Student and Exchange Visitor Information System (SEVIS). SEVIS allows the DHS to maintain up-to-date information (e.g., enrollment status, current address) on exchange visitors. As of January 30, 2002, SEVIS Form DS-2019 will be used for visa applications, admission, and change of status. Non-SEVIS forms such as Form IAP-66 issued prior to January 30, 2003, will be accepted until August 1, 2003. Procedural details for this new legislation are still being hammered out, so contact your SRP or check the DHS Web site (*www.immigration.gov*) for the most current information.

Duration of Participation. The duration of a resident's participation in a program of graduate medical education or training is limited to the time normally required to complete such a program. If you would like to get an idea of the typical training time for the various medical subspecialties, you may consult the *Directory of Medical Specialties,* published by Marquis Who's Who for the American Board of Medical Specialties. The authority charged with determining the duration of time required by an individual IMG is the State Department.

The maximum amount of time for participation in a training program is ordinarily limited to seven years unless the IMG has demonstrated to the satisfaction of the ECFMG and the State Department that his or her home country has an exceptional need for the specialty in which he or she will receive further training. An extension of stay may be granted in the event that an IMG needs to repeat a year of clinical medical training or needs time for training or education to take an exam required for board certification.

Requirements After Entry into the United States. Each year, all IMGs participating in a residency program on a J1 visa must furnish the Attorney General of the United States with an affidavit (Form I-644) attesting that they are in good standing in the program of graduate medical education or training in which they are participating and that they will return to their home countries upon completion of the education or training for which they came to the United States.

Restrictions Under the J1 Visa. No later than two years after the date of entry into the United States, an IMG participating in a residency program on a J1 visa is allowed one opportunity to change his or her designated program of graduate medical education or training if his or her director approves that change.

The J1 visa includes a condition called the "two-year foreign residence requirement." The relevant section of the Immigration and Nationality Act states:

> Any exchange visitor physician coming to the United States on or after January 10, 1977, for the purpose of receiving graduate medical education or training is automatically subject to the two-year home-country physical presence requirement of section 212(e) of the Immigration and Nationality Act, as amended. Such physicians are not eligible to be considered for section 212(e) waivers on the basis of 'No Objection' statements issued by their governments.

The law thus requires that a J1 visa holder, upon completion of the training program, leave the United States and reside in his or her home country for a period of at least two years. Currently, there is pressure from the American Medical Association (AMA) to extend this period to five years.

An IMG on a J1 visa is ordinarily not allowed to change from a J1 to most other types of visas or (in most cases) to change from J1 to permanent residence while in the United States until he or she has fulfilled the "foreign residence requirement." The purpose of the foreign residence requirement is to ensure that an IMG uses the training he or she obtained in the United States for the benefit of his or her home country. The U.S. government may, however, waive the two-year foreign residence requirement under the following circumstances:

- If you as an IMG can prove that returning to your country would result in "exceptional hardship" to you or to members of your immediate family who are U.S. citizens or permanent residents;
- If you as an IMG can demonstrate a "well-founded fear of persecution" due to race, religion, or political opinions if forced to return to your country;
- If you obtain a "no objection" statement from your government; or
- If you are sponsored by an "interested governmental agency" or a designated state Department of Health in the United States.

Applying for a J1 Visa Waiver. IMGs who have sought a waiver on the basis of the last alternative have found it beneficial to approach the following potentially "interested government agencies":

- **The Department of Health and Human Services.** As of 2003, HHS has expanded its role in reviewing J1 waiver applications. HHS's considerations for a waiver have classically been as follows: (1) the program or activity in which the IMG is engaged is "of high priority and of national or international significance in an area of interest" to HHS; (2) the IMG must be an "integral" part of the program or activity "so that the loss of his/her services would necessitate discontinuance of the program or a major phase of it"; and (3) the IMG "must possess outstanding qualifications, training, and experience well beyond the usually expected accomplishments at the graduate, postgraduate, and residency levels and must clearly demonstrate the capability to make original and significant contributions to the program." Under these criteria, HHS waivers are granted to physicians working in high-level biomedical research.

  New rules will also allow HHS to review J1 waiver applications from community health centers, rural hospitals, and other health care providers. In the past, the U.S. Department of Agriculture (USDA) served as the interested federal government agency that reviewed waiver applications to allow foreign doctors to serve in rural underserved communities outside Appalachia, while the Appalachian Regional Commission played that role for Appalachian communities. The USDA is no longer handling applications for J1 waivers. As such, HHS will now review waiver applications for primary care practitioners and psychiatrists who have completed residency training within one year of application to practice in designated Health Professional Shortage Areas (HPSAs), Medically Underserved Areas and Populations (MUA/Ps), and Mental Health Professional Shortage Areas (MHPSAs).

HHS waiver applications should be mailed to Joyce E. Jones, Executive Secretary, Exchange Visitor Waiver Review Board, Room 639-H, Hubert H. Humphrey Building, Department of Health and Human Services, 200 Independence Avenue, S.W., Washington, D.C. 20201; phone 202-690-6174; fax 202-690-7127.

- **The Veterans Administration.** With more than 170 health care facilities located in various parts of the United States, the VA is a major employer of physicians in this country. In addition, many VA hospitals are affiliated with university medical centers. The VA sponsors IMGs working in research, patient care (regardless of specialty), and teaching. The waiver applicant may engage in teaching and research in conjunction with clinical duties. The VA's latest guidelines (issued on June 22, 1994) provide that it will act as an interested government agency only when the loss of the IMG's services would necessitate the discontinuance of a program or a major phase of it and when recruitment efforts have failed to locate a U.S. physician to fill the position.

  The procedure for obtaining a VA sponsorship for a J1 waiver is as follows: (1) the IMG should deal directly with the Human Resources Department at the local VA facility; and (2) the facility must request that the VA's chief medical director sponsor the IMG for a waiver. The waiver request should include the following documentation: (1) a letter from the director of the local facility describing the program, the IMG's immigration status, the health care needs of the facility, and the facility's recruitment efforts; (2) recruitment efforts, including copies of all job advertisements run within the preceding year; and (3) copies of the IMG's licenses, test results, board certifications, IAP-66 or SEVIS DS-2019 forms, etc. The VA contact person in Washington, D.C., should be contacted by the local medical facility rather than by IMGs or their attorneys.

- **The Appalachian Regional Commission (ARC).** The ARC sponsors physicians in certain places in the eastern and southern United States— namely, in Alabama, Georgia, Kentucky, Maryland, Mississippi, New York, North Carolina, Ohio, Pennsylvania, South Carolina, Tennessee, Virginia, and West Virginia. Since 1992, the ARC has sponsored approximately 200 primary care IMGs annually in counties within its jurisdiction that have been designated as HPSAs by HHS.

  In accordance with its February 1994 revision of its J1 waiver policies, the ARC requires that waiver requests initially be submitted to the ARC contact person in the state of intended employment. Contact information for each state can be found on the ARC Web site (*www.arc.gov*). If the state concurs, a letter from the state's governor recommending the waiver must be addressed to Anne B. Pope, the new federal cochairman of the ARC. The waiver request should include the following: (1) a letter from the facility to Ms. Pope stating the proposed dates of employment, the IMG's medical specialty, the address of the practice location, an assertion that the IMG will practice primary care for at least 40 hours per week in the HPSA, and details as to why the facility needs the services of the IMG; (2) a J1 Visa Data Sheet; (3) the ARC federal cochairman's J1 Visa Waiver Policy and the J1 Visa Waiver Policy Affidavit and Agreement with the notarized signature of the IMG; (4) a contract of at least three years' duration; (5) evidence of the IMG's qualifications, including a résumé, medical diplomas and licenses, and IAP-66 or SEVIS DS-2019 forms; and (6) evidence of unsuccessful attempts to recruit qualified U.S. physicians within the preceding six months. Copies of advertisements, copies of résumés received, and reasons for rejection must also be included. The ARC will not sponsor IMGs who have been out of status for six months or longer.

Requests for ARC waivers are then processed in Washington, D.C. (ARC, 1666 Connecticut Avenue, N.W., Washington, D.C. 20235). The ARC is usually able to forward a letter confirming that a waiver has been recommended to the United States Information Agency (USIA) to the requesting facility or attorney within 30 days of the request.

- **The Department of Agriculture.** At the time of publication, the USDA is no longer sponsoring J1 waivers. The scope of the HHS J1 waiver program has been expanded to fill the gap.

- **State Departments of Public Health.** There is no application form for a state-sponsored J1 waiver. However, USIA regulations specify that an application must include the following documents: (1) a letter from the state Department of Public Health identifying the physician and specifying that it would be in the public interest to grant him a J1 waiver; (2) an employment contract that is valid for a minimum of three years and that states the name and address of the facility that will employ the physician and the geographic areas in which he or she will practice medicine; (3) evidence that these geographic areas are located within HPSAs; (4) a statement by the physician agreeing to the contractual requirements; (5) copies of all IAP-66 or SEVIS DS-2019 forms; and (6) a completed USIA Data Sheet. Applications are numbered in the order in which they are received, since only 30 physicians per year may be granted waivers in a particular state under the Conrad State 30 program. Individual states may choose to participate or not to participate in this program. At the time of publication, nonparticipating states included Idaho, Oklahoma, and Wyoming, while Texas had suspended its J1 waiver program pending new legislation.

The H1B Visa

Since 1991, the law has allowed medical residency programs to sponsor foreign-born medical residents for H1B visas. There are no restrictions to changing the H1B visa to any other kind of visa, including permanent resident status (green card), through employer sponsorship or through close relatives who are U.S. citizens or permanent residents. The overall ceiling for the number of H1B visas issued to professionals in all categories was increased to 195,000 for the years

2002–2003. This ceiling is scheduled to revert to 65,000 visas in 2004. It is advisable for SRPs to apply for H1B visas as soon as possible in the official year (beginning October 1) when the new quota officially opens up.

According to the Web site *www.immihelp.com*, as of October 17, 2000, the following beneficiaries of approved H1B petitions are exempt from the H1B annual cap:

- Beneficiaries who are in J1 nonimmigrant status in order to receive graduate medical education or training, and who have obtained a waiver of the two-year home residency requirement.
- Beneficiaries who are employed at, or who have received an offer of employment at, an institution of higher education or a related or affiliated nonprofit entity.
- Beneficiaries who are employed by, or who have received an offer of employment from, a nonprofit research organization.
- Beneficiaries who are employed by, or who have received an offer of employment from, a governmental research organization.
- Beneficiaries who are currently maintaining, or who have held within the last six years, H1B status, and are ineligible for another full six-year stay as an H1B.
- Beneficiaries who have been counted once toward the numerical limit and are the beneficiary of multiple petitions.

H1B visas are intended for "professionals" in a "specialty occupation." This means that an IMG intending to pursue a residency program in the United States with an H1B visa needs to clear all three USMLE Steps before becoming eligible for the H1B. The ECFMG administers Steps 1 and 2, whereas Step 3 is conducted by the individual states. You will need to contact the FSMB or the medical board of the state where you intend to take the Step 3 for details (see "USMLE Step 3 and the IMG," p. 27).

H1B Application

An application for an H1B visa is filed not by the IMG but rather by his or her employment sponsor—in your case, by the SRP in the United States. If an SRP is willing to do so, you will be told about it at the time of your interview for the residency program.

Before filing an H1B application with the DHS, an SRP must file an application with the U.S. Department of Labor affirming that the SRP will pay at least the normal salary for your job that a U.S. professional would earn. After receiving approval from the Labor Department, your SRP should be ready to file the H1B application with the DHS. The SRP's supporting letter is the most important part of the H1B application package; it must describe the job duties to make it clear that the physician is needed in a "specialty occupation" (resident) under the prevalent legal definition of that term.

Most SRPs prefer to issue a SEVIS Form DS-2019 for a J1 visa rather than file papers for an H1B visa because of the burden of paperwork and the attorney costs involved in securing approval of an H1B visa application. Even so, a sizable number of SRPs are willing to go through the trouble, particularly if an IMG is an excellent candidate or if the SRP concerned finds it difficult to fill all the available residency slots (although this is becoming rarer with continuing cuts in residency slots). If an SRP is unwilling to file for an H1B visa because of attorney costs, you could suggest that you would be willing to bear the burden of such costs. The entire process of getting an H1B visa can take anywhere from 10 to 20 weeks.

H1B Premium Processing Service. According to the Web site *www.my visa.com,* the DHS offers the opportunity to obtain processing of an H1B visa application within 15 calendar days. Within 15 days of receiving Form I-907, the DHS will mail you a notice of approval, request for evidence, intent to deny, or notice of investigation for fraud or misrepresentation. If the notice requires the submission of additional evidence or indicates an intent to deny, a new 15-day period will begin upon delivery to the DHS of a complete response to the request for evidence or notice of intent to deny. The fee for this service is $1,000. With this service, the total time needed to obtain an H1B visa has become significantly shorter than that required for the J1.

Although an H1B visa can be stamped by any U.S. consulate abroad, it is advisable that you have it stamped at the U.S. consulate where you first applied for a visitor visa to travel to the United States for interviews.

A FINAL WORD

IMGs should also be aware of a new program called the National Security Entry-Exit Registration System, which aims to tighten up homeland security by keeping closer tabs on nonimmigrants residing in or entering the United States on temporary visas.

Male citizens or nationals of specific countries who are already residing in the United States may be required to report to a designated DHS office for registration, which includes being fingerprinted, photographed, and interviewed under oath. The official list of countries includes Bangladesh, Egypt, Indonesia, Jordan, Kuwait, Pakistan, Saudi Arabia, Afghanistan, Algeria, Bahrain, Eritrea, Lebanon, Morocco, North Korea, Oman, Qatar, Somalia, Tunisia, the United Arab Emirates, Yemen, Iran, Iraq, Libya, Sudan, and Syria. Different registration deadlines and criteria have been assigned to citizens of the above-mentioned countries, so please refer to the DHS Web site for details (*www.im migration.gov*).

If you are entering the United States, you may be registered at the port of entry if you are (1) a citizen or national of Iran, Iraq, Libya, Sudan, or Syria; (2) a nonimmigrant who has been designated by the State Department; or (3) any other nonimmigrant identified by immigration officers at airports, seaports, and land ports of entry in accordance with new regulation 8 CFR 264.1(f)(2). If you will be staying in the United States for more than 30 days, you will then be required to register in person at a DHS district office within 30 days for an interview and will be required to reregister annually.

Once you are registered, certain special procedures will apply. If you leave the United States for any reason, you must appear in person before a DHS inspecting officer at a preapproved airport, seaport, or land port and leave the United States from that port on the same day. If you change your address, employment, or school, you must report to the DHS in writing within ten days using Form AR-11 SR. If any of these regulations are not followed, you may be considered out of status and subject to arrest, detention, fines, and/or removal from the United States, and any further application for immigration may be affected.

For the most up-to-date information regarding policies and procedures, please consult *www.immigration.gov*.

Summary

Despite some significant obstacles, a number of viable methods are available to IMGs who seek visas to pursue a residency program or eventually practice medicine in the United States.

There is no doubt that the best alternative for an IMG is to obtain an H1B visa to pursue a medical residency. However, in cases where an IMG joins a residency program with a J1 visa, there are some possibilities for obtaining waivers of the two-year foreign residency requirement, particularly for those who are willing to make a commitment to perform primary care medicine in medically underserved areas.

RESOURCES FOR THE IMG

- ECFMG
  3624 Market Street, Fourth Floor
  Philadelphia, PA 19104-2685
  215-386-5900 or 202-293-9320
  Fax: 215-386-9196
  www.ecfmg.org

  The ECFMG telephone number is answered only between 9:00 A.M. and 12:30 P.M. and between 1:30 P.M. and 5:00 P.M. Monday through Friday EST. The ECFMG often takes a long time to answer the phone, which is frequently busy at peak times of the year, and then gives you a long voice-mail message—so it is better to write or fax early than to rely on a last-minute phone call. Do not contact the NBME, as all IMG exam matters are conducted by the ECFMG. The ECFMG also publishes an information booklet on ECFMG certification and the USMLE program, which gives details on the dates and locations of forthcoming USMLE, CSA, and English tests for IMGs together with application forms. It is free of charge and is also available from the public affairs offices of U.S. embassies and consulates worldwide as well as from Overseas Educational Advisory Centers. You may order single copies of the handbook by calling 215-386-5900, preferably on weekends or between 6 P.M. and 6 A.M. Philadelphia time, or by faxing to 215-387-9963. Requests for multiple copies must be made by fax or mail on organizational letterhead. The full text of the booklet is also available on the ECFMG's Web site at *www.ecfmg.org*.

- Federation of State Medical Boards
  P.O. Box 619850
  Dallas, TX 75261-9850
  817-868-4000
  Fax: 817-868-4099
  www.fsmb.org

The FSMB has a number of publications available, including *The Exchange, Section I*, which gives detailed information on examination and licensing requirements in all U.S. jurisdictions. The cost is $30. (Texas residents must add 8.25% state sales tax.) To obtain these publications, submit the online order form. Payment options include Visa or Master-Card. Alternatively, write to Federation Publications at the above address. All orders must be prepaid with a personal check drawn on a U.S. bank, a cashier's check, or a money order payable to the federation. Foreign orders must be accompanied by an international money order or the equivalent, payable in U.S. dollars through a U.S. bank or a U.S. affiliate of a foreign bank. For Step 3 inquiries, the telephone number is 817-868-4041. You may e-mail the FSMB at usmle@fsmb.org or write to Examination Services at the address above.

- Immigration information for IMGs is available from the sites of Siskind, Susser, Haas & Devine, a firm of attorneys specializing in immigration law: *www.visalaw.com/IMG/resources.html.*
- Another source of immigration information can be found on the Web site of the law offices of Carl Shusterman, a Los Angeles attorney specializing in medical immigration law: *www.shusterman.com.*
- The AMA has dedicated a portion of its Web site to information on IMG demographics, residencies, immigration (double-check that the information is up to date), and the like: *www.ama-assn.org/ama/pub/category/17.html.*
- International Medical Placement Ltd., a U.S. company specializing in recruiting foreign physicians to work in the United States, has a site at *www.intlmedicalplacement.com.*
- Two more useful Web sites are *www.myvisa.com* and *www.immihelp.com.*
- *First Aid for the International Medical Graduate*, 2nd ed., by Keshav Chander (2002; 313 pages; ISBN 0071385320), is an excellent resource written by a successful IMG. The book includes interviews with successful IMGs and students gearing up for the USMLE, complete "getting settled" information for new residents, and tips for dealing with possible social and cultural transition difficulties. The book provides useful advice on the U.S. curriculum, the health care delivery system, and ethical issues—and the differences IMGs should expect. Dr. Chander points out the weaknesses often found in IMG hopefuls and suggests ways to improve their performance on standardized tests as well as on academic and clinical evaluations. As a bonus, the guide contains information on how to get good fellowships after residency. The bottom line is that this is a reassuring guide that can help IMGs boost their confidence and proficiency. A great "first of its kind" that will empower IMGs with information that they need to succeed.

Other books that may be useful and of interest to IMGs are as follows:

- *International Medical Graduates in U.S. Hospitals: A Guide for Program Directors and Applicants*, by Faroque A. Khan and Lawrence G. Smith (1995; ISBN 094312641x).
- *Insider's Guide for the International Medical Graduate to Obtain a Medical Residency in the U.S.A.*, by Ahmad Hakemi (1999; ISBN 1929803001).

The USMLE provides accommodations for students with documented disabilities. The basis for such accommodations is the Americans with Disabilities Act (ADA) of 1990. The ADA defines a disability as "a significant limitation in one or more major life activities." This includes both "observable/physical" disabilities (e.g., blindness, hearing loss, narcolepsy) and "hidden/mental disabilities" (e.g., attention deficit hyperactivity disorder [ADHD], chronic fatigue syndrome, learning disabilities).

To provide appropriate support, the administrators of the USMLE must be informed of both the nature and the severity of an examinee's disability. Such documentation is required for an examinee to receive testing accommodations. Accommodations include extra time on tests, low-stimulation environments, extra or extended breaks, and an enlarged typeface.

Who Can Apply for Accommodations?

Students or graduates of a school in the United States or Canada that is accredited by the LCME or the American Osteopathic Association (AOA) may apply for test accommodations directly from the NBME. Requests are granted only if they meet the ADA definition of a disability. If you are a disabled student or a disabled graduate of a foreign medical school, you must contact the ECFMG (see below).

Who Is Not Eligible for Accommodations?

Individuals who do not meet the ADA definition of disabled are not eligible for test accommodations. Difficulties not eligible for test accommodations include test anxiety, slow reading without an identified underlying cognitive deficit, English as a second language, or learning difficulties that have not been diagnosed as a medically recognized disability.

Understanding the Need for Documentation

Although most learning-disabled medical students are all too familiar with the often exhausting process of providing documentation of their disability, you should realize that **applying for USMLE accommodation is different from these previous experiences.** This is because the NBME determines whether an individual is disabled solely on the basis of the guidelines set by the ADA.

Getting the Information

The first step in applying for USMLE special accommodations is to contact the NBME and obtain guidelines and a questionnaire booklet. You can do so by calling or writing to:

Testing Coordinator
Disability Services
National Board of Medical Examiners
3750 Market Street
Philadelphia, PA 19104-3190
215-590-9869

Internet access to this information is available at *www.nbme.org*. This information is also relevant to IMGs.

Foreign graduates should contact the ECFMG to obtain information on special accommodations by calling or writing to:

Test Accommodations Coordinator
ECFMG
3624 Market Street, Fourth Floor
Philadelphia, PA 19104-2685
215-386-5900

When you get this information, take some time to read it carefully. The guidelines are explicit about what you need to do to obtain accommodations.

Applying for Accommodations

Although the accommodation guidelines cited above are self-explanatory, here are some key points to keep in mind:

- **Produce a history.** Send the NBME extensive past records. Since almost all learning disabilities are present from birth, even the earliest records of your disability can be invaluable tools in your assessment. Even if you were diagnosed at a late age, a "paper trail" of your learning disability should still be evident. Grade-school reports, tutoring letters, job reports, previous physician notes, report cards, teacher comments, medication history, and other documents will go a long way toward providing significant evidence of your learning disability.
- **Send your "official" documentation.** Most individuals who were diagnosed with a learning disability were given a specific battery of tests (an extensive list of these tests is given in the guidelines). Contact the physician who administered these tests and have the results sent to you. If you cannot locate that physician, obtain the documentation from the educational institutions you attended (college, high school, etc.). Verify that both the administering physician's clinical impressions and the results of your specific tests are included in your submitted material.

Reevaluating Your Disability

You may want to have your disability reevaluated for the USMLE. As stated previously, obtaining accommodations for the USMLE is different from any other process, as you are being evaluated solely on the basis of how well you meet the criteria specified by the ADA. Your evaluator should bear this in mind when he or she performs the assessment. Sharing the information in the guidelines and questionnaire booklet with your evaluator will ensure that he or she is aware of this.

The purpose of a reevaluation is twofold. First, it is meant to produce further proof of the disability. Second, it is meant to determine the need for accommodation based on the level of current functioning.

Reevaluation is not for everyone. An evaluation represents a considerable time commitment and is difficult to schedule during the hectic second year. An evaluation is also expensive, usually costing anywhere from $500 to

$2,000. Furthermore, since a reevaluation is not being ordered for strictly "medical reasons" and is investigating a "previous condition," your insurance company may not cover it.

If you do decide to get reevaluated, the following is highly recommended:

- **Choose an expert.** You're in medical school. Use it! Most of the leading experts on learning disabilities are associated with medical school faculty, so ask around for the leading learning disabilities expert affiliated with your medical school, and use that physician as your evaluator. Make sure you stress to the evaluator that he or she is functioning independently and not as a school advocate. Using someone at your school is also desirable from a cost perspective, as a faculty member may charge you a lower evaluation fee.
- **Undergo some testing.** If you have undergone previous cognitive testing, this step is probably not that important. However, you might want to undergo some basic tests that assess your current level of cognitive functioning. A purely clinical evaluation is commonly limited in both scope and ability. **If you have never undergone a full evaluation, a comprehensive diagnostic battery is essential.** Make sure your evaluator is looking not just at one or two sessions or subtests but at the entire gestalt.
- **Share your previous history with the evaluator.** Even though the USMLE reviewer will examine your documentation, your evaluator should also have access to your medical history. In that way, he or she can highlight or emphasize certain aspects of your record.
- **Ask for a differential diagnosis.** Evaluators should offer a differential, not just a single diagnosis. Once the differential has been made, evidence for or against any alternative diagnosis should be presented.

Finally, it is highly advisable that you talk from the heart. Part of the application is an essay you write about your disability. This is your opportunity to shine. Even if you have problems with writing, an honest, heartfelt essay will go a long way. No one else but you can truly describe your learning disability, so view this as an opportunity to share your difficulties with a receptive audience.

The Accommodations

A wide variety of accommodations exist for the USMLE. Test accommodations include but are not limited to the following:

- Assistance with keyboard tasks
- Audio rendition
- Extended testing time
- Extra breaks
- Enlarged typeface

By far the most commonly requested and granted accommodation is for extra time. The ADA requires that individuals with a disability be provided with "equal access" to the testing program. Therefore, the purpose of accommodations is to "cancel" the effect of the disability, not to provide extra help in passing an examination.

Because the same types of impairments often vary in severity and frequently restrict different people to different degrees or in different ways, each request is considered individually to determine the effect of the impairment on the life of the applicant and whether a particular accommodation is even appropriate for that person.

The following additional material is excerpted from the NBME Web site (*www.nbme.org*) and is copyright 1996–2002 by the NBME.

If I am requesting an accommodation from the NBME on Step 1 or Step 2, when should I send in my request and documentation?

Mail your request and supporting documentation for test accommodations directly to the NBME Office of Test Accommodations at the *same time* you submit your Step 1 application. Don't submit your test accommodations request with your application.

Can my evaluator or my medical school send in my request for test accommodations?

No. A request for accommodations, by law, must be initiated by the person with a disability. Also, to protect your confidentiality, the NBME does not provide information concerning your request to third parties.

How does the NBME determine what is an appropriate accommodation for USMLE?

As part of the documentation, the examinee's evaluator should recommend appropriate accommodations to ease the impact of the impairment on the testing activity. Professional consultants in learning disabilities, ADHD, and various other psychiatric and physical conditions review the documentation and recommendations of evaluators to help match the type of assistance with the demonstrated need. The NBME consults with the examinee to determine what accommodations have been effectively used in the past.

If I apply for test accommodations on USMLE, does my disability evaluation have to be up to date?

For someone with a continuing history of accommodation, which would likely include high school and college as well as medical school, current testing is usually not necessary if objective documentation of the past accommodations is provided. However, the impact of the disability may change over time, and new testing may be necessary to demonstrate the current level of impairment and resulting need for accommodation. You will be advised if updated testing is needed.

What are some reasons my request for accommodations might not be approved?

- Insufficient documentation of a need for accommodation. Conditions such as learning disabilities and ADHD are permanent and lifelong. A diagnosis requires an objective history of chronic symptoms from childhood to adulthood as well as evidence of significant impairment currently.

- Absence of a moderate to severe level of impairment attributable to the disorder.
- The identified difficulty is not considered to be a disability under the law, i.e., slow reading without evidence of an underlying language processing disorder; language difficulties as a result of English as a second language.

Once my request for accommodations has been approved, do I need to arrange for accommodations the next time I register for a Step?

Yes. An examinee with a disability must request accommodations at the time of registration for each Step. NBME examinees must send a letter requesting accommodations to the Office of Test Accommodations. A repeated request must state whether any change in the accommodations is required, and if so, documentation of the needed change must be provided.

Accommodations are not granted automatically even if they were approved for previous Step administrations.

Miscellaneous Suggestions

- **Get your information to the USMLE early.** The earlier your information is received, the more time the USMLE will have for evaluating and considering your case. They will also have time to ask you for additional material should this prove necessary.
- **Use your winter holiday.** It is a lot easier to get this material ready for the USMLE when you are not in school. It is also immeasurably easier to be evaluated when you are not facing the pressures of the second year.

Approximately 75% of the total number of requests for all Steps are approved.

NOTES

Database of High-Yield Facts

"There comes a time when for every addition of knowledge you forget something that you knew before. It is of the highest importance, therefore, not to have useless facts elbowing out the useful ones."
—Arthur Conan Doyle, "A Study in Scarlet"

"Never regard study as a duty, but as the enviable opportunity to learn."
—Albert Einstein

"Live as if you were to die tomorrow. Learn as if you were to live forever."
—Gandhi

Cardiovascular
Dermatology
Endocrinology
Epidemiology and Preventive Medicine
Ethics
Gastrointestinal
Hematology/Oncology
Infectious Disease
Musculoskeletal
Neurology
Obstetrics
Gynecology
Pediatrics
Psychiatry
Pulmonary
Renal
Selected Topics in Emergency Medicine
Rapid Review

The fourth edition of *First Aid for the USMLE Step 2* contains a revised and expanded database of clinical material that student authors and faculty have identified as high yield for boards review. The facts are organized according to subject matter, whether medical specialty (e.g., Cardiovascular, Renal) or high-yield topic (e.g., Ethics) in medicine. Each subject is then divided into smaller subsections of related facts. Individual facts are generally presented in a logical approach, from basic definitions and epidemiology to **History/Physical Exam, Differential, Evaluation,** and **Treatment.** Lists, mnemonics, and tables are used when helpful in forming key associations.

The content is mostly useful for reviewing material already learned. This section is not ideal for learning complex or highly conceptual material for the first time. At the beginning of many sections we list supplementary high-yield review material from ***First Aid for the USMLE Step 1*** to jog your memory about important basic science concepts. Black-and-white images appear throughout the text. In some cases, reference is made to the "clinical image" section at the end of Section II, which contains full-color glossy plates of histology and patient pathology by topic. Selected topics have embedded references to the eight titles in the ***Underground Clinical Vignettes*** (UCV) ***Step 2*** series, second edition (Blackwell Science). These annotations link the high-yield fact to a corresponding vignette, illustrating how that fact may appear in a Step 2 clinical scenario. The following annotation, for example, refers to cases 23 and 45 from *UCV Pediatrics:* Ped.23, 45

UCV REFERENCE LEGEND	
UCV Title	**Abbreviation**
Emergency Medicine, 3rd ed.	EM
Internal Medicine, Vol. 1, 3rd ed.	IM1
Internal Medicine, Vol. 2, 3rd ed.	IM2
Neurology, 3rd ed.	Neuro
Obstetrics and Gynecology, 3rd ed.	OB
Pediatrics, 3rd ed.	Ped
Psychiatry, 3rd ed.	Psych
Surgery, 3rd ed.	Surg

At the end of each chapter we include boards-type clinical case scenarios extracted from the McGraw-Hill *PreTest* series. Multiple-choice question-and-answer explanations are provided. At the end of Section II, we also feature a Rapid Review chapter of key facts and classic associations to cram a day or two before the exam.

The Database of High-Yield Facts is not comprehensive. Use it to complement your core study material and not as your primary study source. The facts and notes have been condensed and edited to emphasize the essential material. Work with the material, add your own notes and mnemonics, and recognize that not all memory techniques work for all students.

We update Section II biannually to keep current with new trends in boards content as well as to expand our database of high-yield information. However, we must note that inevitably many other very high-yield entries and topics are not yet included in our database.

We actively encourage medical students and faculty to submit entries and mnemonics so that we may enhance the database for future students. We also solicit recommendations of alternate tools for study that may be useful in preparing for the examination, such as diagrams, charts, and computer-based tutorials (see How to Contribute, page xv).

Disclaimer

The entries in this section reflect student opinions of what is high yield. Owing to the diverse sources of material, no attempt has been made to trace or reference the origins of entries individually. We have regarded mnemonics as essentially in the public domain. All errors and omissions will be gladly corrected if brought to the attention of the authors, either through the publisher or directly by e-mail.

Cardiovascular

Coronary artery anatomy

In the majority of cases, the SA and AV nodes are supplied by the RCA. 80% of the time, the RCA supplies the inferior portion of the left ventricle via the PD artery (= right dominant).

Coronary artery occlusion occurs most commonly in the LAD, which supplies the anterior interventricular septum.

Coronary arteries fill during diastole.

Right coronary artery (RCA)

Left main coronary artery (LCA)

Circumflex artery (CFX)

Left anterior descending artery (LAD)

Acute marginal artery

Posterior descending artery (PD)

(Adapted, with permission, from Ganong WF. *Review of Medical Physiology*, 19th ed. Stamford, CT: Appleton & Lange, 1999:592.)

Diagnosis of MI

In the first 6 hours, ECG is the gold standard.

Cardiac troponin I is used within the first 4 hours up to 7–10 days; more specific than other protein markers.

CK-MB is test of choice in the first 24 hours post-MI.

LDH_1 (former test of choice) is also elevated from 2 to 7 days post-MI.

AST is nonspecific and can be found in cardiac, liver, and skeletal muscle cells.

ECG changes can include ST elevation (transmural ischemia) and Q waves (transmural infarct).

Troponin CK-MB AST LDH_1

Pain Days 1 2

Cardiac cycle

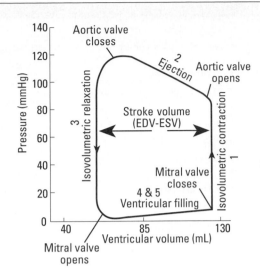

Phases:

1. Isovolumetric contraction—period between mitral valve closure and aortic valve opening; period of highest oxygen consumption
2. Systolic ejection—period between aortic valve opening and closing
3. Isovolumetric relaxation—period between aortic valve closing and mitral valve opening
4. Rapid filling—period just after mitral valve opening
5. Slow filling—period just before mitral valve closure

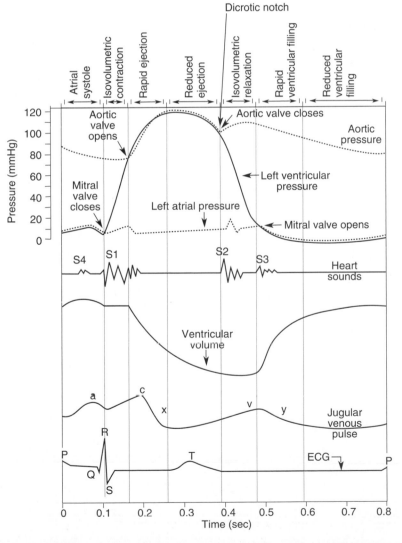

Sounds:

S1—mitral and tricuspid valve closure.
S2—aortic and pulmonary valve closure.
S3—at end of rapid ventricular filling.
S4—high atrial pressure/stiff ventricle.

S3 is associated with dilated CHF.
S4 ("atrial kick") is associated with a hypertrophic ventricle.

a wave—atrial contraction.
c wave—RV contraction (tricuspid valve bulging into atrium).
v wave—increased atrial pressure due to filling against closed tricuspid valve.

Jugular venous distention is seen in right heart failure.

(Adapted, with permission, from Ganong WF. *Review of Medical Physiology*, 19th ed. Stamford, CT: Appleton & Lange, 1999:541.)

Cardiac output (CO)

Cardiac output = (stroke volume) × (heart rate).

Fick principle

$$CO = \frac{\text{rate of } O_2 \text{ consumption}}{\text{arterial } O_2 \text{ content} - \text{venous } O_2 \text{ content}}$$

$$\begin{pmatrix}\text{Mean arterial} \\ \text{pressure}\end{pmatrix} = \begin{pmatrix}\text{cardiac} \\ \text{output}\end{pmatrix} \times \begin{pmatrix}\text{total peripheral} \\ \text{resistance}\end{pmatrix}$$

Similar to Ohm's law:
  Voltage = (current) × (resistance)
MAP = ⅓ systolic + ⅔ diastolic.
Pulse pressure = systolic − diastolic.
Pulse pressure ≈ stroke volume.

$$SV = \frac{CO}{HR} = EDV - ESV$$

$$EF = \frac{SV}{EDV} \times 100\% \ (\text{normal} \approx 55\text{--}80\%)$$

During exercise, CO ↑ initially as a result of an ↑ in SV. After prolonged exercise, CO ↑ as a result of an ↑ in HR.
If HR is too high, diastolic filling is incomplete and CO ↓ (e.g., ventricular tachycardia).

Cardiac output variables

Stroke volume affected by **C**ontractility, **A**fterload, and **P**reload. Increased SV when ↑ preload, ↓ afterload, or ↑ contractility.
Contractility (and SV) ↑ with:
  1. Catecholamines (↑ activity of Ca^{2+} pump in sarcoplasmic reticulum)
  2. ↑ intracellular calcium
  3. ↓ extracellular sodium
  4. Digitalis (↑ intracellular Na^+, resulting in ↑ Ca^{2+})
Contractility (and SV) ↓ with:
  1. β_1 blockade
  2. Heart failure
  3. Acidosis
  4. Hypoxia/hypercapnea

SV **CAP**.

Stroke volume ↑ in anxiety, exercise, and pregnancy.
A failing heart has ↓ stroke volume.
Myocardial O_2 demand is ↑ by:
  1. ↑ afterload (∝ diastolic BP)
  2. ↑ contractility
  3. ↑ heart rate
  4. ↑ heart size (↑ wall tension)

HIGH-YIELD FACTS

Cardiovascular

Electrocardiogram

P wave—atrial depolarization.

PR segment—conduction delay through AV node (normally < 200 msec).

QRS complex—ventricular depolarization (normally < 120 msec).

Q-T interval—mechanical contraction of the ventricles.

T wave—ventricular repolarization.

Atrial repolarization is masked by QRS complex.

ST segment—isoelectric, ventricles depolarized.

U wave—caused by hypokalemia.

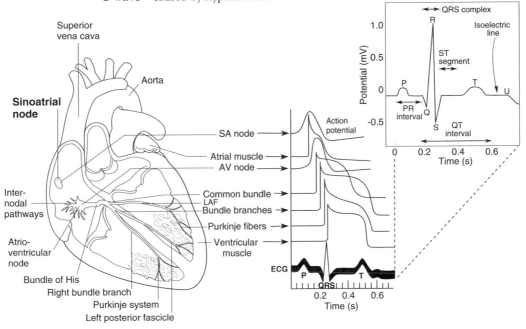

SA node "pacemaker" inherent dominance with slow phase of upstroke
AV node - 100-msec delay - atrioventricular delay

(Adapted, with permission, from Ganong WF. *Review of Medical Physiology,* 20th ed. New York: McGraw-Hill, 2001.)

Myocardial action potential

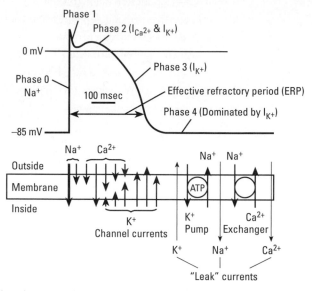

Occurs in atrial and ventricular myocytes and Purkinje fibers.

Phase 0 = rapid upstroke—voltage-gated Na^+ channels open.

Phase 1 = initial repolarization—inactivation of voltage-gated Na^+ channels. Voltage-gated K^+ channels begin to open.

Phase 2 = plateau—Ca^{2+} influx through voltage-gated Ca^{2+} channels balances K^+ efflux. Ca^{2+} influx triggers another Ca^{2+} release from SR and myocyte contraction.

Phase 3 = rapid repolarization—massive K^+ efflux due to opening of voltage-gated slow K^+ channels and closure of voltage-gated Ca^{2+} channels.

Phase 4 = resting potential—high K^+ permeability through K^+ channels.

Lipid-lowering agents

Drug	Effect on LDL "bad cholesterol"	Effect on HDL "good cholesterol"	Effect on triglycerides	Side effects/problems
Bile acid resins (cholestyramine, colestipol)	↓↓	No effect	Slightly ↑	Patients hate it—tastes bad and causes GI discomfort
HMG-CoA reductase inhibitors (lovastatin, pravastatin, simvastatin, atorvastatin)	↓↓↓	↑	↓	Expensive, reversible ↑ LFTs, myositis
Niacin	↓↓	↑↑	↓	Red, flushed face, which is ↓ by aspirin or long-term use
Lipoprotein lipase stimulators (gemfibrozil, clofibrate)	↓	↑	↓↓↓	Myositis, ↑ LFTs

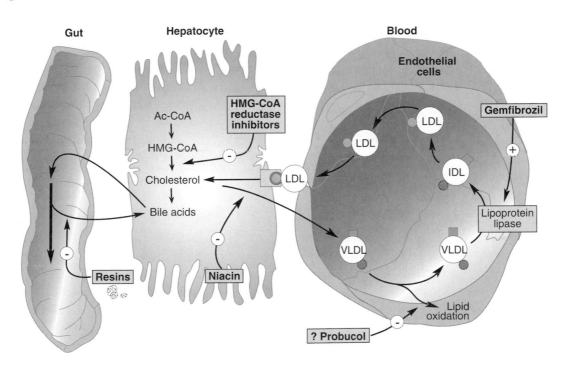

(Adapted, with permission, from Katzung BG, Trevor AJ. *Examination & Board Review: Pharmacology*, 5th ed. Stamford, CT: Appleton & Lange, 1998:267.)

Cardiovascular

Abnormalities of cardiac rhythm can be asymptomatic, symptomatic, or lethal (Tables 2.1–1 to 2.1–3 and Figures 2.1–1 to 2.1–3).

HIGH-YIELD FACTS

Cardiovascular

		TABLE 2.1–1. Bradyarrhythmias		
Type	**Etiology**	**Signs/ Symptoms**	**ECG Findings**	**Treatment**
Sinus bradycardia	Normal response to cardiovascular (CV) conditioning. Can arise due to sinus node dysfunction.	Asymptomatic or light-headedness, syncope, and hypotension.	Ventricular rate < 60 bpm. Normal P waves before every QRS complex.	None necessary if asymptomatic. Atropine may be used to increase HR. Pacemaker placement is definitive treatment.
Right bundle branch block (RBBB)	Can occur in normal individuals. Can arise as a result of COPD, valvular disease, chronic CAD, or after surgical repair of a VSD.	Asymptomatic.	QRS duration > 0.12 sec. rSR complex with a wide R wave in V_1. QRS pattern with a wide S wave in V_6.	None necessary.
Left bundle branch block (LBBB)	Usually a sign of organic heart disease. HTN, valvular disease, cardio-myopathy, CAD.	Often asymptomatic.	QRS duration > 0.12 sec. Wide, entirely negative QS complex in V_1. Wide, tall R wave with no Q wave in V_6.	Usually none necessary. Ventricular pace-maker is defini-tive therapy in post-MI LBBB patients with conduction defects.
AV block				
Primary (first-degree) heart block	Can occur in normal individuals. Increased vagal tone.	Asymptomatic.	PR interval > 0.2 sec.	None necessary.
Secondary (second-degree) heart block (Mobitz I)	Drug effect (digoxin, β-blockade, Ca^{2+} channel blockers). Increased vagal tone.	Usually asymptomatic.	Increasing PR interval until a dropped beat occurs (Wenckebach); PR then resets.	Stop the offending drug.

TABLE 2.1–1. Bradyarrhythmias (continued)

Type	Etiology	Signs/Symptoms	ECG Findings	Treatment
AV block (*continued*) Secondary (second-degree) heart block (Mobitz II)	Fibrotic disease of the conduction system or previous septal MI.	Occasionally syncope or progression to third-degree AV block.	Unexpected dropped beat without a change in PR interval.	Pacemaker placement.
Tertiary (third-degree, complete) heart block	No electrical communication between the atria and ventricles.	Syncope, dizziness, acute heart failure, hypotension, cannon A waves.	No relationship between P waves and QRS complexes.	Pacemaker placement.

TABLE 2.1–2. Supraventricular Tachyarrhythmias

Type	Etiology	Signs/Symptoms	ECG Findings	Treatment
Sinus tachycardia	Normal physiologic response to fear, pain, exercise.	Palpitations, shortness of breath (SOB).	Ventricular rate > 100 bpm. Normal P waves before every QRS complex.	None necessary.
Atrial fibrillation (AF)	**PIRATES:** **P**ulmonary disease **I**schemia **R**heumatic heart disease **A**nemia/atrial myxoma *(IM1.3)* **T**hyrotoxicosis **E**thanol **S**epsis	Often asymptomatic. May have SOB, chest pain, or palpitations. Irregularly irregular pulse.	Wavy baseline without discernible P waves. Variable and irregular QRS response.	Anticoagulation (to prevent stroke) and rate control (Ca^{2+} channel blockers, β-blockers, digoxin). Cardioversion (electrical or pharmacologic) only if new onset (< 36 hours), if transesophageal echocardiogram (TEE) shows no clot in the left atrium, or after six weeks of warfarin treatment.

HIGH-YIELD FACTS

Cardiovascular

57

TABLE 2.1–2. Supraventricular Tachyarrhythmias *(continued)*

Type	Etiology	Signs/Symptoms	ECG Findings	Treatment
Atrial flutter	Circular movement of electrical activity around atrium at rate of 300 times/minute. Associated with CAD, CHF, COPD, valvular disease, pericarditis.	Asymptomatic or palpitations, syncope, and light-headedness.	Regular rhythm. "Sawtooth" appearance of P waves.	Anticoagulation and rate control. Cardioversion (electrical, pharmacologic) only if new onset (< 36 hours), if TEE shows no clot in the left atrium, or after six weeks of warfarin treatment.
Multifocal atrial tachycardia	Multiple atrial pacemakers or reentrant pathways. COPD, hypoxemia	May be asymptomatic.	Three or more P-wave morphologies. Rate > 100.	Treat underlying disorder. Verapamil.
Paroxysmal supraventricular tachycardia (PSVT) Atrioventricular nodal reentry tachycardia	Reentry circuit in AV node depolarizes atrium and ventricle simultaneously.	Palpitations, SOB, angina, syncope, light-headedness.	Rate 150–250 bpm. P wave often buried in **normal QRS** or shortly after.	Carotid massage, Valsalva, or adenosine (to slow AV node for diagnosis). Cardioversion if hemodynamically unstable.
Atrioventricular reentry tachycardia	Circular movement of impulse down AV node and back up to atrium through a bypass tract *(IM1.15)*.	Palpitations, SOB, angina, syncope, light-headedness.	Retrograde P wave often seen after a **normal QRS.**	Carotid massage, Valsalva, or adenosine. Cardioversion if hemodynamically unstable.
Paroxysmal atrial tachycardia	Rapid ectopic pacemaker in atrium (not sinus node).	Palpitations, SOB, angina, syncope, light-headedness.	Rate > 100 bpm. P wave with unusual axis before each **normal QRS.**	Carotid massage, Valsalva, or adenosine. Cardioversion if hemodynamically unstable.

TABLE 2.1–3. Ventricular Tachyarrhythmias

Type	Etiology	Signs/ Symptoms	ECG Findings	Treatment
Premature ventricular contraction (PVC)	Ectopic beats arise from ventricular foci. Common and often benign. Causes include hypoxia, electrolyte abnormalities, hyperthyroidism.	Usually asymptomatic, but may cause palpitations.	Early, wide QRS complexes that are not preceded by a P wave. PVCs are followed by a compensatory pause.	No treatment if asymptomatic. If symptomatic, give β-blockers or other antiarrhythmics. Treat underlying cause.
Ventricular tachycardia (VT)	Associated with CAD and MI.	Nonsustained VT (NSVT) is often asymptomatic. Sustained VT can cause palpitations, hypotension, angina, and VF (if untreated).	Three or more consecutive PVCs. Wide QRS complexes in a regular rapid rhythm. AV dissociation.	Antiarrhythmics (amiodarone, lidocaine, procainamide). If hemodynamically unstable, treat as VF.
Ventricular fibrillation (VF) (EM.6)	Associated with CAD and MI.	Syncope, hypotension, pulselessness.	Totally erratic tracing.	Immediate electrical cardioversion and ACLS protocol.

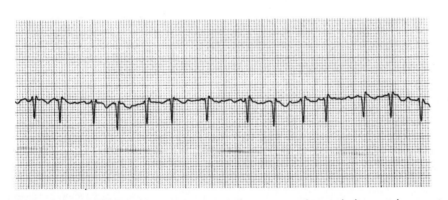

FIGURE 2.1–1. Atrial fibrillation. Note the absence of P waves and irregularly irregular ventricular rhythm. (Reproduced, with permission, from Stobo J et al. *The Principles and Practice of Medicine*, 23rd ed. Stamford, CT: Appleton & Lange, 1996:78, Fig. 1–9–3B.)

HIGH-YIELD FACTS

Cardiovascular

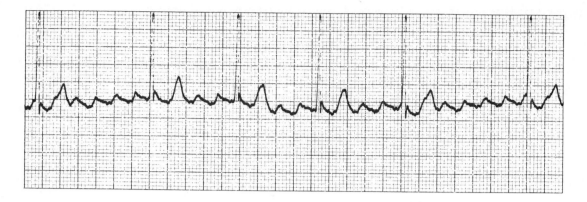

FIGURE 2.1–2. Atrial flutter. The "sawtooth" baseline of rapid but organized atrial activity (usually between 250 and 350 bpm) is characteristic. (Reproduced, with permission, from Ochs G. *Recognition and Interpretation of ECG Rhythms,* 3rd ed. Stamford, CT: Appleton & Lange, 1997:34, Fig. 2–17.)

A. Ventricular tachycardia

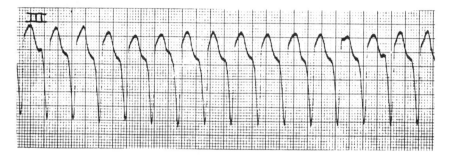

B. Ventricular fibrillation

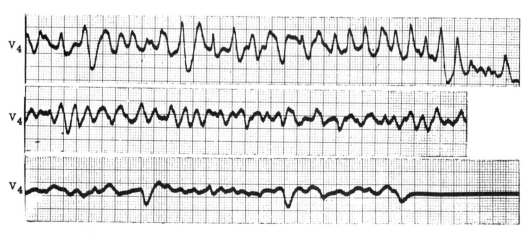

FIGURE 2.1–3. (A) Ventricular tachycardia. Note the regular, wide-complex rhythm with no discernible P waves. **(B) Ventricular fibrillation.** Note the erratic nature of the tracing. (Reproduced, with permission, from Saunders CE. *Current Emergency Diagnosis & Treatment,* 4th ed. Stamford, CT: Appleton & Lange, 1992:515, 517, Figs. 29–30, 29–34.)

Intrinsic disease of the myocardium that is categorized as dilated, hypertrophic, or restrictive. Strictly speaking, this excludes myocardial dysfunction attributable to ischemic, valvular, or hypertensive disease.

PRIMARY DILATED CARDIOMYOPATHY

Comprises 90% of all cardiomyopathies. Generally presents with symptoms of CHF. **LV dilation** and **systolic dysfunction** must be present for diagnosis. Most cases are idiopathic, although known causes include alcohol, wet beriberi, coxsackievirus, Chagas disease, parasites, cocaine, myocarditis, **doxorubicin,** HIV, and AZT.

History/PE

Signs of heart failure develop gradually. Exam may reveal cardiomegaly, an **S3,** and tricuspid and mitral regurgitation. Fever may be present if an infectious cause is responsible.

Evaluation

ECG may show nonspecific ST-T changes, low-voltage QRS, sinus tachycardia, and ectopy. LBBB is common. CXR shows an enlarged, **balloon-like heart** and pulmonary congestion. Echocardiography is diagnostic.

Treatment

Stop all **alcohol usage.** Treat symptoms of CHF (e.g., diuretics, ACE inhibitors [ACEIs], β-blockers). Consider anticoagulation. Consider an implantable cardiac defibrillator (ICD) if ejection fraction (EF) is < 35%.

UCV *IM1.6*

> **The ABCDs of dilated cardiomyopathy:**
>
> **A**lcohol
> **B**eriberi
> **C**oxsackie (B)
> **C**hagas disease
> **C**ocaine
> **D**oxorubicin

HYPERTROPHIC CARDIOMYOPATHY

Also known as idiopathic hypertrophic subaortic stenosis (IHSS). It is inherited as an autosomal-dominant trait in 50% of patients and is the most common cause of sudden death in young healthy athletes. Ventricular hypertrophy with a thickened intraventricular septum results in decreased filling and diastolic dysfunction, while LV outflow tract obstruction results in systolic dysfunction. Obstruction is worsened by increased myocardial contractility or decreased LV filling (e.g., exercise, Valsalva maneuvers, vasodilators, dehydration).

Hypertrophic cardiomyopathy is the most common cause of sudden death in young healthy athletes.

History/PE

The most common symptoms are **syncope** (after exertion), dyspnea, palpitations, and chest pain. Poor prognostic signs include arrhythmias, AF, and elevated LA pressures. The exam may reveal mitral regurgitation, a sustained apical impulse, an S4, and a **systolic ejection murmur.**

Evaluation

ECG shows LVH and abnormal Q waves. CXR may show a boot-shaped heart (more common in RVH). Echocardiogram is diagnostic and shows thickened LV walls and dynamic obstruction of blood flow.

Treatment

Beta-blockade is the initial treatment in symptomatic individuals. Calcium channel blockers (e.g., verapamil) also help. Surgical options include dual-chamber pacing, partial excision of the myocardial septum, or an ICD. Patients should avoid intense athletic competition and training.

UCV *IM1.7*

RESTRICTIVE CARDIOMYOPATHY

> *Restrictive cardiomyopathy is caused by infiltrative disease or scarring and fibrosis.*

Characterized by **impaired diastolic filling** without significant contractile dysfunction. Caused by infiltrative disease (e.g., sarcoidosis, hemochromatosis, amyloidosis) or by scarring and fibrosis (due to radiation or a drug such as adriamycin).

History/PE

Signs/symptoms of left heart failure (LHF) and right heart failure (RHF) occur, but right heart symptoms (e.g., JVD, edema, ascites) often predominate.

Evaluation/Treatment

Cardiac biopsy is diagnostic. Treat the underlying cause and heart failure symptoms (e.g., sodium restriction, diuretics for fluid overload). Differentiate from **constrictive pericarditis,** which is characterized by thickened pericardium on CT or MRI and is **treatable.**

CONGESTIVE HEART FAILURE (CHF)

> **Causes of recurrent CHF—**
>
> **FAILURE**
> **F**orgot medication
> **A**rrhythmia/**A**nemia
> **I**schemia/**I**nfarct/
>   **I**nfection
> **L**ifestyle (most common cause, e.g., high Na⁺ intake, low/no exercise)
> **U**pregulation (increased CO; e.g., pregnancy, hyperthyroidism)
> **R**enal failure (fluid overload)
> **E**mbolus (pulmonary)

Occurs when the heart is unable to pump enough blood to meet the oxygen requirements of the heart and other body tissues. Nearly 10% of Americans > 70 years of age will have CHF; there are ~ 400,000 new cases per year. Overall mortality approaches 20%, while those with the most severe CHF sustain a 50% annual mortality. CHF risk factors include CAD (causes 50–75% of cases), HTN, valvular heart disease (e.g., mitral stenosis, right-sided endocarditis), pericardial disease, cardiomyopathy, and pulmonary HTN.

CHF classification systems include functional (severity), systolic versus diastolic, and left versus right. The New York Heart Association has defined the functional classification for CHF:

- **Class I:** No limitation of activity; no symptoms with normal activity.
- **Class II:** Slight limitation of activity; comfortable at rest or with mild exertion.

- **Class III:** Marked limitation of activity; comfortable only at rest.
- **Class IV:** Confined to complete rest in bed or chair, as any physical activity brings on discomfort; symptoms present at rest.

UCV *IM1.4*

SYSTOLIC DYSFUNCTION

Defined by an EF < 50%; results from reduced LV contractile function. Decreased EF results in increased preload (increased left ventricular end-diastolic pressure [LVEDP]) and, ultimately, increased systolic contractility according to the Frank-Starling law. Compensatory mechanisms are temporarily effective but ultimately lead to hypertrophy, ventricular dilation, and increased myocardial work. Most cases of CHF arise from systolic dysfunction, but diastolic dysfunction (discussed below) is also becoming recognized as an important component.

Diastolic dysfunction is an increasingly recognized cause of heart failure.

History/PE

Presents with **dyspnea on exertion** (DOE) or at rest if severe, as well as with chronic cough, fatigue, lower extremity edema, **orthopnea, paroxysmal nocturnal dyspnea,** and/or abdominal fullness. Exam may reveal sinus tachycardia and laterally displaced PMI. Look for signs of RHF (**JVD,** hepatomegaly, **hepatojugular reflux,** bipedal **edema**) *(IM1.5)* and LHF (bilateral **basilar rales, S3** gallop).

Differential

MI, angina, pericarditis, nephrotic syndrome/renal failure, cirrhosis, pneumonia.

Evaluation

Includes ECG, **echocardiography,** and CXR (look for **cardiomegaly, cephalization of pulmonary vessels,** pleural effusions, vascular indistinctness, and prominent hila). Diagnose on the basis of the clinical picture and an echocardiogram showing impaired cardiac function (hypertrophic or dilated cardiomyopathy may be present). Rule out MI in acute exacerbations. If amyloid or viral myocarditis is suspected (e.g., previous viral prodrome, young age), a myocardial biopsy may be performed. AF is a common comorbid condition and carries a high risk for stroke (~ 3–6% per year).

Treatment

- **Correct treatable causes** (e.g., arrhythmias, alcohol-induced failure, thyroid and valvular disease).
- **Acute:** For worsening symptoms, diurese aggressively with a **loop diuretic** (e.g., furosemide) and a non-loop diuretic (monitor K⁺ with potassium-sparing agents). Use **ACEIs** in all patients who can tolerate them. Hospital admission and intubation may be necessary. Dobutamine for inotropy (aka "dobutamine holiday") and nitroprusside for afterload reduction may help.
- **Chronic:** β-blockers are becoming first-line agents. Also use **ACEIs**/angiotensin receptor blockers (which have been shown to decrease mor-

tality), **diuretics** (furosemide), and **digoxin.** Together these agents block neurohormonal remodeling of the heart. Treat arrhythmias as they arise, and limit dietary Na$^+$ and fluid intake. Consider **warfarin** for severe dilated cardiomyopathy, AF, or previous embolic episodes. Consider an ICD in patients with EF < 35%.

- Low-dose **spironolactone** has been shown to decrease mortality risk by 30% when given with ACEIs, digoxin, and diuretics in patients with **LV systolic dysfunction.**
- CHF unresponsive to maximal medical therapy may require mechanical ventricular assist devices and cardiac transplantation.

DIASTOLIC DYSFUNCTION

Characterized by **decreased ventricular compliance with normal contractile function.** The ventricle is unable either to actively relax or to passively fill properly (i.e., increased stiffness, decreased recoil, and concentric hypertrophy). LVEDP is increased, cardiac output remains essentially normal, and EF is normal or slightly increased. Activation of the renin-angiotensin-aldosterone system (RAAS) is not prominent, but increased hydrostatic pressure can cause pulmonary congestion and other CHF symptoms. Although diastolic and systolic dysfunction have similar causes and workup, there are some differences (see Table 2.1–4). Treatment centers on β-blockers, ACEIs, diuretics, rate control, and BP management. **Avoid digoxin in these patients.**

CORONARY ARTERY DISEASE (CAD)

Continues to be a leading cause of morbidity and mortality in the United States. Clinical manifestations include stable and unstable angina, SOB, DOE, arrhythmias, MI, heart failure, and sudden death.

UCV *EM.2*

HYPERCHOLESTEROLEMIA

Elevated blood cholesterol increases the incidence of CAD.

> **Major risk factors for CAD:**
>
> Age
> Gender
> Hypercholesterolemia
> Diabetes mellitus
> Hypertension
> Smoking
> Family history

Table 2.1–4. Differences Between Systolic and Diastolic Dysfunction

	Systolic Dysfunction	Diastolic Dysfunction
Patient age	Often < 65 years old.	Often > 65 years old.
Comorbid/contributing illnesses	Ischemic heart disease, HTN, dilated cardiomyopathy, diabetes, valvular heart disease.	Ischemic heart disease, HTN, hypertrophic and restrictive cardiomyopathy, renal disease, diabetes.
Pulmonary embolism	Displaced PMI, S3 gallop.	Sustained PMI, S4 gallop.
CXR	Pulmonary congestion, cardiomegaly.	Pulmonary congestion, normal heart size.
ECG/echo	Q waves, decreased EF (< 40%).	LVH, normal EF (> 50%).

History/PE

Most patients have **no specific signs or symptoms.** Patients with extremely elevated triglycerides or LDL may have xanthomas (eruptive and/or tendinous), xanthelasmas, and lipemia retinalis (creamy appearance of retinal vessels). These manifestations are usually related to a familial hypercholesterolemia.

Hypercholesterolemia is generally asymptomatic.

Etiologies

Obesity, diabetes mellitus (DM), alcoholism, hypothyroidism, nephrotic syndrome, hepatic disease, Cushing's disease, OCP use, diuretic use, and familial hypercholesterolemia.

Evaluation

Conduct a fasting lipoprotein profile for patients > 20 years of age and repeat every five years. Treatment is based on CAD risk factors, which include **diabetes (CAD risk equivalent),** smoking, HTN, HDL < 40 mg/dL, age ≥ 45 (males), age ≥ 55 (females), and early CAD in first-degree relatives (males ≤ 55 and females ≤ 65). See Table 2.1–5 for treatment guidelines.

- **Diet:** A 10–15% reduction in cholesterol results in a 15–30% reduction in cardiovascular events.
- **HMG-CoA reductase inhibitors ("stains"):** The most effective cholesterol-lowering drugs. May cause LFT abnormalities, warfarin potentiation, and/or myositis. The risk of myositis is increased if "stains" and lipoprotein lipase inhibitors (e.g., gemfibrozil) are taken together.
- **Bile acid sequestrants (cholestyramine):** May interfere with absorption of other drugs (e.g., digoxin, warfarin, thiazides). Constipation and gas are common.
- **Niacin:** Cheap and effective. Compliance is a problem because of facial flushing and pruritic side effects. Aspirin (ASA) can be used to ameliorate flushing.

ANGINA PECTORIS

Refers to substernal chest pain due to myocardial ischemia (increased O_2 demand or decreased O_2 supply). In addition to the major risk factors identified

Table 2.1–5. Risk Stratification and Treatment Based on LDL

Risk Category	Target LDL	Treatment
0–1 RF[a]	< 160	TLC[b] at ≥ 160 Drug therapy at ≥ 190
≥ 2 RFs	< 130	TLC or drug therapy at ≥ 130–160
CHD or risk equivalent	< 100	TLC at ≥ 100 Drug therapy at ≥ 130

[a]RF = risk factor.
[b]TLC = therapeutic lifestyle changes, which include a 12-week trial of diet, exercise, and weight loss.

above, CAD risk factors include cocaine and/or amphetamine use, history of prior MI, obesity, elevated homocysteine, and lipoprotein (a). Having a "type A" personality may play a role. Males are affected more often than females. **Prinzmetal's (variant) angina** mimics angina pectoris but is caused by vasospasm of coronary vessels. It often affects young women and classically occurs at rest in the early morning.

History/PE

The classic triad includes **substernal chest pain** or pressure **precipitated by exertion** and **relieved by rest or nitrates.** Pain can radiate to the arms, jaw, and neck and be associated with SOB, diaphoresis, nausea/emesis, or lightheadedness. Symptoms vary significantly among patients. Exam may reveal diaphoresis, HTN, tachycardia, and apical systolic murmur or gallop.

Differential

Tension pneumothorax, aortic dissection, pulmonary embolism, unstable angina, MI, costochondritis, varicella zoster neuropathy, GERD (may worsen with nitrates or Ca^{2+} blockers), esophageal spasm, PUD, cholecystitis, pericarditis, and pneumonia.

Evaluation

ECG may show **ST-segment depression** or T-wave flattening. Check **cardiac enzymes** to rule out MI. Risk stratify with **cardiac stress testing** (exercise versus pharmacologic stress and ECG/echo/nuclear medicine perfusion scan) or coronary **catheterization,** if highly suspicious.

Treatment

- Patients with suspected MI must be admitted and monitored by ECG/telemetry until acute MI is ruled out by serial cardiac enzymes.
- Treat acute symptoms with O_2, sublingual **nitroglycerin, ASA, IV β-blockers,** and clopidogrel (for acute coronary syndrome). Start heparin drip in patients with ECG changes, multiple attacks, or unstable angina.
- Treat chronic symptoms with nitrates (for further attacks), β-blockers, and ASA. Discuss **risk factor reduction** (e.g., smoking, cholesterol, HTN). Consider stress test. Check lipid panel and consider starting a statin.
- If pain increases in frequency, is unrelieved with nitroglycerin, or occurs at rest **(unstable angina),** proceed to **heparinization, angiography,** and possible **revascularization** (PTCA versus CABG). Indications for revascularization depend on the angiogram results. If there is single- or double-vessel disease with discrete lesions, the patient is a candidate for PTCA. If there is three-vessel disease, left main disease, discrete lesions not amenable to PTCA, or diffuse disease with good targets, the patient is a candidate for CABG.

UNSTABLE ANGINA

Angina is considered "unstable" if it is new, is accelerating (i.e., occurs with less exertion, lasts longer, or is less responsive to medications), or occurs at rest. This is worrisome because it often signifies a transient vessel occlusion (i.e., disruption of an atherosclerotic plaque and/or vasospasm in the area of a plaque) and an area of myocardial ischemia that can acutely progress to complete occlusion and MI.

Patients should be hospitalized for aggressive management similar to that for MI. Therapy includes nitrates, β-blockers, morphine, O_2, ASA, clopidogrel, and heparin. After stabilization, evaluate the coronary vasculature using the diagnostic methods discussed above. If angina persists, consider urgent coronary angiography and revascularization. Patients should also receive an ACEI and lipid-lowering therapy.

MYOCARDIAL INFARCTION (MI)

Usually caused by an occlusive thrombus or prolonged vasospasm in a coronary artery. The most common cause is an **acute thrombus on a ruptured atherosclerotic plaque.** Time course and extent of vessel occlusion are key, as collateral circulation may help preserve some myocardial function. Risk factors are similar to those for angina. Males are affected more often than females, although **incidence increases in postmenopausal women.** Twenty percent of MI patients present with sudden death from a lethal arrhythmia (often VF). The best predictor of survival is left ventricular EF. A Q-wave MI involves the full thickness of the myocardium (transmural); a non-Q-wave MI involves only the subendocardium (not full thickness) and increases the risk for a transmural MI in that region.

History/PE

Presents with **acute-onset substernal chest pain,** often described as a **pressure or tightness,** that can **radiate to the left arm,** neck, or jaw. Pain lasts for > 30 minutes and does not completely resolve with nitroglycerin. **Diaphoresis,** SOB, light-headedness, anxiety, **nausea/emesis,** and syncope may be present. On exam, look for tachycardia, bradycardia, arrhythmias, **new mitral regurgitation** (ruptured papillary muscle), hypotension (cardiogenic shock), rales **(pulmonary edema),** and VF. Be alert to atypical presentations; elderly, diabetic, and post-orthotopic heart transplant patients are particularly likely to have "silent" MIs.

Elderly, diabetic, and post-orthotopic heart transplant patients are particularly likely to have "silent" MIs.

Differential

Angina, pulmonary edema, aortic dissection, pneumothorax, pericarditis, GERD, costochondritis, varicella zoster, esophageal spasm, peptic ulcer, pneumonia, cholecystitis.

Evaluation

- **ECG:** Look for ST-segment changes or new LBBB (see Figures 2.1–4 and 2.1–5). ECG changes typically follow a specific sequence in acute MI: Peaked T waves → T-wave inversion → ST-segment elevation → Q waves → ST-segment normalization → T waves return to upright position. Changes in anterior leads (V_1–V_4) usually indicate an **anterior** MI. Changes in leads II, III, and aVF are consistent with an **inferior** MI.

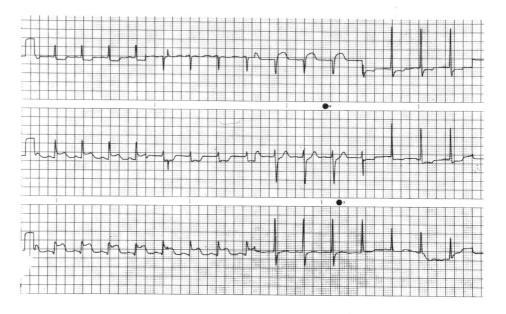

FIGURE 2.1–4. Inferior wall myocardial infarction. In this patient with acute chest pain, the ECG demonstrated acute ST elevation in leads II, III, and aVF with reciprocal ST depression and T-wave flattening in leads I, aVL, and V_4–V_6. (Reproduced, with permission, from Stobo J et al. *The Principles and Practice of Medicine*, 23rd ed. Stamford, CT: Appleton & Lange, 1996:20, Fig. 1–3–3A.)

- **Serial cardiac enzymes:** Check troponin I and T, CK with CK-MB fraction, and LDH. Death of myocardium releases enzymes into the blood that can be measured. Troponin I appears first and is the most sensitive and specific; CK-MB appears next. LDH appears last, and levels remain elevated for 3–6 days.
- MI is also associated with **arrhythmias,** including AF, SVT, VT, or VF. CXR may show signs of CHF.

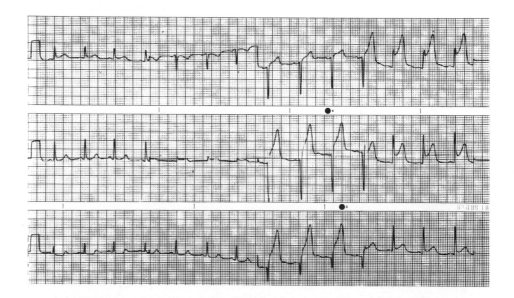

FIGURE 2.1–5. Anterior wall myocardial infarction. This patient presented with acute chest pain. ECG showed ST elevation in leads aVL and V_1–V_6 and hyperacute T waves. (Reproduced, with permission, from Stobo J et al. *The Principles and Practice of Medicine*, 23rd ed. Stamford, CT: Appleton & Lange, 1996:19, Fig. 1–3–2A.)

Treatment

- **Acute:** Give **O₂, ASA, β-blockers** (hold in the presence of bradycardia, hypotension, or pulmonary edema), **nitroglycerin** (can cause hypotension), and **morphine** (for pain and dyspnea). Consider emergent angiography with potential revascularization. If this is not available, consider **thrombolysis** with tissue plasminogen activator (tPA), urokinase, or streptokinase (if the patient presents within six hours of onset). In hypotensive patients, start IV fluids and stop nitroglycerin. Patients with suspected MI require hospitalization in a cardiac-monitored bed to watch for continuing ischemia and arrhythmias, especially in the first 24 hours post-MI.
- **Inpatient:** Treat with **ASA, heparin, β-blockers,** and **ACEIs;** perform a **stress test** and/or echo after five days to assess future risk. If the stress test is positive, **catheterize** to assess vessel patency. Consider PTCA or CABG for significant occlusions.
- **Long term:** Give **ASA, β-blockers,** and **ACEIs** if tolerated (especially in patients with pulmonary edema). **Modify risk factors** with lipid-lowering agents, antihypertensives, dietary modifications, and exercise as indicated.

Time is myocardium.

Complications

Reinfarction, LV wall rupture, pericarditis, **Dressler's syndrome** (autoimmune process with fever, pericarditis, pleural effusion, leukocytosis, and increased ESR at 2–4 weeks post-MI), papillary muscle rupture (with mitral regurgitation), aneurysmal LV dilatation, and mural thrombi. **Lethal arrhythmia** is the most common cause of death following acute MI. More than six PVCs/minute indicate a poor prognosis.

HYPERTENSION

Usually defined as **systolic BP > 140** and/or **diastolic BP > 90** based on three measurements separated by two weeks time (see Table 2.1–6). It is classified as primary (essential) or secondary.

PRIMARY (ESSENTIAL) HYPERTENSION

High blood pressure from an unidentified cause **accounts for > 95% of cases.** Risk factors include **family history** of HTN or heart disease, **high-sodium diet, smoking, obesity,** and **advanced age;** blacks are affected more often than whites.

Primary hypertension is the most common cause of high blood pressure.

History/PE

BP elevation is **asymptomatic** until complications develop. Retinal changes (copper wires, AV nicking; see Clinical Images, Plate 6), an S4, and a systolic click and/or loud S2 may be present.

Differential/Evaluation

Rule out NSAID use, pregnancy, or secondary causes (discussed below) if the clinical picture is consistent with secondary HTN. Conduct periodic tests for

Table 2.1–6. Classification and Interpretation of Blood Pressure Measurements[a]

Category[b]	Systolic BP	Diastolic BP	Follow-up Recommended
Normal	< 130	< 85	Recheck in two years.
High normal	130–139	85–89	Recheck in one year.[c]
Hypertension			
Stage 1 (mild)	140–159	90–99	Confirm within two months.
Stage 2 (moderate)	160–179	100–109	Evaluate or refer within one month.
Stage 3 (severe)	180–209	110–119	Evaluate or refer within one week.
Stage 4 (very severe)	≥ 210	≥ 120	Evaluate or refer immediately.

[a]Reproduced from the sixth report of the Joint National Committee on Detection, Education, and Treatment of High Blood Pressure (JNCVI), *Arch Intern Med* 157:243, 1997. Updated guidelines (JNC VII) are due out in late 2003.
[b]When systolic and diastolic pressures fall into different categories, select the higher category to classify the BP.
[c]Consider offering counseling about lifestyle modifications.

BP goal in uncomplicated HTN is <140/<90.

end-organ complications, including renal (BUN, Cr, microalbumin-to-creatinine ratio) and cardiac (ECG).

Treatment

Begin with lifestyle management (e.g., diet, exercise). The BP goal in uncomplicated HTN is < 140/< 90. The goal in patients with renal disease with proteinuria is < 130/< 85 (< 125/< 75 if possible). The goal in diabetic patients is < 130/< 75. Diuretics (inexpensive and particularly effective in African-Americans) and β-blockers (beneficial for patients with CAD) have been shown to reduce mortality in uncomplicated HTN. They are first-line agents unless a comorbid condition requires another medication (see Tables 2.1–7 and 2.1–8). See "Topics in Emergency Medicine," p. xxx, for a discussion of individual diuretic agents.

Table 2.1–7. Hypertension Management Indications

Manifestation	Treatment
DM with proteinuria	ACEIs.
CHF	β-blockers, ACEIs, and diuretics (including spironolactone; see CHF section).
Isolated systolic HTN	Diuretics are preferred; long-acting dihydropyridine Ca^{2+} channel blockers.
MI	Non–intrinsic sympathomimetic activity (ISA) β-blockers, ACEIs.
Osteoporosis	Thiazide diuretics.
Benign prostatic hypertrophy	α-antagonists.
Peripheral vascular disease	Ca^{2+} channel blockers.

Table 2.1–8. Major Classes of Antihypertensive Agents

Class	Agents	Mechanism of Action	Side Effects
Diuretics	Thiazide, loop, K^+-sparing, other (e.g., spironolactone)	Reduce extracellular fluid volume and thereby reduce vascular resistance.	Hypokalemia, hyperglycemia, hyperlipidemia, hyperuricemia (problematic in gout), azotemia.
β-adrenergic blockers	Propranolol, metoprolol, nadolol, atenolol, timolol, carvedilol, labetalol	Reduce cardiac contractility and renin release.	Bronchospasm (in severe asthma), bradycardia, CHF exacerbation, impotence, fatigue, depression.
Centrally acting adrenergic agonists	Methyldopa, clonidine, guanabenz	Inhibit sympathetic nervous system via central α_2-adrenergic receptors.	Somnolence, orthostasis, impotence, rebound HTN.
α_1-adrenergic blockers	Prazosin, terazosin, phenoxybenzamine	Cause vasodilation by blocking actions of norepinephrine on vascular smooth muscle.	Orthostasis.
Ca^{2+} channel blockers	Dihydropyridines (nifedipine, felodipine, amlodipine), diltiazem, verapamil	Reduce smooth muscle tone and cause vasodilation; may also reduce cardiac output.	Dihydropyridines: headache, flushing, peripheral edema. Verapamil/diltiazem: reduced contractility.
Vasodilators	Hydralazine, minoxidil	Decrease peripheral resistance by dilating arteries/arterioles.	Hydralazine: headache, lupus-like syndrome. Minoxidil: orthostasis, facial hirsutism.
ACEIs	Captopril, enalapril, fosinopril, benazepril, lisinopril	Block aldosterone formation, reducing peripheral resistance and salt/water retention.	**Cough,** rashes, leukopenia, hyperkalemia.
Angiotensin II receptor antagonists	Losartan, valsartan, irbesartan	Block aldosterone effects, reducing peripheral resistance and salt/water retention.	Rashes, leukopenia, and hyperkalemia but **no cough.**

Complications

The best way to prevent stroke is to control hypertension.

CAD, renal disease, **cerebrovascular disease,** aortic aneurysm, aortic dissection, LVH, CHF.

SECONDARY HYPERTENSION

HTN due to an **identifiable** organic cause. **Surgically correctable** causes (< 5%) include **renal artery stenosis** (most common), obstructive sleep apnea, coarctation of the aorta (especially in children), pheochromocytoma, Conn's syndrome (primary hyperaldosteronism), Cushing's syndrome, unilateral renal parenchymal disease, hyperthyroidism, and hyperparathyroidism. Also consider alcohol and medication use. Diagnosis and treatment of common causes include:

Causes of secondary hypertension—

CHAPS
Cushing's syndrome
Hyperaldosteronism
Aortic coarctation
Pheochromocytoma
Stenosis of renal arteries

- **Primary renal disease:** Treat with **ACEIs,** which will slow the progression of renal disease.
- **Renal artery stenosis:** Especially common in patients < 25 and > 50 years of age with recent-onset HTN. Etiologies include **fibromuscular dysplasia** (usually in **younger** patients [IM2.38]) and **atherosclerosis** (usually in older patients). Screen with the captopril provocation test or nuclear perfusion scan. Diagnose with magnetic resonance angiography (MRA) and renal vein renin ratio (RVRR). Treat with **angioplasty** and **stenting** if possible. Consider ACEIs as adjunctive or temporary therapy in unilateral disease **(in bilateral disease, ACEIs can accelerate kidney failure by preferential vasodilation of the efferent arteriole).** Open surgery is a secondary option if angioplasty is not effective or feasible.
- **OCP use:** Common in women > 35 years old, obese women, and those with long-standing use. Discontinue OCP (it can take time to see an effect).
- See Endocrine section for a discussion of pheochromocytoma and hyperaldosteronism.

HYPERTENSIVE URGENCY AND EMERGENCY

Hypertensive emergency includes signs and symptoms of end-organ damage.

Urgency consists of **BP > 200/> 120** that is asymptomatic or moderately symptomatic (headache, chest pain, syncope). **Emergency** includes **symptoms** and **signs** of impending **end-organ damage.** This includes acute renal failure or **hematuria, altered mental status** or evidence of neurologic disease, intracranial hemorrhage (see Clinical Images, Plate 6), ophthalmologic findings suggesting retinal damage **(papilledema,** vascular changes), unstable angina/MI, or pulmonary edema. "Malignant hypertension" (EM.5) is defined as progressive **renal failure** and/or encephalopathy with papilledema.

Evaluation

Cardiovascular, neurologic, ophthalmologic, and abdominal exams. Obtain head and/or abdominal CT, UA, BUN/Cr, CBC, and electrolytes to assess the extent of end-organ damage.

Treatment

- **Hypertensive urgency:** To prevent cerebral hypoperfusion or coronary insufficiency, lower BP slowly (over a few hours) with **oral agents** such as β-blockers, clonidine, and ACEIs. Avoid short-acting Ca^{2+} channel blockers. If oral therapy is insufficient, try IV agents (see below).
- **Hypertensive emergency:** Use **IV agents** to reduce BP by approximately 25% **within one hour.** Treat with **nitroprusside** (very potent; use carefully), nitroglycerin, labetalol, nicardipine, or hydralazine. Add a **diuretic** if there are signs of fluid overload.

PERICARDIAL DISEASE

Results from acute or chronic pericardial insult and can lead to pericardial effusion. Important diseases include pericarditis and cardiac tamponade.

PERICARDITIS

Inflammation of the pericardial sac, often with an effusion. Causes include viral infection, TB, systemic lupus erythematosus (SLE), uremia, drugs, and neoplasms. Pericarditis may also occur after MI (Dressler's syndrome), open heart surgery, or radiotherapy.

History/PE

May present with **pleuritic chest pain,** dyspnea, cough, and **fever.** Pain is often **positional** (i.e., worsens in the supine position and improves with shallow breathing or leaning forward). Exam may reveal a pericardial **friction rub** (best heard with the patient leaning forward). In tamponade, **elevated JVP (neck veins)** and/or **pulsus paradoxus** (a fall in systolic BP > 10 mmHg on inspiration) may be seen.

Differential/Evaluation

Obtain CXR and echocardiogram to rule out MI/angina, cardiac tamponade, heart failure, pneumonia, and pneumothorax. **Low-voltage, diffuse ST-segment elevation** or PR-segment depression on ECG (see Figure 2.1–6) suggests the diagnosis. Pericardial thickening or effusion on echocardiography supports the diagnosis.

Treatment

- Treat the underlying cause (e.g., **steroids**/immunosuppressants for SLE or ASA/**NSAIDs** for viral pericarditis).
- Small effusions can be followed, but tamponade or large effusions require **pericardiocentesis** with continuous drainage if necessary.

UCV *IM1.12*

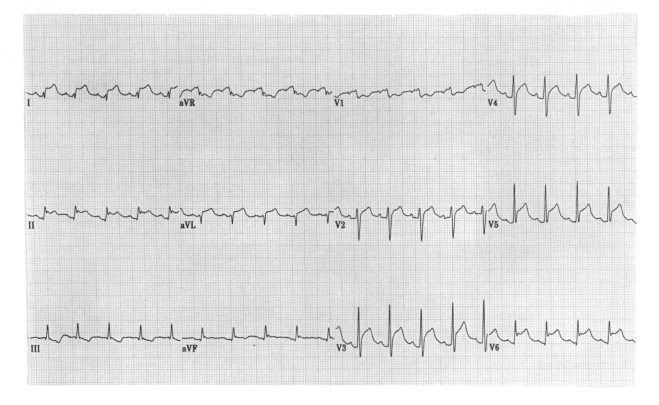

FIGURE 2.1–6. Pericarditis. There is characteristic ST elevation in all leads and PR depression in the precordial leads. (Reproduced, with permission, from Stobo J et al. *The Principles and Practice of Medicine,* 23rd ed. Stamford, CT: Appleton & Lange, 1996:85, Fig.1–10–1.)

CARDIAC TAMPONADE

Tamponade should be suspected in any hemodynamically unstable patient who does not respond to initial resuscitative measures.

Fluid in the pericardial sac results in compromised ventricular filling and decreased cardiac output. Tamponade is more closely related to the rate of fluid formation than to the size of the effusion. Risk factors include pericarditis, malignancy, SLE, TB, and trauma (commonly stab wounds medial to the left nipple).

History/PE

Presents with severe **chest pain, fatigue, dyspnea, tachycardia,** and **tachypnea** that can rapidly lead to shock and death. Exam may reveal **Beck's triad (hypotension, distant heart sounds,** and **distended neck veins).** Other symptoms include a narrow pulse pressure, **pulsus paradoxus,** and **Kussmaul's sign** (JVD on inspiration).

Differential/Evaluation

Rule out severe MI, tension pneumothorax, and decompensated CHF. Obtain an immediate **echocardiogram** if time permits. CXR may demonstrate an enlarged, globular heart. ECG may show decreased amplitude and/or electrical alternans.

Treatment

Treat with urgent **pericardiocentesis** (aspirate will be **nonclotting** blood); balloon pericardotomy and pericardial window may be required. **Volume expansion** with aggressive IV fluids is also helpful.

UCV *EM.3*

VALVULAR HEART DISEASE

Lesions can be divided into stenotic and regurgitant. Most valvular disease presents after age 70 with the exception of mitral stenosis, which often presents in the fourth and fifth decades. Until recently, rheumatic fever *(IM1.13)* was the most common cause in adults; owing to treatment of streptococcal infections and decreased incidence of rheumatic fever in the United States, the leading cause is now mechanical degeneration due to normal "wear and tear." Childhood valvular lesions are mainly caused by congenital abnormalities. Table 2.1–9 summarizes the major valvular lesions.

VASCULAR DISEASE

AORTIC ANEURYSM

Atherosclerosis is the most common cause (whereas aortic dissection is most commonly due to HTN). Most are abdominal, and > 90% originate below the renal arteries. Risk factors include **HTN,** other vascular disease (atherosclerosis), family history, and smoking. **Males** are affected more often than females, and risk increases with age.

Atherosclerosis is the most common cause of aortic aneurysm.

History/PE

Usually **asymptomatic** and discovered incidentally on exam or radiologic study. However, a ruptured aneurysm can cause hypotension and severe, tearing abdominal pain radiating to the back. Many individuals with rupture die before they reach the hospital. Exam often demonstrates a **pulsatile abdominal mass,** abdominal bruits, and hypotension (if ruptured).

Differential

Pancreatitis/pseudocyst, neoplasms (e.g., pancreatic, colonic), orthopedic causes of back pain, appendicitis, gallbladder disease, gastritis, nephrolithiasis.

Evaluation

Abdominal U/S for diagnosis or to follow an aneurysm over time. CT may be a useful adjunct to determine the precise anatomy.

Table 2.1–9. Valvular Heart Lesions

Valvular Lesion	Risk Factors	Symptoms	Murmur	Physical Exam	Treatment
Aortic stenosis	Rheumatic heart disease, congenital aortic stenosis, bicuspid valve.	Classic triad: **exertional dyspnea, angina, and syncope.** Can lead to CHF and death.	Midsystolic crescendo-decrescendo murmur heard best at second intercostal space, radiates to neck.	"Pulsus parvus et tardus" (weak, delayed carotid upstroke), sustained apical beat. Paradoxically split S2.	Avoid afterload reducers. Valve replacement is curative.
Aortic regurgitation *(IM1.1)*	Rheumatic heart disease, VSD, infective endocarditis (IE), congenital bicuspid valve, Marfan's syndrome.	LVH, angina, LHF due to volume overload.	Three murmurs: 1. High-pitched, blowing diastolic murmur at left sternal border. 2. Austin Flint → low-pitched mid-diastolic rumble. 3. Midsystolic murmur at base.	Widened pulse pressure, laterally displaced PMI.	Aortic valve replacement is curative. If not possible, treat with afterload reducers (ACEIs, vasodilators), diuretics, and/or digitalis.
Mitral stenosis *(IM1.10)*	Rheumatic heart disease.	Symptoms of left-sided and right-sided failure.	Mid-diastolic rumble with opening snap at apex.	AF, pulmonary rales, increased intensity of S1 and P2, RV heave.	Avoid inotropic agents. Use diuretics, anticoagulants, digitalis, balloon valvuloplasty.
Mitral valve prolapse	Found in 7% of the population, especially in young women.	Usually benign and asymptomatic.	Late systolic murmur with midsystolic click.	Can progress to mitral regurgitation.	Generally unnecessary unless symptomatic or progressing to mitral regurgitation.
Mitral regurgitation	Rheumatic heart disease, MI, IE, severe mitral valve prolapse.	LHF that can progress to RHF.	High-pitched, holosystolic murmur at apex radiates to axilla.	Laterally displaced PMI with LV heave, AF, fatigue, signs of LHF and possibly RHF.	ACEIs, vasodilators, diuretics, digitalis, anticoagulation, and valve repair/replacement.

Treatment

- In asymptomatic patients, **monitoring** is appropriate for lesions < 5 cm. **Surgical repair is indicated if the lesion is > 5 cm (abdominal) or > 6 cm (thoracic) or is enlarging rapidly.**
- Emergent surgery is indicated for symptomatic or ruptured aneurysms.

UCV *EM.15*

DEEP VENOUS THROMBOSIS (DVT)

Arises when a blood clot forms in large veins of the extremities or pelvis. Predisposing factors include venous stasis due to immobilization (e.g., plane flights, bed rest), incompetent venous valves in the lower extremities, CHF, traumatic injury to the lower extremities, hypercoagulable states (e.g., malignancy, HRT), obesity, and indwelling venous catheters.

History/PE

Generally presents with unilateral lower extremity pain, erythema, and swelling. There may be a positive **Homans' sign** (calf tenderness with palpation).

Evaluation

Noninvasive diagnostics include Doppler U/S and impedance plethysmography. A more invasive test (contrast venography) can then be employed to demonstrate the area of the blood clot.

Treatment

The goal is to prevent further thrombosis with **anticoagulants** (IV heparin or low-molecular-weight heparin, followed by PO warfarin for a total of 3–6 months) and allow the body's fibrinolytic system to dissolve existing clot(s). Hospitalized patients should receive DVT prophylaxis (e.g., rapid mobilization, antithromboembolic stockings, leg exercises, and/or subcutaneous heparin). Consider an IVC filter in patients with contraindications to anticoagulation.

PERIPHERAL VASCULAR DISEASE (PVD)

Defined as occlusion of the blood supply to the extremities by atherosclerotic plaques. The lower extremities are most commonly affected. Clinical manifestations depend on the vessels involved, extent and rapidity of obstruction, and presence of collateral blood flow.

History/PE

Initially presents with **intermittent claudication** (reproducible leg pain that occurs with walking and is always relieved with rest). As disease worsens, there is progression to rest pain and ischemia that affects the distal aspects of the extremities. A painful, cold, numb foot is characteristic of severe ischemia. Dorsal foot ulcerations may develop.

Claudication is reproducible leg pain that occurs with walking and is relieved with rest.

- **Aortoiliac disease:** Buttock claudication is present and femoral pulses are absent; **impotence** is common in males.
- **Femoropopliteal disease:** Calf claudication is present; pulses below the femoral are absent.
- **Small vessel disease:** Foot pulses are absent.
- **Acute ischemia:** Most often caused by **embolization** from the heart; acute occlusions commonly occur at bifurcations distal to the last palpable pulse.
- **Severe chronic ischemia:** Lack of blood perfusion results in muscle atrophy, pallor, cyanosis, hair loss, and gangrene/necrosis.

Differential

Thromboangiitis obliterans, Raynaud's phenomenon, arterial embolism, acrocyanosis, erythromelalgia.

Evaluation

Careful **palpation of pulses and auscultation for bruits** are necessary. Measurement of ankle and brachial systolic BP **(ankle-brachial index [ABI])** can provide objective evidence of atherosclerosis (rest pain occurs with ABIs < 0.4). **Doppler U/S** helps identify stenosis and occlusion; Doppler ankle systolic pressure readings that are > 90% of brachial readings are normal. Arteriography and digital subtraction angiography are necessary for surgical evaluation.

Treatment

Exercise (as tolerated) helps develop collateral circulation. Eliminate tobacco and follow careful hygiene and foot care. Control of underlying causes (e.g., DM) is crucial. **Pentoxifylline,** calcium antagonists, and thromboxane inhibitors may improve symptoms. PTCA has a variable success rate that is dependent on the area of occlusion. Surgery (arterial bypass) or amputation can be employed when conservative treatment fails.

Questions 1, 2, and 5: Reproduced, with permission, from Berk SL, *PreTest: Medicine*, 9th ed., New York: McGraw-Hill, 2001.
Questions 3 and 4: Reproduced, with permission, from Reteguiz J, *PreTest: Physical Diagnosis*, 4th ed., New York: McGraw-Hill, 2001.

Questions

1. A 36-year-old white female nurse comes to the ER due to a sensation of fast heart rate, slight dizziness, and vague chest fullness. The following rhythm strip is obtained which shows

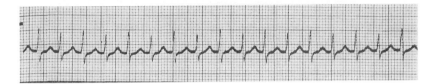

   a. Atrial fibrillation
   b. Atrial flutter
   c. Supraventricular tachycardia
   d. Ventricular tachycardia

2. The initial therapy of choice in this stable patient is
   a. Adenosine 6 mg rapid IV bolus
   b. Verapamil 2.5 to 5 mg IV over 1 to 2 minutes
   c. Diltiazem 0.25 mg/kg IV over 2 minutes
   d. Digoxin 0.5 mg IV slowly
   e. Lidocaine 1.5 mg/kg IV bolus
   f. Electrical cardioversion at 50 joules

3. A 71-year-old man complains of occasional lower back pain. His blood pressure is 150/85 mm Hg and his pulse is 80/min. Cardiac examination reveals an S4 gallop. Abdominal examination reveals a pulsatile mass approximately 5.0 cm in diameter palpable in the epigastric area. Peripheral pulses are normal. Which of the following is the most likely diagnosis?
   a. Abdominal aortic aneurysm
   b. Cancer of the proximal colon
   c. Peptic ulcer disease
   d. Chronic pancreatitis
   e. Lipoma of the abdominal wall

4. A 47-year-old man has been at home recovering from an anterior myocardial infarction that occurred 10 days ago. He presents to your office complaining of persistent chest pain that is worse on inspiration and that is different from his "heart attack" pain. The pain radiates to both clavicles. The pain is worse when the patient is lying down and improves with sitting up and leaning forward. The patient has a temperature of 101.2°F and a normal blood pressure. Heart auscultation reveals a pericardial rub. Lung examination is positive for dullness and diminished breath sounds at the right base. Chest radiograph reveals a small right-sided pleural effusion. Laboratory data reveal that the patient has a mild leukocytosis and an increased erythrocyte sedimentation rate (ESR). Which of the following is the most likely diagnosis?

HIGH-YIELD FACTS

Cardiovascular

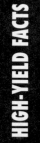

a. Extension of the myocardial infarction
b. Unstable angina
c. Prinzmetal's angina
d. Pulmonary embolus
e. Postmyocardial infarction syndrome

5. A 55-year-old obese woman develops pressure-like substernal chest pain of one-hour duration. Her EKG is shown below. The most likely diagnosis is

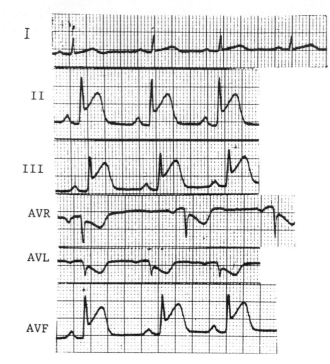

a. Costochondritis
b. Acute anterior myocardial infarction
c. Acute inferior myocardial infarction
d. Pericarditis
e. Esophageal reflux
f. Cholecystitis

Answers

1. **The answer is c.** Paroxysmal supraventricular tachycardia typically displays a narrow QRS complex without clearly discernible P waves, with rate in the 160 to 190 range. The rate is faster in atrial flutter. Atrial fibrillation would show an irregularly irregular rate. Wide QRS complexes would be expected in ventricular tachycardia.

2. **The answer is a.** Adenosine is the drug of choice for supraventricular tachycardia, with verapamil the next alternative. Adenosine has an excellent safety profile, making it the preferred drug for supraventricular tachycardia.

3. **The answer is a. Abdominal aortic aneurysms (AAAs)** are usually due to atherosclerosis and > 90% originate below the renal arteries. The aneurysms are typically asymptomatic until they rupture, but patients may complain of lower back or hypogastric pain. The aneurysms may be associated with emboli to the feet and kidneys. Normal diameter of the aorta is < 2 cm. **When the diameter of the AAA is > 5 cm, repair is generally suggested.** Risk of rupture is 1–2% over 5 years when the AAA is < 5 cm, but 20–40% when the AAA reaches 6 cm in diameter. The best method of evaluating the AAA is by **ultrasound or CT scan.**

4. **The answer is e.** Postmyocardial infarction syndrome or **Dressler syndrome** is an autoimmune complication of myocardial infarction. It occurs from two to four weeks after the infarction and usually responds quickly to salicylates. The fever, pericarditis, leukocytosis, elevated ESR, and pleural effusion are all part of the autoimmune process.

5. **The answer is c.** The ECG shows ST-segment elevation in inferior leads II, III, and aVF with reciprocal ST-depression in aVL, consistent with an acute inferior MI. An anterior MI would give ST-segment elevation in the precordial leads. Pericarditis classically causes pleuritic chest pain and diffuse ST-segment elevation (except aVR) on ECG. Costochondritis, esophageal reflux, cholecystitis, and duodenal ulcer disease can all cause the symptoms of substernal chest pain, but not these ECG findings.

HIGH-YIELD FACTS

Cardiovascular

HIGH-YIELD FACTS

Cardiovascular

Dermatology

HIGH-YIELD FACTS

Dermatology

Hypersensitivity

Type I

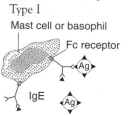

Mast cell or basophil

Fc receptor

Ag

IgE

Ag

Anaphylactic and atopic—Ag cross-links IgE on presensitized mast cells and basophils, triggering release of vasoactive amines (i.e., histamine). Reaction develops rapidly after Ag exposure due to preformed Ab. Examples include anaphylaxis, asthma, local wheal and flare.

First and Fast (anaphylaxis). I, II, and III are all antibody mediated.

Type II

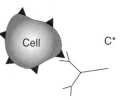

Cell   C*

Cytotoxic—IgM, IgG bind to Ag on "enemy" cell, leading to lysis (by complement) or phagocytosis. Examples include autoimmune hemolytic anemia, Rh disease (erythroblastosis fetalis), Goodpasture's syndrome, rheumatic fever.

Cy-**2**-toxic. Antibody and complement lead to membrane attack complex (MAC).

Type III

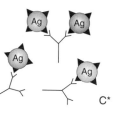

Ag   Ag

Ag

Ag

C*

Immune complex—Ag-Ab complexes activate complement, which attracts neutrophils; neutrophils release lysosomal enzymes. Examples include PAN, immune complex GN, SLE, rheumatoid arthritis.

Serum sickness—an immune complex disease (type III) in which Abs to the foreign proteins are produced (takes 5 days). Immune complexes form and are deposited in membranes, where they fix complement (leads to tissue damage). More common than Arthus reaction.

Arthus reaction—a local subacute Ab-mediated hypersensitivity (type III) reaction. Intradermal injection of Ag induces antibodies, which form Ag-Ab complexes in the skin. Characterized by edema, necrosis, and activation of complement. Examples include hypersensitivity pneumonitis, thermophilic actinomycetes.

Imagine an immune complex as **3** things stuck together: Ag-Ab-complement.

Most serum sickness is now caused by drugs (not serum). Fever, urticaria, arthralgias, proteinuria, lymphadenopathy 5–10 days after Ag exposure.

Ag-Ab complexes cause the Arthus reaction.

Type IV

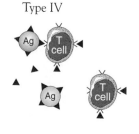

Ag   T cell

Ag   T cell

Delayed (cell-mediated) type—sensitized T lymphocytes encounter antigen and then release lymphokines (leads to macrophage activation). Examples include TB skin test, transplant rejection, contact dermatitis (e.g., poison ivy, poison oak).

4th and last—delayed. Cell mediated; therefore, it is not transferable by serum.

ACID:
   Anaphylactic and **A**topic (type I)
   Cytotoxic (type II)
   Immune complex (type III)
   Delayed (cell-mediated) (type IV)

C* = complement

Cutaneous mycoses

Tinea versicolor	Caused by *Malassezia furfur*. Causes hypopigmented skin lesions. Occurs in hot, humid weather. Treat with topical miconazole, selenium sulfide (Selsun).
Tinea nigra	Caused by *Cladosporium werneckii*. Infection of keratinized layer of skin. Appears as brownish spot. Treat with topical salicylic acid.
Tinea pedis, tinea cruris, tinea corporis, tinea capitis	Pruritic lesions with central clearing resembling a ring, caused by dermatophytes (*Microsporum*, *Trichophyton*, and *Epidermophyton*). See mold hyphae in KOH prep, not dimorphic. Pets are a reservoir for *Microsporum* and can be treated with topical azoles. Tinea capitis must be treated with systemics.

Common drugs causing hyperpigmentation of the skin:

Minocycline

Amiodarone

Chloroquine

Gold

Chlorpromazine

Bleomycin

5-FU

Daunorubicin

ACANTHOSIS NIGRICANS

Diffuse hyperpigmentation of the skin associated with heredity, endocrine disorders, obesity, drugs, and malignancy. Dark, thickened, **dirty-appearing, velvety** plaques are found predominantly on the **axillae, neck,** groin, and anogenital region (see Figure 2.2–1). Evaluation should include a fasting glucose to rule out diabetes mellitus (DM). Treatment should be aimed at the underlying disorder.

ACNE VULGARIS

Inflammation of pilosebaceous units and abnormal keratinization associated with changes in androgen levels (e.g., polycystic ovarian syndrome) and *Propionibacterium acnes.* Drug-related acne is associated with lithium, steroids, OCPs, and androgens. Acne vulgaris is found primarily during puberty and in males. Open comedones (blackheads) and closed comedones (whiteheads) are commonly found on the face, neck, arms, back, and buttocks. Treatment includes:

- **Mild:** Topical clindamycin or erythromycin, benzoyl peroxide, topical retinoids.
- **Moderate:** The above regimen plus oral antibiotics such as tetracycline.
- **Severe:** Oral isotretinoin (treatment of choice for nodulocystic acne).

ATOPIC DERMATITIS/ECZEMA

A relapsing inflammatory skin disorder that is common in infancy, is characterized by **pruritus,** and causes persistent scratching leading to **lichenification.**

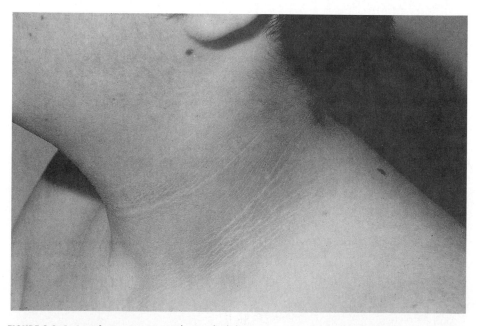

FIGURE 2.2–1. Acanthosis nigricans. Velvety, dark brown epidermal thickening of the neck with prominent skin fold and feathered edges. (Reproduced, with permission, from Fitzpatrick TB. *Color Atlas & Synopsis of Clinical Dermatology,* 4th ed. New York: McGraw-Hill, 2001:83, Fig. 3–17.)

History/PE

Patients present with dry, scaly, itchy patches and plaques with excoriations in the **flexural areas and neck** (see Figure 2.2–2). Triggers include foods (e.g., eggs, milk, peanuts, seafood, wheat, soybeans), airborne allergens (e.g., dust mites, pollen), stress, dry skin, winter season, and wool clothing. **Associated with asthma** and **allergic rhinitis.** Patients are at **increased risk of cellulitis.** A personal or family history of the "allergic triad" is common.

Differential

Seborrheic dermatitis, contact dermatitis, pityriasis rosea, drug eruption.

Evaluation/Treatment

This is a clinical diagnosis. IgE levels may be elevated. Treat with emollients, topical steroids, topical tacrolimus, PUVA, methotrexate. Biopsy if not responsive.

Eczema is an "itch that rashes."

Allergic triad:
  Atopic dermatitis
  Asthma
  Hay fever

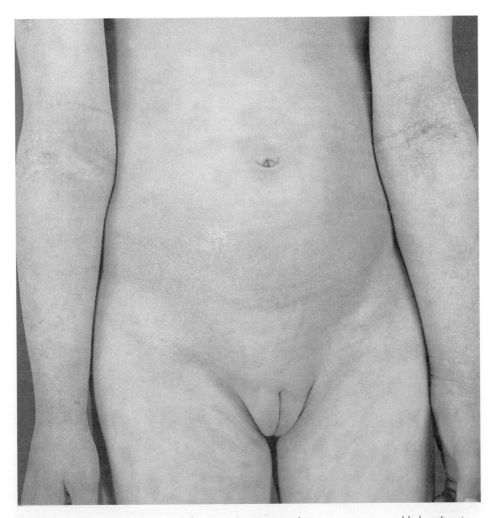

FIGURE 2.2–2. Atopic dermatitis. Ill-defined erythema, papules, excoriations, and lichenification (thickening of the skin with accentuation of the skin lines) in the antecubital fossae, with less severe changes on the trunk and thighs. (Reproduced, with permission, from Fitzpatrick TB. *Color Atlas & Synopsis of Clinical Dermatology,* 4th ed. New York: McGraw-Hill, 2001:35, Fig. 2–10.)

HIGH-YIELD FACTS

Dermatology

An autoimmune disorder with chronic blistering eruptions.

History/PE

Onset typically occurs in patients > **60** years of age. Prodromal erythematous, **urticarial,** papular lesions progress to localized, **large, tense, pruritic bullae** filled with serous to bloody fluid (see Figure 2.2–3). Pressure on bullae does not cause lateral extension. Erosions and crusts result from collapsed bullae. **Negative Nikolsky's sign.** Commonly found on the axillae, medial thigh, abdomen, and lower legs; **rarely involves the mucous membranes.** Constitutional symptoms are minimal.

Differential

Pemphigus vulgaris, erythema multiforme, dermatitis herpetiformis.

Evaluation

Biopsy shows neutrophils in "indian-file" alignment at the **dermal-epidermal** junction, along with **subepidermal bullae.** CBC may show **eosinophilia.**

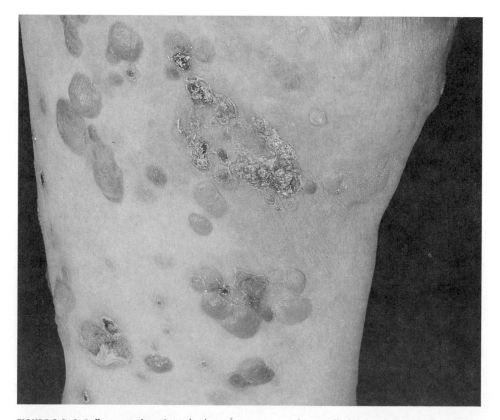

FIGURE 2.2–3. Bullous pemphigoid. Multiple tense serous and partially hemorrhagic bullae. (Reproduced, with permission, from Fitzpatrick TB. *Color Atlas & Synopsis of Clinical Dermatology,* 4th ed. New York: McGraw-Hill, 2001:100, Fig. 4–10.)

Treatment

Oral prednisone for severe cases, tapered to the lowest tolerated dose. Azathioprine and dapsone may also be used. Potent topical glucocorticoids for mild cases.

CELLULITIS

A primary skin infection commonly caused by group A streptococci or staphylococci. Risk factors include diabetes, IV drug use, venous stasis, and immune-compromised states.

History/PE

Presents with red, hot, swollen, tender skin lesions. Fever and chills may be present. Tinea pedis with resultant skin fissures is a common portal of bacterial entry (often not apparent on physical exam).

Differential

Necrotizing fasciitis, osteomyelitis, abscess, urticaria, allergic contact dermatitis, phlebitis.

Evaluation

Wound culture may aid diagnosis. Blood cultures should be obtained when bacteremia is suspected. Otherwise, this is a clinical diagnosis.

Treatment

For mild to moderate cases, prescribe oral antibiotics (cephalexin or dicloxacillin for penicillinase-producing organisms) for 7–10 days. Hospitalization and IV antibiotics (e.g., oxacillin) are necessary if there are any signs of systemic toxicity, comorbid conditions, DM, extremes of age, hand or orbital involvement, or other concerns.

CONTACT DERMATITIS

A delayed (type IV—cell-mediated) hypersensitivity reaction in the form of a skin rash that develops from contact with a substance to which the patient has previously been sensitized. Common offending agents include poison ivy, poison oak, nickel, perfumes, soaps and detergents, and cosmetics.

History

Patients most commonly present with pruritus and rash. Rarely, they may present with edema, fever, lymphadenopathy, and generalized malaise.

PE

Presents with **erythematous, weepy, crusted patches, plaques,** or **papulovesicles** grouped in **linear arrays** or **geometric shapes** with sharp angles and straight borders (see Figure 2.2–4). Characteristic locations are where makeup, clothing, perfume, jewelry, and plants contact the skin.

Differential

Impetigo, herpes simplex, herpes zoster, seborrheic dermatitis, eczema.

Evaluation

Clinical impression and, if necessary, skin patch testing.

Treatment

- **Mild cases:** **Cool compresses** or oatmeal preparation; **topical steroids** 3–4 times a day to reduce pruritus.
- **Severe cases:** **Systemic corticosteroids** may be required; **antihistamines** to reduce pruritus.

UCV *IM2.4*

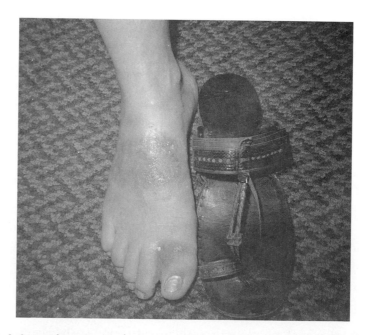

FIGURE 2.2–4. Contact dermatitis. Erythematous papules, vesicles, and serous weeping localized to areas of contact with the offending agent are characteristic. (Reproduced, with permission, from Hurwitz RM. *Pathology of the Skin: Atlas of Clinical-Pathological Correlation,* 2nd ed. Stamford, CT: Appleton & Lange, 1998:3, Fig. 1–5.)

An **immune-mediated disorder** that is due to drugs (e.g., penicillin, sulfon-amides, phenytoin), infection (especially herpes simplex and *Mycoplasma*), vaccination, or malignancy. The severe form of the disease is known as Stevens-Johnson syndrome or toxic epidermal lysis syndrome.

History

May present with a mild **prodrome** of malaise and myalgias. Lesions may be associated with pain and fever. Mucosal involvement may result in dysphagia and dysuria.

PE

Pink-red to red-blue **macules, papules, gyrate erythematous plaques, target lesions,** and bullae are found on physical exam (see Figure 2.2–5). Lesions may be found anywhere but are most commonly seen on the **extremities, palms, and soles.**

Differential

Urticaria, viral exanthem, staphylococcal scalded skin syndrome, bullous pemphigoid, pemphigus vulgaris.

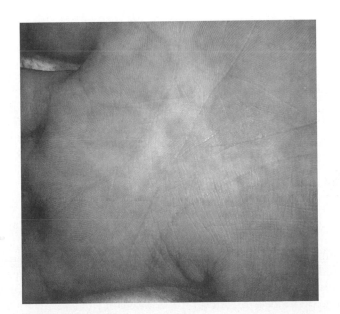

FIGURE 2.2–5. Erythema multiforme. Evolving erythematous plaques and papules with a target appearance: dull red center, pale zone, and darker outer ring. This acute self-limited reaction may occur with infection, antibiotic use, exposure to radiation or chemicals, or malignancy. (Reproduced, with permission, from Hurwitz RM. *Pathology of the Skin: Atlas of Clinical-Pathological Correlation,* 2nd ed. Stamford, CT: Appleton & Lange, 1998:24, Fig. 2–2.)

HIGH-YIELD FACTS

Dermatology

Evaluation

Look for a clinical history of **exposure** to causative agents. Eosinophilia or positive serologic tests for hepatitis, infectious mononucleosis, histoplasmosis, or mycoplasma may be seen. Skin biopsy may show perivascular lymphocytes and necrotic keratinocytes.

Treatment

Think HSV infection with recurrent erythema multiforme.

Mild cases resolve spontaneously. If the condition is drug-induced, **discontinue the inciting agent** immediately. If due to herpes simplex, acyclovir should be given.

ERYTHEMA NODOSUM

An inflammation of the subcutaneous fat that produces tender erythematous nodules, usually on the **anterior tibial areas,** most commonly in young women. Lesions result from hypersensitivity reactions to drugs (OCPs, NSAIDs) or infections (including α-hemolytic strep, coccidioidomycosis, histoplasmosis, TB, and rarely syphilis), sarcoid, rheumatic fever, or inflammatory bowel disease.

History/PE

Lesions are usually **painful,** erythematous bilateral pretibial nodules without ulceration. Lesions rarely occur on the face, arms, or trunk. Malaise, arthralgias, and fever may precede the rash (see Figure 2.2–6).

Differential

Polyarteritis nodosa, other types of panniculitis, furunculosis.

Evaluation

Incisional wedge biopsy provides a definitive diagnosis. Other helpful laboratory findings include an elevated ESR, mild leukocytosis, a high antistreptolysin O (ASO) titer, and a false-positive VDRL. CXR, cultures, and a Gram stain of the lesion may also be performed. Gram stain should be negative, since erythema nodosum is a reactive lesion.

Treatment

NSAIDs are both a precipitating factor and a treatment for erythema nodosum.

Therapy is supportive and includes elevation of the leg, bed rest, and **NSAIDs.** **Potassium iodide** may be given as well. Systemic corticosteroids may be necessary for persistent cases. Before steroid therapy is initiated, a thorough evaluation should be performed to confirm the etiology of the lesion.

UCV *IM2.6*

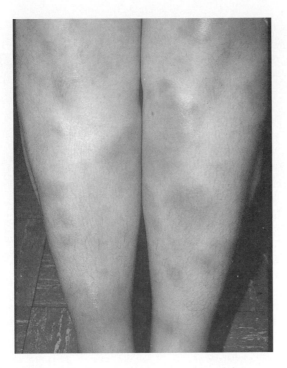

FIGURE 2.2–6. Erythema nodosum. Erythematous plaques and nodules are commonly located on pretibial areas. Lesions are painful and indurated and heal spontaneously without ulceration. (Reproduced, with permission, from Hurwitz RM. *Pathology of the Skin: Atlas of Clinical-Pathological Correlation*, 2nd ed. Stamford, CT: Appleton & Lange, 1998:132, Fig. 10–1A.)

HERPES SIMPLEX

A painful, **recurrent** vesicular eruption of the mucocutaneous surfaces due to HSV infection. The **oral-labial** form is usually due to HSV-1. The **genital** form is usually due to HSV-2.

History

Primary eruptions are longer and more severe than recurrent eruptions. **Primary** outbreaks may be accompanied by **lymphadenopathy, fever,** discomfort, **malaise,** and edema of the involved tissue. **Recurrent** infections are limited to the mucocutaneous area innervated by the **involved nerve.** Onset is preceded by prodromal **tingling,** burning, or frank pain.

PE

Physical exam reveals **grouped vesicles on an erythematous base** (see Figure 2.2–7A).

Evaluation

Multinucleated giant cells and acantholytic cells on **Tzanck smear** yield a presumptive diagnosis (see Figure 2.2–7B). However, varicella-zoster virus (VZV) has the same appearance on the Tzanck, so definitive diagnosis requires culture or direct fluorescent antibody testing.

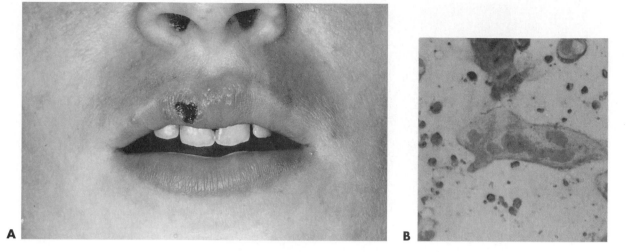

FIGURE 2.2–7. Herpes simplex. (A) Primary infection. Grouped vesicles on an erythematous base on the patient's lips and oral mucosa may progress to pustules before resolving. (B) Tzanck smear. The multinucleated giant cells from vesicular fluid provide a presumptive diagnosis of HSV infection. The Tzanck smear cannot distinguish between HSV and VZV infection. (Reproduced, with permission, from Hurwitz RM. *Pathology of the Skin: Atlas of Clinical-Pathological Correlation,* 2nd ed. Stamford, CT: Appleton & Lange, 1998:145, Fig. 11–9.)

Treatment

Acyclovir ointment is somewhat effective in reducing the duration of viral shedding but not in preventing recurrence. The mainstay of therapy is oral or IV acyclovir (use IV acyclovir for severe cases or immune-compromised patients), which reduces both the frequency and the severity of recurrences. Daily acyclovir suppressive therapy may be used in patients with > 6 outbreaks per year.

IMPETIGO

A contagious and autoinoculable skin infection that is caused by **staphylococcal or streptococcal organisms** and is more common in **children** than in adults. Bullous impetigo is due to coagulase-positive staphylococci that produce exfoliatin, a toxin that leads to vesicle or bulla formation. Nonbullous impetigo is caused by group A streptococci, which produce superficial pustular lesions.

History

Patients often present with **pruritic facial lesions** that develop over a few days.

PE

Classically, **honey-colored crusts** are seen on the lesions, which often involve the face. Common sites of distribution are the **face, neck,** and **extremities**

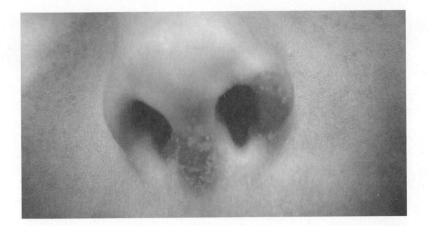

FIGURE 2.2–8. Impetigo. Dried pustules with superficial golden-brown crust are most commonly found around the nose and mouth. (Reproduced, with permission, from Hurwitz RM. *Pathology of the Skin: Atlas of Clinical-Pathological Correlation,* 2nd ed. Stamford, CT: Appleton & Lange, 1998:165, Fig. 12–12.)

(see Figure 2.2–8). **Bullous impetigo** begins as small, erythematous macules that develop into thin-walled vesicles or bullae on an erythematous base. **Nonbullous impetigo** is characterized by superficial pustules with surrounding erythema.

Differential

Ecthyma (thick crust overlying a deep ulcer), allergic contact dermatitis, candidal intertrigo (in warm, moist, intertriginous areas).

Evaluation/Treatment

Affected areas should be gently washed with a mild soap. Obtain bacterial cultures for sensitivities. Topical mupirocin is effective only against coagulase-positive *Staphylococcus aureus*. **Systemic antibiotics** should have activity against both staphylococcus and streptococcus, since the distinction may at times be difficult to make. Because of contagion, the patient's towels and washcloths should be segregated from those of other household members.

LICHEN PLANUS

An inflammatory dermatosis involving the skin and mucous membranes. It is often induced by drugs and is strongly associated with **hepatitis C.**

History

Presents with acute or chronic pruritic, purple lesions. Ulcers are common on mucous membranes.

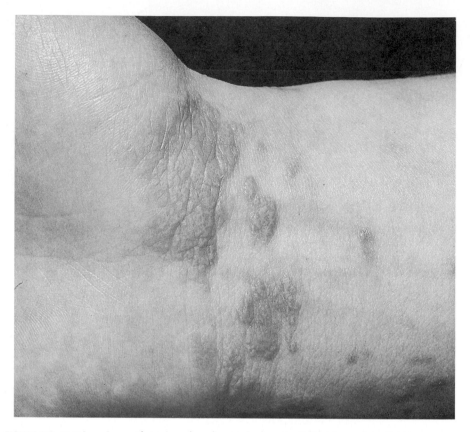

FIGURE 2.2–9. Lichen planus. Flat-topped, polygonal, sharply defined papules of violaceous color, grouped and confluent. The surface is shiny and reveals fine white lines (Wickham's striae). (Reproduced, with permission, from Fitzpatrick TB. *Color Atlas & Synopsis of Clinical Dermatology,* 4th ed. New York: McGraw-Hill, 2001:115, Fig. 5–5.)

PPPP for lichen planus:

Polygonal
Purple
Pruritic
Papules

PE

Flat-topped, purple, polygonal, pruritic papules with white lines (Wickham's striae) (see Figure 2.2–9) are commonly found on the wrist, eyelids, scalp, penis, and shins. Reticulate white hyperkeratosis on buccal mucosa is also common.

Evaluation

Biopsy shows inflammation with hyperkeratosis, an increased granular layer, and bandlike mononuclear infiltrate in the superficial dermis.

Treatment

Topical glucocorticoids for skin lesions. Severe cases may require cyclosporine, oral prednisone, oral retinoids, and PUVA.

A chronic atrophic disorder commonly affecting **skin in the anogenital area.**

History

Age of onset is 40s–50s with a female predominance. Often asymptomatic, but may be pruritic and painful and may also cause dysuria. May rarely develop into squamous cell carcinoma.

PE

Exam reveals white, sharply demarcated, confluent macules and papules (see Figure 2.2–10). **Dilated sweat ducts with keratin plugs** (dells) are characteristic. Lesions are most often found in the **anogenital region** but may also be found on the trunk, neck, and oral mucosa. Follows a waxing and waning course.

Differential

Scleroderma, lichen planus, candida, discoid lupus, extramammary Paget's disease, vitiligo.

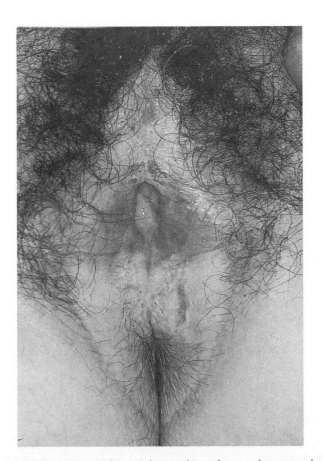

FIGURE 2.2–10. Lichen sclerosus et atrophicus. A large white sclerotic plaque involving the anogenital region. Ecchymoses are noted with atrophy. (Reproduced, with permission, from Fitzpatrick TB. *Color Atlas & Synopsis of Clinical Dermatology,* 4th ed. New York: McGraw-Hill, 2001:999, Fig. 30–12.)

HIGH-YIELD FACTS

Dermatology

Evaluation

Early **biopsy** shows a hyperkeratotic epidermis with follicular plugging, progressing to atrophy. **Homogeneous collagen bands** are found in the dermis.

Treatment

Short-term topical glucocorticoids, topical androgens, oral hydrochloroquine.

MOLLUSCUM CONTAGIOSUM

A poxvirus infection that is most common in **young children** and is also among the most common cutaneous findings in **AIDS patients.**

History/PE

If you see giant molluscum contagiosum, think HIV.

Physical exam reveals 2- to 5-mm discrete, **dome-shaped, shiny papules,** frequently with central **umbilication** (see Figure 2.2–11). In children, the lesions are commonly found on the trunk, extremities, and face. In adults they are more frequently found in the perianal and perigenital areas. If lesions are found in other areas, suspect immune compromise. Lesions are **asymptomatic** unless inflamed or irritated.

Evaluation

Expressing and staining the contents confirms the diagnosis. Giemsa or Wright's stain allows for the identification of large inclusion or molluscum bodies. Ask adults about HIV risk factors.

Treatment

Treatment consists of **curetting the lesion,** liquid nitrogen cryotherapy, or application of trichloroacetic acid. Lesions resolve spontaneously over months to years and are often left untreated in children.

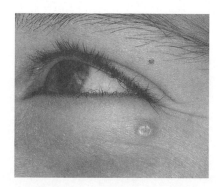

FIGURE 2.2–11. Molluscum contagiosum. The dome-shaped, fleshy, umbilicated papule on the child's eyelid is characteristic. (Reproduced, with permission, from Hurwitz RM. *Pathology of the Skin: Atlas of Clinical-Pathological Correlation,* 2nd ed. Stamford, CT: Appleton & Lange, 1998:149, Fig. 11–19.)

PEMPHIGUS VULGARIS

A serious autoimmune disease of **skin and mucous membranes.** It is often fatal without appropriate immunosuppressive drugs.

History

Onset is usually between the ages of **40 and 60 years.** Erosions often start in the **oral mucosa** (causing decreased food intake secondary to pain), progressing from localized skin blisters to generalized bullae. Lesions are **not pruritic** but are often painful. Associated with epistaxis, hoarseness, weakness, malaise, and weight loss.

PE

Flaccid vesicles and bullae containing serous fluid with a predilection for the **scalp, face, axillae, groin,** and **back.** Oral erosions are common. **Positive Nikolsky's sign**—pressure on bullae causes lateral extension of blisters.

Differential

Pemphigus foliaceus, bullous pemphigoid, bullous impetigo, VZV.

Evaluation

Biopsy shows **intraepidermal** bullae and acantholysis. Direct immunofluorescence shows **IgG and C3 deposits** in the intercellular substance of the epidermis. Indirect immunofluorescence shows autoantibodies directed against desmoglein 3.

Treatment

Oral prednisone to control new bulla formation. Taper to the lowest tolerated dose. **Immunosuppressive agents** such as azathioprine, methotrexate, and cyclophosphamide can help in resistant cases.

PITYRIASIS ROSEA

A mild, self-limited cutaneous eruption seen primarily in children and adolescents. It is associated with human herpesvirus 7 (HHV7).

History/PE

Patients present with moderate to severe pruritus. Exam reveals a diffuse eruption of round to **oval erythematous papules** and plaques covered with a fine "cigarette paper" white scale, distributed on the trunk following skin lines in a **Christmas-tree pattern** (see Figure 2.2–12). A **herald patch**—a solitary patch 2–6 cm in diameter that precedes the rest of the rash—is pathognomonic.

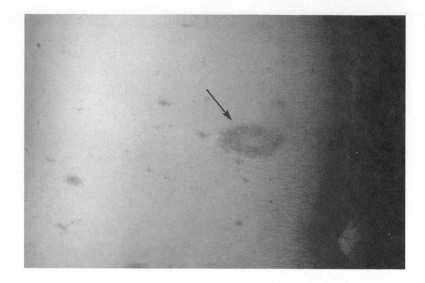

FIGURE 2.2–12. Pityriasis rosea. The round to oval erythematous plaques are often covered with a fine white scale ("cigarette paper") and are often found on the trunk and proximal extremities. Plaques are often preceded by a larger herald patch (arrow). (Reproduced, with permission, from Hurwitz RM. *Pathology of the Skin: Atlas of Clinical-Pathological Correlation,* 2nd ed. Stamford, CT: Appleton & Lange, 1998:13, Fig. 1–42.)

Evaluation

A **skin biopsy** is required if the lesions do not resolve in two months. A serologic test is indicated to rule out secondary syphilis.

Treatment

Lesions are **self-limited.** A mild topical steroid or talc may be used for relief of pruritus. Natural sunlight or daily UVB treatments may hasten healing.

PITYRIASIS VERSICOLOR

A common superficial fungal infection caused by *Malassezia furfur.* Also called **tinea versicolor.** Lesions are usually asymptomatic but may cause mild itching. Physical exam reveals **small, scaling macules** that tend to enlarge and sometimes coalesce. They can be pinkish, lightly pigmented, or **hypopigmented.** The usual sites are the chest and back, but lesions can be found anywhere. **KOH examination** reveals **short, blunt hyphae and small spores** ("spaghetti and meatballs"). Wood's light examination helps evaluate the extent of the disease. Initial treatment is with a topical antifungal agent and selenium sulfide shampoo.

A T-cell-mediated inflammatory disorder resulting in **epidermal hyperprolif-eration.**

History/PE

Presents with dark **red plaques with silvery-white scales** and **sharp margins** (see Figure 2.2–13), classically found over the **extensor surfaces.** Characteristic nail findings include **nail pitting,** "oil spots," and **onycholysis** (lifting of the nail plate). **Pruritus,** pain, tenderness, and joint stiffness may occur with **psoriatic arthritis** (classically, DIP joints). **Generalized toxicity,** fever, and malaise may occur with the generalized pustular form.

Differential

Systemic lupus erythematosus (possibly without systemic symptoms), syphilis, allergic contact dermatitis, fungal infections, seborrheic dermatitis, cutaneous T-cell lymphoma, eczema.

Evaluation

Diagnosis is based on the **gross appearance** and pattern of distribution of the lesions. **Skin biopsy** shows a **thickened epidermis** with an absent granular cell layer and preservation of the nuclei within the hyperkeratotic stratum corneum. **Neutrophils** in the stratum corneum **(Munro microabcesses)** are classic. Blood tests may show elevated uric acid levels, increased ESR, and mild anemia.

Treatment

Topical steroids and intralesional corticosteroid therapy for mild to moderate disease. Phototherapy and methotrexate for severe or generalized disease.

UCV *IM2.8*

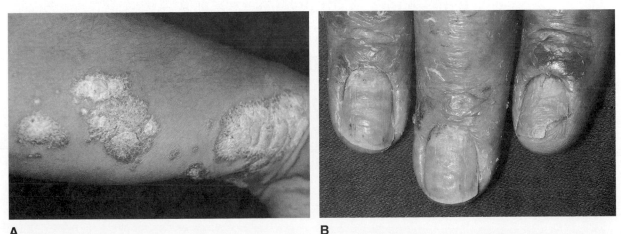

A

B

FIGURE 2.2–13. Psoriasis. (A) Skin changes. The classic sharply demarcated plaques with silvery scales are commonly located on extensor surfaces (e.g., elbows, knees). These plaques are fully developed. (B) Nail changes. Note the pitting, onycholysis, and "oil spots." (Reproduced, with permission, from Hurwitz RM. *Pathology of the Skin: Atlas of Clinical-Pathological Correlation,* 2nd ed. Stamford, CT: Appleton & Lange, 1998:15 and 18, Figs. 1–55 and 1–64.)

ROSACEA

A chronic disorder of pilosebaceous units and increased reactivity of capillaries to heat. Facial flushing is worsened by hot liquids, spicy foods, alcohol, heat, caffeine, and sun exposure. Onset occurs between the ages of 40 and 50 years and exhibits a female predominance. More common in fair-skinned individuals; associated with rhinophyma (large nose) in males. Rosacea typically presents with small papules and pustules distributed symmetrically on the face, predominantly on the cheeks, chin, and forehead. Treatment includes avoiding precipitating factors, topical metronidazole, and sulfur lotions. Oral tetracycline may be added. Oral isotretinoin may be used for severe cases.

SCABIES

A common pruritic rash that develops when *Sarcoptes scabiei,* the human itch mite, burrows into the skin to lay its eggs. Pruritus is worse at night and after a hot shower. Symptoms result from a hypersensitivity reaction against the mite feces. Mites are passed from person to person. Infection is associated with **crowded and dirty living conditions.** Exam reveals excoriations, papules and vesicles, and sometimes **mite burrows** on the wrists and **between the fingers,** elbows, and intertriginous areas. First-line treatment consists of **5% permethrin cream.** Treat close contacts. Antihistamines for symptomatic relief. Wash bedding and clothing in hot water to prevent reinfestation.

SEBORRHEIC DERMATITIS

Suspect HIV in a young person with severe seborrheic dermatitis.

A chronic, superficial inflammatory disorder, commonly involving the **face,** that is thought to be a reaction to *Pityrosporum* yeast. It most commonly presents with **pruritis** during the neonatal and postpubertal periods. **Yellowish, greasy,** and **erythematous scaling patches and plaques** are seen on the **scalp ("cradle cap"), ears,** and face. Treat the face, body, and intertriginous areas with **1% hydrocortisone** and/or topical antifungals. Treat the scalp with **medicated shampoos** with selenium sulfide or zinc pyrithione.

UCV *IM2.9*

SEBORRHEIC KERATOSIS

A common, benign epithelial tumor that rarely appears before age 30. Has a **"stuck-on"** appearance of a wartlike papule or plaque, usually brown in color (see Figure 2.2–14). Lesions are often found on the face, trunk, and upper extremities. Beware of pigmented actinic keratosis and melanoma, which may look like seborrheic keratosis. These are benign lesions that do not require further treatment. When seborrheic keratosis acutely erupts, it is known as the "sign of Leser-Trélat" and is indicative of underlying malignancy (e.g., gastric cancer).

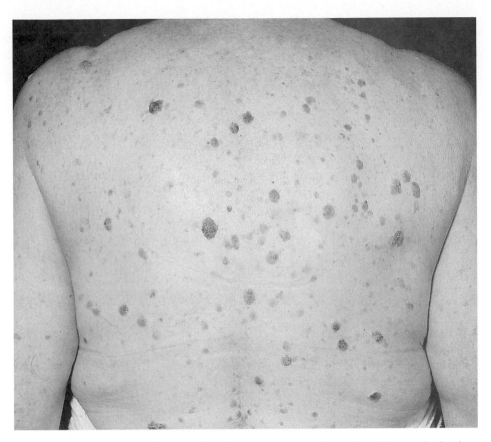

FIGURE 2.2–14. Seborrheic keratoses. Multiple brown, warty papules and nodules on the back, characterized by a "stuck-on" appearance. (Reproduced, with permission, from Fitzpatrick TB. *Color Atlas & Synopsis of Clinical Dermatology,* 4th ed. New York: McGraw-Hill, 2001:195, Fig. 7–32.)

STEVENS-JOHNSON SYNDROME/TOXIC EPIDERMAL LYSIS SYNDROME

A life-threatening exfoliative mucocutaneous disease often caused by a drug-induced reaction. The most commonly implicated drugs are sulfa drugs, allopurinol, carbamazepine, hydantoins, phenylbutazone, cephalosporins, and aminopenicillins. Also known as erythema multiforme major.

History

Patients present with fever with a flu-like prodrome, increasing skin tenderness, painful mouth lesions, and a history of **new-drug exposure,** often within 1–3 weeks of initial exposure.

PE

A **morbilliform rash** evolves into coalescing red macules and **flaccid blisters** along with full-thickness epidermal loss. **Positive Nikolsky's sign.** Lesions usually start on the face and spread downward. Painful erosive lesions on the **mucous membranes** are common.

Evaluation/Treatment

Biopsy shows full-thickness epidermal necrosis. Early diagnosis and **elimination of the offending agents,** analgesia, systemic steroids, IVIG and burn ICU hospitalization to manage skin and fluid losses.

TINEA CORPORIS

A fungal infection on the body. Pruritic, **ring-shaped,** erythematous, and **scaling plaques** are seen, often with central clearing and elevated borders. Lesions are usually few. Diagnosis is based on physical findings and on **hyphae** seen on **KOH preparation.** Culture is not necessary. Treatment includes **topical antifungal cream.**

VARICELLA

Infection by VZV (a member of the herpesvirus family). Transmission is via **respiratory droplet contamination** or contact with **skin lesions.** Varicella has an incubation period of 10–20 days. Contagion begins **24 hours** before the eruption appears and continues until crusting has occurred.

History/PE

A **prodrome** of malaise, fever, headache, and myalgia commonly occurs 24 hours before the onset of the rash. **Pruritic lesions appear in crops** over a period of 3–4 days. Lesions start as pink to red macules and then progress to grouped central vesicles, giving the classic appearance of a **"dewdrop on a rose petal,"** and then crust over. Lesions are commonly found on the **trunk, face,** and **scalp.**

Evaluation/Treatment

Requires clinical evaluation. The disease is **self-limited** in healthy children. For healthy adults with uncomplicated primary varicella, **oral acyclovir** is the appropriate therapy. For adults with severe disease, immune-compromised patients, and those with primary varicella pneumonia, **IV acyclovir** may be required. A **vaccine** is available for infants, children, and adults (immune-compromised patients and adults without previous infection). Recurrent infection can present as **shingles (varicella zoster),** which can be quite painful and serious (see Figure 2.2–15).

UCV *IM2.20*

ACTINIC KERATOSIS

A **premalignant lesion** resulting from **sun exposure** that can lead to squamous cell carcinoma. Also known as solar keratosis.

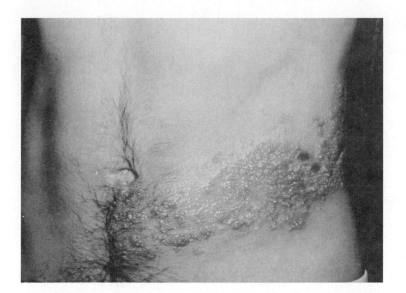

FIGURE 2.2–15. Varicella zoster. The unilateral dermatomal distribution of the grouped vesicles on an erythematous base is characteristic. (Reproduced courtesy of the Yale Department of Dermatology.)

History/PE

Exam reveals **asymptomatic, discrete, rough, scaling patches** and papules 1–5 mm in diameter. Lesions usually have a poorly demarcated erythematous base with an area of rough, **white superficial scaling.** Generally found in sun-exposed areas (see Figure 2.2–16).

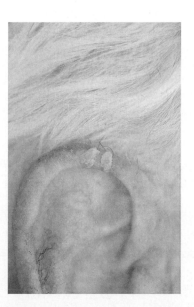

FIGURE 2.2–16. Actinic keratosis. The discrete patch has an erythematous base and rough white scale. Actinic keratosis is a premalignant lesion that may progress to squamous cell carcinoma. It is most commonly found in sun-exposed areas. (Reproduced, with permission, from Hurwitz RM. *Pathology of the Skin: Atlas of Clinical-Pathological Correlation,* 2nd ed. Stamford, CT: Appleton & Lange, 1998:359, Fig. 31–3.)

Differential

Squamous cell carcinoma, eczema.

Evaluation

Skin biopsy shows areas of **dysplastic squamous epithelium** (hyperkeratosis, with cells of the lower epidermis showing loss of polarity, pleomorphism, and hyperchromatic nuclei) **without invasion into the dermis.**

Treatment

Treat with **cryosurgery,** topical 5-FU, curettage, and chemical peel. **Prevent with UVA/UVB sunscreens** and by minimizing sun exposure.

UCV *IM2.3*

BASAL CELL CARCINOMA

The **most common skin cancer.** Associated with excessive sun exposure. Lesions take many forms, including nodular, ulcerative, pigmented, superficial, and sclerosing/morpheaform subtypes.

History/PE

Exam reveals a **pearly-colored papule** of variable size. The external surface is frequently covered with fine **telangiectasias** and appears **translucent** (see Figure 2.2–17). Lesions may be anywhere on the body but are most commonly on sun-exposed areas. Large ulcers are described as **"rodent ulcers."**

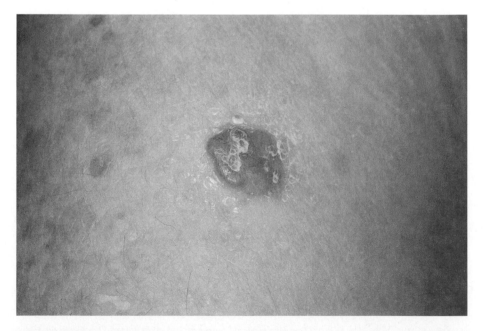

FIGURE 2.2–17. Basal cell carcinoma. Erythematous, fleshy, telangiectatic nodule with translucent surface. (Reproduced, with permission, from Hurwitz RM. *Pathology of the Skin: Atlas of Clinical-Pathological Correlation,* 2nd ed. Stamford, CT: Appleton & Lange, 1998:362, Fig. 31–24.)

Differential

Squamous cell carcinoma, actinic keratosis, seborrheic keratosis.

Evaluation

Skin biopsy shows characteristic basophilic **palisading cells with retraction.**

Treatment

Therapy depends on the size and location of the tumor, the histologic type, the history of prior treatment, the underlying health of the patient, and cosmetic considerations. Options include curettage, surgical excision, Mohs' micrographic surgery (serial excisions with fresh-tissue microscopic examination to maximize cosmesis), cryosurgery, and radiation. **Prevent with UVA/UVB sunscreens** and by avoiding prolonged and unnecessary sun exposure.

SQUAMOUS CELL CARCINOMA

Risk factors include **exposure** to sun and ionizing radiation, actinic keratosis, immunosuppression, arsenic, and industrial carcinogens.

History/PE

Usually slowly evolving and **asymptomatic;** occasionally, bleeding or pain may develop. Exam reveals small, red, **exophytic nodules** with varying degrees of scaling or crusting (see Figure 2.2–18). Lesions are commonly found in **sun-exposed areas,** including the ears, cheeks, lower lip, and dorsum of the hands.

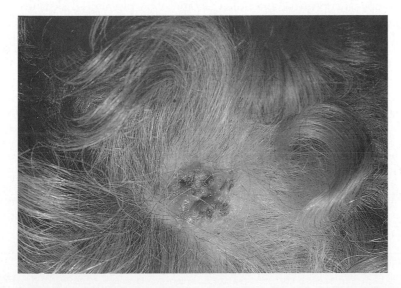

FIGURE 2.2–18. Squamous cell carcinoma. Note the crusting and ulceration of this erythematous plaque. Most lesions are exophytic nodules with erosion or ulceration. (Reproduced, with permission, from Hurwitz RM. *Pathology of the Skin: Atlas of Clinical-Pathological Correlation,* 2nd ed. Stamford, CT: Appleton & Lange, 1998:360, Fig. 31–20.)

Differential

Basal cell carcinoma, warts, actinic keratosis.

Evaluation

Biopsy shows irregular masses of anaplastic epidermal cells proliferating down to the dermis.

Treatment

Surgical excision is necessary for larger lesions and for those involving the periorbital, periauricular, perilabial, genital, and perigenital areas. **Mohs' micrographic surgery** may be performed for recurrent lesions and on areas of the face that are difficult to reconstruct, as well as for poorly differentiated tumors and those with ill-defined margins. **Radiation** may be necessary in cases where surgery is not a viable option. **Prevent with UVA/UVB sunscreens** and by avoiding prolonged and unnecessary sun exposure.

UCV *IM2.10*

MELANOMA

An **aggressive** skin malignancy of melanocytic origin. Risk factors include **sun exposure,** fair skin, a family history (e.g., dysplastic nevus syndrome), xeroderma pigmentosum, a large number of nevi, and the presence of dysplastic nevi. Melanoma is the leading cause of death from skin disease and carries a 1.7% lifetime risk (see Tables 2.2–1 to 2.2–3).

History

Melanoma is usually **asymptomatic** until late in the disease process. Patients may present with pruritus and mild discomfort. **A pigmented skin lesion that has recently changed in size or appearance should raise concern.** Lesions may be seen on sun-exposed areas as well as on the plantar aspect of the feet.

PE

> **The ABCDs of melanoma:**
>
> **A**symmetric shape
> **B**orders irregular
> **C**olor variegated
> **D**iameter > 6 mm

Lesions are characterized by the **ABCDs** of melanoma (see mnemonic) and may occur anywhere on the body (see Figure 2.2–19). They are most commonly found **on the trunk for men** and on the **legs for women.**

Differential

Nevi, seborrheic keratosis, freckles, pigmented basal cell carcinoma, atypical nevus.

TABLE 2.2–1. Types of Malignant Melanoma

	Superficial Spreading	Nodular	Acral-Lentiginous	Lentigo Maligna
Appearance	Dark brown, variegated, irregular borders; asymmetric shape.	Uniform, dark, "blueberry-like" nodule.	Marked variegation of brown/black macule or papule.	Flat, "geographic" shape; brown/black with "stain-like" appearance.
Distribution	Back, legs.	Any area; arises rapidly.	Palms, soles, mucous membranes, nails.	Head, neck, hands, sun-exposed areas.
Epidemiology	30s–50s, M = F, fair-skinned, 70% of all melanomas.	50s, M = F.	60s, M > F, more common in Asians and African-Americans.	60s, M = F, fair-skinned.

Evaluation

Skin biopsy shows **melanocytes with marked cellular atypia** (vacuolated cytoplasm, hyperchromatic nuclei with prominent nucleoli, and pleomorphism) and melanocytic invasion (Clark and Breslow staging) into the dermis.

Treatment

Surgical excision is the treatment of choice. Advanced disease may not respond to therapy. **The thickness of the melanoma (depth of invasion)** is the most important prognostic factor. Depending on depth, lymph node dissection may be necessary. Systemic chemotherapy is used for metastatic disease.

MYCOSIS FUNGOIDES

Cutaneous T-cell lymphoma of unknown etiology. Associated with HTLV in some patients.

History

Intractable pruritus. Look for previous diagnoses of skin diseases such as psoriasis and nummular dermatitis that have been refractory to treatment.

TABLE 2.2–2. Prognosis of Melanoma Based on Thickness (Breslow)

Risk	Thickness (mm)	Five-Year Survival (%)
Minimum	< 0.76	96–99
Low	0.76–1.5	87–94
Intermediate	1.51–4.0	66–77
High	> 4.0	< 50

HIGH-YIELD FACTS

Dermatology

TABLE 2.2–3. Prognosis of Melanoma Based on Histology (Clark)

Level	Depth	Five-Year Survival (%)
I	Intraepidermal (in situ)	100
II	Penetrates papillary dermis	95
III	Fills papillary dermis	82
IV	Penetrates reticular dermis	71
V	Penetrates subcutaneous fat	49

PE

Randomly distributed red plaques may progress to nodules. Scaling may be present. Extensive infiltration is associated with **lion-like facies** (see Figure 2.2–20). Lymphadenopathy can be present.

Differential

Psoriasis, atopic dermatitis, dermatophytosis.

Evaluation

Biopsy shows band-like infiltrate in the upper dermis with atypical lymphocytes with convoluted cerebriform nuclei and **microabscesses in the epidermis** (Pautrier's microabscesses). Immunostaining will show T cells (CD3+, CD4+), not B cells. CBC shows eosinophilia. LDH is often increased.

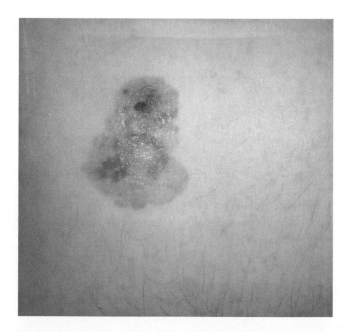

FIGURE 2.2–19. Melanoma. Note the asymmetry, border irregularity, color variation, and large diameter of this plaque. (Reproduced, with permission, from Hurwitz RM. *Pathology of the Skin: Atlas of Clinical-Pathological Correlation,* 2nd ed. Stamford, CT: Appleton & Lange, 1998:432, Fig. 36–8.)

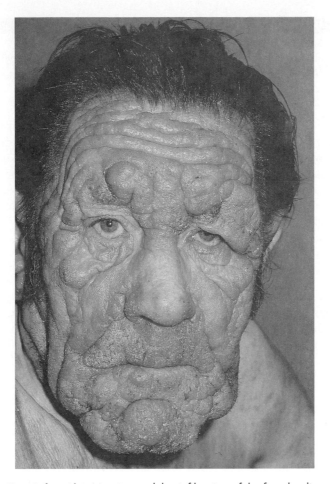

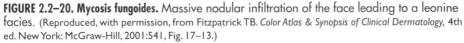

FIGURE 2.2–20. Mycosis fungoides. Massive nodular infiltration of the face leading to a leonine facies. (Reproduced, with permission, from Fitzpatrick TB. *Color Atlas & Synopsis of Clinical Dermatology,* 4th ed. New York: McGraw-Hill, 2001:541, Fig. 17–13.)

Treatment

PUVA photochemotherapy; topical nitrogen mustard; total body electron-beam irradiation, ultra-high-potency topical steroids, systemic and topical retinoids.

Complications

Sézary's syndrome (advanced form with generalized erythroderma, lymphadenopathy, and peripheral blood involvement); sepsis secondary to skin infection; transformation to high-grade lymphoma.

Dermatology

The following clinical questions and accompanying answers are reproduced, with permission, from Reteguiz J, *PreTest: Physical Diagnosis*, 4th ed., New York: McGraw-Hill, 2001.

Questions

1. A 16-year-old student with a history of herpetic gingivostomatitis develops a generalized and symmetric rash. The lesions are 1–2 cm in diameter and look like round patches. They consist of two concentric rings surrounding a central disk. The rash is burning and pruritic. A few erosive lesions are visible in the oral mucosa. Which of the following is the most likely diagnosis?
   a. Erythema multiforme
   b. Secondary syphilis
   c. Systemic lupus erythematosus
   d. Pemphigus vulgaris
   e. Urticaria

2. A 17-year-old patient presents with severe pruritus that is worse at night. Upon examination of the skin, areas of excoriated papules are observed in the interdigital area. Family members report similar symptoms. Which of the following is the most likely diagnosis?
   a. Scabies
   b. Cutaneous larva migrans
   c. Contact dermatitis
   d. Dermatitis herpetiformis
   e. Impetigo

3. A 6-year-old child presents complaining of patchy hair loss on the back of the scalp. Examination reveals well-demarcated areas of erythema and scaling, and although there are still some hairs in the area, they are extremely short and broken in appearance. Which of the following is the most likely diagnosis?
   a. Androgenic hair loss
   b. Psoriasis of the scalp
   c. Seborrheic dermatitis
   d. Tinea capitis
   e. Carbuncle

4. Five days after going on a nature walk, a 13-year-old boy develops well-demarcated, erythematous plaques and vesicles over his arms and face. The plaques are arranged in a linear fashion and are crusting. The boy has some facial edema. He has no history of fever or chills but complains of pruritus. Which of the following is the most likely diagnosis?
   a. Rubeola
   b. Atopic dermatitis
   c. Acute contact dermatitis
   d. Impetigo
   e. Erythema infectiosum

5. A 6-year-old child presents with flesh-colored papules on the hand that are not pruritic. Examination reveals lesions that are approximately 4 mm in diameter with central umbilication. A halo is seen around those lesions undergoing regression. Which of the following is the most likely diagnosis?
   a. Verruca vulgaris
   b. Molluscum contagiosum
   c. Keratoacanthoma
   d. Herpetic whitlow
   e. Hemangioma

Answers

1. **The answer is a.** Erythema multiforme (EM) **minor** due to the herpes infection is the most likely diagnosis in this patient. The lesions of EM are classically target lesions; they are burning and pruritic. They are generalized and often involve the oral mucosa. Etiologies of **EM major** include drugs such as phenytoin, sulfonamides, barbiturates, and allopurinol. Finger pressure in the vicinity of a lesion in EM major leads to a sheetlike removal of the epidermis **(Nikolsky sign).** Pemphigus vulgaris is a chronic, bullous, autoimmune disease usually seen in middle-aged adults. The Nikolsky sign is positive in pemphigus vulgaris. **Secondary syphilis** appears 2–6 months after a primary infection and consists of round to oval, maculopapular lesions 0.5–1.0 cm in diameter. The eruptions typically involve the palms and soles. Secondary syphilis lesions that are flat and soft with a predilection for the mouth, perineum, and perianal areas are called **condylomata lata.** The skin lesions of SLE range from the classic butterfly malar rash to the discoid plaques of chronic cutaneous lupus erythematosus (CCLE). Urticaria is characterized by pruritic wheals typically lasting several hours.

2. **The answer is a.** The history is classic for scabies. Scabies is an infestation by the mite *Sarcoptes scabiei* that is spread by skin-to-skin contact. Although there are few skin findings on physical examination, patients usually complain of intense pruritus. Contact dermatitis is unlikely in this location, and cutaneous larva migrans (most commonly from *Ancylostoma braziliense* due to the dog and cat hookworm) typically has large, erythematous, serpiginous tracks. **Dermatitis herpetiformis** is associated with a gluten-sensitive enteropathy and is characterized by tiny papules, vesicles, and urticarial wheals. **Impetigo** is an infectious skin disease due to either *Staphylococcus aureus* or *Streptococcus pyogenes* seen typically on the face and characterized by discrete vesicles that rupture to form a yellowish crust.

3. **The answer is d.** The history is most consistent with tinea capitis due to either *Trichophyton tonsurans* or *Microsporum canis*. It is usually seen in school-age children and may be transmitted from person to person. **Psoriasis** is a hereditary disorder characterized by scaling patches and plaques appearing in specific areas of the body, such as the scalp, elbows, lumbosacral region, and knees. The lesions are "salmon pink" with a silver-colored scale that on removal produces blood **(Auspitz sign).** The **Koebner phenomenon** (with trauma, the lesion jumps to a new location) is also elicited in patients with psoriasis. **Seborrheic dermatitis** is a common chronic dermatosis occurring in areas with active sebaceous glands (face, scalp, and body folds) and may occur either in infancy or in people over the age of 20. The eczematous plaques of seborrheic dermatitis are yellowish red and are often greasy with a sticky crust. Androgenic hair loss is a progressive hereditary bitemporal, frontal, or vertex balding that may begin any time after puberty. A **carbuncle** is a deep infectious collection of interconnecting abscesses **(furuncles)** arising from several hair follicles.

4. **The answer is c.** Contact dermatitis can be due to an allergen causing a type IV, cell-mediated, delayed hypersensitivity reaction. It may also be due to a nonallergen such as a chemical irritant. This patient presents with typical symptoms of acute contact dermatitis due to **poison ivy** resin. This results in sensitization within a week of exposure. Contact dermatitis due to poison ivy is usually pruritic, localized to one region, and often linear. **Impetigo** is an epidermal bacterial infection seen on the face characterized

by vesicles that rupture and crust. Erythema infectiosum or **fifth disease** is a childhood disease due to parvovirus B19 and is characterized by edematous, erythematous plaques on the cheeks **("slapped cheek" disease).** Atopic dermatitis or eczema is an autosomal dominant pruritic inflammation with a predilection for the neck, face, flexor areas, feet, wrists, and hands. Usually there is a personal or family history of asthma, allergic rhinitis, or hay fever. **Rubeola (measles)** is a viral infection characterized by conjunctivitis and cough and a confluent erythematous maculopapular rash that spreads centrifugally. **Koplik spots** (bright red spots with blue-white specks in the center), which appear on the buccal mucosa opposite the premolar teeth, are pathognomonic for rubeola.

5. **The answer is b.** The description of the skin lesions is most consistent with **molluscum contagiosum.** This is a self-limited viral infection due to a pox virus (molluscum contagiosum virus) seen in children, sexually active adults, and HIV-infected patients. These lesions characteristically have a central keratotic plug that gives them the appearance of being dimpled (umbilication). The lesions resolve spontaneously. Common **warts or verrucae vulgaris** are due to human papillomavirus (HPV). Warts are firm, hyperkeratotic, round papules that are 1–10 mm in diameter. They have no umbilication but have a predilection for sites of trauma, including hands, fingers, and knees. A **keratoacanthoma** is a skin-colored, isolated, dome-shaped nodule with a central hyperkeratotic core usually found on the face. A **herpetic whitlow,** due to herpes simplex virus, consists of a painful group of vesicles on the volar finger. Capillary **hemangiomas** are bright red or purple nodules or plaques that develop at birth and spontaneously disappear by the fifth year.

Endocrinology

Type 1 vs. type 2 diabetes mellitus

Variable	Type 1—juvenile onset (IDDM)	Type 2—adult onset (NIDDM)
Incidence	15%	85%
Insulin necessary in treatment	Always	Sometimes
Age (exceptions commonly occur)	< 30	> 40
Association with obesity	No	Yes
Genetic predisposition	Weak, polygenic	Strong, polygenic
Association with HLA system	Yes (HLA-DR 3 and 4)	No
Glucose intolerance	Severe	Mild to moderate
Ketoacidosis	Common	Rare
β cell numbers in the islets	$\downarrow$	Variable
Serum insulin level	$\downarrow$	Variable
Classic symptoms of polyuria, polydipsia, thirst, weight loss	Common	Sometimes
Theorized cause	Viral or immune destruction of β cells	$\uparrow$ resistance to insulin

Diabetic ketoacidosis

One of the most important complications of type 1 diabetes. Usually due to an $\uparrow$ in insulin requirements from an $\uparrow$ in stress (e.g., infection). Excess fat breakdown and $\uparrow$ ketogenesis from the $\uparrow$ in free fatty acids, which are then made into ketone bodies.

Signs/symptoms
Kussmaul respirations (rapid/deep breathing), hyperthermia, nausea/vomiting, abdominal pain, psychosis/dementia, dehydration. Fruity breath odor.

Labs
Hyperglycemia, $\uparrow$ H+, $\downarrow$ HCO$_3^-$ (anion gap metabolic acidosis), $\uparrow$ blood ketone levels, leukocytosis.

Complications
Life-threatening mucormycosis, *Rhizopus* infection, cerebral edema, cardiac arrhythmias, heart failure.

Treatment
Fluids, insulin, and potassium; glucose if necessary to prevent hypoglycemia.

HIGH-YIELD FACTS

Endocrinology

Diabetes mellitus

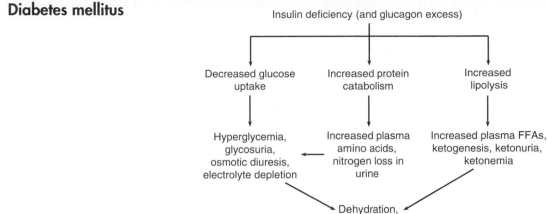

Insulin deficiency (and glucagon excess)

- Decreased glucose uptake → Hyperglycemia, glycosuria, osmotic diuresis, electrolyte depletion
- Increased protein catabolism → Increased plasma amino acids, nitrogen loss in urine
- Increased lipolysis → Increased plasma FFAs, ketogenesis, ketonuria, ketonemia

→ Dehydration, acidosis

→ Coma, death

Adrenal cortex and medulla

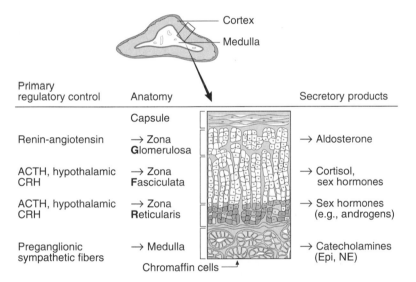

Cortex
Medulla

Primary regulatory control	Anatomy	Secretory products
	Capsule	
Renin-angiotensin	→ Zona **G**lomerulosa	→ Aldosterone
ACTH, hypothalamic CRH	→ Zona **F**asciculata	→ Cortisol, sex hormones
ACTH, hypothalamic CRH	→ Zona **R**eticularis	→ Sex hormones (e.g., androgens)
Preganglionic sympathetic fibers	→ Medulla	→ Catecholamines (Epi, NE)

Chromaffin cells →

GFR corresponds with salt (Na⁺), sugar (glucocorticoids), and sex (androgens).

"The deeper you go, the sweeter it gets."

Pheochromocytoma—most common tumor of the adrenal medulla in adults. *Bio.26*

Neuroblastoma—most common in children. *Path3.26*

Pheochromocytoma causes episodic hypertension; neuroblastoma does not.

PTH

Source	Chief cells of parathyroid.
Function	1. ↑ bone resorption of calcium and phosphate
	2. ↑ kidney reabsorption of calcium in DCT
	3. ↓ kidney reabsorption of phosphate
	4. ↑ 1,25-(OH)$_2$ vitamin D (cholecalciferol) production by stimulating kidney 1α-hydroxylase
Regulation	↓ in free serum Ca²⁺ ↑ PTH secretion.

PTH ↑ serum Ca²⁺, ↓ serum (PO₄)³⁻, ↑ urine (PO₄)³⁻.

PTH stimulates both osteoclasts and osteoblasts.

PTH = **P**hosphate **T**rashing **H**ormone.

Thyroid hormones (T_3/T_4)

Iodine-containing hormones that control the body's metabolic rate.

Source	Follicles of thyroid.	T_3 functions—**4B's:**
Function	1. Bone growth (synergism with GH)	**B**rain maturation
	2. CNS maturation	**B**one growth
	3. β-adrenergic effects	**B**eta-adrenergic effects
	4. ↑ basal metabolic rate via ↑ Na^+/K^+ ATPase activity = ↑ O_2 consumption, ↑ body temp	**B**MR ↑
	5. ↑ glycogenolysis, gluconeogenesis, lipolysis	
	6. CV— ↑ CO, HR, SV, contractility, RR	
Regulation	TRH (hypothalamus) stimulates TSH (pituitary), which stimulates follicular cells. Negative feedback by T_3 to anterior pituitary ↓ sensitivity to TRH. TSI, like TSH, stimulates follicular cells (Graves' disease).	

Cushing's syndrome

↑ cortisol due to a variety of causes.
Etiologies include:
1. Cushing's disease (1° pituitary adenoma); ↑ ACTH
2. 1° adrenal (hyperplasia/neoplasia); ↓ ACTH
3. Ectopic ACTH production (e.g., small cell lung cancer); ↑ ACTH
4. Iatrogenic; ↓ ACTH

The clinical picture includes hypertension, weight gain, moon facies, truncal obesity, buffalo hump, hyperglycemia (insulin resistance), skin changes (thinning, striae), osteoporosis, and immune suppression.

Multiple endocrine neoplasias (MEN)

MEN type I (Wermer's syndrome)—pancreas (e.g., ZE syndrome, insulinomas, VIPomas), parathyroid, and pituitary tumors.	MEN I = 3 "**P**" organs (**P**ancreas, **P**ituitary, and **P**arathyroid).
MEN type II (Sipple's syndrome)—medullary carcinoma of the thyroid, pheochromocytoma, parathyroid tumor or adenoma.	All MEN syndromes have autosomal-dominant inheritance.
MEN type III (formerly MEN IIB)—medullary carcinoma of the thyroid, pheochromocytoma, and oral and intestinal ganglioneuromatosis (mucosal neuromas).	

Propylthiouracil (PTU)

Mechanism	Inhibits organification and coupling of thyroid hormone synthesis. Also ↓ peripheral conversion of T_4 to T_3.
Clinical use	Hyperthyroidism.
Toxicity	Skin rash, agranulocytosis (rare), aplastic anemia.

CUSHING'S SYNDROME

Results from high levels of cortisol **(hypercortisolism).** The most common etiology is iatrogenic (excessive corticosteroid administration). **Cushing's disease is central,** due to hypersecretion of ACTH from a pituitary adenoma. Other causes include ectopic ACTH production due to neoplasia (e.g., carcinoid tumor, small cell lung cancer) and excess adrenal secretion of cortisol (e.g., bilateral adrenal hyperplasia, adrenal cancer).

High ACTH: ectopic or pituitary source.
Low ACTH: adrenal or exogenous source.

History

Depression, oligomenorrhea, growth retardation, weakness, acne, and **excessive hair growth.** Symptoms of **diabetes** (e.g., polydipsia, polyuria, polyphagia) may also be present secondary to glucose intolerance.

PE

HTN, central obesity, muscle wasting, thin skin with easy **bruisability** and purple **striae,** psychological disturbances, **hirsutism, moon facies,** and "buffalo hump."

Differential

Chronic alcoholism, depression, diabetes mellitus (DM), exogenous steroid administration, adrenogenital syndrome.

Evaluation

- **Screen: Low-dose dexamethasone suppression test:** abnormal if cortisol is persistently elevated after suppression the previous night.
- **Confirm: 24-hour free urine cortisol.**
- **Differentiate: High-dose dexamethasone suppression test:** Cortisol is suppressed in patients with ACTH-secreting pituitary adenomas, but not in patients with ectopic ACTH production or adrenal cortisol secreting tumors.
- CT (adrenal) or MRI (sphenoid) to further localize lesions.
- Hyperglycemia, glycosuria, and **hypokalemia** are also consistent with Cushing's.

Table 2.3–1 lists the important differences in laboratory findings between the various causes of Cushing's syndrome.

TABLE 2.3–1. Laboratory Findings in Cushing's Syndrome

	Iatrogenic Hypercortisolism	Pituitary ACTH Hypersecretion	Adrenal Cortisol Hypersecretion	Ectopic ACTH Production
ACTH	↓	↑	↓	↑
Urinary free cortisol	↑	↑	↑	↑
DHEA	↓	↑	↑	↑

Treatment

Surgical resection of the hypersecretory source (pituitary, adrenal). Irradiation is also possible for pituitary disease. **Mitotane** and adrenal enzyme inhibitors **(ketoconazole, metyrapone, aminoglutethimide)** are used as medical therapy.

Complications

Increased susceptibility to infection, vertebral compression fractures, avascular necrosis of the femoral head.

UCV *IM1.17*

ADRENAL INSUFFICIENCY

Can be primary (Addison's disease) or secondary (due to decreased ACTH production by the pituitary). **Addison's disease** is caused by destruction of the adrenal cortices, leading to deficiencies of both mineralocorticoids and glucocorticoids. **Autoimmune destruction** is the most common etiology. May occur as part of a polyglandular autoimmune syndrome (hypothyroidism, type 1 DM, vitiligo, premature ovarian failure, testicular failure, and pernicious anemia). Other causes of primary adrenal insufficiency include congenital enzyme deficiencies, adrenal hemorrhage (often as part of DIC, as in Waterhouse-Friderichsen syndrome), TB, and other infections. Secondary adrenal insufficiency is most often due to **abrupt cessation of chronic glucocorticoid treatment.**

History

Presenting symptoms include **weakness, weight loss, nausea,** and **vomiting.** **Addisonian crisis** presents with nausea, vomiting, hypoglycemia, dehydration, and CV collapse.

PE

Hypotension; anorexia; **skin hyperpigmentation** with **Addison's disease** (due to increased ACTH; no pigmentation changes with secondary insufficiency).

Differential

Anorexia nervosa, malabsorption disorders, occult malignancy, panhypopituitarism, hemochromatosis.

Evaluation

Hyponatremia, hyperkalemia, and **eosinophilia** are consistent with either primary or secondary adrenal insufficiency. Table 2.3–2 lists important differences in the laboratory evaluation of primary and secondary adrenal insufficiency.

Treatment

Treat with replacement **glucocorticoids** and **mineralocorticoids.** Increase steroids during periods of stress (e.g., major surgery, trauma, infection). Avoid

	Addison's Disease	Secondary Adrenal Insufficiency
TABLE 2.3–2. Primary vs. Secondary Adrenal Insufficiency		
ACTH	High	Low
Cortisol after ACTH challenge	Low	High

secondary adrenal insufficiency by tapering off glucocorticoids, allowing endogenous production of ACTH to return to normal.

UCV *IM1.16*

HYPERALDOSTERONISM

Primary hyperaldosteronism most commonly results from a unilateral adrenal adenoma **(Conn's syndrome).** Most remaining cases result from bilateral adrenocortical hyperplasia.

History/PE

HTN, headache, polyuria (secondary to hypokalemic nephropathy), **muscle weakness** (secondary to hypokalemia). Tetany and/or paresthesias, and, in severe cases, peripheral edema.

Differential

Essential HTN, diuretic toxicity, nephrogenic diabetes insipidus (DI), secondary hyperaldosteronism (renal artery stenosis, CHF, cirrhosis, renal failure associated with high plasma renin).

Evaluation

Hypokalemia, hypernatremia, metabolic alkalosis, **low plasma renin,** and elevated **24-hour urine aldosterone;** CT or MRI may reveal an adrenal mass.

In Conn's syndrome, renin levels are low.

Treatment

Treat with laparoscopic or open **adrenalectomy** for adrenal tumor after correcting BP and potassium. Treat with **spironolactone** (an aldosterone receptor antagonist) for bilateral hyperplasia.

CONGENITAL ADRENAL HYPERPLASIA (CAH)

A congenital disorder that commonly results in a deficiency of cortisol. The majority of cases are due to an autosomal-recessive defect in **21-hydroxylase,**

The majority of CAH cases are due to 21-hydroxylase deficiency.

a crucial cortisol synthesis enzyme. Other causes include 11-hydroxylase and 17-hydroxylase deficiencies. Cortisol deficiency stimulates ACTH synthesis and leads to overproduction of other adrenal steroids that are not affected by the enzyme deficiency (mainly adrenal androgens). Severe 21-hydroxylase deficiency causes mineralocorticoid deficiency with salt wasting, a serious complication requiring mineralocorticoid replacement (e.g., fludricortisone).

History/PE

Ambiguous genitalia in female infants; **virilization** (if manifested later in life). **Macrogenitosomia** in male infants; precocious puberty (if manifested later in life); and HTN (with 11- and 17-hydroxylase deficiencies). Cortisol deficiency is usually minimized owing to adrenal hyperplasia.

Evaluation

High levels of cortisol precursors and androgens in blood and urine.

Treatment

- **Medical:** Cortisol administration reduces ACTH and adrenal androgens.
- **Surgical:** May be required in the case of ambiguous genitalia in female infants.

PHEOCHROMOCYTOMA

The most common primary tumor of the adrenal gland in adults. Pheochromocytomas arise from **chromaffin cells** and secrete epinephrine and norepinephrine, thus mimicking activation of the sympathetic nervous system. May be associated with von Hippel-Lindau syndrome, neurofibromatosis, or MEN II/III syndromes.

Rule of 10's:

10% bilateral
10% malignant
10% extra-adrenal
10% calcify
10% occur in kids
10% familial

The 5 P's:

Pressure (↑ BP)
Pain (headache)
Perspiration
Palpitations
Pallor/diaphoresis

History/PE

Intermittent tachycardia, palpitations, chest pain, diaphoresis, HTN, headache, tremor, anxiety.

Evaluation

CT or MRI often demonstrates a suprarenal mass. Measurement of 24-hour **urinary catecholamine metabolites** (e.g., VMA, HVA) offer the most useful screening test.

Treatment

Definitive treatment involves surgical removal of the tumor. Prior to surgery, implement α and β blockade. Use α-antagonists first (phentolamine and phenoxybenzamine) to avoid unopposed α stimulation (which causes extreme HTN). Use propranolol for β-blockade and consider metyrosine.

UCV *Surg.7*

TYPE 1 DIABETES MELLITUS

Thought to be due to autoimmune destruction of the β cells of the pancreas. Type 1 DM manifests as hyperglycemia secondary to insulin deficiency, ultimately requiring exogenous insulin therapy. It is usually diagnosed in children or adolescents. Type 1 DM is associated with **HLA-DR3** and **-DR4.**

History/PE

Patients commonly present with **polyuria** (including nocturia), **polydipsia, polyphagia,** and rapid or unexplained weight loss.

Differential

Pancreatic disease (e.g., chronic pancreatitis), glucagonoma, Cushing's disease, iatrogenic factors (e.g., corticosteroids), gestational diabetes, DI.

Evaluation

At least one of the following is required to make the diagnosis:

- Random plasma glucose concentration > 200 mg/dL with classic symptoms of diabetes.
- Fasting plasma glucose > 126 mg/dL on two separate occasions.
- Two-hour postprandial glucose > 200 mg/dL after 75-g oral glucose tolerance test (on two separate occasions).

The presence of urine glucose and urine ketones supports the diagnosis. HbA_{1c} is used to monitor the efficacy of and compliance with treatment, since it reflects glucose levels over the three months prior to measurement. **The goal is to maintain $HbA_{1c} < 7$,** as near-normalization of blood glucose has been shown to slow the development and progression of microvascular disease, including retinopathy, nephropathy, and neuropathy (but not macrovascular disease).

Treatment

Treat with a regular regimen of insulin injections (see Table 2.3–3). Patients must be taught to monitor their glucose levels at home. Patients should be carefully monitored for diabetes-related complications; including annual dilated eye exams, annual testing for microalbuminuria, and frequent foot checks (see Table 2.3–4).

UCV *IM1.18*

TYPE 2 DIABETES MELLITUS

In contrast to type 1 DM, hyperglycemia here is secondary to end-organ insulin resistance. Type 2 DM is most commonly diagnosed in obese patients > 40 years of age. It often has a family history, but there is no known HLA linkage.

> **The 3 P's of type 1 DM:**
>
> **P**olyuria
> **P**olydipsia
> **P**olyphagia

HIGH-YIELD FACTS

Endocrinology

TABLE 2.3–3. Insulin Formulations

Type	Time of Onset of Action	Peak Effect
Aspart	10–15 minutes	0.5–1.5 hours
Lispro	10–15 minutes	1–2 hours
Regular	45 minutes	2–5 hours
NPH	2–4 hours	6–10 hours
Glargine	4 hours	None (lasts 16–20 hours)

History/PE

Presentation is similar to that of type 1 DM, including polyuria, polydipsia, and polyphagia. However, type 2 DM is typically characterized by an **insidious onset,** so patients may initially present with symptoms of diabetic complications such as blurry vision or recurrent infections. Patients with type 2 DM rarely develop DKA, but with very poor glycemic control, **hyperosmolar nonketotic** coma may occur.

Differential

Same as for type 1 DM. Additionally, blurry vision may be due to primary visual disorders such as glaucoma, cataracts, or macular degeneration.

Evaluation

Same as for type 1 DM.

Treatment

LDL goal for patients with DM is < 100; BP goal is < 130/< 75.

- Diet, weight loss, and exercise.
- Oral agents (monotherapy or combination if uncontrolled):
  - **Metformin:** Inhibits hepatic gluconeogenesis, increases peripheral sensitivity to insulin, and may decrease intestinal absorption of carbohydrates. May cause GI symptoms and, very rarely, lactic acidosis.
  - **Thiazolidinediones** (the "glitazones"): Increase peripheral sensitivity to insulin. The main side effect is edema.
  - **Sulfonylureas** (tolbutamide, glyburide, glipizide): Increase pancreatic secretion of insulin. The main side effects are hypoglycemia and weight gain.
  - **Alpha-glucosidase inhibitors:** Decrease intestinal absorption of carbohydrates. The main side effect is GI upset.
- Insulin (alone or in conjunction with oral agents).
- Statin for hyperlipidemia.
- **Strict BP control.**

COMPLICATIONS OF DIABETES MELLITUS

Table 2.3–4 lists the acute, chronic, and treatment-related complications of DM.

TABLE 2.3–4. Complications of Diabetes Mellitus

Complication	Description
Complications of treatment	
Somogyi effect	Rebound A.M. hyperglycemia in response to early morning (3 A.M.) hypoglycemia, causing release of counterregulatory hormones. Treat by reducing P.M. insulin dose (**reduce insulin to treat**).
Dawn phenomenon	Early-morning hyperglycemia caused by reduced effectiveness of insulin at that time. Treat by increasing P.M. NPH insulin dose.
Acute complications	
DKA	Hyperglycemia-induced crisis that occurs most commonly in **type 1 DM.** Often precipitated by stress, including infections, MI, alcohol, drugs (e.g., corticosteroids, thiazide diuretics), or pancreatitis, or by noncompliance with insulin therapy. Patients often present with **abdominal pain, vomiting, Kussmaul respirations** (rapid, deep breaths), and a **fruity, acetone breath odor.** Patients are severely dehydrated with many electrolyte abnormalities (e.g., hypokalemia, hypophosphatemia, **increased anion gap metabolic acidosis**) and may also develop mental status changes. Treatment includes fluids, potassium, insulin, and treatment of initiating event or underlying disease process.
Hyperosmolar hyperglycemic nonketotic coma (HHNK)	Presents as **profound dehydration,** mental status changes, hyperosmolarity and an extremely high plasma glucose (> 600 mg/dL) without acidosis; occurs most commonly in **type 2 DM,** is precipitated by acute stress (dehydration, infections), and is often fatal. Treatment includes **aggressive fluid and electrolyte replacement** and insulin. Treat initiating event.
Chronic complications	
Retinopathy (non-proliferative, proliferative)	Appears when diabetes has been present for at least **3–5 years.** Preventive measures include control of hyperglycemia and HTN, annual eye exams, and **laser photocoagulation therapy for retinal neovascularization.**
Diabetic nephropathy	Characterized by glomerular hyperfiltration followed by **microalbuminuria.** Preventive measures include **ACE inhibitors** and BP and glucose control.
Neuropathy	Peripheral, symmetric, sensorimotor neuropathy leading to burning pain, foot trauma, infections, and diabetic ulcers. Treat with preventive **foot care** and **analgesics.** Some respond to tricyclic antidepressants or gabapentin. Late complications due to automatic dysfunction include delayed gastric emptying, esophageal dysmotility, impotence, and orthostatic hypotension.
Macrovascular complications	Cardiovascular, cerebrovascular, peripheral vascular disease. Cardiovascular disease is the most common cause of death in diabetic patients. Goal BP is < 130/< 75; lower LDL to < 100 mg/dL; lower triglycerides to < 150 mg/dL. Patients with evidence of macrovascular complications should also be started on low dose ASA.

UCV *IM1.19,26*

Osteoporosis is the most common cause of pathologic fractures in elderly, thin women.

OSTEOPOROSIS

A common metabolic bone disease characterized by osteopenia with normal bone mineralization. Most often affects thin, Caucasian, postmenopausal women. Bone mass peaks at age 30–35 and then progressively declines. **Smoking** and long-term administration of heparin and **glucocorticoids** are associated with an increased risk of osteoporosis.

History/PE

Commonly asymptomatic. Patients may present with **hip fractures, vertebral compression fractures** (resulting in loss of height and progressive thoracic kyphosis), and/or distal radius fractures after minimal trauma.

Differential

Osteomalacia (inadequate bone mineralization), hyperparathyroidism, multiple myeloma, metastatic carcinoma (pathologic fracture).

Evaluation

Lab tests are normal; radiographs show global demineralization after > 30% of bone density is lost. Dual-energy x-ray absorptiometry (DEXA) scanning shows significant osteopenia (bone mineral density < 2.5 standard deviations from normal), most commonly in the vertebral bodies, proximal femur, and distal radius.

Treatment

Prevention is key. The risks of HRT may limit its long-term use for treatment of osteoporosis. **Calcium supplementation** and vitamin D should be taken throughout adulthood to maintain bone density. Smoking cessation and weight-bearing exercises help maintain bone density, while bisphosphonates (alendronate, etidronate), selective estrogen receptor modulators (raloxifene), and intranasal calcitonin can increase bone density.

PARATHYROID GLAND DISORDERS

HYPERPARATHYROIDISM

Occurs in 0.1% of the population. Ninety percent of cases result from a single **adenoma;** 10% result from parathyroid hyperplasia. Parathyroid carcinoma accounts for < 1% of all cases.

History/PE

Seventy percent of cases are **asymptomatic.** Symptoms and signs may include: **stones** (nephrolithiasis or nephrocalcinosis), **bones** (bone pain, muscle aches, arthralgias, fractures [osteitis fibrosa cystica]), abdominal **groans** (PUD, pancreatitis), and **psychiatric overtones** (fatigue, depression, anxiety, irritability, sleep/concentration disturbances).

Signs and symptoms of hyperparathyroidism:
Stones
Bones
Groans
Psychiatric overtones

Differential

Consider all major causes of hypercalcemia (see Renal section).

Evaluation

Hypercalcemia, hypophosphatemia, and hypercalciuria are the hallmarks. PTH is inappropriately elevated relative to ionized calcium. "Brown tumors," may be present.

Treatment

Treat with **parathyroidectomy** if symptomatic; administer bisphosphonates preoperatively. For acute hypercalcemia, give **IV fluids** and **loop diuretics** (once adequately hydrated).

UCV *IM1.22*

PITUITARY GLAND DISORDERS

ACROMEGALY

An adult condition due to a benign pituitary growth hormone adenoma. Children with excess growth hormone production present with **gigantism.**

History/PE

Enlargement of the jaw, hands, and feet; coarsening of facial features (see Figure 2.3–1). May lead to carpal tunnel syndrome, diastolic HTN, and arthritis. **Bitemporal hemianopsia** due to compression of the optic chiasm by a pituitary adenoma. Excess growth hormone may also lead to **glucose intolerance or frank diabetes.**

Evaluation

MRI of the pituitary shows a sellar lesion. Serum growth hormone levels may be elevated, but this finding is unreliable. Screen by measuring insulin-like growth factor I (IGF-I) levels (elevated), and confirm diagnosis with an oral glucose tolerance test (GH levels will remain elevated despite glucose stimulation).

Treatment

Transsphenoidal surgical resection or irradiative ablation of the tumor. Octreotide can be used for symptomatic management of refractory cases.

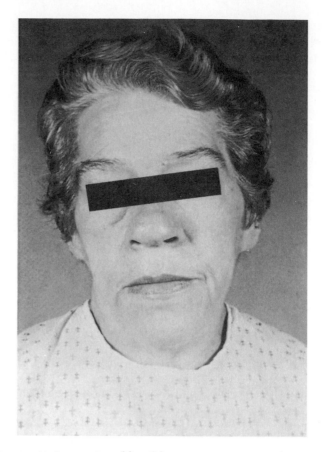

FIGURE 2.3–1. Acromegaly. Coarsening of facial features in a woman with active disease. (Reproduced, with permission, from Stobo JD et al. *The Principles and Practice of Medicine,* 23rd ed. Stamford, CT: Appleton. & Lange, 1996:276, Fig. 4.2–1.)

THYROID DISORDERS

THYROID FUNCTION TESTS

Free T_4 is a better measure of thyroid hormone than total T_4 because it is not affected by changes in TBG.

- **Radioactive iodine uptake and scan:** Determines level of iodine uptake by the thyroid. Very useful in differentiating thyrotoxic states, but not useful in hypothyroidism.
- **Total T_4 measurement:** Not an adequate screening test because results are highly dependent on thyroid-binding globulin (TBG) levels, which fluctuate as a result of a number of factors, including pregnancy and liver disease.
- **T_3 resin uptake (T_3RU):** Used in conjunction with total T_4 or T_3 to correct for changes in TBG levels (e.g., the Free Thyroxine Index: total $T_4 \times T_3RU$). T_3RU is inversely proportional to the number of open binding sites on TBG. If total T_4 is high due to increased TBG (not increased T_4 production), there will be more open binding sites and T_3RU will be low. If total T_4 is high due to increased T_4 production, there will be fewer open binding sites and T_3RU will be high (hyperthyroidism).
- **Free T_4 measurement:** The preferred screening test to directly identify elevation or depletion of thyroid hormone.
- **TSH measurement:** High TSH levels are highly sensitive for hypothyroidism. Low TSH levels are highly sensitive for hyperthyroidism.

HYPOTHYROIDISM

A condition characterized by low levels of thyroid hormone. Most commonly caused by **Hashimoto's thyroiditis;** other causes include subacute or postpartum thyroiditis, drugs (e.g., iodide, amiodarone, sulfonamides, lithium), iatrogenic factors (radioactive thyroid ablation or excision with inadequate supplementation), and pituitary dysfunction (with low TSH). Myxedema refers to severe hypothyroidism with deposition of mucopolysaccharides in the myocardium and dermis. **Cretinism** refers to untreated congenital hypothyroidism leading to cognitive defects and physical abnormalities.

History

Weakness, fatigue, **cold intolerance, constipation,** weight gain, **depression,** menstrual irregularities, and **hoarseness.**

PE

Dry, cold, puffy skin; edema; thin eyebrows; **bradycardia;** and delayed relaxation of DTRs.

Differential

Chronic fatigue, malnutrition, CHF, primary amyloidosis, depression.

Evaluation

Elevated TSH is the most sensitive measure for primary hypothyroidism. Also look for decreased total T_4, **free T_4,** and free T_3. ESR will be elevated in thyroiditis. Antimicrosomal and antithyroglobulin antibodies are seen in patients with Hashimoto's thyroiditis.

Treatment

- **Uncomplicated hypothyroidism** (e.g., Hashimoto's disease): Administer levothyroxine.
- **Subacute thyroiditis:** Usually self-limited; treat with ASA and add cortisol in severe cases.
- **Myxedema coma:** IV levothyroxine and IV hydrocortisone (unless the patient is known to have normal adrenal function prior to the coma).

UCV *IM1.24*

HYPERTHYROIDISM

Graves' disease is the most common etiology of hyperthyroidism. It is most often seen in **women** 20–40 years of age. Other etiologies include toxic nodular goiter, toxic adenomas, and subacute thyroiditis (initial phase). Less common etiologies include pituitary TSH hypersecretion, exogenous iodide (Jod-Basedow phenomenon), struma ovarii, and Hashimoto's thyroiditis.

History

Weight loss and increased appetite as well as **heat intolerance, nervousness,** weakness, **increased bowel frequency,** and menstrual abnormalities.

PE

Warm, moist skin; goiter; sinus **tachycardia** or **atrial fibrillation;** thyroid bruit; fine **tremor;** and hyperactive reflexes. **Exophthalmos** and pretibial myxedema are seen only in Graves' disease (see Figure 2.3–2).

Differential

Anxiety, neurosis, mania, **pheochromocytoma,** malignancy, chronic alcoholism, primary myopathy.

Evaluation

TSH receptor antibodies are seen in patients with Graves' disease.

Suppressed TSH is the most sensitive test for primary hyperthyroidism; also look for elevated total T_4, **free T_4,** and free T4 index. Thyroid stimulating antibodies that compete for the TSH receptor are present in Graves' disease.

Treatment

Administer **propranolol** for catecholamine symptoms and **antithyroid drugs** (methimazole, carbimazole, propylthiouracil [PTU]) for patients with mild thyrotoxicosis or goiter. More severe cases are treated with radioactive ^{131}I thyroid ablation. **Thyroidectomy** is indicated for large goiters or pregnant patients. Patients who have undergone ablation or surgery are given levothyroxine to prevent hypothyroidism.

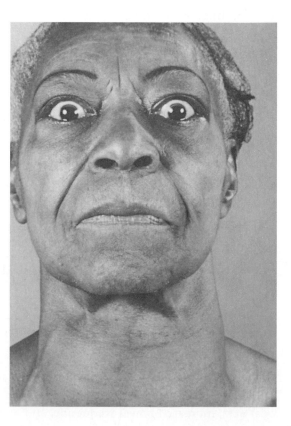

FIGURE 2.3–2. Graves' ophthalmopathy. Proptosis with lid retraction that results from lymphocytic infiltration and edema of the extraocular muscles. May progress to fibrosis with limited eye movement and blindness from optic nerve compression. The patient also demonstrates an impressive goiter. (Reproduced, with permission, from Stobo JD et al. *The Principles and Practice of Medicine,* 23rd ed. Stamford, CT: Appleton & Lange, 1996:276, Fig. 4.2–1.)

Complications

Thyroid storm—extreme hyperthyroidism often precipitated by surgery or infection. Symptoms include high fever, dehydration, tachycardia with **high-output cardiac failure,** and coma. Carries a **25% mortality.** Treatment includes a β-blocker (propranolol), PTU, iodine, and cooling measures.

THYROIDITIS

Thyroiditis is inflammation of the thyroid gland. Table 2.3–5 compares the most common types of thyroiditis.

THYROID NODULES

Thyroid nodules are extremely common and show an increasing incidence with age. The vast majority are benign. There is a higher risk of malignancy in patients with a **history of neck irradiation, "cold" nodules** (on radionuclide scan), firm and fixed solitary nodules, and **rapidly growing nodules** with **hoarseness** or **dysphagia.**

Malignant thyroid nodules are usually cold and solid.

History

Usually **asymptomatic** on initial presentation. To differentiate benign from malignant nodules, note the presence of systemic symptoms (e.g., hypo-/hyperthyroidism), local symptoms (dysphagia, dyspnea/respiratory difficulties, odynophagia, hoarse voice), family history (especially **medullary thyroid cancer**), and history of neck irradiation (for thyroid cancer, hyperthyroidism, or salivary gland tumors).

PE

Carcinoma will likely be palpable, **firm, fixed,** and **nontender.** Check for anterior cervical lymphadenopathy.

TABLE 2.3–5. Subacute vs. Hashimoto's Thyroiditis

	Subacute Thyroiditis	Hashimoto's Thyroiditis
Etiology	Viral (possibly mumps, coxsackievirus).	Autoimmune disorder more commonly affecting women (antithyroid antibodies).
History/PE	Malaise, URI symptoms, and fever early on; hyperthyroidism progressing to hypothyroidism. Tender thyroid.	Painless thyroid enlargement, and hyperthyroidism progressing to hypothyroidism.
Evaluation	Low radioactive iodine uptake scan with high T_4 and T_3 levels.	Antithyroid antibody assay is generally positive; TFTs are usually normal.
Treatment	Symptomatic, as the illness is self-limited.	Exogenous thyroid hormone.

Differential

Lymphocytic thyroiditis, multinodular goiter, colloid nodule, benign follicular adenoma, papillary or follicular carcinoma.

Evaluation/Treatment

- TSH and **TFTs.**
- **U/S** can determine if the nodule is cystic; a radioactive scan can determine if it is cold or hot (cancers are usually cold and solid).
- The best method of assessing a nodule for malignancy is **fine-needle aspiration** (FNA) (high sensitivity and moderate specificity).
- If the FNA is benign, treat with thyroid hormone (suppresses TSH and shrinks nodule) and follow with U/S.
- If malignant, perform **surgical resection.**
- If the distinction between benign and malignant is not clear (this is often a difficult diagnosis), perform a lobectomy and wait for final pathology.
- Medullary thyroid cancer/anaplastic carcinomas are aggressive variants with a poorer prognosis. Medullary thyroid carcinoma is associated with multiple endocrine neoplasia (MEN) IIA and IIB cancer syndromes.
- Look for metastases with radioactive iodine scans.

Questions reproduced, with permission, from Berk SL, *PreTest: Medicine*, 9th ed., New York: McGraw-Hill, 2001, and from Reteguiz J, *PreTest: Physical Diagnosis*, 4th ed., New York: McGraw-Hill, 2001.

Questions

1. A 50-year-old obese female is taking oral hypoglycemic agents. While being treated for an upper respiratory infection, she develops lethargy and is brought to the emergency room. On physical exam, there is no focal neurologic finding or neck rigidity. Laboratory results are as follows:

Na^+	134 mEq/L
K^+	4.0 mEq/L
HCO_3	25 mEq/L
glucose	900 mg/dL
BUN	84 mg/dL
creatinine	3.0 mg/dL
BP	120/80 sitting
BP	105/65 lying

The most likely cause of this patient's coma is
a. Diabetic ketoacidosis
b. Hyperosmolar coma
c. Inappropriate ADH
d. Bacterial meningitis

2. The most important treatment in this patient is
a. Large volumes of fluid, insulin; seek concurrent illnesses
b. Bicarbonate infusion 100 mEq/L
c. Rapid glucose lowering with intravenous insulin
d. 30 mEq/hr of KCl.

3. This 30-year-old female complains of palpitations, fatigue, and insomnia. On physical exam, her extremities are warm and she is tachycardic. There is diffuse thyroid gland enlargement and proptosis. There is an orange thickening of the skin in the pretibial area. Which of the following lab values would you expect in this patient?
a. Increased TSH, total thyroxine, total T_3
b. Decreased TSH, increased total thyroxine
c. Increased T_3 uptake, decreased T_3
d. Normal T_4, decreased TSH

4. The cause of this patient's thyrotoxicosis is
a. Autoimmune disease
b. Benign tumor
c. Malignancy
d. Viral infection of the thyroid

Answers

1. **The answer is b.** This obese patient on oral hypoglycemics has developed hyperglycemia and lethargy during an upper respiratory infection. The patient's serum osmolality is as follows:

$$\frac{900}{18}\text{ (glucose)} + 2\text{ (Na}^+ + \text{K}^+) + \frac{84}{2.8} = 50 + 276 + 30 = 356$$

Hence the serum osmolality is greater than 350 mOsm/kg. The serum bicarbonate is too high to be consistent with diabetic ketoacidosis. The hyponatremia is related to hyperglycemia. SIADH could not be diagnosed in this clinical setting. The patient's diabetes likely went out of control due to infection. There is no clinical evidence for meningitis.

2. **The answer is a.** The primary treatment for hyperosmolar nonketotic states is fluid replacement, usually normal saline. Hypotonic saline may be given for severe hypernatremia or congestive heart failure. Hyperglycemia can be corrected slowly. The patient is not acidotic and would not require bicarbonate treatment (used in severe DKA when pH is less than 7.0). The patient's serum potassium is in the normal range and would not be expected to fall rapidly.

3. **The answer is b.** This patient has clinical symptoms of thyrotoxicosis. Most patients with thyrotoxicosis have increases in total and free concentrations of T_3 and T_4. (Some may have isolated T_3 or T_4 increases.) Most thyrotoxicosis results in suppression of pituitary TSH secretion, so low TSH levels can also confirm the diagnosis.

4. **The answer is a.** This patient has, in addition to thyrotoxicosis, orbitopathy as well as the characteristic dermopathy of Graves' disease, called *pretibial myxedema*. Graves' disease is an autoimmune phenomena. Biopsy of the thyroid shows lymphocytic infiltration. Toxic multinodular goiter produces thyrotoxicosis caused by benign, functionally autonomous tumors. It would not produce the protopsis or dermopathy of Graves' disease. Subacute thyroiditis (de Quervain's) is probably caused by a viral infection. It produces a transient hyperthyroidism followed by hypothyroidism.

Epidemiology and Preventive Medicine

Any process that leads to conclusions that are different from the truth. Researchers should design studies and analyze data in a way that minimizes bias. Sources of bias and the implications of this bias in analyzing results should be discussed.

- **Length bias:** The tendency of a screening test to detect a disproportionate number of slowly progressive diseases and to miss rapidly progressive ones, leading to **overestimation of the benefit of screening.**
- **Lead-time bias: Screening advances the time of diagnosis,** thereby prolonging the period of time between diagnosis and death **without actually prolonging true survival.** Since a disease is identified earlier but its natural course is not altered, survival appears to be greater.
- **Enrollment bias:** Subjects are assigned to a study group in a nonrandom fashion. A classic example is the **assignment of healthier patients to the intervention group** than to the placebo group.
- **Measurement bias:** Information is gathered in a way that distorts the data and, ultimately, the results and conclusions.
- **Observational bias:** Participants' responses to subjective questions may be affected by their awareness of the arm of the study in which they were enrolled. The observer's evaluation of a participant's response to treatment may similarly be affected. A **double-blinded** study can eliminate this source of bias.
- **Recall bias: Errors of memory** that occur in retrospective, case-control studies when patients are asked to recall past events and exposures. People who develop a disease or who have a negative outcome may be more likely to remember risk factors or exaggerate their history of exposures than people who do not have a disease.
- **Self-selection bias:** Patients who choose or do not choose (**nonrespondent bias**) to enroll may yield results that are not representative of the diseased population. For example, patients with a disease that is resistant to conventional treatment may be more likely to enroll in an experimental treatment study.
- **Confounding variables:** Variables that are associated with both the exposure of interest and the disease and that may disrupt the true relationship between these two variables and lead to erroneous conclusions. Can be **controlled for by design** (matching for case control) or by analysis type (multivariate analysis).

Confounding variables may lead to erroneous conclusions about the relationship between an exposure and an outcome.

EVALUATION OF SCREENING TEST PERFORMANCE

SENSITIVITY

The probability that a diseased patient will have a positive test result (true positives divided by the total number of people with the disease; see Figure 2.4–1). The false negative ratio is (1 − sensitivity). A sensitive test is good for **ruling out (SnOUT)** a disease; a test with high sensitivity is a good **screening test.**

SPECIFICITY

The probability that a nondiseased person will have a negative test result (true negatives divided by the total number without the disease; (see Figure

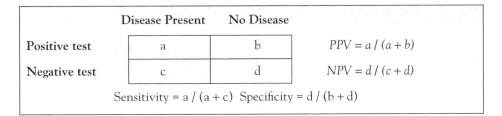

	Disease Present	No Disease	
Positive test	a	b	PPV = a / (a + b)
Negative test	c	d	NPV = d / (c + d)
Sensitivity = a / (a + c) Specificity = d / (b + d)			

FIGURE 2.4–1. Sensitivity, specificity, positive predictive value, and negative predictive value.

2.4–1). The false positive ratio is (1 − specificity). A specific test is good for **ruling in (SpIN)** a disease; a highly specific test is a good **confirmatory test.** For quantitative tests, there is often a **trade-off between sensitivity and specificity.** The ideal test is both sensitive and specific (see Figure 2.4–2), such as serial troponin-I measurements for acute MI.

> **SnOUT: Sen**sitive tests rule **OUT** disease.
>
> **SpIN: Sp**ecific tests rule **IN** disease.

Positive Predictive Value (PPV)

The probability that a patient with a positive test result has the disease (true positives divided by the total number who tested positive). A test will have a higher PPV for diseases with a **high prevalence** (the relative contribution of false positive tests to the total number of positive tests will be smaller).

Negative Predictive Value (NPV)

The probability that a patient with a negative test result is disease free. A test will have a higher NPV for diseases with a **low prevalence** (the relative number of false negative to true negatives will be lower).

Both positive and negative predictive values are affected by the prevalence of the disease.

Incidence and Prevalence

The **incidence** of a disease is the **number of new cases** in a given population that develop over a period of time. The **prevalence** of a disease is the **number of existing cases** at a moment in time.

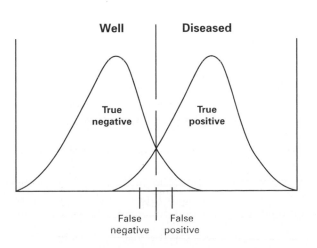

FIGURE 2.4–2. The graphical balance between sensitivity and specificity.

Reliability, or precision, is the reproducibility of results. **Inter-rater reliability** measures the similarity of results when tests are interpreted by different people; **test-retest probability** assesses the similarity when a single person interprets a test repeatedly. **Validity,** or accuracy, measures how well a test measures what it intends to measure. New diagnostic tests are compared to a **gold standard test,** which is considered the most valid and reliable (although typically not the most convenient or safe) test available.

STUDY DESIGNS

CASE-CONTROL STUDY

An observational study, usually **retrospective,** in which cases (with disease) and controls (without disease) are identified. Information collected about past exposure to possible etiologic factors is used to calculate an odds ratio (OR).

- **Advantages:** Studies use small study groups, are inexpensive, focus on **rare diseases,** and examine multiple potential etiologic factors.
- **Limitations:** Data may be inaccurate owing to **recall bias** and **survivorship bias** (those with disease have already died); cannot calculate prevalence, incidence, or relative risk (RR).

COHORT STUDY

An observational study, usually **prospective,** in which a sample group (cohort) is matched to controls also with the presence or absence of a particular risk factor. The groups are **followed to determine if disease develops.**

- **Advantages:** Data are often more accurate than in case-control studies, as they are collected as the exposure occurs (recall bias is not present). Studies can examine the effects of **rare exposures** and multiple outcomes for the same exposure. **RR and incidence** can be determined.
- **Limitations:** Studies require a long time, many subjects, and sometimes significant funds to complete. **Selection bias** and confounding variables may complicate result interpretation (exposure is not randomly distributed); rare diseases cannot be studied (a high prevalence required), and some cases are lost to follow-up.

CROSS-SECTIONAL SURVEY

A survey of the population at **a single point in time.**

- **Advantages:** Can be used to **estimate disease prevalence** and to form hypotheses.
- **Limitations:** Because risk factors and presence of disease are collected simultaneously, causal relationships cannot be established (unlike case-control and cohort studies). Chi-square analyses may estimate these relationships.

Meta-Analysis

A statistical combination of data from several studies (often via a literature search).

- **Advantages:** Can increase the statistical power of a study to allow evaluation of small differences. May resolve controversial issues between conflicting studies in the literature.
- **Limitations:** Cannot overcome limitations of individual studies. One must make sure that the pooled data evaluate similar populations and interventions. Analyses are complicated because errors are introduced when means and variances from different studies are combined.

Randomized Controlled Clinical Trial (RCT)

An experimental, **prospective** study in which subjects are assigned to a treatment or a control group. Studies are usually **randomized** to account for selection bias and to balance prognostic factors. The studies may also be **blinded** (i.e., the patient does not know to which group he is assigned) or **double-blinded** (i.e., neither the patient nor the care provider knows to which group the patient is assigned) to further minimize bias. New therapies should be compared to the accepted standard of care if this standard of care has been shown to be preferable to placebo.

Randomization minimizes for bias and confounding variables; double-blinded studies prevent observation bias.

- **Advantages: Highest-quality** study; can minimize the impact of bias and confounding variables. Can potentially demonstrate a causal relationship.
- **Limitations:** Very costly and time-intensive; informed consent is required; may be difficult to blind some interventions (e.g., education, exercise programs, surgeries). For ethical reasons, may be difficult to compare a new treatment to an accepted treatment.

STUDY ANALYSES

Different analyses are discussed in Table 2.4–1.

TABLE 2.4–1. Descriptions of Study Analyses

Analysis	Analysis Description
Attributable risk (AR)	Used in **prospective, cohort studies,** AR is the absolute difference in incidence rate (IR) of a disease in the exposed versus the unexposed groups: (IR of disease in exposed − IR of disease in unexposed).
Relative risk (RR)	Used in **prospective, cohort studies** to determine the likelihood of developing a disease when exposed to a risk factor, RR is the IR of a disease in a population exposed to a particular factor divided by the IR of those not exposed to the factor (see Figure 2.4–3).
Odds ratio (OR)	Used in **retrospective, case-control studies,** the OR determines the likelihood of exposure to a risk factor in individuals with and without the disease (see Figure 2.4–3). For rare diseases, OR approaches RR.
Number needed to treat (NNT)	The number of people in the general population that must be treated to prevent disease in one patient. Calculated as the inverse of IR.

*A type I (α) error is the
rejection of a true null
hypothesis; a type II (β)
error is the acceptance of a
false null hypothesis.*

*Power ($\beta = [1 - power]$) is
the ability to detect a
significant difference if one
exists and is related to the
number of subjects.*

	Disease Develops	No Disease	
Exposure	a	b	$RR = \dfrac{a\,/\,(a+b)}{c\,/\,(c+d)}$
No exposure	c	d	$OR = ad/bc$

FIGURE 2.4–3. Relative risk and odds ratio.

PUBLIC HEALTH

DISEASE PREVENTION

Disease prevention can be divided into three categories:

- **Primary prevention:** Health-promoting measures to reduce the development (i.e., reduce incidence) of disease.
- **Secondary prevention:** Detection of a disease when asymptomatic or mild.
- **Tertiary prevention:** Reduction of morbidity associated with the presence of a disease.

LEADING CAUSES OF MORTALITY

Table 2.4–2 summarizes the leading causes of mortality in different age groups. Prostate and breast cancer are the most common cancers in men and women, respectively. Lung and colorectal cancers are the second and third most common types in both genders. **Lung cancer is the most common cause of death from cancer in all groups except black women,** for whom death from breast cancer is slightly more common. Since the 1950s, deaths from lung cancer have increased, while deaths from gastric, colorectal, and cervical cancer have decreased.

TABLE 2.4–2. Leading Causes of Death by Age[a]

Age	Most Common Causes of Death
Birth – 18 months	Perinatal conditions, congenital anomalies, injuries, pneumonia.
2–6 years	Injuries, motor vehicle accidents (MVAs), congenital anomalies, cancers, homicide, heart disease.
7–12 years	MVAs, injuries, leukemia, homicide, congenital abnormalities, heart disease.
13–39 years	MVAs, suicide, homicide, injuries, heart disease, HIV.
40–60 years	Heart disease, breast cancer, lung cancer, CVA, COPD.
> 60 years	Heart disease, lung cancer, cerebrovascular disease, COPD, pneumonia, colorectal cancer.

[a]Adapted from the U.S. Preventive Services Task Force, 1996.

Table 2.4–3 summarizes recommended screening measures by age.

TABLE 2.4–3. Health Care Screening[a]	
Age	**Screening Measures**
Birth – 10 years	Height and weight, BP, vision screening, hemoglobinopathy screen (at birth), phenylalanine level (at birth), TSH and/or T_4 (at birth), lead level (at least one time before 6 years old).
11–24 years	Height and weight, BP, Pap smear, chlamydia and gonorrhea (GC) screen (if sexually active), rubella serology or vaccination (women only); screen for risky behaviors, including alcohol abuse.
25–64 years	Height and weight, BP (q 2 years), cholesterol (q 5 years), Pap smear and bimanual pelvic exam, fecal occult blood test (FOBT) and digital rectal exam (DRE), sigmoidoscopy or colonoscopy, breast self-exam (BSE), clinical breast exam, mammography, rubella serology or vaccination (women only); screen for alcohol abuse and depression.
≥ 65 years	Height and weight, BP, FOBT, DRE, sigmoidoscopy or colonoscopy, breast exams continued as above (if reasonable life expectancy), Pap smear, vision and hearing screening; screen for alcohol abuse and depression.

[a]Refer to Table 2.4–4 for specific screening recommendations.

CANCER SCREENING

Table 2.4–4 summarizes recommended cancer screening measures.

TABLE 2.4–4. Recommended Cancer Screening Measures[a]	
Screening Measure	**Screening Recommendations**
Flexible sigmoidoscopy	q 5 years ≥ 50 years; screening ≥ 40 years for high-risk patients.
FOBT	q 1 year ≥ 50 years.
DRE	q 1 year ≥ 50 years.
Prostate examination	q 1 year ≥ 50 years.
Pap smear	q 1 year if sexually active or ≥ 18 years; q 3 years after three normal smears.
Bimanual pelvic exam	q 1–3 years at 20–40 years; q 1 year ≥ 40 years.
Endometrial tissue sampling	Not recommended as screening test; indicated for postmenopausal bleeding.
BSE	q month ≥ 20 years.
Breast exam by clinician	q 1–3 years from 20–40 years; q 1 year ≥ 40 years.
Mammography	q 1–2 years ≥ 40 years; q 1 year ≥ 50 years (controversial).
Skin exam	Self-exam q month; clinical exam q 3 years from 20 to 40 years and q 1 year ≥ 40 years.
CXR	Not recommended as a screening test.

[a]Different medical societies have various recommendations regarding cancer screening. Refer to the National Cancer Institute's Web site for a recent summary of recommendations: *www.nci.nih.gov/cancer_information/testing/*.

CXRs are not effective for lung cancer screening.

Pap smears are an expensive but effective method of decreasing mortality from cervical cancer.

The influenza vaccine is dead and encouraged for pregnant women in their second or third trimester; the measles and varicella vaccines are alive and are contraindicated in pregnancy.

COLORECTAL CANCER SCREENING

- Currently, screening recommendations vary (e.g., sigmoidoscopy +/– FOBT versus colonoscopy +/– FOBT versus combined sigmoidoscopy with barium enema +/– FOBT). Screening of the general population should begin at age 50.
- All polyps identified on endoscopy should be removed entirely and reviewed by pathology.
- Patients with **large or multiple adenomas** on endoscopy should have a follow-up colonoscopy within three years.
- Patients with a **first-degree relative** with a history of colorectal cancer should begin sigmoidoscopy screening at 40 years or 10 years before the earliest diagnosis of cancer.
- Patients with **inflammatory bowel disease of eight years' duration** should consider surveillance with colonoscopy.
- Patients with a family history of **familial adenomatous polyposis (FAP)** should be screened by genetic analysis; if the mutation is present, screening with colonoscopy starting at age 10 is recommended.
- Patients with **FAP** or long-standing **ulcerative colitis** (≥ 10 years) should consider prophylactic colectomy.

INFLUENZA A VACCINE

A trivalent killed virus vaccine recommended for all persons ≥ 65 years old (especially in **chronic care facilities**), pregnant women (second and third trimester), health care workers, and patients with cardiopulmonary disease, diabetes mellitus (DM), hemoglobinopathies, renal dysfunction, or an immune-compromised status.

PNEUMOCOCCAL VACCINE

Recommended for all persons ≥ 65 years old, Native Americans and Alaskans, and patients with cardiopulmonary disease, DM, nephrotic syndrome, cirrhosis, or asplenia (e.g., sickle cell disease). The standard pneumococcal vaccine (PPV23) is not effective in children < 2 years old. A new conjugate vaccine (PPV7) has been approved for these children.

REPORTABLE DISEASES

There are many diseases that must be reported to the CDC, including: HIV, AIDS, syphilis, gonorrhea, chlamydia, measles, mumps, rubella, diphtheria, tetanus, pertussis, viral hepatitis, TB, Lyme disease, cholera, varicella, salmonella, shigella, coccidioidomycosis, and cryptosporidiosis.

POSTMENOPAUSAL RISK FACTOR MODIFICATION

Caucasian women > 50 years old have an increased risk of CAD, hip fractures, breast cancer, and endometrial cancer. The leading causes of death in women 50–75 years old are, in descending order, CAD, cancer, and CVA. HRT is recommended for the reduction of menopausal symptoms, osteoporosis and hip fractures, and, possibly, colorectal cancer and Alzheimer's disease. However, the benefit of HRT in reducing CAD risk is controversial. HRT increases the risk of endometrial cancer (risk is decreased with combined estrogen and progesterone) and thromboembolic disease. A personal history of breast cancer is a contraindication to HRT use.

The following clinical questions and accompanying answers are reproduced, with permission, from Ratelle S, *PreTest: USMLE Step 2: Preventive Medicine and Public Health*, 9th ed., New York: McGraw-Hill, 2001.

Questions

Lou Stewells, a pioneer in the study of diarrheal disease, has developed a new diagnostic test for cholera. When his agent is added to the stool, the organisms develop a characteristic ring around them. (He calls it the "Ring-Around-the-Cholera" [RAC] test.) He performs the test on 100 patients known to have cholera and 100 patients known not to have cholera with the following results:

	Cholera	No Cholera
RAC test +	91	12
RAC test –	9	88
Totals	100	100

1. Which of the following statements is INCORRECT about the RAC test?
   a. The sensitivity of the test was about 91%
   b. The specificity of the test was about 12%
   c. The false negative rate was about 9%
   d. The predictive value of a positive result cannot be determined from the preceding information
   e. The predictive value of a negative result cannot be determined from the preceding information

2. In a study of the cause of lung cancer, patients who had the disease were matched with controls by age, sex, place of residence, and social class. The frequency of cigarette smoking was then compared in the two groups. What type of study was this?
   a. Prospective cohort
   b. Retrospective cohort
   c. Clinical trial
   d. Case-control
   e. Correlation

3. For which patient is pneumococcal vaccine PPV23 not beneficial?
   a. A 15-month-old HIV-infected infant
   b. A 20-year-old about to undergo a splenectomy for ITP
   c. A 70-year-old healthy female
   d. A 5-year-old with sickle cell disease
   e. A 10-year-old with nephrotic syndrome who received the vaccine five years ago

A 53-year-old woman presents to your office with questions about hormonal replacement therapy (HRT). She has been experiencing hot flashes and night sweats. She has not menstruated for one year. She has no risk factors for cardiovascular disease. She is 5'6" and weighs 120 lbs. Her gynecological examination and Pap smear are normal. Her breast examination and mammography are also normal. She wonders about the risks and benefits of HRT given her health status.

4. HRT most increases her risk of developing which of the following conditions?
   a. Hypertension
   b. Thrombosis
   c. Alzheimer's disease
   d. Gallbladder disease
   e. Endometrial cancer

Answers

1. **The answer is b.** Sensitivity and specificity are measures of how often a diagnostic test gives the correct answer. Sensitivity reflects the test's performance in people who have the disease, and specificity measures the test's performance in people who do not have the disease. These definitions can be illustrated as follows:

	Disease Present	**Disease Absent**
Test positive	True positive (TP)	False positive (FP)
Test negative	False negative (FN)	True negative (TN)
	Sensitivity = TP/(TP + FN)	Specificity = TN/(TN + FP)

Among people who have the disease, there are two possibilities: either the test correctly identifies them (TP), or it falsely classifies them as negative (FN). Thus, among those with disease, sensitivity measures how often the test gives the right answer. (A good way to remember sensitivity is by the initials PID: positive in disease.) Similarly, among people who do not have the disease, there are also two possibilities: either the test will correctly identify them as not having disease (TN), or it will falsely classify them as diseased (FP). Thus, specificity measures how often the test gives the right answer among those who do not have the disease. (A good way to remember specificity is by the initials NIH: negative in health.)

As opposed to sensitivity and specificity, which measure the test's performance in groups of patients who do and do not have the disease, predictive value measures how often the test is right in patients grouped another way: by whether the test result is positive or negative. Thus, predictive value of a positive test is the proportion of positive tests that are true positives [TP/(TP + FP)], and predictive value of a negative result is the proportion of negative test results that are true negatives [TN/(TN + FN)].

But predictive value is a little tricky because it also depends on the prevalence of the disease in the population tested. In this case, Dr. Stewells assembled groups of 100 patients with and without cholera, and the prevalence is not given. Therefore, predictive value cannot be calculated in this question, and the correct answer is B, since specificity is 88%, not 12%.

2. **The answer is d.** The study described was a case-control study. In this type of study, people who have a disease (cases) are compared with people whom they closely resemble except for the presence of the disease under study (controls). Cases and controls are then studied for the frequency of exposure to a suspected risk factor. In case-control studies, the validity of inferences about the causal relationship between the exposure (cigarette smoking) and the disease (lung cancer) depends on how comparable the cases and controls are for all variables that may be related to both the risk factor and disease under study (e.g., age, sex, race, place of residence, and occupation). Matching is a method to control for confounding in case-control studies to eliminate the effect of any extraneous variable that is not under study but may have an effect on the results. In clinical trials, or experimental/intervention studies, the investigators allocate the exposure. Correlation studies are used to compare disease frequencies between entire populations (as opposed to individuals). For example, a correlation study could examine the consumption of animal fat and the rates of colon cancer among 20 different countries.

3. **The answer is a.** Pneumococcal vaccine PPV23 is not effective in children < 2 years of age. A heptavalent pneumococcal conjugate vaccine PPV7 can be used for children 23 months and younger. PPV7 is now recommended for universal use for all children under 23 months, including those at high risk (which includes HIV infection). Other indications for pneumococcal vaccine include persons over the age of 65 and those with anatomical or functional asplenia, nephrotic syndrome, sickle cell disease, chronic heart and lung disease, cirrhosis of the liver, and diabetes. As this is a rapidly evolving field and includes more complicated regimens for children, consultation with local health departments should be made for the latest recommendations for immunization series and boosters.

4. **The answer is e.** Menopause is associated with substantial rises in total and LDL cholesterol. Some studies have suggested that HRT appears to decrease the incidence of Alzheimer's disease. HRT has no effect on gallbladder disease and hypertension. Unopposed estrogen therapy particularly increases the risk of endometrial cancer. Adding progesterone to the regimen significantly reduces this risk, but does not eliminate it. Thin, white women are particularly at risk of osteoporosis. HRT may increase the risk of developing breast cancer and may slightly increase the risk of deep venous thrombosis (DVT). On a population basis, the benefits of HRT (reduction in cardiovascular diseases and osteoporosis) are of greater magnitude than the risks (DVT, endometrial, and breast cancer). On an individual basis, risks and benefits should be assessed based on risk profile.

Ethics and Legal Issues

GENERAL PRINCIPLES

- **Autonomy:** Clinicians are obligated to respect patients as individuals and to honor their preferences in medical care (Psych.32).
- **Beneficence:** Physicians have a responsibility to act in the patient's best interest ("physician is a fiduciary"). Patient autonomy may conflict with beneficence. If the patient makes an informed decision, he/she has the ultimate right to decide.
- **Nonmaleficence:** "Do no harm." However, if the benefits of an intervention outweigh the risks, a patient may make an informed decision to proceed.

DISCLOSURE

Patients have a right to know about their medical status, prognosis, and treatment options (full disclosure). **Physicians are obligated to inform patients of mistakes made in their medical treatment.** A patient's family cannot require that a doctor withhold information from the patient. A doctor may withhold information only if the patient requests not to be told or in the rare case when a physician determines that disclosure would severely harm the patient or undermine informed decision-making capacity **(therapeutic privilege).**

CONFIDENTIALITY

When in doubt, always maintain patient confidentiality.

Information disclosed by a patient to his/her physician and information about a patient's medical condition is confidential and cannot be divulged without express patient consent. However, a patient may waive the right to confidentiality (e.g., with insurance companies). In addition, it is ethically and legally necessary to override confidentiality in the following situations:

- Patient intent to commit a violent crime. The **Tarasoff decision** set a precedent that if a patient presents a **serious, credible danger of violence** to a third party, physicians have a **duty to protect** the intended victim through reasonable means (e.g., warn victim, notify police) (Psych.34).
- Suicidal patients.
- Child and elder abuse.
- Infectious diseases (duty to warn public officials and identifiable people at risk).
- Gunshot and knife wounds.
- Impaired automobile drivers.

UCV Psych.33

INFORMED CONSENT

Defined by willing acceptance (without coercion) of a medical intervention by a patient after adequate discussion with a physician about the **nature** of the intervention, **indications, risks, benefits,** and potential **alternatives** (including no treatment). **Patients may change their minds at any time.** Exceptions include:

- **Consent is implied** when emergency treatment is required.
- Consent can be obtained from a surrogate decision maker when patients lack decision-making capacity.
- Patients who sign waivers to the right of informed consent.

COMPETENCE AND DECISION-MAKING CAPACITY

Competence is a legal term referring to a patient's **authority to make personal and medical choices. Decision-making capacity** is a medical term referring to a patient's **capacity to accept or refuse treatment.** It is determined by a medical provider and is defined as the ability to understand relevant information, appreciate the medical situation and its consequences, communicate a choice, and deliberate rationally about one's values in relation to the decision.

REFUSAL OF TREATMENT

All competent patients have the right to refuse or discontinue treatment as long as this will not harm other parties (e.g., Jehovah's Witnesses can refuse blood products). An incompetent or decisionally incapacitated patient (e.g., an intoxicated patient with altered mental status) cannot refuse treatment.

Incompetent people cannot refuse treatment.

MINORS

- **Consent for treatment:** Consent is implied in life-threatening situations when parents cannot be contacted. Emancipated minors (e.g., those who are living independently of parents, married, or in the armed services) and minors requesting care for pregnancy *(Psych.30)*, STDs, and drug/alcohol abuse do not require parental consent. Even if a parent requests information, confidentiality can be broken only with the patient's permission or if the minor is a danger to him/herself or others.
- **Refusal of treatment:** A parent has the right to make treatment decisions for his/her child as long as those decisions do not pose a serious threat to the child's well-being (e.g., refusing immunizations). If a decision is not in the best interest of the child, a physician may seek a court order to provide treatment against parental wishes. In emergent situations, if withholding treatment jeopardizes the child's safety, treatment can be initiated on the basis of legal precedent.

Parental consent is not required if minors request treatment for pregnancy, STDs, or substance abuse.

END-OF-LIFE ISSUES

WRITTEN ADVANCE DIRECTIVES

- **Living will:** Addresses a patient's wishes to withhold or withdraw life sustaining treatment in the event of terminal disease or a persistent vegetative state. Examples include **DNR** (do not resuscitate) and **DNI**

DNR/DNI orders do not mean "do not treat."

(do not intubate) orders. Patients should still receive maximum medical intervention short of these specific procedures.

- **Durable power of attorney (DPOA):** Legally designates a **surrogate** health care decision maker if a patient becomes decisionally incapacitated. This is **more flexible** than a living will. Surrogates should make decisions consistent with the person's stated wishes. If no living will or DPOA exists, decisions should be made by close family members (spouse, adult children, parents, and adult siblings), friends, or personal physicians, in that order.

UCV *Psych.29*

It is ethical to provide palliative treatment even though it may hasten a patient's death.

WITHDRAWAL OF CARE

Patients and their decision makers have the right to forgo life-sustaining treatment. There is **no ethical distinction between withholding and withdrawing life-sustaining interventions.** This includes ventilation, fluids, nutrition, and medications (e.g., antibiotics). It is ethical to provide palliative treatment to relieve pain and suffering even if it may hasten a patient's death.

UCV *Psych.35*

EUTHANASIA AND PHYSICIAN-ASSISTED SUICIDE

Euthanasia is the administration of a lethal agent with the intent to relieve suffering. It is opposed by the AMA Code of Medical Ethics and **is illegal.** Patients who request euthanasia should be evaluated for inadequate pain control and comorbid depression. **Physician-assisted suicide** is prescribing a lethal agent to a patient who will self-administer it to end his/her own life. This is currently legal only in the state of Oregon.

FUTILITY

Physicians are not ethically obligated to provide treatment and may **refuse** a family's request for further intervention on the grounds of futility when:

- There is no pathophysiological rationale for treatment.
- Maximal intervention is currently failing.
- A given intervention has already failed.
- Treatment will not achieve the goals of care.

CONFLICT OF INTEREST

Occurs when physicians find themselves having two interests in a given situation. For example, a physician may own stock in a pharmaceutical company (financial interest) that produces a drug he is prescribing to his patient (patient care interest). Patients, research participants, supporting institutions, and readers (i.e., of journal articles and books) have the right to know about any existing conflicts of interest.

The essential elements of a civil suit under negligence include the **four D's:**

1. The physician has a **D**uty to the patient.
2. **D**ereliction of duty occurs.
3. There is **D**amage to the patient.
4. **D**ereliction is the **D**irect cause of damage.

Unlike a criminal suit, in which the burden of proof is "beyond a reasonable doubt," the burden of proof in a malpractice suit is "more likely than not."

The 4 D's of Malpractice

Duty
Dereliction
Damage
Direct cause

HIGH-YIELD FACTS

Ethics

Gastrointestinal

Portal-systemic anastomoses

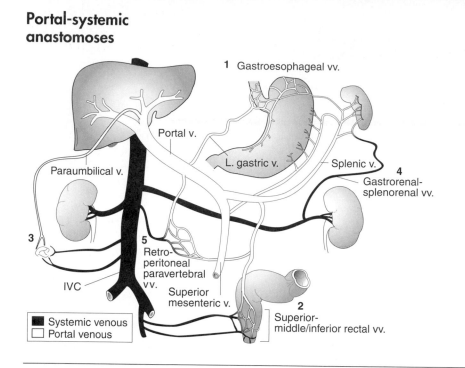

1. Gastroesophageal vv.

Portal v.

Paraumbilical v.

L. gastric v.

Splenic v.

4

Gastrorenal-splenorenal vv.

3

5

Retro-peritoneal paravertebral vv.

IVC

Superior mesenteric v.

2

Superior-middle/inferior rectal vv.

■ Systemic venous
□ Portal venous

1. Left gastric–azygos → **esophageal varices.**
2. Superior–middle/inferior rectal → **hemorrhoids.**
3. Paraumbilical–inferior epigastric → **caput medusae** (navel).
4. Retroperitoneal → renal.
5. Retroperitoneal → paravertebral.

Gut, butt, and caput, the 3 anastomoses. Commonly seen in alcoholic cirrhosis.

GI blood supply

Artery	Gut region	Structures supplied
Celiac	Foregut	Stomach to duodenum; liver, gallbladder, pancreas
SMA	Midgut	Duodenum to proximal $^2/_3$ of transverse colon
IMA	Hindgut	Distal $^1/_3$ of transverse colon to upper portion of rectum

Heart

Esophageal regions

Gastric and duodenal regions

Celiac artery

Primordium of liver

Superior mesenteric artery to midgut

Hindgut

Inferior mesenteric artery

HIGH-YIELD FACTS

Gastrointestinal

Cirrhosis/ portal hypertension

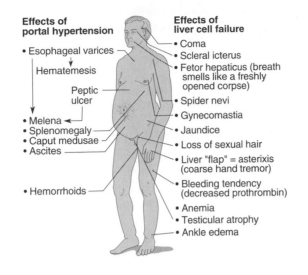

Effects of portal hypertension

- Esophageal varices
  - ↓ Hematemesis
- Peptic ulcer
- Melena ←
- Splenomegaly
- Caput medusae
- Ascites

- Hemorrhoids

Effects of liver cell failure

- Coma
- Scleral icterus
- Fetor hepaticus (breath smells like a freshly opened corpse)
- Spider nevi
- Gynecomastia
- Jaundice
- Loss of sexual hair
- Liver "flap" = asterixis (coarse hand tremor)
- Bleeding tendency (decreased prothrombin)
- Anemia
- Testicular atrophy
- Ankle edema

(Adapted, with permission, from Chandrasoma P, Taylor CE. *Concise Pathology*, 3rd ed. Stamford, CT: Appleton and Lange, 1998:654.)

Cirrho (Greek) = tawny yellow. Diffuse fibrosis of liver, destroys normal architecture.
Nodular regeneration.
Micronodular—nodules < 3 mm, uniform size. Due to metabolic insult (e.g., alcohol).
Macronodular—nodules > 3 mm, varied size. Usually due to significant liver injury leading to hepatic necrosis (e.g., postinfectious or drug-induced hepatitis).
↑ risk of hepatocellular carcinoma.

Common serologic patterns in hepatitis B virus infection

HBsAg	Anti-HBs	Anti-HBc	HBeAg	Anti-HBe	Interpretation
+	−	IgM	+	−	Acute hepatitis B
−	−	IgM	+ / −	−	Acute hepatitis B, window period
+	−	IgG	+	−	Chronic hepatitis B with active viral replication
+	−	IgG	−	+	Chronic hepatitis B with low viral replication
+	+	IgG	+ / −	+ / −	Chronic hepatitis B with heterotypic anti-HBs (10% of cases)
−	+	IgG	−	+ / −	Recovery from hepatitis B (immunity)
−	+	−	−	−	Vaccination (immunity)

Hepatocellular carcinoma

Also called hepatoma. Most common 1° malignant tumor of the liver in adults. ↑ incidence of hepatocellular carcinoma is associated with hepatitis B and C, Wilson's disease, hemochromatosis, α_1-antitrypsin deficiency, alcoholic cirrhosis, and carcinogens (e.g., aflatoxin B1).

Hepatocellular carcinoma, like renal cell carcinoma, is commonly spread by hematogenous dissemination.
Elevated AFP.

Gallstones

Form when solubilizing bile acids and lecithin are overwhelmed by ↑ cholesterol and/or bilirubin.
Three types of stones:
1. Cholesterol stones (radiolucent with 10–20% opaque due to calcifications)—associated with obesity, Crohn's disease, cystic fibrosis, advanced age, clofibrate, estrogens, multiparity, rapid weight loss, and Native American origin.
2. Mixed stones (radiolucent)—have both cholesterol and pigment components. Most common type.
3. Pigment stones (radiopaque)—seen in patients with chronic RBC hemolysis, alcoholic cirrhosis, advanced age, and biliary infection.

Diagnose with ultrasound. Treat with cholecystectomy.

Risk factors (5 F's):
1. Female
2. Fat
3. Fertile
4. Forty
5. Flatulent

May present with Charcot's triad of epigastric/RUQ pain, fever, jaundice.

Cystic duct
Hepatic duct
Stone in the common bile duct
Fibrosed gallbladder with gallstones
Pancreatic duct

Pancreatic adenocarcinoma

Prognosis averages 6 months or less; very aggressive; usually already metastasized at presentation; tumors more common in pancreatic head (obstructive jaundice).
Often presents with:
1. Abdominal pain radiating to back
2. Weight loss
3. Anorexia
4. Migratory thrombophlebitis (Trousseau's syndrome)
5. Pancreatic duct obstruction (malabsorption with palpable gallbladder)

H₂ blockers
Mechanism
Clinical use
Toxicity

Cimetidine, ranitidine, famotidine, nizatidine.
Reversible block of histamine H_2 receptors.
Peptic ulcer, gastritis, esophageal reflux, Zollinger-Ellison syndrome.
Cimetidine is a potent inhibitor of P450; it also has an antiandrogenic effect and ↓ renal excretion of creatinine. Other H_2 blockers are relatively free of these effects.

Proton pump inhibitors (PPIs)
Mechanism
Clinical use

Omeprazole, lansoprazole
Irreversibly inhibits H^+/K^+ ATPase in stomach parietal cells.
Peptic ulcer, gastritis, esophageal reflux, Zollinger-Ellison syndrome.

CHOLELITHIASIS AND BILIARY COLIC

Colic results from transient cystic duct blockage from impacted stones. Risk factors include the **5 F's: F**emale, **F**at, **F**ertile, **F**orty, and **F**latulent—although the disorder is common and can occur in any patient. Other risk factors include OCP use, rapid weight loss, family history, chronic hemolysis (pigment stones), small bowel resection, and TPN.

Pigmented gallstones result from hemolysis.

History/PE

Patients present with **postprandial abdominal pain** (usually in the **RUQ**) that radiates to the right subscapular area or epigastrium. Pain is abrupt, is followed by gradual relief, and is often associated with **nausea and vomiting,** fatty food intolerance, dyspepsia, and flatulence. Gallstones may be asymptomatic in up to 80% of patients. Exam may reveal RUQ tenderness and a palpable gallbladder.

Differential

Acute cholecystitis, PUD, MI, acute pancreatitis, GERD, hepatitis, appendicitis, irritable bowel syndrome (IBS).

Evaluation

Plain x-rays are rarely diagnostic, as only 10–15% of stones are radiopaque. **RUQ U/S** may show gallstones (95% sensitive). Consider an upper GI series to rule out a hiatal hernia or ulcer.

Only 10–15% of gallstones are radiopaque.

Treatment

Cholecystectomy is both definitive and curative and can be performed on an elective basis. Patients may require preoperative ERCP for common bile duct stones. For patients who are not surgical candidates, treat with **dietary modification** (avoid triggering substances such as fatty foods). **Bile salt dissolution** with or without **lithotripsy** is an experimental treatment.

Complications

Recurrent biliary colic, acute cholecystitis, choledocholithiasis, acute cholangitis, gallstone ileus, gallstone pancreatitis.

UCV *Surg. 24*

ACUTE CHOLECYSTITIS

Prolonged blockage of the cystic duct, usually by an impacted stone, resulting in postobstructive distention, inflammation, superinfection, and, in extreme cases, gangrene of the gallbladder (acute gangrenous cholecystitis). In chronically debilitated patients, those on TPN, and trauma or burn victims, acute cholecystitis may occur in the absence of cholelithiasis (**acalculous cholecystitis**).

History/PE

Patients present with **RUQ pain, nausea, low-grade fever, and vomiting** similar to that seen in biliary colic, but typically more severe and of longer duration. RUQ tenderness, inspiratory arrest during deep palpation of the RUQ **(Murphy's sign),** low-grade fever, leukocytosis, mild icterus, and possibly guarding or rebound tenderness may be present on examination.

Differential

Biliary colic, acute cholangitis, GERD, hepatitis, acute pancreatitis, MI, acute appendicitis, renal colic, Fitz-Hugh–Curtis syndrome (acute perihepatitis), PUD, pneumonia.

Evaluation

CBC, amylase, lipase, LFTs, and bilirubin (possibly elevated) should be obtained. U/S may demonstrate stones, bile sludge, pericholecystic fluid, a thickened gallbladder wall, gas in the gallbladder, and an ultrasonic Murphy's sign (see Figure 2.6–1). Obtain a **HIDA scan** when U/S is equivocal (see Figure 2.6–2); absence of the gallbladder on HIDA scan suggests acute cholecystitis.

Treatment

In patients with significant medical problems (including DM), delay cholecystectomy until acute inflammation resolves.

Hospitalize patients, administer **IV antibiotics** and **IV fluids,** and replete electrolytes. Perform **early cholecystectomy** (within 72 hours of onset of symptoms) along with either a preoperative ERCP or an **intraoperative cholangiogram** to rule out common bile duct stones in patients without significant operative risk factors. Since 50% of cases resolve spontaneously, hemodynamically stable patients with significant medical problems (e.g., diabetes mellitus [DM]) can be initially treated medically with a four- to six-week delay in surgical treatment.

Complications

Gangrene, empyema, perforation, gallstone ileus, fistulization, sepsis, abscess formation.

UCV *Surg.17*

CHOLEDOCHOLITHIASIS

Gallstones in the common bile duct. Although it is sometimes asymptomatic, presenting symptoms often include biliary pain, jaundice, episodic colic, and pancreatitis. Symptoms vary according to the degree of obstruction, the duration of the obstruction, and the extent of bacterial infection. Choledocholithiasis should be considered in patients with a history of fever, jaundice, and biliary colic. Its hallmark is **elevated alkaline phosphatase** and **total bilirubin,** which may be the only abnormal lab values. Management generally consists of operative stone removal by common bile duct exploration or ERCP with sphincterotomy.

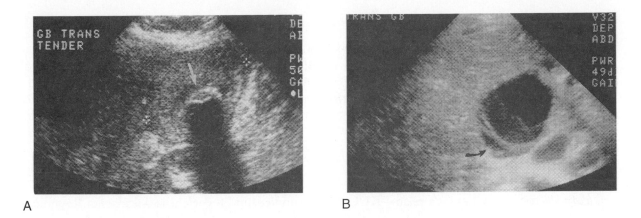

A

B

FIGURE 2.6–1. Acute cholecystitis, U/S. (A) Note the sludge-filled, thick-walled gallbladder with a hyperechoic stone and acoustic shadow (arrow). (B) This patient exhibits sludge and pericholecystic fluid (arrow) but no gallstones. (Reproduced, with permission, from Grendell J. *Current Diagnosis and Treatment in Gastroenterology,* 1st ed. Stamford, CT: Appleton & Lange, 1996:212, Fig. 15–14A and B.)

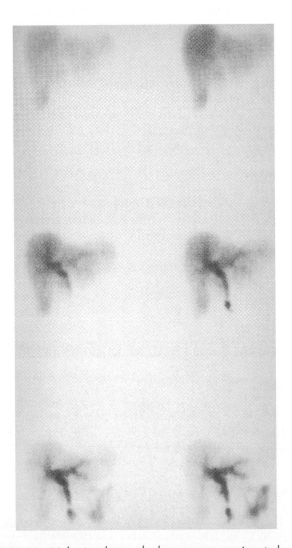

FIGURE 2.6–2. Acute cholecystitis, HIDA scan. IV dye is taken up by hepatocytes, conjugated, and excreted into the common bile duct. The gallbladder is not visualized, although activity is present in the liver, common duct, and small bowel, suggesting cystic duct obstruction due to acute cholecystitis. (Reproduced, with permission, from Grendell J. *Current Diagnosis and Treatment in Gastroenterology,* 1st ed. Stamford, CT: Appleton & Lange, 1996:217, Fig. 15–18.)

ACUTE CHOLANGITIS

An acute bacterial infection of the biliary tree that commonly occurs secondary to **obstruction,** usually from **gallstones (choledocholithiasis)** or primary sclerosing cholangitis (progressive inflammation of the biliary tree associated with ulcerative colitis). Other risk factors include bile duct stricture, ampullary carcinoma, and pancreatic pseudocyst. Gram-negative enterics (e.g., *Escherichia coli, Enterobacter, Pseudomonas*) are the commonly identified pathogens.

History/PE

Charcot's triad = RUQ pain, jaundice, and fever/chills.

Reynold's pentad = RUQ pain, jaundice, fever/chills, shock, and altered mental status.

Charcot's triad—**RUQ pain, jaundice,** and **fever/chills**—is classic. **Reynold's pentad**—Charcot's triad plus **shock** and **altered mental status**—may be present in acute suppurative cholangitis.

Differential

Pancreatic cancer, cholangiocarcinoma, metastatic carcinoma, hepatitis, primary biliary cirrhosis, acute cholecystitis, pancreatitis, sepsis, liver abscess.

Evaluation

Look for **leukocytosis, increased bilirubin,** and **increased alkaline phosphatase.** Obtain blood cultures to rule out sepsis, **U/S** or **CT** may be a useful adjunct, but diagnosis is often clinical. **ERCP** is both diagnostic and therapeutic (biliary drainage).

Treatment

This is a serious, life-threatening disease, and the diagnosis must not be missed. Patients often require **ICU admission** for monitoring, hydration, pressor support, and aggressive **IV antibiotic treatment.** Patients with acute suppurative cholangitis require **emergent bile duct decompression** via ERCP sphincterotomy, percutaneous transhepatic drainage, or open decompression.

UCV *EM.13*

DISORDERS OF THE SMALL BOWEL

DIARRHEA

Production of **> 200 g of feces per day.** Risk factors include viral/bacterial gastrointestinal infection, systemic infection, sick contacts, immunosuppression, and recent travel.

History/PE

Acute diarrhea is generally infectious and self-limited.

- **Acute diarrhea:** Acute onset with < 3 weeks of symptoms; usually infectious and self-limited. Causes include *E. coli, Salmonella, Shigella, Staphylococcus aureus, Campylobacter,* cholera, *Giardia,* postantibiotic pseudomembranous colitis (*Clostridium difficile*), and HIV-related dis-

TABLE 2.6–1. Causes of Infectious Diarrhea

Infectious Agent	History	PE	Comments
Campylobacter	**Most common etiology of infectious diarrhea.** Ingestion of contaminated food or water. Affects young children and young adults. Generally lasts 7–10 days.	Fecal RBCs and WBCs.	Rule out appendicitis and inflammatory bowel disease (IBD).
C. difficile	Recent treatment with antibiotics (cephalosporins, **clindamycin**). Affects hospitalized adult patients. **Watch for toxic megacolon.**	Fever, abdominal pain, possible systemic toxicity. Fecal RBCs and WBCs.	Most commonly in the large bowel, but can involve the small bowel. Identify *C. difficile* toxin in the stool. Avoid antimotility agents.
Entamoeba histolytica	Ingestion of contaminated food or water, history of travel in developing countries. Incubation period can last up to three months.	Severe abdominal pain, fever. Fecal RBCs and WBCs.	Chronic amebic colitis mimics IBD. Steroids can cause fatal perforation.
E. coli 0157:H7	Ingestion of contaminated food (raw meat). Affects children and the elderly. Generally lasts 5–10 days.	Severe abdominal pain, low-grade fever, vomiting. Fecal RBCs and WBCs.	Important to rule out GI bleed and ischemic colitis. Treatment is supportive; **avoid antibiotics.**
Salmonella	Ingestion of contaminated poultry or eggs. Affects young children and elderly patients. Generally lasts 2–5 days.	Prodromal headache, fever, myalgia, abdominal pain. Fecal WBCs.	Sepsis is a concern as 5–10% of patients become bacteremic; sepsis is a concern.
Shigella	Extremely contagious; transmitted between people by fecal-oral route. Affects young children and institutionalized patients.	Fecal RBCs and WBCs.	May cause severe dehydration. Can lead to febrile seizures in the very young.

eases (*Cryptosporidium, Isospora*). Table 2.6–1 summarizes the presentation of common infectious diarrheas.

- **Chronic diarrhea:** Insidious onset with > 6 weeks of symptoms; usually due to disrupted secretion (e.g., carcinoid, VIPomas), absorption (e.g., lactose intolerance, celiac sprue, bacterial overgrowth, IBD), or motility.
- **Pediatric diarrhea:** Most commonly due to **rotavirus infection (winter),** but can also be due to any adult causes.

HIGH-YIELD FACTS

Gastrointestinal

Evaluation

Acute diarrhea usually does not require laboratory investigation unless the patient has a high fever, bloody diarrhea, or diarrhea lasting > 4–5 days. Send stool for fecal leukocytes, bacterial culture, *C. difficile* toxin, and ova and parasites (O&P). Consider sigmoidoscopy in patients with bloody diarrhea. See Figure 2.6–3 for the evaluation of chronic diarrhea.

Treatment

Avoid antimotility agents in patients with bloody diarrhea, high fever, or systemic toxicity.

- **Acute diarrhea:** Treat symptomatically with antidiarrheals (e.g., loperamide, bismuth salicylate) and oral **fluids** with electrolyte replacement. If the patient has evidence of systemic infection (e.g., fever, chills, malaise), avoid antimobility agents and start antibiotics after stool studies have been sent.
- **Chronic diarrhea:** Identify the underlying cause and treat symptomatically with loperamide, opioids, clonidine, octreotide, or cholestyramine.
- **Pediatric diarrhea:** For a child who cannot take medication or PO fluids, hospitalize, give IV fluids, and treat the underlying cause.

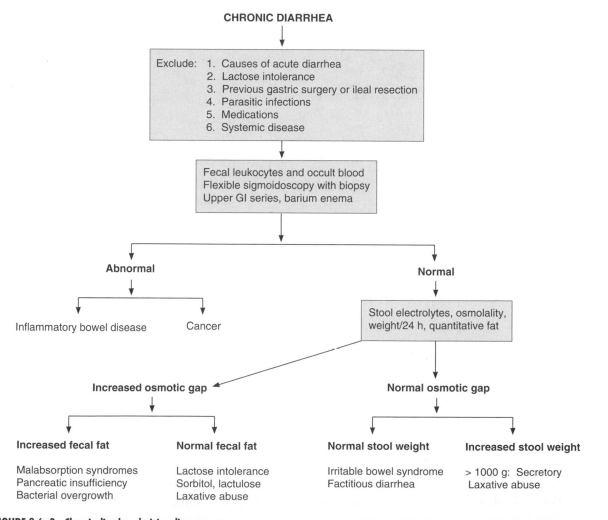

FIGURE 2.6–3. Chronic diarrhea decision diagram. (Reproduced, with permission, from Tierney LM. *Current Medical Diagnosis & Treatment,* 39th ed. New York: McGraw-Hill, 2000:566, Fig. 14–1.)

IRRITABLE BOWEL SYNDROME

An idiopathic **functional disorder** characterized by abdominal pain and changes in bowel habits that increase with stress and are **relieved by bowel movements.** Most common in the second and third decades, but since this syndrome is chronic, patients may present at any age. Half of all patients with this condition who seek medical care have **comorbid psychiatric disorders** (e.g., depression, anxiety).

Half of all patients with IBS have comorbid psychiatric disturbances.

History/PE

Patients present with **abdominal pain,** a change in bowel habits **(diarrhea and/or constipation),** abdominal distention, stools with mucus, and **relief of pain with a bowel movement.** IBS rarely awakens patients from sleep: vomiting, significant weight loss, and constitutional symptoms are also uncommon. Exam is usually **unremarkable** except for mild abdominal tenderness.

Differential

Crohn's disease, ulcerative colitis, mesenteric ischemia, diverticulitis, PUD, colonic neoplasia, infectious/pseudomembranous colitis, gynecologic disorders.

Evaluation

IBS is a **diagnosis of exclusion** based on clinical history and evaluation. Tests to rule out other GI causes include CBC and electrolytes, stool cultures, abdominal films, and barium contrast studies. Manometry can assess sphincter function.

IBS is a diagnosis of exclusion.

Treatment

- **Psychological:** Patients need **assurance** from their physicians. Patients should not be told that their symptoms are "all in their head."
- **Dietary: Fiber supplements** (psyllium) may help.
- **Pharmacologic:** Treat with tricyclics, **antidiarrheals** (loperamide), **antispasmodics** (dicyclomine, anticholinergics), alosetron (for diarrheal type) as needed.

UCV *IM1.37*

SMALL BOWEL OBSTRUCTION (SBO)

Blocked passage of bowel contents through the small bowel. Fluid and gas can build up proximal to the obstruction, resulting in fluid and electrolyte imbalances and significant abdominal discomfort. The obstruction can be complete or partial and may be very dangerous if strangulation of the bowel occurs. SBO may arise from adhesions from a prior abdominal surgery (60% of cases), hernias (10–20%), neoplasms (10–20%), intussusception, gallstone ileus, stricture due to IBD, volvulus, and cystic fibrosis (CF).

#1 cause of SBO in adults = adhesions.

#1 cause of SBO in children = hernias.

History/PE

Patients typically experience cramping abdominal pain with a recurrent **crescendo-decrescendo pattern** at 5- to 10-minute intervals. Early emesis is nonfeculent if the obstruction is proximal; vomiting typically follows the pain and is **feculent** in nature in distal obstruction. In partial obstruction there is continued passage of flatus but no stool, whereas in complete obstruction no flatus or stool is passed **(obstipation).** Abdominal exam often reveals distention, tenderness, prior surgical scars, or hernias. Rebound tenderness suggests more advanced disease. Bowel sounds are characterized by **high-pitched tinkles** and **peristaltic rushes.** Later in the disease, peristalsis may disappear. Fever, hypotension, and tachycardia are not uncommon and suggest a surgical emergency.

Differential

- **Acute appendicitis:** This should **always** be near the top of your differential for an acute abdomen.
- **Adynamic ileus:** Postoperative ileus after abdominal surgery, hypokalemia, anesthesia, pain medications.
- **Large bowel obstruction (LBO):** Colorectal cancer, diverticulitis, and sigmoid volvulus.
- Less commonly: IBD, mesenteric ischemia, renal colic/pyelonephritis.

Evaluation

Never let the sun rise or set on a complete SBO.

CBC may demonstrate leukocytosis if there is strangulation of bowel. Chemistries often reflect dehydration and metabolic alkalosis due to vomiting. The presence of acidosis is particularly worrisome, as it suggests necrotic bowel and an emergent need for surgical intervention. Abdominal films often demonstrate a **stepladder pattern** of **dilated small-bowel loops** and **air-fluid levels** (see Figure 2.6–4) and a paucity of gas in the colon. The presence of radiopaque material at the cecum is suggestive of gallstone ileus.

Treatment

For a partial obstruction, supportive care may be sufficient and should include NPO status, NG suction, IV hydration, correction of electrolyte abnormalities, and Foley catheterization to monitor fluid status. Surgery is required in cases of complete SBO, vascular compromise (i.e., necrotic bowel), or symptoms lasting > 3 days without resolution. Exploratory laparotomy may be performed with lysis of adhesions, resection of necrotic bowel, and evaluation for stricture, IBD, and hernias. There is a 2% mortality risk for a nonstrangulated SBO and, depending on the time between diagnosis and treatment; strangulated SBO carries up to a 25% mortality. A second-look laparotomy or laparoscopy may be performed 18–36 hours after initial surgical treatment to reevaluate bowel viability.

UCV *Surg.30*

ILEUS

Anticholinergics, opioids, and hypokalemia slow GI motility.

Loss of peristalsis **without structural obstruction.** Risk factors include recent surgery/GI procedures, severe medical illness, **hypokalemia** or other electrolyte imbalances, **hypothyroidism,** DM, or medications that slow GI motility (e.g., **anticholinergics, opioids**).

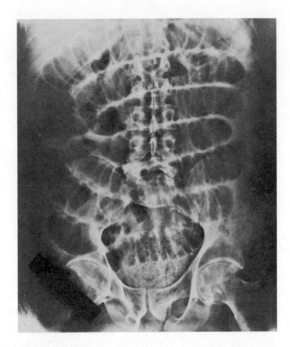

FIGURE 2.6–4. Small bowel obstruction. Supine abdominal x-ray reveals dilated loops of small bowel in a ladder-like pattern. Air-fluid levels may be apparent on an upright x-ray. (Reproduced, with permission, from Way L. *Current Surgical Diagnosis & Treatment,* 10th ed. Stamford, CT: Appleton & Lange, 1994:626, Fig. 30–6.)

History/PE

Presenting symptoms include diffuse, constant, moderate abdominal discomfort, **nausea/vomiting** (especially with feeding), **abdominal distention,** and an absence of **flatulence or bowel movements.** Exam may reveal diffuse tenderness and **abdominal distention** with a lack of **peritoneal signs** and **reduced or absent bowel sounds.** A **rectal examination is required** to rule out fecal impaction in elderly patients.

Differential

Partial or complete obstruction of the small intestine or colon, appendicitis, gastroenteritis, pancreatitis, neoplasm.

Evaluation

Diffusely **distended loops of small and large bowel** with air-fluid levels on supine and upright abdominal x-rays (AXRs) will confirm the diagnosis. A Gastrografin study can rule out partial obstruction; a CT can rule out neoplasms.

Look for air throughout the small and large bowel on AXR.

Treatment

- Decrease use of narcotics and any other drugs that reduce **bowel motility.**
- Temporarily reduce or discontinue oral feeds.
- Initiate **NG suction/parenteral feeds** as necessary.
- Replete electrolytes as needed.

MALABSORPTION

Inability to absorb nutrients as a result of an underlying condition such as **celiac disease, Whipple's disease, short bowel syndrome, pancreatic insufficiency, lactose intolerance, and infection.** The small bowel is most commonly involved. Reduced absorption of protein, fat, carbohydrates, and the smaller vitamins and minerals can be present. Symptoms include **frequent, loose, watery stools** and/or **pale, foul-smelling, bulky stools** associated with abdominal pain, **flatus, bloating,** weight loss, **nutritional deficiencies,** and fatigue. Treatment is etiology-dependent, but severely affected patients may receive total parental nutrition (TPN), immunosuppressants, and anti-inflammatory medications.

CARCINOID SYNDROME

Cutaneous flushing, diarrhea, wheezing, and cardiac valvular lesions are the most common manifestations of carcinoid tumors.

Due to liver metastasis of **carcinoid tumors** (from hormone-producing enterochromaffin cells) that most commonly arise from the ileum and appendix. **Cutaneous flushing, diarrhea, wheezing,** and **cardiac valvular lesions** are the most common manifestations of these tumors and result from tumor production of serotonin and substance P. Symptoms usually follow eating, exertion, or excitement. High urine levels of the serotonin metabolite 5-HIAA are diagnostic. Chest and abdominal CT scans can localize the tumor. Treatment includes **octreotide** (for symptoms) and reduction of tumor mass. Carcinoid tumors are slow growing, and patients often survive for a decade or more after diagnosis.

DISORDERS OF THE LARGE BOWEL

DIVERTICULAR DISEASE

Diverticular disease is the most common cause of acute lower GI bleeding in patients > 40 years old.

Outpouchings of mucosa and submucosa (false diverticula) that herniate through the colonic muscle layers at areas of high intraluminal pressure; most common in the sigmoid colon. **Diverticulosis is the most common cause of acute lower GI bleeding in patients > 40 years of age.** Risk factors include a **low-fiber and high-fat diet,** advanced age (65% occur in those > 80 years old), and connective tissue disorders (e.g., Ehlers-Danlos, Marfan's). **Diverticulitis** is due to inflammation and, potentially, perforation of a diverticulum.

History/PE

Diverticulosis is often **asymptomatic** but can manifest with constipation, **left lower quadrant abdominal pain,** and **abnormal bowel habits.** Bleeding is painless and sudden and generally presents as hematochezia with symptoms of anemia (fatigue, light-headedness, dyspnea on exertion). Uncomplicated diverticular disease will present with a benign exam. Diverticulitis presents as an acute, mild to severe, steady or cramping pain commonly localized to the **LLQ** with fever, nausea, and vomiting. Generalized abdominal tenderness with peritoneal signs in the presence of free perforation suggest diverticulitis.

Differential

Colon cancer with perforation, Crohn's disease, mesenteric ischemia, appendicitis, gynecologic disease (e.g., ovarian cyst, PID, ectopic pregnancy).

Diverticular disease must be distinguished from colon cancer with perforation.

Evaluation

CBC can show **leukocytosis.** Diagnosis is based on AXR, colonoscopy, or barium enema. However, invasive techniques must be avoided in the early diverticulitic due to perforation risk. In patients with severe disease or in those who show lack of improvement, CT scan may reveal abscess or free air.

Treatment

Avoid flexible sigmoidoscopy and barium enemas in the initial stages of diverticulitis because there is a risk of perforation.

- **Uncomplicated diverticular disease:** Patients can be followed and placed on a **high-fiber diet** or fiber supplements.
- **Diverticular bleeding:** Bleeding usually stops spontaneously; transfuse and hydrate as needed. If bleeding does not stop, angiography with embolization or **surgery** is indicated.
- **Diverticulitis:** Treat with **bowel rest** (NPO), NG tube, and **broad-spectrum antibiotics** (metronidazole and a fluoroquinolone or second- or third-generation cephalosporin) if the patient is stable. For perforation, perform immediate surgical resection of diseased bowel with primary anastomosis or temporary colostomy with a Hartmann's pouch and mucous fistula.

Complications

Abscess formation, intestinal perforation, **fistula formation,** hepatic abscess, retroperitoneal fibrosis, sepsis.

UCV *IM1.31, Surg.11*

LARGE BOWEL OBSTRUCTION

Table 2.6–2 describes features that distinguish SBO from LBO. Figure 2.6–5 demonstrates the classic radiographic findings of LBO.

COLON AND RECTAL CANCER

The second-leading cause of cancer mortality in the United States after lung cancer. It affects approximately 150,000 new patients per year and accounts for 50,000–60,000 deaths annually. There is an increasing incidence with age with a peak incidence at 70–80 years. Risk factors and screening protocols are summarized in Table 2.6–3.

History/PE

Without screening, colon and rectal cancer typically presents with symptoms after a prolonged period of silent growth. Abdominal pain is the most common presenting complaint. Other features depend on location:

- **Right-sided lesions:** Often bulky, ulcerating masses that cause **anemia from chronic occult blood loss.** Patients may complain of weight loss,

TABLE 2.6–2. Characteristics of Small and Large Bowel Obstruction

Variable	SBO	LBO
History	Moderate to severe acute abdominal pain; **copious emesis.** Cramping pain with distal SBO. Fever, signs of dehydration, and hypotension may be seen.	Constipation/obstipation, deep and cramping abdominal pain, nausea/vomiting (less than SBO but more commonly **feculent**).
PE	**Abdominal distention** (distal SBO), abdominal tenderness, visible peristaltic waves, fever, hypovolemia. Look for **surgical scars/hernias;** perform a rectal exam. **High-pitched "tinkly" bowel sounds;** later, absence of bowel sounds.	Significant **distention,** tympany, tenderness; examine for peritoneal irritation or mass; fever or signs of shock suggest perforation/peritonitis or ischemia/strangulation. **High-pitched "tinkly" bowel sounds;** later, absence of bowel sounds.
Causes	**Adhesions** (postsurgery), hernias, neoplasm, volvulus, intussusception, gallstone ileus, foreign body, Crohn's disease, CF, stricture, hematoma.	**Colon cancer,** diverticulitis, volvulus, fecal impaction, benign tumors. **Assume colon cancer until proven otherwise.**
Differential	LBO, paralytic ileus, gastroenteritis.	SBO, paralytic ileus, appendicitis, IBD.
Evaluation	CBC, lactic acid, electrolytes, AXR (see Figure 2.6–4); contrast studies (determine if it is partial or complete), CT scan.	CBC, electrolytes, lactic acid, AXR (see Figure 2.6–5), CT scan; water contrast enema (if perforation is suspected); sigmoidoscopy/colonoscopy if stable.
Treatment	Hospitalize. Partial SBO can be treated conservatively with **NG decompression** and NPO status. Patients with complete SBO should be managed aggressively with NPO status, NG decompression, IV fluids, and **surgical correction.**	Hospitalize. In some cases, obstruction can be with a Gastrografin enema, colonoscopy, or a **rectal tube;** however, **surgery** is usually required. Gangrenous colon usually requires partial colectomy with a diverting colostomy. Treat the underlying cause (e.g., neoplasm).

anorexia, diarrhea, weakness, or vague abdominal pain. Obstructive symptoms are rare.

- **Left-sided lesions:** Typically **"apple-core" obstructing** masses (see Figure 2.6–6). Patients complain of a **change in bowel habits** (e.g., decreasing stool caliber, constipation, obstipation) and/or blood-streaked stools. Obstruction is often present.
- **Rectal lesions:** Usually present with bright red blood per rectum (BRBPR) and may have tenesmus and/or rectal pain. Can coexist with hemorrhoids, so rectal cancer must be ruled out in all patients with rectal bleeding.

Differential

IBD, diverticulitis, ischemic colitis, hemorrhoids, PUD, other intra-abdominal malignancies.

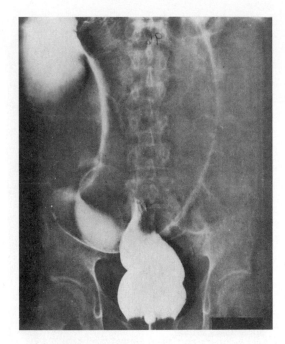

FIGURE 2.6–5. Large bowel obstruction. Barium study shows the "bird-beak" sign, with juxtaposed adjacent bowel walls in the dilated loop pointing toward the site of obstruction. (Reproduced, with permission, from Way L. *Current Surgical Diagnosis & Treatment*, 10th ed. Stamford, CT: Appleton & Lange, 1994:676, Fig. 31–15.)

Evaluation

- Order a CBC (often shows microcytic anemia) and stool occult blood.
- Perform sigmoidoscopy to evaluate rectal bleeding and all suspicious left-sided lesions. Rule out synchronous right-sided lesions with colonoscopy. Rule out missed lesions after incomplete colonoscopy with

TABLE 2.6–3. Risk Factors and Screening for Colorectal Cancer

Risk Factors	Screening
Age.	A digital rectal exam should be performed yearly for patients ≥ 50 years. Up to 10% of all lesions are palpable with DRE.
Hereditary syndromes—familial adenomatous polyposis (100% risk), Gardner's disease, hereditary nonpolyposis colorectal cancer (HNPCC).	Stool guaiac should be performed every year for patients ≥ 50 years. Up to 50% of positive guaiac tests are due to colorectal cancer.
Family history.	
IBD—ulcerative colitis carries a higher risk than does Crohn's disease.	Sigmoidoscopy performed every 3–5 years for those ≥ 50 years of age can be used to identify and biopsy 50–75% of lesions.
Adenomatous polyps—villous polyps progress more often than tubular polyps and sessile more than pedunculated polyps. Lesions > 2 cm carry an increased risk.	Perform colonoscopy every 10 years in patients ≥ 40 years with a family history of colon cancer or polyps, or 10 years prior to the age at diagnosis of the youngest family member with colorectal cancer.
Past history of colorectal cancer.	
High-fat, low-fiber diet.	Colonoscopy every 10 years > 50 years of age can be performed instead of sigmoidoscopy.

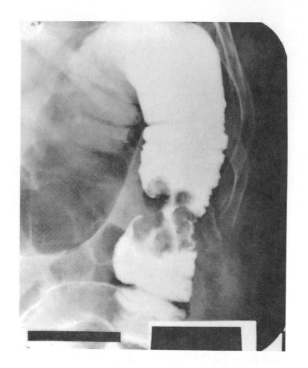

FIGURE 2.6–6. Colon carcinoma. The encircling carcinoma appears as an "apple-core" filling defect in the descending colon on barium enema x-ray. (Reproduced, with permission, from Way L. *Current Surgical Diagnosis & Treatment,* 10th ed. Stamford, CT: Appleton & Lange, 1994:658, Fig. 31–8.)

Iron-deficiency anemia in an elderly male is colorectal cancer until proven otherwise.

an air-contrast barium enema. Determine the degree of invasion in **rectal cancer** with an endoscopic U/S.

- Abdominal CT/MRI is used to stage colon cancer according to Dukes' staging criteria.
- Order CXR, LFTs, and an abdominal CT for metastatic workup. Metastases may arise from direct extension (to local viscera), hematogenous spread (40–50% go to the liver, but may also spread to the bone, lungs, and brain), and lymphatic spread (to pelvic lymph nodes).

Treatment

- **Preoperative bowel prep:** Mechanical cleaning (e.g., GoLytely) and oral antibiotics (neomycin, erythromycin).
- **Colonic lesions:** Surgical resection of the lesion with 3- to 5-cm margins. The lymphatic drainage and mesentery at the origin of the arterial supply are also resected. Primary anastomosis of bowel can usually be performed. Prognosis is determined by the extent of disease, as defined by Dukes' staging criteria.
- **Rectal lesions:** The resection technique depends on the proximity of the lesion to the anal verge.
  - **Abdominoperineal resection:** For low-lying lesions < 10 cm from the anal verge, the rectum and anus are resected and a permanent colostomy placed.
  - **Low anterior resection:** For proximal lesions > 10 cm from the anal verge, a primary anastomosis between the colon and rectum is created.

- **Wide local excision:** For small, low-stage, well-differentiated tumors in the lower third of the rectum.
  - **Adjuvant chemotherapy:** Used in cases of colon cancer with positive nodes. Radiation is ineffective for colon cancer but is a useful adjuvant in rectal cancer.
  - Follow with serial CEA levels (nonspecific, but useful for monitoring recurrence), colonoscopy, LFTs, CXR, and abdominal CT (for metastasis).

UCV *Surg.21*

Management of colon cancer depends on lymph node status.

ESOPHAGEAL DISEASE

DYSPHAGIA

Pain with swallowing (odynophagia) or difficulty swallowing due to abnormalities of the oropharynx or esophagus.

History/PE

Oropharyngeal dysphagia usually involves **liquids** more than solids and may be accompanied by dysarthria or dysphonia. Esophageal dysphagia usually involves **both** liquids and solids and is generally progressive. Examine for masses (e.g., goiter, tumor) and anatomical defects.

Differential

- **Oropharyngeal dysphagia:** Neurologic disorders (e.g., cranial nerve disease or bulbar injury), muscular disease, thyroid disease, sphincter dysfunction, Zenker's diverticulum, neoplasm, postsurgery, postradiation.
- **Esophageal dysphagia:** Schatzki's rings, esophageal webs, neoplasm, achalasia (abnormal peristalsis with decreased LES relaxation), diffuse esophageal spasm ("nutcracker esophagus"), peptic stricture, scleroderma.
- **Odynophagia:** Infectious agents (in HIV patients, consider *Candida*, CMV, and HSV), caustic agents.

Squamous esophageal cancer = tobacco and EtOH use.

Esophageal webs = iron-deficiency anemia.

Candidal esophagitis = AIDS.

Evaluation

- **Oropharyngeal dysphagia:** Videoesophagography.
- **Esophageal dysphagia:** Barium swallow followed by endoscopy, manometry, and/or pH monitoring. If an obstructive lesion is suspected, proceed directly to endoscopy with biopsy.
- **Odynophagia:** Barium study or endoscopy.

Treatment

Treatment is etiology-dependent. For achalasia, consider botulinum toxin injection, calcium channel blockers, or balloon dilatation as temporizing measures or esophageal myotomy for long-term treatment.

171

ESOPHAGEAL CANCER

Squamous cell carcinoma is the most common cancer of the upper esophagus (90%). Risk factors include alcohol, male gender, smoking, and age > 50 years. Approximately 10% of esophageal cancers are **adenocarcinomas,** which are associated with Barrett's esophagus (columnar metaplasia of the distal esophagus secondary to chronic GERD). Progressive dysphagia, initially to solids and later to liquids, is commonly seen, as are weight loss, odynophagia, GERD, GI bleeding, and vomiting. Barium study shows narrowing of the esophagus with an irregular border protruding into the lumen. Esophagogastroduodenoscopy (EGD) and biopsy confirm the diagnosis. MRI or CT are used to evaluate for metastases. Chemoradiation therapy is used, but the prognosis is poor. Surgical resection can be beneficial in some cases. Patients may require an endoscopically placed esophageal stent for palliation and improved quality of life.

UCV *Surg.22*

GASTROESOPHAGEAL REFLUX DISEASE (GERD)

Risk factors for GERD include hiatal hernia, and increased intra-abdominal pressure.

Symptomatic reflux of gastric contents into the esophagus, most commonly due to **transient LES relaxation.** Can be due to an incompetent LES, abnormally acidic gastric contents, or hiatal hernias. Risk factors include increased intra-abdominal pressure (e.g., obesity, pregnancy), scleroderma, alcohol, caffeine, nicotine, chocolate, and fatty foods.

History/PE

GERD may mimic asthma.

Patients present with **heartburn** that commonly occurs 30–90 minutes **after a meal, worsens with reclining,** and often improves with antacids, sitting, or standing. Sour taste ("water brash"), laryngitis, dysphagia, and cough or wheezing can be present. Exam is usually **normal** unless a systemic disease (e.g., Raynaud's disease/scleroderma) is present.

Differential

PUD, CAD, infectious (CMV, candidal) or chemical esophagitis, gallbladder disease, asthma, achalasia, esophageal spasm, pericarditis.

Evaluation

Diagnosis is based primarily on history. Evaluation may include an AXR, CXR, barium swallow (of limited usefulness, but can diagnose hiatal hernia), esophageal manometry, and 24-hour pH monitoring. **EGD** with biopsies should be performed if the patient has long-standing symptoms (to rule out Barrett's esophagus and adenocarcinoma).

Treatment

Patients with GERD should avoid caffeine, alcohol, chocolate, garlic, onions, mints, and nicotine.

- **Lifestyle:** Includes weight loss, head-of-bed elevation, and avoidance of nocturnal meals and substances that reduce LES tone.
- **Pharmacologic:** Start with **antacids** in patients with mild to moderate disease; use **H₂ receptor antagonists** (cimetidine, ranitidine) or **proton pump inhibitors (PPIs;** omeprazole; lansoprazole) in patients with severe or refractory disease.

- **Surgical:** For refractory or severe disease, **Nissen fundoplication** may offer significant relief.
- **Health maintenance:** Monitor for Barrett's esophagus and esophageal adenocarcinoma with **serial EGD and biopsy.**

Complications

Esophageal ulceration, esophageal stricture, aspiration of gastric contents, upper GI bleeding, **Barrett's esophagus.**

UCV *IM1.32*

GASTRIC DISEASE

HIATAL HERNIA

A condition in which a portion of the stomach herniates upward into the chest through a diaphragmatic opening. There are two common types: 95% are **sliding hiatal hernias** in which the gastroesophageal junction and a portion of the stomach are displaced; 5% are **paraesophageal hiatal hernias** in which the gastroesophageal junction remains below the diaphragm while a neighboring portion of the fundus herniates into the mediastinum.

History/PE

Patients may be asymptomatic. Those with sliding hernias may present with GERD.

Evaluation

May be an incidental finding on CXR but is more commonly diagnosed by barium swallow or EGD.

Treatment

- **Sliding hernias:** Medical therapy and lifestyle modifications reduce GERD symptoms.
- **Paraesophageal hernias:** Surgical gastropexy (attachment of the stomach to the rectus sheath and closure of the hiatus) is recommended to prevent torsion and ensuing complications.

GASTRITIS

Inflammation of the stomach lining.

- **Acute (stress) gastritis:** Rapidly developing superficial lesions often due to **NSAIDs,** alcohol, and stress from severe illness (e.g., burns, CNS injury).
- **Chronic gastritis: Type A** (~10%) occurs in the fundus and is due to **autoantibodies to parietal cells.** Associated with other autoimmune disorders, including pernicious anemia and thyroiditis. **Type B** (~90%) occurs in the antrum and may be caused by NSAID use or *Helicobacter*

pylori **infection.** Often asymptomatic, but is associated with an increased risk for PUD and gastric cancer.

History/PE

Patients may be asymptomatic or may complain of indigestion, nausea, vomiting, hematemesis, or melena.

Evaluation

Upper endoscopy can help visualize the gastric lining. *H. pylori* infection can be detected by urease breath test, serum IgG antibody (indicating exposure, not current infection), or endoscopic biopsy.

Treatment

Treatment is etiology-dependent. Decrease intake of offending agents; antacids, sucralfate, H$_2$ blockers, and/or PPIs may help. Use triple therapy (metronidazole, clarithromycin, bismuth salicylate/amoxicillin) with or without a PPI to treat *H. pylori.* Give a prophylactic H$_2$ blocker for patients at risk for stress ulcers (e.g., ICU patients).

GASTRIC CANCER

The most common malignant tumor of the stomach (90–95% of all gastric neoplasms). They are generally adenocarcinomas, which exhibit two morphologic types:

- **Intestinal type:** Thought to arise from intestinal metaplasia of **gastric mucosal cells.** Risk factors include a diet high in nitrites and salt and low in fresh vegetables (antioxidants), *H. pylori* colonization, and chronic gastritis.
- **Diffuse type:** Tends to be poorly differentiated and is not associated with *H. pylori* infection or chronic gastritis. Risk factors are largely unknown.

Early gastric carcinoma is largely asymptomatic and is discovered serendipitously with endoscopic examination of high-risk individuals. Advanced cases generally present with abdominal pain, early satiety, and weight loss. Five-year survival is < 10%; thus, successful treatment rests entirely on early detection and surgical removal of the tumor.

UCV *Surg. 25*

PEPTIC ULCER DISEASE

Damage to the gastric or duodenal mucosa caused by impaired mucosal defense and/or increased acidic gastric contents. **H. pylori** plays a causative role in > 90% of duodenal ulcers and in 70% of gastric ulcers. Other risk factors include **corticosteroid, NSAID, alcohol,** and **tobacco** use. Males are affected more often than females.

History/PE

Classically presents with chronic or periodic **dull, burning, aching epigastric pain** that **improves with meals** (especially duodenal ulcers), that worsens 2–3 hours after eating, and that can radiate to the back. Patients may also complain of nausea, hematemesis ("coffee-ground" emesis), or blood in the stool (melena or hematochezia). Exam may reveal varying degrees of **epigastric tenderness** and, if there is active bleeding, **positive stool guaiac.** An acute perforation can present with a rigid abdomen, rebound tenderness, guarding, or other signs of peritoneal irritation.

Differential

GERD, CAD, gastritis, pancreatitis, cholecystitis, Zollinger-Ellison syndrome, aortic aneurysm, and other causes of acute abdomen, depending on the severity of the pain and other physical findings.

Evaluation

AXR to **rule out perforation** (free air under the diaphragm) and CBC to assess for GI bleeding (low or falling HCT). Do an **upper endoscopy** with biopsy to confirm PUD and to rule out active bleeding or gastric adenocarcinoma (10% of gastric ulcers); barium swallow is an alternative. *H. pylori* testing includes urease breath test, serum IgG (less expensive but less sensitive and indicates exposure, not active infection), or endoscopic biopsy. In recurrent or refractory cases, serum gastrin can be used to screen for Zollinger-Ellison syndrome (patients must discontinue PPI use prior to testing).

Rule out Zollinger-Ellison syndrome with serum gastrin levels in cases of GERD and PUD that are refractory to medical management.

Treatment

- **Acute:** Rule out active bleeding with serial HCTs, rectal exam with stool guaiac, and NG lavage. Monitor the patient's HCT and BP and initiate IV hydration, transfusion, endoscopy, and surgery as needed. If perforation is likely, **emergent surgery** is indicated.
- **Pharmacologic:** Involves protecting the mucosa, decreasing acid production, and eradicating *H. pylori* infection. Treat mild disease with antacids or with sucralfate, bismuth, and misoprostol (a prostaglandin analog) for mucosal protection. PPIs or H_2 receptor antagonists may be used to reduce acid secretion. Patients with confirmed *H. pylori* infection should receive triple therapy. Discontinue use of exacerbating agents. Patients with recurrent or severe disease may require chronic symptomatic therapy.
- **Endoscopy and surgery:** All patients with symptomatic gastric ulcers for **> 2 months** and who are **refractory** to medical therapy should have either an endoscopy or an upper GI series with barium to rule out gastric adenocarcinoma. Refractory cases may require a surgical procedure such as **parietal cell vagotomy** (the most selective and preferred surgical approach).

Misoprostol can help patients with PUD who require NSAID therapy (e.g., patients with arthritis).

Complications

Hemorrhage (posterior ulcers that erode into the gastroduodenal artery), gastric outlet obstruction, perforation (usually anterior ulcers), intractable disease.

`UCV` *IM1.38, Surg.14*

ZOLLINGER-ELLISON SYNDROME

A rare condition characterized by **gastrin-producing tumors** in the duodenum and/or pancreas, leading to oversecretion of gastrin. This high level of gastrin in turn stimulates production of high levels of **gastric acid** by the gastric mucosa, leading to recurrent/intractable **ulcers** in the stomach and duodenum. In 25–50% of cases, gastrinomas are associated with multiple endocrine neoplasia type I (MEN I). Patients may present with unresponsive, recurrent **gnawing, burning abdominal pain, diarrhea,** nausea, vomiting, fatigue, weakness, weight loss, and **GI bleeding.** Diagnostic workup includes measurement of serum gastrin level and endoscopic examination of the gastric mucosa. Treatment requires **reduction of acid production.** H_2 blockers are typically ineffective, but a moderate- to high-dose PPI often controls the symptoms. Surgical repair of peptic ulcers and/or removal of tumor can be beneficial in refractory cases. Since roughly 50% of gastrinomas tumors are malignant, close **follow-up** is mandatory.

Zollinger-Ellison syndrome is associated with MEN I syndrome in roughly 25–50% of cases.

GASTROINTESTINAL BLEEDING

Bleeding from the GI tract may present as hematemesis, hematochezia, and/or melena. Table 2.6–4 presents the features of upper and lower GI bleeding.

INFLAMMATORY BOWEL DISEASE

Consists of **Crohn's disease and ulcerative colitis** (see Figure 2.6–7). Most common in whites and **Ashkenazi Jews,** during their teens to early 20s or in their 50s. Table 2.6–5 summarizes the features of IBD.

INGUINAL HERNIAS

An abnormal **protrusion of abdominal contents** (usually the small intestine) into the inguinal region through a weakness or defect in the abdominal wall. They are defined as **direct** or **indirect** on the basis of their relationship to the inguinal canal.

- **Indirect: Most common hernia in both genders.** Herniation of abdominal contents through the **internal,** and then **external, inguinal rings** and eventually into the scrotum (in males); due to a **congenital patent processus vaginalis.**
- **Direct:** Herniation of abdominal contents through the floor of **Hesselbach's triangle** (see Figure 2.6–8). Hernial sac contents do not traverse

TABLE 2.6–4. Features of Upper and Lower GI Bleeding

Variable	Upper GI Bleeding *(Surg.27)*	Lower GI Bleeding *(Surg.26)*
History/PE	Hematemesis, melena > hematochezia, depleted volume status (e.g., tachycardia, light-headedness, hypotension).	Hematochezia > melena, but can be either.
Evaluation	NG tube and NG lavage; endoscopy if stable.	Rule out upper GI bleed with NG tube and NG lavage. Colonoscopy if stable.
Common causes	**Gastritis,** PUD, Mallory-Weiss tear, esophageal varices, vascular abnormalities, neoplasm, esophagitis.	**Diverticulosis** (most common), arteriovenous malformations, neoplasm, IBD, anorectal disease, mesenteric ischemia.
Initial management	Protect the airway (may need intubation). Stabilize the patient with IV fluids, blood (HCT is not an accurate measure of acute blood loss).	Similar to upper GI bleed.
Long-term management	Endoscopy followed by therapy directed at underlying cause (e.g., H₂ blockers or PPI for PUD; sclerotherapy or banding for varices).	Rule out upper GI source; anoscopy or sigmoidoscopy; colonoscopy; manage etiology (e.g., surgical resection for tumor or diverticula, medical therapy for IBD).

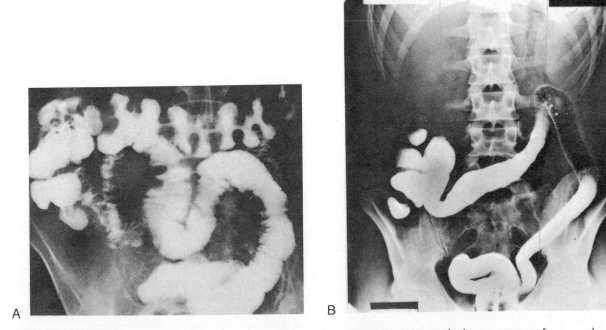

A   B

FIGURE 2.6–7. Inflammatory bowel disease. (A) Crohn's disease. Barium enema x-ray reveals deep transverse fissures, ulcers, and edema of the bowel. (B) Ulcerative colitis. Barium enema x-ray demonstrates shortening of the colon, loss of haustra ("lead pipe" appearance), and fine serrations at the bowel edges from small ulcers. (Reproduced, with permission, from Stobo JD et al. *The Principles and Practice of Medicine,* 23rd ed. Stamford, CT: Appleton & Lange, 1996:135, Fig. 23–2.)

TABLE 2.6–5. Features of Ulcerative Colitis and Crohn's Disease

Variable	Ulcerative Colitis (IM1.40)	Crohn's Disease (IM1.30)
Site of involvement	The **rectum** is always involved. May extend proximally in a **continuous fashion.** Inflammation and ulceration are **limited to the mucosa and submucosa.**	May involve **any portion** of the GI tract, particularly the **ileocecal region,** in a **discontinuous pattern** ("skip lesions"). The rectum is often spared. **Transmural inflammation.**
Symptoms and signs	**Bloody diarrhea,** lower abdominal cramps, tenesmus, urgency. Exam may reveal orthostatic hypotension, tachycardia, abdominal tenderness, frank blood on rectal exam, and extraintestinal manifestations.	Abdominal pain, abdominal mass, low-grade fever, weight loss, watery diarrhea. Exam may reveal fever, abdominal tenderness or mass, **perianal fissures, fistulas,** and extraintestinal manifestations.
Extraintestinal manifestations	Aphthous stomatitis, episcleritis/uveitis, arthritis, **primary sclerosing cholangitis, toxic megacolon,** erythema nodosum, and pyoderma gangrenosum.	Same as ulcerative colitis, as well as nephrolithiasis and fistulas to the skin, biliary tract, or urinary tract or between bowel loops.
Workup	CBC, AXR, stool cultures, O&P, stool assay for *C. difficile*. Colonoscopy can show diffuse and continuous rectal involvement, friability, edema, and **pseudopolyps.** Definitive diagnosis can be made with biopsy.	Same laboratory workup as ulcerative colitis. Colonoscopy may show aphthoid, linear, or stellate ulcers, strictures, **"cobblestoning,"** and **"skip lesions."** "Creeping fat" may also be present. Definitive diagnosis can be made with biopsy.
Treatment	**Sulfasalazine** or **5-ASA** (mesalamine); corticosteroids and immunosuppressants for refractory disease. **Total colectomy is curative** for long-standing or fulminant colitis or toxic megacolon.	**Sulfasalazine;** corticosteroids and immunosuppression indicated if no improvement. Surgical resection may be necessary for suspected perforation; **may recur** anywhere in the GI tract.
Incidence of cancer	**Markedly increased risk of colorectal cancer** in long-standing cases (monitor with frequent fecal occult blood screening and colonoscopy after eight years of disease).	Incidence of secondary malignancy is much lower than in ulcerative colitis.

the internal **inguinal ring;** they herniate directly through the abdominal wall and are contained within the **aponeurosis** of the **external oblique muscle.** Most often due to an acquired defect in the **transversalis fascia** from mechanical breakdown. This increases with age.

Treatment

Because of the risk of **incarceration** and **strangulation,** surgical management (open or laparoscopic) is indicated unless specific contraindications are pres-

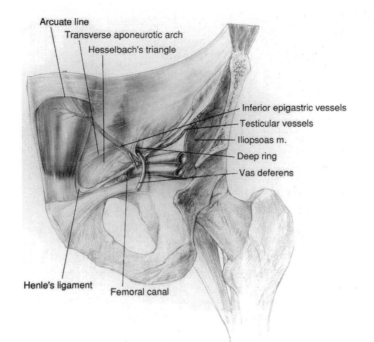

FIGURE 2.6–8. Hesselbach's triangle. (Reproduced, with permission, from Schwartz LS. *Principles of Surgery*, 7th ed. New York: McGraw-Hill, 1999:1588.)

ent. Repair of a direct inguinal hernia involves correcting the defect in the transversalis fascia. Indirect inguinal hernias are repaired by isolating and ligating the hernia sac and reducing the size of the internal inguinal ring to allow only the spermatic cord structures in males to pass through.

UCV *Surg. 23, 29*

LIVER DISEASE

HEPATITIS

History/PE

Acute hepatitis often starts with a viral prodrome of nonspecific symptoms (e.g., **malaise**, fever, joint pain, fatigue, URI symptoms, **nausea, vomiting**, changes in bowel habits) followed by **jaundice** and RUQ tenderness. There is a convalescent period followed by recovery. Exam often reveals **jaundice**, scleral icterus, **tender hepatomegaly**, possible splenomegaly, and lymphadenopathy. Chronic hepatitis usually gives rise to symptoms indicative of chronic liver disease (jaundice, cirrhosis, fatigue). At least 80% of those infected with HCV and 10% of those with HBV will develop chronic hepatitis. Other etiologies of chronic hepatitis include HDV (with HBV), autoimmune hepatitis, alcoholic hepatitis, drug-induced disease (e.g., INH, methyldopa, acetaminophen), Wilson's disease, hemochromatosis, α_1-antitrypsin deficiency, and neoplasms.

Eighty percent of patients infected with HCV will develop chronic hepatitis.

Differential

Mononucleosis and other systemic viral illnesses (CMV), toxoplasmosis, rickettsial disease (Q fever, Rocky Mountain spotted fever), drug-induced hepatitis, autoimmune hepatitis, "shock liver" secondary to hypoperfusion (e.g., MI, sepsis, or trauma), neoplasm, alcohol use.

Evaluation

An AST/ALT ratio > 2 suggests alcoholic hepatitis.

Normal WBC (with relative leukcytosis), dramatically **elevated ALT/AST,** and elevated bilirubin/alkaline phosphatase are present in the acute form. In chronic hepatitis, ALT and AST are increased for > 6 months with concurrent alkaline phosphatase/bilirubin elevations. In severe cases, PT will be prolonged, as all clotting factors except Factor VIII are produced by the liver. Diagnosis is made by **hepatitis serology** and in chronic or severe cases, liver biopsy. ANA (autoimmune hepatitis), anti–smooth muscle antibody, and antimitochondrial antibody can identify other causes.

Treatment

- Monitor for resolution of symptoms over time.
- Steroids for severe alcoholic hepatitis.
- **Immunosuppression** with steroids and other agents (azathioprine) for autoimmune hepatitis.
- **IFN-α and lamivudine (3TC)** for chronic HBV infection; **IFN-β and ribavirin** for chronic HCV infection.
- **Liver transplantation** is the treatment of choice for patients with end-stage liver failure, if possible.
- ICU management and emergent transplant for fulminant hepatic failure.

Complications

Sequelae of chronic hepatitis include cirrhosis, liver failure, and HCC.

Cirrhosis, liver failure, hepatocellular carcinoma (HCC; 3–5%), death within five years (50%).

UCV *IM1.35, 36*

PORTAL HYPERTENSION

Portal pressure > 5 mmHg the pressure in the IVC. Causes are divided into presinusoidal (splenic or portal vein thrombosis, schistosomiasis, granulomatous), sinusoidal (cirrhosis, granulomatous disease), and postsinusoidal (right heart failure, constrictive pericarditis, hepatic vein thrombosis). **Budd-Chiari syndrome** is hepatic vein thrombosis secondary to hypercoagulability. Treatment includes clot lysis, TIPS, or hepatic transplantation and has a poor prognosis.

Alcoholism, chronic hepatitis, and other chronic liver diseases most commonly cause cirrhosis.

History/PE

Patients may present with **jaundice, ascites, spontaneous bacterial peritonitis, hepatic encephalopathy** (e.g., asterixis, altered mental status), **esophageal varices,** and renal dysfunction. Exam may reveal icteric sclera, an **abdominal**

fluid wave, shifting dullness, splenomegaly, easy bruising, spider angiomata, dilated abdominal veins **(caput medusae),** palmar erythema, gynecomastia, and testicular atrophy. Jaundice arises when excess bilirubin circulating in the blood dissolves in the subcutaneous fat. With the exception of physiologic jaundice of the newborn, jaundice is pathological, indicating either overload or damage to the liver or an inability to excrete bilirubin through the biliary system. Causes of jaundice are numerous and include obstruction of the biliary system (by infection, stone, stricture, or tumor), hepatitis (viral, drug-induced, autoimmune), alcoholic cirrhosis, pancreatic cancer, hemolytic anemia, and congenital disorders of bilirubin metabolism (Gilbert's syndrome, Dubin-Johnson syndrome, Crigler-Najjar syndrome).

Evaluation

Evaluation includes LFTs, alkaline phosphatase, bilirubin, albumin, and PT/PTT to assess hepatic function; serum ferritin, ceruloplasmin, α_1-antitrypsin, and U/S may help identify additional causes such as hemochromatosis, Wilson's disease, α_1-antitrypsin deficiency, and Budd-Chiari syndrome, respectively. Indirect hepatic vein wedge pressure (a measure of portal pressure) is increased. The etiology of ascites can be established by measurement of the **serum-ascites albumin gradient (SAAG;** see Table 2.6–6)

Treatment

Treatment is aimed at ameliorating the complications of portal hypertension.

- **Ascites: Sodium restriction** and **diuretics** (furosemide and spironolactone); rule out infectious/neoplastic causes (perform paracentesis to obtain the SAAG, CBC, and cultures); treat underlying liver disease if possible.
- **Spontaneous bacterial peritonitis:** Check peritoneal fluid if there is a possibility of infection. The fluid is positive if there are > 250 PMNs/mL or > 500 WBCs. Treat with **IV antibiotics** (e.g., third-generation cephalosporin) to cover both gram-positive (*Enterococcus*) and gram-negative (*E. coli, Klebsiella*) organisms until a causative organism is identified.
- **Hepatorenal syndrome:** Diagnosis of exclusion; difficult to treat and often requires dialysis. May be fatal.
- **Hepatic encephalopathy:** Decrease protein consumption; treat with **lactulose** and/or **neomycin.**

Spontaneous bacterial peritonitis is diagnosed by > 250 PMNs/mL or > 500 WBCs in the ascitic fluid.

TABLE 2.6–6. Serum-Ascites Albumin Gradient

SAAG > 1.1	SAAG < 1.1
Ascites is due to an imbalance between hydrostatic and oncotic pressures:	Ascites is due to protein leakage:
Chronic liver disease	Nephrotic syndrome
Massive hepatic metastases	Tuberculosis
CHF	Malignancy (e.g., ovarian cancer)

- **Esophageal varices:** Monitor for GI bleeding; treat medically (β-blockers), endoscopically (sclerotherapy), or surgically (portocaval shunt).

UCV *IM1.34, Surg.16*

HEPATOCELLULAR CARCINOMA

Complications of HCC include GI bleeding, liver failure, and metastasis.

One of the most common cancers worldwide despite its relatively low incidence in the United States. The primary risk factors for the development of HCC in the United States are **cirrhosis** and **chronic hepatitis** (HBV or HCV). In developing countries, **aflatoxins** (in various food sources) are also major risk factors. Patients commonly present with **RUQ tenderness, abdominal distention,** and signs of chronic liver disease such as **jaundice, bruisability,** and **coagulopathy.** Exam reveals a **tender, enlarged liver.** Diagnosis is often suggested by the presence of a mass on **U/S** or **CT** as well as by elevated LFTs and significantly elevated α-fetoprotein (AFP) levels. Definitive diagnosis is made with liver biopsy. For cases of small tumors that are detected early, aggressive resection of tumor or **orthotopic liver transplantation** may be successful. Chemotherapy and radiation are generally not effective, although they may be used to shrink large tumors prior to surgery **(neoadjuvant therapy).** Monitor tumor recurrence with serial AFP levels. Prevent exposure to hepatic carcinogens and vaccinate against hepatitis in high-risk individuals.

HEMOCHROMATOSIS

An **autosomal-recessive** disease that usually occurs in males of northern European descent and is rarely recognized before the fifth decade. Hemochromatosis is caused by hyperabsorption of iron with parenchymal hemosiderin accumulation in the liver, pancreas, heart, adrenals, testes, pituitary, and kidneys. Secondary hemochromatosis may occur with iron overload and is common in patients receiving **chronic transfusion therapy,** in **alcoholics** (alcohol increases iron absorption), and in patients with β-thalassemia. Patients may present with abdominal pain or **symptoms of DM, hypogonadism,** or cirrhosis. Exam may reveal **bronze skin pigmentation,** pancreatic dysfunction **cardiac dysfunction** (CHF), hepatomegaly, and testicular atrophy. Evaluate for **elevated serum iron,** percent saturation of iron, and ferritin with decreased serum transferrin. Fasting transferrin saturation (serum iron divided by transferrin level) > 45% is the most sensitive diagnostic test. **Glucose intolerance** and mildly elevated AST and alkaline phosphatase can be present. Perform a **liver biopsy** (to determine hepatic iron index), hepatic MRI, or hemochromatosis mutation C282Y screen. Treat with **weekly phlebotomy;** when serum iron levels decline, perform maintenance phlebotomy every 2–4 months. **Deferoxamine** can be used for maintenance therapy. Complications include **cirrhosis, HCC,** cardiomegaly leading to CHF and/or conduction defects, DM, impotence, arthropathy, and hypopituitarism.

UCV *IM1.33*

WILSON'S DISEASE (HEPATOLENTICULAR DEGENERATION)

Decreased ceruloplasmin and **excessive deposition of copper** in the liver and brain due to a deficient copper-transporting protein linked to an autosomal-recessive defect on chromosome 13. Wilson's disease usually occurs in patients ≤ 30 years old; half of patients are symptomatic by age 15. Patients present with **liver abnormalities** (jaundice secondary to hepatitis/cirrhosis) as well neurologic (loss of coordination, **tremor,** dysphagia) and **psychiatric** (psychosis, anxiety, mania, depression) **abnormalities.** Exam may reveal **Kayser-Fleischer rings** in the cornea (green-to-brown deposits of copper in Descemet's membrane), jaundice, hepatomegaly, choreiform movements, parkinsonian tremor, and rigidity. Evaluation reveals **decreased serum ceruloplasmin,** elevated urinary copper excretion, and elevated hepatic copper. Treatment includes **dietary copper restriction** (avoid shellfish, liver, legumes), **penicillamine** (a copper chelator that increases urinary copper excretion; administer with pyridoxine), and possibly oral zinc (increases fecal excretion).

PANCREATIC DISEASE

PANCREATITIS

Table 2.6–7 lists the important features of acute and chronic pancreatitis. Table 2.6–8 lists Ranson's criteria for predicting mortality associated with acute pancreatitis.

PANCREATIC CANCER

Most commonly a pancreatic head adenocarcinoma (90%). Risk factors include smoking, chronic pancreatitis, a first-degree relative with pancreatic cancer, and a high-fat diet. Pancreatic cancer is most commonly seen in men in their 60s. Abdominal pain radiating toward the back, jaundice, loss of appetite, nausea, vomiting, weight loss, weakness, fatigue, and indigestion are classic complaints. Exam may reveal a palpable, nontender gallbladder **(Courvoisier's sign)** or migratory thrombophlebitis **(Trousseau's sign;** in 10% of patients due to ectopic production of procoagulants). Use CT scan to detect a pancreatic mass, dilated pancreatic and bile ducts, the extent of vascular involvement, and metastases. If a mass is not visualized, use ERCP or endoscopic U/S for better visualization and possibly fine-needle aspiration. Ten to twenty percent of pancreatic head tumors have no evidence of metastasis and may be resected using the Whipple procedure (pancreaticoduodenectomy). However, the majority present with metastatic disease, and treatment for this is palliative. Chemotherapy with 5-FU and gemcitabine may help prolong survival temporarily, but long-term prognosis is poor (< 5% survive > 5 years after diagnosis).

UCV *Surg.33*

TABLE 2.6–7. Features of Acute and Chronic Pancreatitis

Variable	Acute Pancreatitis (Surg.13)	Chronic Pancreatitis (IM1.29)
Pathophysiology	Leakage of pancreatic enzymes into pancreatic and peripancreatic tissue, often secondary to gallstone disease or alcoholism.	Irreversible parenchymal destruction leading to pancreatic dysfunction.
Time course	Abrupt onset of severe pain.	Persistent, recurrent episodes of severe pain.
Risk factors	**Gallstones, alcoholism,** hypercalcemia, hypertriglyceridemia, trauma, drug side effects (thiazide diuretics), viral infections, post-ERCP, scorpion bites.	**Alcoholism (90%),** gallstones, hyperparathyroidism, congenital malformation (pancreas divisum). May also be idiopathic.
Symptoms/signs	**Severe epigastric pain (radiating to the back),** nausea, vomiting, weakness, fever, shock. Flank discoloration (**Grey Turner sign**) and periumbilical discoloration (**Cullen's sign**) may be evident on exam.	Recurrent episodes of **persistent epigastric pain,** anorexia, nausea, constipation, flatulence, **steatorrhea,** DM.
Evaluation	↑ **amylase,** ↑ **lipase,** ↓ **calcium** if severe; "**sentinel loop**" or "**colon cutoff**" **sign** on AXR. U/S or CT may show enlarged pancreas with stranding, abscess, hemorrhage, necrosis, or pseudocyst.	Increased or normal amylase and lipase, **glycosuria, pancreatic calcifications,** and mild ileus on AXR and CT (**"chain of lakes"**).
Management	Removal of offending agent, if possible. Standard supportive measures: IV fluids/electrolyte replacement, analgesia, bowel rest, NG suction, nutritional support, O_2, "tincture of time." IV antibiotics, respiratory support, and surgical debridement if necrotizing pancreatitis is present.	Analgesia, exogenous lipase/trypsin and medium-chain fatty-acid diet for exocrine dysfunction, avoidance of causative agents (EtOH), surgery for intractable pain or structural causes.
Prognosis	85–90% mild, self-limited; 10–15% severe, requiring ICU admission; mortality may approach 50% in severe cases.	Can have chronic pain and pancreatic exocrine and endocrine dysfunction.
Complications	**Pancreatic pseudocyst, fistula formation,** hypocalcemia, renal failure, pleural effusion, chronic pancreatitis, sepsis. Mortality secondary to acute pancreatitis can be predicted with Ranson's criteria (see Table 2.6–8) (Surg.12).	**Chronic pain,** malnutrition, PUD.

TABLE 2.6–8. Ranson's Criteria for Acute Pancreatitis[a]

On Admission	After 48 Hours
"GA LAW":	**"C HOBBS":**
Glucose > 200 mg/dL	Ca^{2+} < 8.0 mg/dL
Age > 55 years	HCT decrease by > 10%
LDH > 350 IU/L	O_2 PaO_2 < 60 mmHg
AST > 250 IU/dL	Base excess > 4 mEq/L
WBC > 16,000/mL	BUN increase > 5 mg/dL
	Sequestered fluid > 6 L

[a]The risk of mortality is 20% with 3–4 signs, 40% with 5–6 signs, and 100% with ≥ 7 signs.

HIGH-YIELD FACTS

Gastrointestinal

The following clinical questions and accompanying answers are reproduced, with permission, from Reteguiz J, *PreTest: Physical Diagnosis*, 4th ed., New York: McGraw-Hill, 2001.

Questions

1. A 40-year-old man presents to the emergency room complaining of severe abdominal pain that radiates to his back accompanied by several episodes of vomiting. He drinks alcohol daily. On physical examination, the patient is found on the stretcher lying in the fetal position. He is febrile and appears ill. The skin of his abdomen has an area of bluish periumbilical discoloration. Abdominal examination reveals decreased bowel sounds. The patient has severe midepigastric tenderness on palpation and complains of exquisite pain when your hands are abruptly withdrawn from his abdomen. Rectal examination is normal. Which of the following is the most likely diagnosis?
    a. Acute cholecystitis
    b. Pyelonephritis
    c. Necrotizing pancreatitis
    d. Chronic pancreatitis
    e. Diverticulitis
    f. Appendicitis

2. A 32-year-old man presents with severe abdominal pain, which he describes as sharp and diffuse. He does not drink alcohol or take any medications. He has a past medical history significant for PUD over five years ago. He has stable vital signs and has no orthostatic changes. You observe the patient to be lying very still on the emergency room stretcher. On physical examination, he has a rigid abdomen and decreased bowel sounds. He has localized left upper quadrant guarding and rebound tenderness. He has referred rebound tenderness on palpation of the right upper quadrant. Rectal examination is fecal occult blood test (FOBT) negative. Which of the following is the best method of confirming the diagnosis in this patient?
    a. Barium swallow
    b. Leukocytosis
    c. Upper endoscopy
    d. Abdominal radiograph
    e. Colonoscopy

3. A 74-year-old man presents with the abrupt onset of pain in the left lower abdomen, which has been progressively worsening over the last two days. He states that the pain is unremitting. He has some diarrhea but no nausea or vomiting. He has no dysuria or hematuria. His temperature is 102°F. Bowel sounds are decreased. The patient has involuntary guarding. There is rebound tenderness when the LLQ is palpated. The referred rebound test is positive. A fixed sausage-like mass is palpable in the area of tenderness. There is no costovertebral angle (CVA) tenderness. Rectal examination reveals brown stool, which is FOBT positive. Bloodwork demonstrates a leukocytosis. Which of the following is the most likely diagnosis?
    a. Colon cancer
    b. Diverticulitis
    c. Pancreatitis
    d. Pyelonephritis
    e. Appendicitis

4. A 42-year-old morbidly obese woman complains of a nonproductive cough for eight months. She denies abdominal discomfort after eating and has never "suffered" from heartburn. Rarely, she has regurgitation, and when she does it has a sour taste to it. Abdominal examination is normal. Rectal examination is FOBT negative. Which of the following is the most likely diagnosis?
   a. Carcinoma of the lung
   b. Gastroesophageal reflux disease
   c. Chronic obstructive lung disease
   d. Lactose deficiency
   e. Chronic cholestasis

5. A 45-year-old patient presents with altered mental status. His wife states that over the last week her husband has been taking acetaminophen for some abdominal discomfort. He uses no illicit drugs but drinks 4–5 beers daily. Over the last 24 hours, the patient has become progressively lethargic. Vital signs reveal a temperature of 97°F, a blood pressure of 100/70 mmHg, a heart rate of 120/min, and a respiratory rate of 26/min. The patient is jaundiced with RUQ abdominal tenderness on palpation. He has no rebound tenderness or splenomegaly but has an enlarged liver. There is no ascites or peripheral edema. Heart and lung examinations are normal. The patient responds to painful stimuli and has asterixis. He has no focal neurologic deficit. Which of the following is the most likely diagnosis?
   a. Alcohol intoxication
   b. Alcohol withdrawal
   c. Delirium tremens
   d. Acetaminophen toxicity
   e. Wilson's disease

Answers

1. **The answer is c.** The patient most likely has **necrotizing pancreatitis,** which is a complication of **acute pancreatitis.** Other complications of pancreatitis include **pseudocyst, abscess,** and **phlegmon.** The periumbilical discoloration **(Cullen sign)** suggests a hemoperitoneum. Discoloration of the flanks would be a positive **Turner sign.** When the patient experiences pain as the hands of the examiner are abruptly withdrawn from the abdomen, he or she is said to have **rebound tenderness** (a sign of peritonitis). Decreased bowel sounds are another sign of peritonitis. Risk factors for acute pancreatitis include alcohol use, trauma, hyperlipidemia, gallstones, and medications. An abdominal radiograph in acute pancreatitis might show a **sentinel loop** (air-filled small intestine in the LUQ) and colon **cutoff sign** (air in the transverse colon). Patients with **chronic pancreatitis** present with bouts of abdominal pain and signs of pancreatic insufficiency (weight loss, steatorrhea, and diabetes). The abdominal radiograph in patients with chronic pancreatitis demonstrates **calcifications** in the pancreas (pathognomonic).

2. **The answer is d.** Guarding, rigidity, absent or diminished bowel sounds, rebound and referred rebound tenderness, and lying perfectly still are all signs of peritonitis. A plain film of the abdomen in this patient with a probable perforated ulcer might show free intraperitoneal air under the diaphragm (in up to 75% of patients). The free air establishes the diagnosis, and no further studies are needed. Barium studies are contraindicated in perforation.

3. **The answer is b.** Complications of diverticular disease include diverticulitis and gastrointestinal bleeding. **Diverticulitis** is an acute inflammatory process caused by bacteria in a diverticulum (outpouching of the mucosa or submucosa). It may occur in up to 50% of patients with diverticulosis. The patient most likely has diverticulitis, which is usually **left-sided** since the diameter of the sigmoid colon is the smallest of the colon (higher wall tension and intraluminal pressure in this area are probably responsible for the diverticular formation). The palpable mass reflects adherent loops of bowel. **Peritonitis** often results in involuntary guarding (abdominal rigidity due to reflex muscle spasm from the peritoneal irritation). Decreased bowel sounds may be heard in peritonitis or in any condition that causes an ileus (absence of peristalsis). Tenderness upon abrupt withdrawal of the hand **(rebound tenderness or Blumberg sign)** occurs because when the abdominal wall passively springs back into place, it carries with it the inflamed peritoneum. The **referred rebound test** is conducted in the same way but in a location away from the area of tenderness. The patient will experience pain in the area of stated tenderness rather than the site where the test is performed.

4. **The answer is b.** The risk factors for gastroesophageal reflux disease (GERD) include obesity, pregnancy, scleroderma, and diet (caffeine, alcohol, nicotine, chocolate, fatty foods). The most common etiology of GERD is transient lower esophageal sphincter (LES) relaxation, but it may also be due to hiatal hernia and acidic gastric contents. The sour taste of GERD is often referred to as **"water brash."** A complication of GERD is Barrett's esophagus. Atypical symptoms of GERD may include asthma, chronic cough, chronic laryngitis, sore throat, and chest pain. **PUD** produces epigastric pain that typically improves with eating. Patients with **lactose intolerance** present with bloating, cramps, and diarrhea after ingesting a milk product.

5. **The answer is d.** This patient with underlying liver disease probably has **fulminant hepatitis from acetaminophen toxicity.** Because of his alcohol use, he has insufficient glutathione stores and induced P450 enzymatic activity and is at greater risk for developing toxicity. Patients who survive the complication of fulminant hepatic failure will begin to recover over the following week, but some require liver transplantation. A serum acetaminophen level should be sent and immediate treatment with *N*-acetylcysteine (NAC), which provides cysteine for glutathione synthesis, is indicated. Signs of **alcohol intoxication** include euphoria, dysarthria, ataxia, labile mood, lethargy, coma, respiratory depression, and death. Patients with **alcohol withdrawal** present with a hyperexcitable state (e.g., hypertension, tachycardia, flushing, sweating, and mydriasis) and have tremors, disordered perceptions, seizures, and delirium tremens (DTs). DTs occur 2–4 days after alcohol abstinence and are characterized by hallucinations, which may be dangerous, combative, and/or destructive.

Hematology/Oncology

Blood cell differentiation

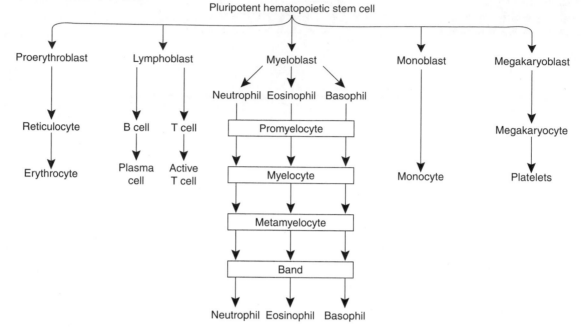

Clotting cascade

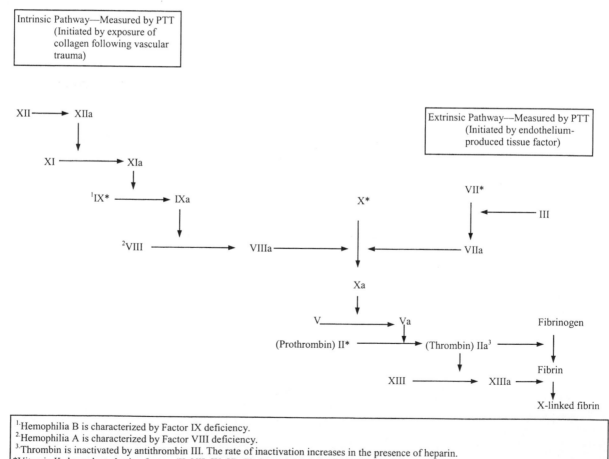

1. Hemophilia B is characterized by Factor IX deficiency.
2. Hemophilia A is characterized by Factor VIII deficiency.
3. Thrombin is inactivated by antithrombin III. The rate of inactivation increases in the presence of heparin.
*Vitamin K-dependent clotting factors (II, VII, IX, X). Their synthesis is inhibited by warfarin.

Diseases associated with neoplasms	Condition	Neoplasm
	1. **Down** syndrome	1. **Acute Lymphoblastic Leukemia**—"We will **ALL** go **DOWN** together"
	2. Xeroderma pigmentosum	2. Squamous cell and basal cell carcinomas of skin
	3. Chronic atrophic gastritis, pernicious anemia, postsurgical gastric remnants	3. Gastric adenocarcinoma
	4. Tuberous sclerosis (facial angiofibroma, seizures, mental retardation)	4. Astrocytoma and cardiac rhabdomyoma
	5. Actinic keratosis	5. Squamous cell carcinoma of skin
	6. Barrett's esophagus (chronic GI reflux)	6. Esophageal adenocarcinoma
	7. Plummer-Vinson syndrome (atrophic glossitis, esophageal webs, anemia; all due to iron deficiency)	7. Squamous cell carcinoma of esophagus
	8. Cirrhosis (alcoholic, hepatitis B or C)	8. Hepatocellular carcinoma
	9. Ulcerative colitis	9. Colonic adenocarcinoma
	10. Paget's disease of bone	10. 2° osteosarcoma and fibrosarcoma
	11. Immunodeficiency states	11. Malignant lymphomas
	12. AIDS	12. Aggressive malignant lymphomas (non-Hodgkin's) and Kaposi's sarcoma
	13. Autoimmune diseases (e.g., Hashimoto's thyroiditis, myasthenia gravis)	13. Benign and malignant thymomas
	14. Acanthosis nigricans (hyperpigmentation and epidermal thickening)	14. Visceral malignancy (stomach, lung, breast, uterus)
	15. Dysplastic nevus	15. Malignant melanoma

ANEMIA

Low HCT and Hb relative to the gender and age of the patient. The chronologic low point for normal HCT is 35%, which occurs at two months of age. By age 18, the normal HCT in males is 47% and in females 41%.

History/PE

Symptoms include weakness, and dyspnea on exertion, and high-output congestive heart failure (CHF). Severe anemia can predispose patients to angina or syncope. Iron-deficient patients may have pica (craving for clay, ice chips). Exam might show **pallor** of skin and conjunctiva, tachycardia, tachypnea, increased pulse pressure, systolic flow murmur, jaundice (hemolytic anemia), and positive stool guaiac (GI bleed).

Differential

Anemias can be organized either by the size of the red cell (MCV) or by the number of reticulocytes (see Figure 2.7–1).

Evaluation

Anemia labs include CBC, MCV, reticulocyte count, ferritin, iron, total iron-binding capacity (TIBC), stool occult blood, folate, serum B_{12}, LDH, bilirubin, haptoglobin, Coombs' test, and DIC panel (e.g., D-dimer, fibrinogen, fibrin split products). Characteristic iron study results are summarized in Table 2.7–1. Characteristic cells on a peripheral smear may be useful in identifying the etiology (see Table 2.7–2).

Treatment

- Identify and treat the underlying disease.
- If iron-deficiency anemia is the cause, identify the site of blood loss or reason for poor intake and replace with oral iron supplements. **Suspect colorectal cancer in an elderly male patient with anemia.**
- Treat B_{12} deficiency with monthly B_{12} shots.
- Exogenous erythropoietin is indicated for patients with anemia due to chronic renal disease and may be used to treat anemia of chronic disease.
- Transfusions are indicated for patients with severe symptoms or worsening status and may be used to suppress abnormal Hb production in patients with sickle cell disease (SCD). A lower threshold for transfusion is used in patients with CAD, as anemia may provoke or worsen cardiac ischemia.

G6PD DEFICIENCY

An **X-linked recessive** disease in which deficient or unstable G6PD causes episodic hemolytic anemia. African-American and Mediterranean men are most often affected.

> **Causes of microcytic anemia—**
>
> **TICS**
> **T**halassemia
> **I**ron deficiency
> **C**hronic disease
> **S**ideroblastic anemia

Serum Fe = iron available for heme production.

TIBC = amount of protein not bound to iron.

Serum ferritin = Fe-protein complex that regulates iron stores and transport.

Indirect Coombs'—tests for antibodies to RBCs in the patient's serum.

Direct Coombs'—tests for sensitized erythrocytes.

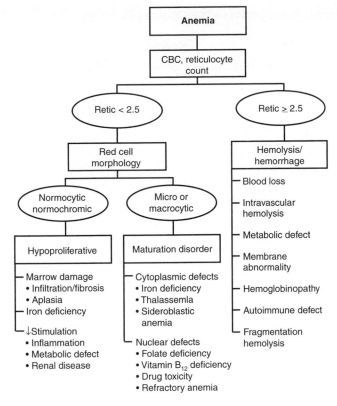

FIGURE 2.7–1. Classification of anemia. Reprinted, with permission, from Braunwald E et al. *Harrison's Principles of Internal Medicine,* 15th ed. New York: McGraw-Hill, 2001:352.

History/PE

Usually asymptomatic, but may present as an acute, self-limited hemolytic anemia (e.g., fatigue, **jaundice, dark urine**). Hemolysis results from RBC oxidative stress due to viral or bacterial infection, metabolic acidosis, or exposure to **fava beans, antimalarials,** dapsone, sulfonamides, or nitrofurantoin. Patients may cite a family history of similar presentations.

Most macrocytic anemias are caused by processes that interfere with normal DNA synthesis and replication.

Iron-deficiency anemia in an elderly patient is colorectal cancer until proven otherwise.

TABLE 2.7–1. Iron Studies in Patients with Microcytic Anemia

	Serum Fe	TIBC (transferrin)	Serum Ferritin	Other
Iron deficiency	↓	↑	↓	Look for blood loss.
Anemia of chronic disease	↓	↓	Normal/↑	May be normocytic.
Sideroblastic anemia	↑	Normal/↑	↑	Give pyridoxine (B$_6$) to see if responsive.
Thalassemia	Normal/↑	Normal/↑	Normal/↑	Check HbA$_2$, HbF levels.

The classic case of G6PD deficiency is an African-American male soldier in Vietnam who took quinine.

Evaluation

During hemolytic episodes, look for a low HCT, a high reticulocyte count, high indirect bilirubin, low serum haptoglobin, and **Heinz bodies** and spherocytes on blood smear. A quantitative G6PD enzyme test is diagnostic but may yield a false negative result during or shortly after a hemolytic episode (as most G6PD-deficient RBCs will be hemolyzed at this time, leaving young RBCs/neocytes with normal enzyme activity).

Treatment

Symptoms are usually self-limited. Patients should avoid exposure to drugs that cause hemolytic episodes. Transfuse RBCs if anemia is severe.

MICROANGIOPATHIC HEMOLYTIC ANEMIAS

Pentad of TTP—

FAT RN
Fever
Anemia
Thrombocytopenia
Renal dysfunction
Neurologic abnormalities

A group of disorders—including thrombotic thrombocytopenic purpura (TTP), hemolytic-uremic syndrome (HUS), and disseminated intravascular coagulation (DIC)—in which a coagulopathy is associated with a platelet deficiency and RBC hemolysis. The disorders are summarized in Table 2.7–3.

TABLE 2.7–2. Blood Cell Morphologies and Associated Diseases

Cell Type	Associated Disease
Spherocytes	G6PD deficiency, membranopathy (immune and nonimmune)
Blister cell	G6PD deficiency
Burr cell	Acute renal failure (ARF), uremia
Heinz body	Thalassemia, hemoglobinopathies, and enzymopathies (G6PD deficiency) as well as post-splenectomy
Schistocyte	Artificial heart valves and microangiopathic hemolytic anemias
Target cell	Splenectomy

In DIC, activation of the clotting cascade leads to increased PT and PTT, but in TTP and HUS, platelet aggregation plays a larger role and PT and PTT are often normal.

TABLE 2.7–3. Microangiopathic Hemolytic Anemias

Disease	Causes	Manifestations	Laboratory Findings	Treatment
HUS	Mild viral illness or gastroenteritis with *Escherichia coli* **0157:H7.**	**Triad** of anemia, thrombocytopenia (TCP), and ARF.	Anemia, TCP; as with TTP, PT/PTT are often normal.	Dialysis for ARF.
TTP *(IM1.54)*	HIV infection, pregnancy, OCP use, individuals < 50 years of age.	**Pentad** of fever, anemia/ splenomegaly, TCP, ARF, and neurologic abnormalities.	Anemia, TCP, **schistocytes,** increased indirect bilirubin, increased LDH, negative Coombs' test, hyaline thrombi in small vessels without inflammatory changes.	Large-volume **plasmapheresis,** corticosteroids, ASA, splenectomy.
DIC *(IM1.47)*	Sepsis, transfusion reaction, neoplasia, trauma, obstetric complications (e.g., amniotic embolus, septic abortion).	Bleeding from venipuncture sites, epistaxis, hematemesis, digital gangrene, hypotension.	Anemia, TCP, ↑ **PT/ PTT,** ↑ **bleeding time,** ↑ **d-dimer,** ↑ **fibrin split products,** ↓ **fibrinogen.**	Treat the underlying condition; transfuse with **platelets and cryoprecipitate.**

SICKLE CELL DISEASE

An autosomal-recessive disease resulting from substitution of valine for glutamic acid at the sixth position in the globin chain. SCD carriers are asymptomatic and common (8% of African-Americans). In the United States, most SCD patients are identified during neonatal screening. Homozygous patients suffer from various crises most commonly precipitated by infection, dehydration, and hypoxia.

- **Aplastic crisis:** Often due to **parvovirus B19** infection.
- **Hemolytic crisis:** Associated with G6PD deficiency.
- **Pain crisis:** Also associated with bone and lung pain due to vaso-occlusion or infarction.
- **Sequestration crisis:** RBCs pool in the spleen and may result in shock and death.
- **Splenic crisis:** Autoinfarction of the spleen increases the risk of osteomyelitis and infections by encapsulated organisms, including *Streptococcus pneumoniae, Haemophilus influenzae, and Neisseria meningitides*.

Treatment

- **Hydration** and O_2 to decrease the amount of RBC sickling.
- Analgesia.

SCD = qualitative defect in the β-globin chain.

Thalassemia = reduced quantity of an α- or β-globin chain.

Porphyria = defect in heme synthesis.

HIGH-YIELD FACTS

Hematology/Oncology

Sickle cell crises are precipitated by infection, dehydration, and hypoxia.

- RBC transfusions for severe anemia and attacks of acute chest syndrome with respiratory distress.
- Long-term **hydroxyurea** to increase (PPV23) HbF production and decrease symptoms.
- 23-valent pneumococcal vaccine to protect against pneumococcal sepsis.
- Prophylactic penicillin for children < 5 years old.
- Antibiotics during acute chest syndrome, as patients often have respiratory infections.

UCV *Peds.21, EM.23*

THALASSEMIA

A group of disorders resulting from reduced synthesis of α- or β-globin protein subunits.

- **α-thalassemia:** Most common in Asians and African-Americans. The severity of the disease depends on the number of affected α-globin alleles. If **all four** α alleles are affected, the baby is stillborn with **hydrops fetalis** or dies shortly after birth. If three alleles are affected, unstable β4 Hb (called HbH in adults) forms; manifestations include **chronic hemolytic anemia** and **splenomegaly.** Carriers of one or two α-globin allele mutations are usually asymptomatic.
- **β-thalassemia:** Most common in people of Mediterranean origin, Asians, and African-Americans. There are only two alleles for β-globin production. **Thalassemia major (Cooley's anemia,** homozygote, no β-globin production) presents in the first year of life as the fraction of HbF declines. By six months, HbF has dropped from 75% to 5% of total Hb. Manifestations include growth retardation, **bony deformities,** hepatosplenomegaly, and jaundice.

Treatment

Use deferoxamine to prevent iron overload complications in thalassemia patients.

Treatment includes transfusions, splenectomy, folic acid, and bone marrow transplant. Subcutaneous **deferoxamine** increases urinary excretion of iron and decreases iron toxicity, the most serious complication of which is cardiac toxicity.

POLYCYTHEMIA VERA (PCV)

A **myeloproliferative disease** marked by increased production of RBCs. Individuals > 60 years old are at highest risk, and males are affected more frequently than females. The most common cause of erythrocytosis is **chronic hypoxia** secondary to lung disease rather than primary PCV. Patients present with malaise, fever, **pruritus (especially after a warm shower),** and signs of vascular sludging (e.g., stroke, angina, MI, claudication, hepatic vein thrombosis, headache, blurred vision). Exam might reveal **plethora,** large retinal veins on funduscopy, and **splenomegaly.** Assessment should include O_2 saturation (normal), **HCT** (> 50%), **RBC mass** (increased), and **erythropoietin level** (decreased). WBCs and platelets are normal or increased; basophilia is associated with the proliferative myelopoiesis. A peripheral blood smear shows normal RBCs; bone marrow biopsy shows hypercellular marrow. Sec-

ondary polycythemia due to hypoxia is associated with elevated erythropoietin. An erythropoietin-producing cyst or mass (e.g., renal cell carcinoma) is associated with elevated erythropoietin and a lack of hypoxia. Treatment includes **serial phlebotomy** to decrease HCT and diminish the risk of vascular accidents from sludging. **Daily ASA** can prevent thrombotic complications; anagrelide can lower platelets. Myelosuppressive agents (e.g., hydroxyurea) may be used if necessary. PCV is associated with an increased **risk of conversion** to chronic myelogenous leukemia (CML), myelofibrosis, or acute myelogenous leukemia (AML).

TRANSFUSION REACTIONS

Acute hemolysis during RBC transfusions occurs as a result of preformed recipient antibodies causing lysis of donor RBCs. Causes include **ABO incompatibilities due to clerical errors (most common),** mislabeled specimens, or reactions to antigens not commonly tested. Patients with **IgA deficiency** who are sensitized to this class of antibodies may have an anaphylactic reaction during plasma transfusions. Although rare, viruses can be transmitted through blood transfusions, including HBV, HCV, HIV, HTLV-1 and -2, and CMV.

History/PE

Hypotension, tachypnea, tachycardia, fevers, chills, hemoglobinuria, chest pain, and discomfort begin shortly after transfusion is administered.

Differential

Leukoagglutination reaction, anaphylaxis, gram-negative bacterial contamination, MI, selective IgA deficiency producing anaphylaxis on subsequent blood transfusions.

Treatment

Stop the transfusion, retype the patient's blood against that of the donor to confirm the diagnosis, culture blood, and check DIC labs (D-dimer, PT, PTT). Assess for free Hb in the blood and urine. Administer **IV fluids** and **mannitol** in efforts to prevent oliguric renal failure. Additional treatment is organ-dependent.

Hemoglobinuria may lead to acute tubular necrosis and subsequent renal failure.

COAGULATION DISORDERS

HEMOPHILIAS

X-linked recessive coagulopathies due to decreased **factor VIII** (hemophilia A) or **factor IX** (hemophilia B).

History/PE

Patients present with soft tissue hemorrhage, including **hemarthroses,** intramuscular bleeding, GI bleeding, and excessive bleeding from **mild trauma** and **surgical/dental procedures.**

The classic case of hemophilia is the boy (X-linked) from the Imperial Russian family (recessive) who presents with hemarthroses following minimal or no trauma.

Evaluation

Table 2.7–4 presents the coagulation study results for various coagulopathies. Heparin can also increase PTT.

Treatment

Factor VIII (hemophilia A) or factor IX (hemophilia B) concentrate should be given if needed during bleeding episodes and as prophylaxis before surgical/dental procedures. In mild hemophilia A, **desmopressin** may be administered before minor surgical procedures to increase endogenous factor VIII activity.

UCV *Peds.18*

IDIOPATHIC THROMBOCYTOPENIC PURPURA (ITP)

An **autoimmune** platelet disorder that includes pediatric (postviral, self-limited) and adult (chronic) forms. Females are affected twice as often as males, and individuals < 50 years of age are at greatest risk. **Evans' syndrome** is ITP with autoimmune hemolytic anemia. ITP may be associated with Hodgkin's and non-Hodgkin's lymphoma (NHL), chronic lymphocytic leukemia (CLL), HIV, systemic lupus erythematosus (SLE), and rheumatoid arthritis (RA).

History/PE

Unlike TTP, patients are **afebrile** and **splenomegaly is absent.** Exam reveals **petechiae, purpura,** ecchymoses, mucosal bleeding (epistaxis, oral bleeding, menorrhagia), and oral hemorrhagic bullae.

Differential

CLL, low-grade lymphoma myelodysplastic syndromes, SLE, drug side effects (e.g., ranitidine), TTP, DIC, alcoholism, HIV, aplastic anemia.

Evaluation

CBC shows very low platelets, possibly with anemia. A normal PT and PTT, prolonged bleeding time, a normal DIC panel, and a **positive platelet-associated IgG test** may be present. A peripheral blood smear will show megathrombocytes **without schistocytes;** bone marrow aspiration will show either normal or increased megakaryocytes.

TABLE 2.7–4. Lab Findings with Various Bleeding Disorders

Disease	PT	PTT	Bleeding Time	Platelets	Ristocetin Cofactor Assay
von Willebrand's	Normal	Normal/↑	↑	Normal	Normal/↓
Hemophilia A/B	Normal	↑	Normal	Normal	Normal
DIC	↑	↑	↑	↓	Normal

Treatment

The condition will resolve spontaneously in most pediatric patients. Most adults are initially treated with corticosteroids. Platelets should be given for severe, uncontrollable bleeding. **IVIG** and **anti-Rho(D)** (for Rh-positive patients) are given for life-threatening hemorrhage or for severe TCP (< 10,000/μL). **Splenectomy** provides effective treatment for two-thirds of patients who are refractory to medical treatment. Treatment with steroids may mask a leukemia that is masquerading as ITP, so consider bone marrow aspiration before treatment.

> **P**etechiae suggest
> **P**latelet deficiency.
> Bleeding into body

> **C**avities or joints
> suggest
> **C**lotting factor
> deficiency.

VON WILLEBRAND'S DISEASE

An **autosomal-dominant** condition resulting in deficient or defective von Willebrand's factor (vWF), von Willebrand's disease is the **most common inherited bleeding disorder.** It is characterized by **decreased platelet adhesion** with a concurrent deficiency of **factor VIII.** Patients present with **easy bruising, mucosal bleeding** (e.g., epistaxis, oral bleeding, menorrhagia, GI bleeding), and postincisional bleeding. The decreased platelet function is usually not sufficiently severe to produce petechiae. Symptoms worsen with ASA use. Suspect this diagnosis in a woman with **heavy menstrual bleeding,** especially if she has a family history of bleeding disorder. Platelet number is normal, PT is usually normal, and PTT may be either normal or increased owing to a deficiency of factor VIII (see Table 2.7–4). Treatment includes desmopressin for mild disease, OCPs for menorrhagia, and FFP or cryoprecipitate for major bleeding. ASA and ASA-containing products should be avoided. Transfusions should be minimized to decrease the risk of transmitted viral infections.

Ristocetin cofactor assay measures the ability of vWF to agglutinate platelets, in vitro, in the presence of ristocetin.

ASA increases the risk of bleeding in patients with von Willebrand's disease.

UCV *Peds.22*

HYPERCOAGULABLE STATES

A group of conditions that predispose patients to **thromboembolic disease,** including **DVTs, pulmonary emboli,** and **CVAs.** Patients often present with venous thrombosis or recurrent thromboembolism in adolescence or early adult life. The major causes of hypercoagulable states are listed in Table 2.7–5. **Factor V Leiden is the most common inherited hypercoagulable disorder.**

Suspect pulmonary embolism in a patient with rapid onset of hypoxia, hypocapnia, and an increased A-a gradient without another obvious explanation.

HEMATOLOGIC NEOPLASMS

LEUKEMIAS

Malignant proliferations of hematopoietic cells; leukemias are the **most common cancer in children.** Categorization is based on cellular origin (promyeloid, myeloid, lymphoid) and on the level of differentiation of neoplastic cells. **Acute leukemias** are proliferations of minimally differentiated blast cells, whereas **chronic leukemias** are proliferations of more mature, differentiated cells. **Lymphocytic leukemias** are neoplasms of lymphoid cells (e.g., B- and T-lymphocytes). **Myelogenous leukemias** are neoplasms of myeloid cells (e.g., granulocytes, monocytes, platelets, and erythrocytes). Tumor invasion of the bone marrow results in pancytopenia. Thus, the major complications of end-stage leukemia are **bleeding** (from TCP), **infection** (from leukopenia), and **anemia.**

TABLE 2.7–5. Causes of Hypercoagulable States

Inherited	Acquired
Factor V Leiden mutation	Prolonged bed rest or immobilization
Protein C or S deficiency	MI
Antithrombin III deficiency	Tissue damage (surgery, fracture)
Homocystinemia	DIC
Fibrinolysis defects	Hyperlipidemia
	Vasculitis
	Multiple myeloma
	Lupus anticoagulant (anti-phospholipid syndrome)
	Nephrotic syndrome
	Smoking
	Cancer
	Warfarin (on initiation of therapy)
	OCPs
	Pregnancy

Factor V Leiden mutation is the most common inherited cause of a hypercoagulable state and causes activated protein C resistance.

ACUTE LYMPHOCYTIC LEUKEMIA

Most common in children; whites are affected more frequently than blacks.

History/PE

Children may present with limp, refusal to walk, **bone pain,** easy bruising, and **fever.** Exam may reveal pallor, widespread **petechiae/purpura,** adenopathy, **hepatosplenomegaly,** multiple ecchymoses, and bleeding.

Differential

Aplastic anemia, mononucleosis or other viral infection, rheumatic disease, ITP, TTP, other neoplasms.

Evaluation

Look for depression of bone marrow elements (e.g., anemia, TCP), **elevated LDH and uric acid,** and cytogenetic changes (CALLA +, TdT +). Diagnosis is based on bone marrow aspirate. Obtain a CXR, LP, and CT scan to rule out mediastinal involvement and brain metastasis.

Treatment

Eighty-five percent of children with ALL achieve complete remission with chemotherapy.

There is a **good prognosis** with **chemotherapy:** 99% of children achieve complete remission and 80% achieve long-term leukemia-free survival. For adults, these numbers are 80% and 30%, respectively.

UCV *Peds.16*

Acute Myelogenous Leukemia

Affects children and adults, with the incidence of the adult form increasing with age. AML is subdivided into eight different types based on the neoplastic cell type and cytogenetics.

History/PE

Adults present with **fatigue, easy bruising, dyspnea due to anemia,** fever, skin disease (leukemia cutis), CNS symptoms, and a history of **frequent infections.** AML M3 may present with **DIC;** AML M5 may present with **gingival hyperplasia** and CNS involvement. Exam will show fever, lethargy, bleeding, **petechiae/purpura,** and hepatosplenomegaly.

Evaluation

In addition to increased myelocytic cell lines, there is **decreased leukocyte alkaline phosphatase (LAP). Auer rods** and **myeloperoxidase** may be present and are diagnostic for AML.

Differential

CML, myelodysplastic syndromes, lymphoma, hairy cell leukemia, mononucleosis, leukemoid reaction. Leukemoid reactions due to infection, stress, chronic inflammation, and certain neoplasms can cause WBC counts of 40,000–100,000 cells/μL but lack the cytogenetic changes and decreased LAP seen with AML and CML.

Leukemoid reactions can cause elevated WBC counts without decreased LAP.

Treatment

Treat with multiagent **chemotherapy,** transfusions, antibiotics as needed, and allogeneic/autogeneic **bone marrow transplant (BMT). Retinoic acid** may induce remission of the promyelocytic form (AML M3). The prognosis depends on subtype, but generally 70–80% of adults < 60 years of age achieve complete remission. **Neutropenic fever,** defined as fever in patients with a neutrophil count < 500 cells/μL, is treated with broad-spectrum antibiotics and antifungals to protect against infections by normal flora. As with NHL, treatment of acute leukemia may be complicated by **tumor lysis syndrome.**

UCV *IM1.41*

Chronic Lymphocytic Leukemia

Primarily affects patients > **65 years old.** CLL is slowly progressive and is associated with good short-term but poor long-term survival.

History/PE

Lymphadenopathy, fatigue, and hepatosplenomegaly may be present on exam. This is usually an **indolent disease,** and many patients are diagnosed by incidental lymphocytosis.

Differential

Viral disease, other leukemias, myelodysplastic disorders.

Evaluation

Isolated lymphocytosis on CBC (HCT and platelets are often normal on presentation). Bone marrow will be infiltrated with lymphocytes. Aberrant CD5+ expression is characteristic, and **smudge cells** may be present on peripheral smear.

Treatment

CLL may be complicated by autoimmune hemolytic anemia.

Most patients are **managed supportively.** Treatment with chemotherapy (e.g., chlorambucil, fludarabine) may be instituted when patients develop fatigue, lymphadenopathy, anemia, or TCP. Splenectomy and steroids are used to treat associated autoimmune hemolytic anemia and TCP.

UCV *IM1.45*

CHRONIC MYELOGENOUS LEUKEMIA

An overproduction of myeloid cells, CML is often stable for several years until it transforms into an overtly malignant form known as a **blast crisis.** CML is associated with prior radiation exposure and most commonly affects people 40–60 years old.

History/PE

In its early stages, CML is asymptomatic or presents with mild, nonspecific symptoms (**fatigue, fever, malaise,** decreased exercise tolerance, weight loss, night sweats). At a later stage, patients present with early satiety and LUQ fullness due to massive **splenomegaly** as well as bleeding due to TCP. All patients eventually suffer from blast crisis with progressive pancytopenia and disseminated disease. **Blast crisis** presents as fever, bone pain, weight loss, and increasing **splenomegaly.**

Evaluation

The presence of the Philadelphia chromosome (t[9,22]) is diagnostic for CML.

Peripheral smear reveals a very high WBC count (median of 150,000 cells/μL at the time of diagnosis) and prominent myeloid cells with basophilia. **LAP is low;** vitamin B_{12} levels are often markedly elevated. Definitive diagnosis is based on cytogenetics that reveal the **Philadelphia chromosome (bcr-abl gene fusion product** from a **9,22 translocation**) in most patients.

Treatment

CML is associated with a poor prognosis, exhibiting a median survival of 3–4 years. Treatment in the chronic phase is palliative; myelosuppressive agents such as α-interferon and hydroxyurea are used. Imatinib mesylate (Gleevec) is therapy directed at the molecular lesion of CML. Although its long-term efficacy is unknown at this time, it is highly effective, rapidly producing hematologic and even cytogenetic remission. **Allogeneic BMT** is curative in roughly 60% of cases, but successfully treated patients often suffer from graft-versus-host disease. Blast crisis is difficult to treat and is rapidly fatal in most patients.

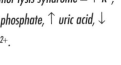 UCV _IM1.46_

LYMPHOMAS

Neoplasms of cells from lymphoid tissue (e.g., lymphocytes, histiocytes, and their precursors and derivatives). Despite the name, all of these disorders are malignant. Hodgkin's lymphomas are distinguished from NHLs by the presence of **Reed-Sternberg giant cells** (see Figure 2.7–2) and by a large number of non-neoplastic inflammatory cells seen on biopsy. Other differences are summarized in Table 2.7–6. The treatment of **high-grade NHL** may be complicated by **tumor lysis syndrome,** in which rapid tumor cell death releases intracellular contents, leading to **hyperkalemia, hyperphosphatemia, hyperuricemia, and hypocalcemia.**

Tumor lysis syndrome = ↑ *K^+,* ↑ *phosphate,* ↑ *uric acid,* ↓ *Ca^{2+}.*

MULTIPLE MYELOMA

A malignancy of **plasma cells** resulting from the expansion of cells within bone marrow, often with unbalanced, excessive production of immunoglobulin heavy/light chain. Radiation, chemical exposure, and monoclonal gammopathy of undetermined significance (MGUS) are risk factors. Patients > 50 years old are most commonly affected; blacks are affected more frequently than whites.

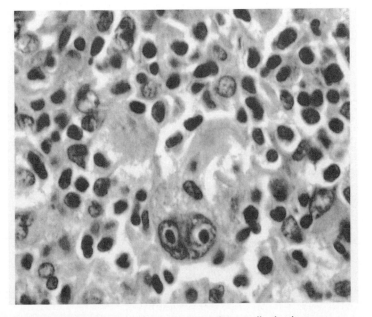

FIGURE 2.7–2. Reed-Sternberg cells. Binucleate Reed-Sternberg cells displaying prominent inclusion-like nucleoli surrounded by lymphocytes. The Reed-Sternberg cell is a necessary but insufficient pathologic finding for the diagnosis of Hodgkin's disease. (Reprinted, with permission, from Bhushan V. *First Aid for the USMLE Step 1.* New York: McGraw-Hill, 1999:266.)

History/PE

The CBC of a patient with multiple myeloma often shows anemia but rarely shows plasmacytosis.

Symptoms include **back pain, hypercalcemic symptoms** ("stones, bones, abdominal moans, and psychiatric overtones"), **pathologic fractures,** fatigue, and frequent infections (secondary to dysregulation of antibody production). Exam may reveal pallor, fever, bone tenderness, bone deformities, and lethargy.

Differential

Because multiple myeloma is an osteoclastic process, a bone scan, which detects osteoblastic activity, may be negative, but plain bone films may show lytic disease or osteoporosis.

MGUS, Waldenström's macroglobulinemia (plasma cell proliferation in which **IgM** is produced), primary amyloidosis, metastatic carcinoma, lymphoma, hyperparathyroidism.

Evaluation

Serum and urine protein electrophoresis (monoclonal gammopathy, most commonly **IgG**), **Bence Jones proteinuria,** CBC (anemia, TCP), peripheral smear (rarely plasmacytosis), electrolytes (decreased anion gap), **full-body skeletal survey** (x-rays showing **punched-out osteolytic lesions** of the skull and long bones), bone scan (negative, as this is an osteoclastic process), and bone marrow biopsy **(plasma cell infiltrate).** Staging is based on the degree of anemia, elevated calcium, x-ray findings, and renal dysfunction.

TABLE 2.7–6. Non-Hodgkin's and Hodgkin's Lymphomas

	Non-Hodgkin's	Hodgkin's
Risk factors	EBV (Burkitt's), HIV, most commonly 7–11 years old.	EBV, bimodal age distribution → 15–45 years old or > 60 years old.
Histology	Varies.	**Reed-Sternberg cells.**
Distribution	**Noncontiguous** lymph node spread.	**Contiguous** lymph node spread.
Variants	Many; separated into low, intermediate, and high grade.	Nodular sclerosis (young females), mixed cellularity, lymphocyte-predominant (most common), or lymphocyte-depleted.
History	Painless adenopathy, B symptoms.[a]	Painless adenopathy, B symptoms, pruritus.
PE	**Systemic** adenopathy, hepatosplenomegaly.	**Regional** adenopathy, hepatosplenomegaly.
Differential	Hodgkin's lymphoma, mononucleosis, cat scratch disease, HIV, sarcoid.	Non-Hodgkin's lymphoma, HIV, sarcoid, lymphadenitis, drug reaction.
Evaluation	**Biopsy** for diagnosis, CXR, whole body CT; consider bone marrow biopsy and LP.	**Biopsy** largest node for diagnosis, then CXR; consider bone marrow biopsy and LP.
Staging	Based on number of nodes, whether disease crosses diaphragm, and B symptoms.	Same.
Treatment	Radiation and chemotherapy (CHOP).[b]	Radiation for localized disease; chemotherapy for advanced/widespread disease (ABVD or MOPP).[c]

[a]B symptoms are defined as fever > 38.5°C, night sweats, or 10% weight loss over six months.
[b]CHOP = Cytoxan, adriamycin, Oncovin (vincristine), and prednisone.
[c]ABVD = adriamycin, bleomycin, vincristine, and dacarbazine. MOPP = mechlorethamine, Oncovin (vincristine), procarbazine, and prednisone.

Treatment

- Multiagent **chemotherapy,** including alkylating agents, melphalan, and prednisone.
- Consider stem cell BMT.
- Fractures may require intramedullary fixation.
- Disease usually recurs and carries a poor prognosis.
- Complications include anemia, infection, neurologic disease, and renal failure.

UCV *IM1.50*

TRANSPLANT MEDICINE

Although current immunosuppressive regimens have decreased the risk of transplant rejection, hyperacute, acute, and chronic rejection must be identified and treated to decrease transplantation-associated morbidity and mortality. Forms include:

- **Hyperacute:** Immediate vascular thrombi from **preformed antibodies.** The organ may show signs of ischemia before completion of the operation. Prevent by **checking ABO compatibility** and giving lymphocytotoxic agents.
- **Acute:** Occurs between five days and three months. Can see increased GGT, alkaline phosphatase, and bilirubin in liver rejection or increased BUN and Cr in kidney rejection. Confirm with biopsy. Treat with steroids and antilymphocyte antibodies (OKT3).
- **Chronic:** Irreversible, gradual loss of organ function occurring months to years after transplant. There is no treatment, but perform biopsy to rule out a late, treatable acute reaction.

Questions 1 and 2: Reproduced, with permission, from Berk SL, *PreTest: Medicine*, 9th ed., New York: McGraw-Hill, 2001.
Questions 3 and 4: Reproduced, with permission, from Reteguiz J, *PreTest: Physical Diagnosis*, 4th ed., New York: McGraw-Hill, 2001.

Questions

1. A 52-year-old man presents with a painless neck mass. He states that after he drinks one to two glasses of wine, the neck mass becomes painful. He also complains of intermittent fever, night sweats, pruritus, and a 10-lb weight loss over the last month. On physical examination he has a 3-cm mass in the left anterior cervical lymph node chain that is hard and tender to deep palpation. Several other cervical nodes and a left axillary node are palpable. The liver is enlarged but there is no splenomegaly. Which of the following is the most likely diagnosis?
   a. Non-Hodgkin's lymphoma
   b. Hodgkin's lymphoma
   c. Mononucleosis
   d. Hairy cell leukemia
   e. Sarcoidosis

2. A 62-year-old man presents for his annual health maintenance visit. The review of systems is positive for occasional fatigue and headache. The patient admits to generalized pruritus following a warm bath or shower. He has plethora and engorgement of the retinal veins. A spleen is palpated on abdominal examination. The patient's hematocrit is 63%, and he has a leukocytosis and thrombocytosis. Peripheral blood smear is normal. The patient does not smoke. Which of the following is the most likely diagnosis?
   a. Spurious polycythemia
   b. Essential thrombocytosis
   c. Myelofibrosis
   d. Polycythemia vera
   e. Secondary polycythemia
   f. Chronic myeloid leukemia
   g. Erythropoietin-secreting renal tumor

3. A 42-year-old woman of Italian descent presents for a preemployment physical examination. She has no past medical problems and takes no medications. Her physical examination is normal except for pale conjunctiva. Fecal occult blood test (FOBT) is negative. Her CBC is remarkable for a hemoglobin of 11.4 g/dL, a mean corpuscular volume (MCV) of 60 fL, and a reticulocyte count of 0.6%. Her white blood cell count and platelets are normal. The peripheral smear reveals microcytosis, hypochromia, acanthocytes (cells with irregularly spaced projections), and occasional target cells. Which of the following is the most likely diagnosis?
   a. Iron-deficiency anemia
   b. Sideroblastic anemia
   c. Anemia of chronic disease
   d. Thalassemia trait
   e. Hemolytic anemia

4. A 32-year-old woman presents with the recent onset of petechiae on her lower extremities. She denies menorrhagia and gastrointestinal bleeding. She has no family history of a bleeding disorder and has been in excellent health her entire life. Physical examination is remarkable for petechiae of both legs. There is no hepatosplenomegaly. The rest of the physical examination is normal. Platelet count is 8000 cells/µL. Hemoglobin and white blood cell count are normal. Peripheral smear reveals reduced platelets and an occasional megathrombocyte. Which of the following is the most likely diagnosis?

   a. Thrombotic thrombocytopenic purpura (TTP)
   b. Hemolytic-uremic syndrome (HUS)
   c. Evans syndrome
   d. Disseminated intravascular coagulation (DIC)
   e. Idiopathic thrombocytopenic purpura (ITP)
   f. Henoch-Schönlein purpura (HSP)

1. **The answer is b.** Patients with **Hodgkin's lymphoma** often present with painless regional lymphadenopathy and the constitutional symptoms of fever, drenching night sweats, and weight loss. Occasionally, patients may present with pruritus or pain in an involved lymph node after ingestion of alcohol. There is a bimodal age distribution with one peak in the twenties and a second peak at over age 50. The diagnosis of Hodgkin's disease is made by lymph node biopsy with the finding of **Reed-Sternberg cells ("owl eyes")**. Patients with non-Hodgkin's lymphoma (a group of cancers variable in presentation and course) often present with disseminated disease such as systemic adenopathy. Patients with hairy cell leukemia present with pancytopenia, massive splenomegaly, and hairy cells on peripheral blood smear.

2. **The answer is d.** The patient most likely has **polycythemia vera.** This is an acquired myeloproliferative disorder characterized by a primary erythrocytosis, but there is overproduction of all three cell lines. Hematocrits are > 54% in males and > 51% in females. Patients present with symptoms related to an increase in blood volume and viscosity. Pruritus after a warm bath or shower is due to histamine release by basophils. Splenomegaly exists in virtually every patient with polycythemia vera. The treatment of choice for polycythemia vera is phlebotomy. **Spurious polycythemia** or **Gaisböck syndrome** is due to a contracted plasma volume (diuretic use); **secondary polycythemia** may be due to smoking, high altitudes, cardiac or pulmonary disease, and erythropoietin-secreting cysts or tumors. Patients with chronic myelogenous leukemia (CML) typically have a leukocytosis and the Philadelphia chromosome. Patients with **essential thrombocythemia** have platelet counts > 2 million/μL. Patients with **myelofibrosis** have splenomegaly, dry bone marrow taps, and peripheral blood smears showing abnormal and bizarre morphologies and immature forms.

3. **The answer is d.** The differential diagnosis for microcytic hypochromic anemia is **TICS** (**T**halassemia, **I**ron deficiency, **C**hronic disease, and **S**ideroblastic). This patient of Mediterranean descent most likely has thalassemia trait. **Thalassemia** generally produces a greater degree of microcytosis for any given level of anemia than does iron deficiency. **Target cells** are seen in this disorder, but these are also seen in lead poisoning, liver disease, hyposplenism, and hemoglobin C disease. The most common cause of a microcytic anemia is iron deficiency, but this is unlikely in this asymptomatic patient with a negative FOBT. The MCV in anemia of chronic disease is usually normal or slightly reduced, and patients typically have a history of chronic infection or inflammation, cancer, or liver disease. Alcoholics, patients taking antituberculosis medication or chloramphenicol, or those with lead poisoning may develop sideroblastic anemia (a failure to incorporate heme into protoporphyrin). Bone marrow staining will demonstrate iron deposits **(ringed sideroblasts)** encircling the nucleus in siderocytes. Coarse **basophilic stippling** of the red blood cells on peripheral smear would be characteristic of lead poisoning.

4. **The answer is e.** Idiopathic thrombocytopenic purpura **(ITP)** is an autoimmune disorder in which an IgG autoantibody binds to platelets. Destruction of the platelets takes place in the spleen, where macrophages bind to the antibody-coated platelets. Fifty percent of patients with ITP have no associated disease, but HIV infection, SLE, or a lymphoproliferative disorder should be considered. ITP is a disease of persons between the ages of 20 and 50 years and occurs in women more than men. There is no splenomegaly in ITP. The diagnosis is one of exclusion, but often megathrombocytes are seen on peripheral smear.

Infectious Disease

Time course of HIV infection

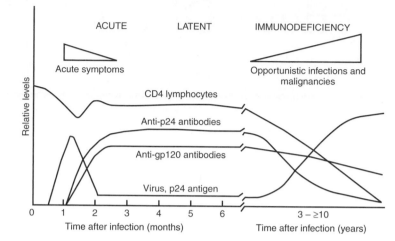

(Adapted, with permission, from Levinson W, Jawetz E. *Medical Microbiology and Immunology: Examination and Board Review*, 6th ed. New York: McGraw-Hill, 2000:276.)

Opportunistic fungal infections

Candida albicans	Thrush in immunocompromised (neonates, steroids, diabetes, AIDS), vulvovaginitis (high pH, diabetes, use of antibiotics), disseminated candidiasis (to any organ), chronic mucocutaneous candidiasis.
Aspergillus fumigatus	Allergic bronchopulmonary aspergillosis, lung cavity aspergilloma ("fungus ball"), invasive aspergillosis. **Mold** with septate hyphae that branch at a V-shaped (45°) angle. Not dimorphic.
Cryptococcus neoformans	Cryptococcal meningitis, cryptococcosis. Heavily encapsulated **yeast.** Not dimorphic. Found in soil, pigeon droppings. Culture on Sabouraud's agar. Stains with India ink. Latex agglutination test detects polysaccharide capsular antigen.
Mucor and *Rhizopus* species	Mucormycosis. **Mold** with irregular nonseptate hyphae branching at wide angles (≥ 90°). Disease mostly in ketoacidotic diabetic and leukemic patients. Fungi also proliferate in the walls of blood vessels and cause infarction of distal tissue.

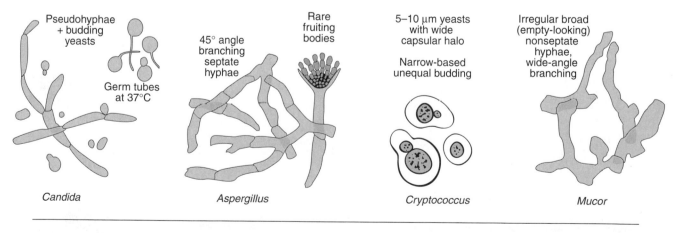

Opportunistic infections in AIDS

Bacterial	Tuberculosis, *Mycobacterium avium–intracellulare* complex.
Viral	Herpes simplex, varicella-zoster virus, cytomegalovirus, progressive multifocal leukoencephalopathy (JC virus).
Fungal	Thrush (*Candida albicans*), cryptococcosis (cryptococcal meningitis), histoplasmosis, *Pneumocystis* pneumonia.
Protozoan	Toxoplasmosis, cryptosporidiosis.

Common causes of pneumonia

Children (6 wks–18 yr) →	Adults (18–40 yr) →	Adults (40–65 yr) →	Elderly
Viruses (RSV)	Mycoplasma	S. pneumoniae	S. pneumoniae
Mycoplasma	C. pneumoniae	H. influenzae	Viruses
Chlamydia pneumoniae	S. pneumoniae	Anaerobes	Anaerobes
Streptococcus pneumoniae		Viruses	H. influenzae
		Mycoplasma	Gram-negative rods

Special groups:

Nosocomial (hospital acquired)	*Staphylococcus*, gram-negative rods
Immunocompromised	*Staphylococcus*, gram-negative rods, fungi, viruses, *Pneumocystis carinii*—with HIV
Aspiration	Anaerobes
Alcoholic/IV drug user	*S. pneumoniae, Klebsiella, Staphylococcus*
Postviral	*Staphylococcus, H. influenzae*
Neonate	Group B streptococci, *E. coli*
Atypical	*Mycoplasma, Legionella, Chlamydia*

Encapsulated bacteria

Examples are *Streptococcus pneumoniae* (pneumococcus), *Haemophilus influenzae* (especially b serotype), *Neisseria meningitidis* (meningococcus), and *Klebsiella pneumoniae*.

Polysaccharide capsule is an antiphagocytic virulence factor.

Positive **Quellung** reaction: If encapsulated bug is present, capsule **swells** when specific anticapsular antisera are added.

IgG_2 necessary for immune response. Capsule serves as antigen in vaccines (Pneumovax, *H. influenzae* b, meningococcal vaccines).

Quellung = capsular **"swellung."**

Pneumococcus associated with "rusty" sputum, sepsis in sickle cell anemia, and splenectomy.

Zoonotic bacteria

Species	Disease	Transmission and source	
Borrelia burgdorferi	Lyme disease	Tick bite; *Ixodes* ticks that live on deer and mice	**B**ugs **F**rom **Y**our **P**et
Brucella spp.	Brucellosis/ Undulant fever	Dairy products, contact with animals	**U**ndulate and **U**npasteurized dairy products give you **U**ndulant fever.
Francisella tularensis	Tularemia	Tick bite; rabbits, deer	
Yersinia pestis	Plague	Flea bite; rodents, especially prairie dogs	
Pasteurella multocida	Cellulitis	Animal bite; cats, dogs	

Hepatitis serologic markers

IgM HAVAb	IgM antibody to HAV; best test to detect active hepatitis A.
HBsAg	Antigen found on surface of HBV; continued presence indicates carrier state.
HBsAb	Antibody to HBsAg; **provides immunity** to hepatitis B.
HBcAg	Antigen associated with core of HBV.
HBcAb	Antibody to HBcAg; positive during **window period.** IgM HBcAb is an indicator of recent disease.
HBeAg	A second, different antigenic determinant in the HBV core. Important indicator of transmissibility. (**BE**ware!)
HBeAb	Antibody to e antigen; indicates low transmissibility.

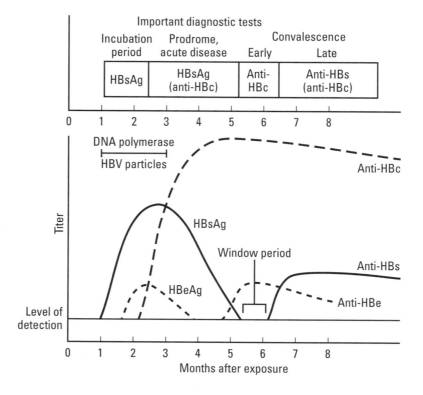

Test	Acute Disease	Window Phase	Complete Recovery	Chronic Carrier
HBsAg	+	–	–	+
HBsAb	–	–	+	–[b]
HBcAb	+[a]	+	+	+

[a]IgM in acute stage; IgG in chronic or recovered stage.

[b]Patient has surface antibody but available antibody is bound to HBsAg.

Causes of meningitis

Newborn (0–6 mos) →	Children (6 mos–6 yrs) →	6–60 yrs →	60 yrs +
Group B streptococci	*Streptococcus pneumoniae*	*N. meningitidis*	*S. pneumoniae*
E. coli	*Neisseria meningitidis*	Enteroviruses	Gram-negative rods
Listeria	*Haemophilus influenzae* B	*S. pneumoniae*	*Listeria*
	Enteroviruses	HSV	

In HIV—*Cryptococcus*, CMV, toxoplasmosis (brain abscess), JC virus (PML).

Note: Incidence of *H. influenzae* meningitis has ↓ greatly with introduction of *H. influenzae* vaccine in last 10–15 years.

Systemic mycoses

Disease	Endemic location	Notes
Coccidioidomycosis	Southwestern United States, California.	San Joaquin Valley or desert (desert bumps) "valley fever."
Histoplasmosis	Mississippi and Ohio river valleys.	Bird or bat droppings; intracellular (frequently seen inside macrophages).
Paracoccidioidomy-cosis	Rural Latin America.	"Captain's wheel" appearance.
Blastomycosis	States east of Mississippi River and Central America.	Big, **B**road-**B**ased **B**udding.

Broad-based budding

All of the above are caused by **dimorphic** fungi, which are mold in soil (at lower temperature) and yeast in tissue (at higher/body temperature: 37°C) except coccidioidomycosis, which is a spherule in tissue. Treat with fluconazole or ketoconazole for local infection; amphotericin B for systemic infection. Systemic mycoses can mimic TB (granuloma formation).

Cold = Mold.
Heat = Yeast.
Culture on Sabouraud's agar.

VDRL false positives

VDRL detects nonspecific Ab that reacts with beef cardiolipin. Used for diagnosis of syphilis, but many biologic false positives, including viral infection (mononucleosis, hepatitis), some drugs, rheumatic fever, rheumatoid arthritis, SLE, and leprosy.

VDRL:
Viruses (mono, hepatitis)
Drugs
Rheumatic fever and rheumatic arthritis
Lupus and leprosy

Bug hints (if all else fails)

Pus, empyema, abscess—*Staphylococcus aureus*.
Pediatric infection—*Haemophilus influenzae* (including epiglottitis).
Pneumonia in CF, burn infection—*Pseudomonas aeruginosa*.
Branching rods in oral infection—*Actinomyces israelii*.
Traumatic open wound—*Clostridium perfringens*.
Surgical wound—*S. aureus*.
Dog or cat bite—*Pasteurella multocida*.
Currant jelly sputum—*Klebsiella*.
Sepsis/meningitis in newborn—Group B strep.

A common URI with inflammation of the pharynx that is generally self-limited. The key is to differentiate streptococcal pharyngitis (**group A β-hemolytic streptococci**) from other causes. Remember that viral causes are more common.

Etiologies

- **Bacterial:** Group A β-hemolytic streptococci, group C β-hemolytic streptococci, *Neisseria gonorrhoeae*, *Corynebacterium diphtheriae*, *Mycoplasma pneumoniae*.
- **Viral:** Rhinovirus, coronavirus, adenovirus, HSV, EBV, CMV, influenza virus, coxsackievirus.

History/PE

- **Typical of strep pharyngitis:** Sudden-onset **sore throat, pharyngeal erythema, tonsillar exudate, fever,** anterior cervical lymphadenopathy, soft palate petechiae, headache, vomiting, scarlatiniform rash (indicates scarlet fever).
- **Atypical of strep pharyngitis:** Coryza, hoarseness, cough, diarrhea, conjunctivitis, anterior stomatitis, ulcerative lesions.

Evaluation

Clinical evaluation, rapid group A strep antigen detection, throat culture.

Treatment

Reduce symptoms with fluids, rest, antipyretics, and salt-water gargles. Prevent complications from strep pharyngitis with penicillin V PO × 10 days or penicillin G benzathine IM × 1 dose.

Complications

Complications of strep pharyngitis include:

- **Nonsuppurative:** Acute rheumatic fever (see Cardiology section), poststreptococcal glomerulonephritis.
- **Suppurative:** Cervical lymphadenitis, mastoiditis, sinusitis, otitis media, retropharyngeal or peritonsillar abscess. Peritonsillar abscess is a commonly tested complication that may present with **odynophagia** (pain with swallowing), **trismus** ("lockjaw"), and muffled voice. Exam reveals unilateral tonsillar enlargement and erythema with the **uvula and soft palate deviated away from the affected side.** Culture abscess fluid and localize the abscess via intraoral U/S or CT. Treat with penicillin or erythromycin and **surgical drainage.** Elective tonsillectomy can be performed after acute infection has resolved.

Signs suggestive of streptococcal pharyngitis include fever, pharyngeal erythema, exudate, and lack of cough.

HIGH-YIELD FACTS

Infectious Disease

Caused by the spore-forming gram-positive bacterium *Bacillus anthracis*. Its natural incidence is rare, but infection is an occupational hazard for veterinarians, farmers, and individuals who handle **animal wool, hair, hides,** or bone meal products. Also a biological weapon. *Bacillus anthracis* can cause cutaneous (most common), inhalation (most deadly), or intestinal anthrax.

History/PE

Cutaneous anthrax occurs 1–7 days after skin exposure and penetration of spores, most commonly affecting the exposed upper extremities. The lesion begins as a **pruritic papule** that enlarges in 24–48 hours to form an ulcer surrounded by a satellite bulbus/lesion with an edematous halo and a round, regular, and raised edge. **Regional lymphadenopathy** is also characteristic. The anthrax ulcer and surrounding edema evolve into a **black eschar** in 7–10 days.

The anthrax-associated pruritic papule forms an ulcer with an edematous halo and then a black eschar.

Differential

Secondary syphilis, tularemia.

Evaluation

Aerobic culture and Gram staining of ulcer exudate shows nonmotile short chains of bacilli.

Treatment

Penicillin (meningeal doses), doxycycline, and chloramphenicol penetrate the CSF, which is important in meningeal anthrax. Use any quinolone for 1–2 weeks for patients who are unable to take penicillin or doxycycline. Postexposure prophylaxis (ciprofloxacin) to prevent inhalation anthrax should be continued for 60 days.

ENCEPHALITIS

Inflammation of the brain. **Arboviruses** and **HSV** are the most common causes of endemic and sporadic encephalitis cases. Children are the most vulnerable. **M. *pneumoniae*** and idiopathic causes are becoming more common in developed countries.

History

Headache, fever, and nuchal rigidity; mild lethargy, confusion, stupor, and coma.

PE

Exam reveals **focal neurologic signs** (motor weakness, accentuated DTRs, extensor plantar responses) and **seizures.** Severe hyperthermia or poikilothermia, diabetes insipidus, and inappropriate ADH secretion are also seen. **Increased intracranial pressure** may cause papilledema and CN III and VI palsies.

Differential

Brain abscess, subdural empyema, brain tumor, subarachnoid hemorrhage (SAH), subdural hematoma, traumatic intracranial hemorrhage.

Evaluation

- **CT scan:** May demonstrate a focal lesion.
- **LP:** Mononuclear cells usually predominate. **RBCs may be found in HSV encephalitis.** Meningoencephalitis caused by *Naegleria, Nocardia, Actinomyces, Candida,* or *Aspergillus* elicits a polymorphonuclear response. CSF protein level is usually increased (increased IgG). Tests for specific IgM in serum to differentiate etiology. Glucose level is usually low in tuberculous, fungal, bacterial, or amebic infections. Direct examination of the CSF by Gram stain for bacteria, by acid-fast stain for mycobacteria, and by India ink for *Cryptococcus* should be performed and may be diagnostic. Wet preparation of CSF may reveal free-living amebae, and Giemsa stain identifies trypanosomes. Perform PCR for herpesviruses.

Treatment

HSV encephalitis requires immediate IV acyclovir. Consider foscarnet in HIV-positive patients in whom there is a high suspicion of resistant HSV. **CMV encephalitis** is treated with a combination of ganciclovir and foscarnet.

MENINGITIS

Infection of the leptomeninges caused by viruses, bacteria, or fungi. Risk factors include recent ear infection, sinusitis, immune deficiencies, recent neurosurgical procedures, and sick contacts.

History/PE

Patients present with **fever,** malaise, **headache, neck stiffness, photophobia,** altered mental status, or seizures. Signs of meningeal irritation (Kernig and Brudzinski) are often absent in infants < 2 years of age.

Differential

Brain abscess, CNS vasculitis, stroke.

Evaluation

A high degree of clinical suspicion is required in children < 2 years of age owing to the possible absence of specific meningeal signs. Evaluation should include **LP** (in the absence of papilledema or focal neurologic deficits) and possibly **CT or MRI** to rule out other diagnoses. CBC may reveal leukocytosis; CSF findings vary (see Table 2.10–1).

TABLE 2.10–1. CSF Profiles.

	RBCs (per mm^3)	WBCs (per mm^3)	Glucose (mg/dL)	Protein (mg/dL)	Opening Pressure (cm H$_2$O)	Appearance	Gamma Globulin (% protein)
Normal	< 10	< 5	~2/3 of serum	15–45	10–20	Clear	3–12
Bacterial meningitis	↔	↑ (PMN)	↓	↑	↑	Cloudy	↔ or ↑
Viral meningitis	↔	↑ (mono)	↔	↔ or ↑	↔ or ↑	Most often clear	↔ or ↑
SAH	↑↑	↑	↔	↑	↔ or ↑	Yellow/red	↔ or ↑
Guillain-Barré syndrome (GBS)	↔	↔	↔ or ↑	↑↑	↔	Clear or yellow (high protein)	↔
Multiple sclerosis	↔	↔ or ↑	↔	↔	↔	Clear	↑↑
Pseudotumor cerebri	↔	↔	↔	↔	↑↑↑	Clear	↔

Treatment

Treat with **antibiotics** (for bacterial infection) and **supportive care.** Viral disease can be treated with supportive care and close follow-up (except HSV meningoencephalitis; treat with acyclovir). The initial choice of antimicrobial agent is based on the most likely organisms involved given the patient's age (see Table 2.10–2). Contacts of patients with meningococcal meningitis should receive rifampin prophylaxis.

Complications

- **Hyponatremia:** Administer fluids and monitor sodium concentration.
- **Seizures:** Treat with benzodiazepines and phenytoin.
- **Subdural effusions:** May be seen on CT scan. Occur in 50% of infants with *Haemophilus influenzae* meningitis. No treatment is necessary.

TABLE 2.10–2. Treatment of Bacterial Meningitis

Age	Causative Organism	Treatment
< 1 month	GBS, *Escherichia coli*, *Listeria*.	**Ampicillin and cefotaxime or gentamicin.**
1–3 months	Pneumococci, meningococci, *H. influenzae*.	**Cefotaxime + vancomycin ± steroids.**
3 months – adulthood	Pneumococci, meningococci.	Ceftriaxone ± vancomycin ± steroids.
> 60 years/alcoholism/ chronic illness	Pneumococci, gram-negative bacilli, *Listeria*.	Ceftriaxone + ampicillin ± steroids.

- **Cerebral edema:** Presents with loss of oculocephalic reflex. Treat with IV mannitol.
- **Subdural empyema:** Presents as intractable seizures. Requires surgical evacuation.
- **Brain abscess:** Requires surgical drainage.
- **Ventriculitis:** Presents as a worsening clinical picture with improved CSF findings. Requires ventriculostomy and possibly intraventricular antibiotics.

UCV *IM2.24, Neuro.26,27*

COCCIDIOIDOMYCOSIS

A pulmonary fungal infection endemic to the **southwestern United States** (e.g., San Joaquin Valley, California). Can present as flu-like illness or acute pneumonia and involve extrapulmonary sites, including bone, CNS, and skin. Known as the "great imitator." The incubation period is 1–4 weeks after exposure.

History/PE

Patients present with **fever,** anorexia, headache, chest pain, **cough,** dyspnea, arthralgias, and **night sweats.**

Differential

Pneumonia, lung carcinoma, sarcoidosis, histoplasmosis, TB, lymphoma.

Evaluation

- **Serology:** Precipitin antibodies (IgM) rise within two weeks and disappear after two months; complement fixation antibodies (IgG) rise at 1–3 months.
- Culture of sputum, wound exudate, joint aspirate.
- CXR findings may be normal or may show infiltrate(s), nodule(s), cavity, mediastinal or hilar adenopathy, or pleural effusion.
- Consider bronchoscopy, fine-needle biopsy, open lung biopsy, or pleural biopsy.

Treatment

Ketoconazole or **fluconazole;** amphotericin B.

UCV *IM2.16*

CONGENITAL INFECTIONS

May occur at any time during pregnancy, labor, and delivery. Common sequelae include **premature delivery, CNS abnormalities,** anemia, **jaundice,** hepatosplenomegaly, and growth retardation. The most common pathogens can be remembered through use of the mnemonic **TORCHeS:**

- Toxoplasmosis: Transplacental transmission, with primary infection via consumption of **raw meat** or contact with **cat feces.** Specific findings include hydrocephalus, **intracranial calcifications,** chorioretinitis, and **ring-enhancing lesions** on head CT.
- Other: **HIV,** parvovirus, varicella, *Listeria*, TB, malaria, fungi.
- Rubella: Transplacental transmission in the first trimester. Specific findings include a purpuric **"blueberry muffin" rash,** cataracts, mental retardation, hearing loss, and **patent ductus arteriosus.**
- CMV: The **most common congenital infection,** primarily transmitted transplacentally. Specific findings include petechial rash (similar to "blueberry muffin" rash) and **periventricular calcifications.**
- Herpes: Intrapartum transmission if mom has **active lesions.** Can cause skin, eye, and mouth infections or life-threatening CNS/systemic infection.
- Syphilis: Primarily intrapartum transmission. Specific findings include **maculopapular skin rash,** lymphadenopathy, hepatomegaly, **"snuffles"** (mucopurulent rhinitis), and osteitis. In childhood, late congenital syphilis is characterized by saber shins, saddle nose, CNS involvement, and Hutchinson's triad: **peg-shaped upper central incisors, deafness, and interstitial keratitis** (photophobia, lacrimation).

Pregnant women should not change the cat's litterbox.

Evaluation

Perform **serologic testing** for rubella, toxoplasmosis, and HSV. Obtain a urine culture for CMV and perform dark-field examination of skin lesions/maternal serology for syphilis. Testing cord blood for elevated IgM may be useful. Other tests include viral isolation, amniocentesis (PCR for CMV), and antigen detection. All ill newborns require blood cultures, LP, and empiric antibiotics.

Treatment

- **Toxoplasmosis:** Pyrimethamine, sulfadiazine, spiramycin (for pregnant women).
- **Syphilis:** Penicillin.
- **HSV:** Acyclovir.
- **CMV:** Ganciclovir.

Prevention

- **Toxoplasmosis:** Avoid exposure to cats and cat feces (e.g., changing litter or gardening) during pregnancy; treat women with primary infection with pyrimethamine and sulfadiazine or spiramycin in the third trimester.
- **Rubella:** Immunize before pregnancy; otherwise, consider abortion if infected or exposed. Vaccinate the mother after delivery if titers remain negative.
- **Syphilis:** Penicillin in pregnant women who test positive for infection.
- **CMV:** Avoid exposure.
- **HSV:** Perform a **C-section if lesions are present at delivery.**
- **HIV:** AZT in pregnant women with HIV; perform a C-section; treat infant with prophylactic AZT; avoid breast-feeding.

First-trimester toxoplasmosis infection is less common and more severe. Third trimester is more common and less severe.

UCV IM2.26

A temperature of > 38.3°C for at least three weeks' duration that remains undiagnosed following three outpatient visits or three days of hospitalization. Risk factors include recent travel, immune deficiency, and drug abuse. In adults, **infections** and **cancer** account for > 60% of cases of FUO, while **autoimmune diseases** account for approximately 15%.

History/PE

Fever, headache, myalgia, malaise.

Differential

- **Infectious: TB** and **endocarditis** (e.g., HACEK organisms; see "Infective Endocarditis," p. 223) are the most common systemic infections causing FUO, while **occult abscess** is the most common localized infection. Also consider osteomyelitis and catheter infections.
- **Neoplastic: Leukemias** and **lymphomas** are the most common neoplasms causing FUO, while **hepatic and renal cell carcinomas** are the most common solid tumors.
- **Autoimmune:** Still's disease, systemic lupus erythematosus (SLE), cryoglobulinemia, and polyarteritis nodosa.
- **Miscellaneous:** Sarcoidosis, Whipple's disease, recurrent pulmonary emboli, alcoholic hepatitis, drug fever, familial Mediterranean fever, and factitious fever.
- Undiagnosed (10–15%).

Evaluation

CXR, CBC with differential, ESR, multiple blood cultures, and PPD should help differentiate likely causes. CT and MRI scans should be done if malignancy or occult abscess is suspected. Specific tests (ANA, RF, viral cultures, viral/fungal antibody/antigen tests) can be obtained if an infectious or autoimmune etiology is suspected.

Treatment

FUO patients without other symptoms do not require empiric antibiotic therapy.

Severely ill patients are usually started empirically on broad-spectrum antibiotics until the precise etiology has been determined. However, antibiotics should be stopped if there is no response.

A retrovirus that targets and destroys CD4$^+$ lymphocytes, leading to AIDS. Risk factors include unprotected sexual intercourse, IVDU, maternal HIV infection, needle sticks and mucocutaneous exposures, and receipt of blood products. Infection is characterized by a high rate of viral replication leading to a progressive decline in the CD4$^+$ count. Broadly stated, the **CD4$^+$ count** is a surrogate marker for the **extent** of disease progression, whereas the **viral load** is an indicator of the **rate** of disease progression.

History/PE

Primary HIV infection is often **asymptomatic;** patients may present with **flu-like symptoms**—e.g., generalized malaise, fever, generalized lymphadenopathy, rash, or even viral meningitis. Later, HIV may present as night sweats, weight loss, thrush, and cachexia. Complications correlate with CD4$^+$ count.

Differential

Flu, lymphoma, hairy leukoplakia, CMV, HSV, syphilis.

Evaluation

- **ELISA test (high sensitivity, moderate specificity)** detects anti-HIV antibodies in the bloodstream (can take up to six months to appear after exposure).
- **Western blot (low sensitivity, high specificity)** is confirmatory.
- Check viral load, PPD with anergy panel, VDRL, and CMV and toxoplasmosis serologies.

Treatment

Currently, **antiretroviral therapy** is initiated for patients with CD4$^+$ counts < 500 or with a detectable viral load. Start patients on two **nucleoside analogs** (e.g., AZT, ddI, 3TC, D4T). Non-nucleoside reverse transcriptase inhibitors and **protease inhibitors** (e.g., saquinavir, ritonavir, indinavir) are added depending on drug-drug interactions, drug tolerance, and patient compliance. See Table 2.10–3 for prophylaxis against opportunistic infections.

INFECTIVE ENDOCARDITIS (IE)

Infection of the endocardial surface of the heart, usually secondary to bacterial or other infectious causes. IE most commonly affects the heart valves, especially the mitral valve. Risk factors include rheumatic, congenital, or valvular heart disease (including mitral valve prolapse), prosthetic heart valves, IVDU, and immunosuppression. **Streptococcus viridans** is the most common pathogen for left-sided subacute bacterial endocarditis; **Staphylococcus aureus** is the causative agent in > 80% of cases of acute bacterial endocarditis in patients with a history of IVDU. Coagulase-negative staphylococcus is the most common infecting organism in prosthetic valve endocarditis. *Streptococcus bovis* endocarditis is associated with coexisting GI malignancy. *Candida* and *Aspergillus* species account for most cases of fungal endocarditis. Predisposing factors for fungal endocarditis include long-term indwelling IV catheters; immunosuppression due to malignancy, AIDS, or organ transplantation; and IVDU. Table 2.10–4 lists the causes of endocarditis.

TABLE 2.10–3. Prophylaxis for HIV-Related Opportunistic Infections

Pathogen	Indication for Prophylaxis	Medication	Comments
Pneumocystis carinii pneumonia (PCP)	$CD4^+ < 200/mm^3$. Persistent unexplained fever. Chronic oropharyngeal candidiasis.	**Trimethoprim-sulfamethoxazole (TMP-SMX)** or dapsone ± pyrimethamine.	SS tablets are effective and may be less toxic than DS.[a]
Mycobacterium avium complex (MAC)	$CD4^+ < 100/mm^3$. Generally, $CD4^+ < 200/mm^3$.	**Clarithromycin** or azithromycin or rifabutin.	Rifabutin increases hepatic metabolism of other drugs.
Toxoplasma	No consensus. Generally, $CD4^+ < 200/mm^3$.	TMP-SMX.	Pyrimethamine alone is not effective.
Mycobacterium tuberculosis	PPD > 5 mm or "high risk."	**Sensitive: INH × 9 mo** or rifampin ± pyrazinamide or rifabutin ± pyrazinamide.	For resistant strains, use two-drug regimens. Include pyridoxine with INH-containing regimens.
Candida	Multiple recurrences.	**Fluconazole** or itraconazole.	—
HSV	Multiple recurrences.	Acyclovir or famciclovir or valacyclovir.	—
Pneumococcus	All patients.	Pneumovax.	—
Influenza	All patients.	Influenza vaccine.	—

[a]DS = double strength; SS = single strength.

(Adapted, with permission, from Mandell GL. *Principles and Practice of Infectious Diseases*, 5th ed. London: Churchill Livingstone, 2000:1507.)

TABLE 2.10–4. Causes of Endocarditis

Acute	Subacute
S. aureus (IVDA)	*S. viridans*
S. pneumoniae	*Enterococcus*
N. gonorrhoeae	*Staphylococcus epidermidis*
	Fungi

Marantic	HACEK (culture-negative)	SLE
Cancer (poor prognosis). Mets seed valves; emboli can cause cerebral infarcts.	*Haemophilus parainfluenzae* *Actinobacillus* *Cardiobacterium* *Eikenella* *Kingella*	Libman-Sacks (autoantibody to valve)

HIGH-YIELD FACTS

Infectious Disease

History

Fever, chills, weakness, dyspnea, sweats, anorexia, skin lesions, and IVDU. In patients with a history of valvular disease or IVDU, fever alone should raise the suspicion of this diagnosis. Also consider endocarditis in cases of FUO.

PE

Exam reveals fever, **heart murmur,** Osler's nodes (small, tender nodules on the finger and toe pads), splinter hemorrhages (subungual petechiae), Janeway lesions (small, peripheral hemorrhages), and Roth's spots (retinal hemorrhages).

Differential

Connective tissue diseases, FUO, glomerulonephritis, intra-abdominal infections, meningitis, MI, osteomyelitis, pericarditis, TB.

Evaluation

Diagnosis is guided by Duke's criteria. Major criteria include: **positive blood cultures** (obtain at least two sets separated in time and location) and **positive echocardiogram** (vegetations, paravalvular abscess, new valvular regurgitation, or new partial dehiscence of a prosthetic valve). Minor criteria include Osler's nodes, Roth's spots, arterial emboli, septic pulmonary infarcts, mycotic aneurysms, conjunctival hemorrhages, and Janeway lesions. Other findings include **CBC** with leukocytosis and left shift and elevated **ESR** and C-reactive protein (CRP) level. Most patients have mild anemia, and 50% have microscopic hematuria as a result of embolic lesions of the kidney. An **ECG** may demonstrate conduction abnormalities if an abscess has formed in the myocardium.

Treatment

Early empiric IV antibiotic treatment includes vancomycin and gentamicin or ceftriaxone and gentamicin. Acute valve replacement is rarely necessary during the active episode of IE. Indications for surgery include severe CHF resulting from valvular incompetence, paravalvular leak around a prosthetic valve, fungal endocarditis, and persistent bacteremia despite antibiotics. In the future, give antibiotic prophylaxis (e.g., amoxicillin or erythromycin) before dental work, as patients now have valvular disease.

UCV *IM2.1,2*

LYME DISEASE

A tick-borne disease caused by the spirochete *Borrelia burgdorferi.* Usually seen during the **summer months** and carried by **Ixodes** ticks, Lyme disease is endemic to the **Northeast,** northern Midwest, and Pacific coast. It is the most common vector-borne disease in North America.

Lyme disease is the most common vector-borne disease in North America.

History/PE

Onset of rash with fever, malaise, fatigue, headache, myalgias, and/or joint pains. Often recent history of camping or hiking in endemic areas. Infection usually occus after ticks feed for > 36 hours.

- **Primary: Erythema migrans** begins as a small erythematous macule or papule that is **found at the tick-feeding site** and expands slowly over days to weeks. The border may be macular or raised, and **central clearing** is often present ("bull's eye"). Median lesion width is 15 cm.
- **Secondary:** Characterized by **migratory polyarthropathies,** neurologic phenomena (e.g., **Bell's palsy**), meningitis, and/or **myocarditis** (presents as conduction abnormalities).
- **Tertiary:** Characterized by arthritis and subacute encephalitis (memory loss and mood change).

Differential

- **Early:** Viral exanthem.
- **Later:** Collagen vascular disease, chronic fatigue syndrome, other causes of neuropathies, encephalitis, aseptic meningitis, myocarditis.

Evaluation

A positive ELISA indicates exposure but does not indicate active disease.

ELISA and **Western blot.** Use Western blot to confirm a positive or indeterminate ELISA. A positive ELISA denotes **exposure** and is not specific for active disease (culture/molecular tests are currently under development).

Treatment

Treat early disease with **doxycycline** and later disease with **ceftriaxone.** Consider empiric therapy for patients with characteristic rash, arthralgias, or a tick bite acquired in an endemic area. Vaccines are available but are < 75% effective.

NEUTROPENIC FEVER

Defined as a single oral temperature of $\geq 38.3°C$ (101°F) or a temperature of $\geq 38.0°C$ (100.4°F) for ≥ 1 hour in a neutropenic patient (i.e., a neutrophil count of < 500 cells/mm³).

History/PE

Common in cancer patients undergoing chemotherapy. Neutropenic nadir occurs at 7–10 days post-chemotherapy. Inflammation may be minimal or absent in severely neutropenic patients. Subtle signs include pain at the most commonly infected sites: the peridontium, pharynx, lower esophagus, abdomen, lung, and perineum (including the anus) as well as the eye and skin.

Differential

Collagen vascular disease, abscess, endocarditis.

Evaluation

Thorough physical examination, but do not perform a rectal exam. CBC with differential, measurement of serum Cr, BUN, and transaminases; culture of blood samples. A CXR is indicated for patients with respiratory signs. **CT scan to evaluate for abscess.**

Never do a rectal exam on a neutropenic patient.

Treatment

Empiric antibiotic therapy (see Figure 2.10–1). The routine use of colony-stimulating factors is not indicated.

OPPORTUNISTIC INFECTIONS

CANDIDAL THRUSH

Candida albicans is a harmless commensal organism that can become an opportunistic pathogen. Risk factors include xerostomia, corticosteroid inhaler use, immune deficiency (e.g., HIV), immunosuppressive treatment, leukemias, lymphomas, cancer, and diabetes. *C. albicans* can also cause skin infections in noncompromised hosts in intertriginous areas (e.g., diaper rash); such infections present with pruritic beefy-red plaques with satellite lesions.

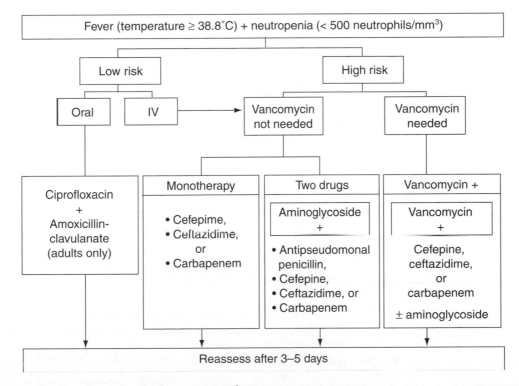

FIGURE 2.10–1. Empiric treatment algorithm for a neutropenic fever patient. (Reproduced, with permission, from Hughes WT. 2002 guidelines for the use of antimicrobial agents in neutropenic patients with cancer. *Clin Infect Dis* 2002;34:730–751.)

History/PE

Presents with **soft white plaques that can be rubbed off,** revealing an erythematous base. Patients frequently complain of mucosal burning.

Differential

Lichen planus, hairy leukoplakia.

Evaluation

The clinical diagnosis may be confirmed with cytologic preparations.

Treatment

Oral nystatin suspension four times a day, swish and swallow. Treatment should be continued for 5–7 days after the lesions disappear. If topical therapy is not effective, fluconazole, oral ketoconazole, or itraconazole may be used. Remove or control predisposing factors.

CRYPTOCOCCOSIS

Cryptococcus neoformans can cause an asymptomatic pulmonary infection followed by meningitis, which is often the first indication of disease. Rarely, invasive infection may occur in the immune-deficient host. Cryptococcal infection is one of the more common AIDS-defining infections in HIV-seropositive patients. *C. neoformans* is found in soil and **bird droppings** (pigeons).

History/PE

- **Meningitis:** Frontal or temporal headache, fever, impaired mentation, absent meningismus.
- **Pneumonia:** Nonproductive cough, shortness of breath, fever.

Differential

- **CNS disease:** Toxoplasmosis, lymphoma, AIDS dementia complex, progressive multifocal leukoencephalopathy, HSV encephalitis, other fungal disease.
- **Pulmonary disease:** TB, PCP, histoplasmosis, coccidioidomycosis, Kaposi's sarcoma, lymphoma.

Evaluation

- **LP:** Elevated opening pressure is associated with poor prognosis; CSF glucose is depressed; protein is elevated; and leukocyte count is high with a lymphocytic predominance.
- **CSF studies: India ink stain,** fungal culture, and latex agglutination test to detect cryptococcal polysaccharide (in serum or CSF).
- CT scan if neurologic deficits are present.

India ink stain is a key study for cryptococcosis.

Treatment

Amphotericin B IV plus flucytosine until the patient clinically improves; then fluconazole or itraconazole until eight weeks of primary therapy have been completed.

UCV *IM2.40*

Cryptococcal infections are fatal if left untreated.

HISTOPLASMOSIS

The fungus exists in mycelial form in nature and in yeast phase when exposed to mammalian temperatures. Histoplasmosis is endemic in the **central United States,** especially around the Mississippi River Valley. Manifestations include a self-limited flu-like syndrome, mediastinal fibrosis, residual scar tissue, chronic cavitary disease in those with obstructive lung disease, and disseminated histoplasmosis, which is more frequent in the immune-compromised host and infants. Risk factors include AIDS, spelunking, and exposure to bird or **bat** excrement.

History/PE

Arthralgia, erythema nodosum, and erythema multiforme are associated with acute infection. Low-grade fever, anorexia, weight loss, night sweats, and productive cough are associated with chronic infection.

Differential

Atypical pneumonia, blastomycosis, coccidioidomycosis, TB, sarcoidosis, pneumoconiosis, lymphoma.

Evaluation

Polysaccharide antigen detection is a rapid test for diagnosis and for monitoring relapse. **Complement fixation antibodies** at titers of 1:8 or 1:16 are presumptive for diagnosis. Identifying organisms by **silver stain** on biopsy (bone marrow, lymph node, liver) or bronchoalveolar lavage is diagnostic. **CXR** may reveal focal midlung field infiltrates, hilar or mediastinal adenopathy, or both. A **chest CT** can differentiate mediastinal fibrosis from mediastinal granuloma.

Polysaccharide antigen detection is a rapid test for the diagnosis of histoplasmosis and for monitoring relapse.

Treatment

Amphotericin B, ketoconazole.

UCV *IM2.21*

PNEUMOCYSTIS CARINII PNEUMONIA

Pneumocystis carinii is an organism of low virulence found in the lungs of humans and a variety of animals in nature. Impaired cellular immunity is an important predisposing factor in the development of pneumocystosis. PCP is one of the more common AIDS-defining infections in HIV-seropositive patients.

History/PE

Shortness of breath, fever, nonproductive cough, tachypnea, tachycardia, impaired oxygenation.

Differential

TB, histoplasmosis, coccidioidomycosis.

Evaluation

CXR classically exhibits **bilateral diffuse perihilar infiltrates.** Silver stain and **immunofluorescence** of induced sputum samples allow for definitive diagnosis. **Fiberoptic bronchoscopy** is diagnostic in > 90% of cases. **Bronchoalveolar lavage** is usually performed instead of washings and brushings because it has greater sensitivity and low morbidity.

Treatment

TMP-SMX, atovaquone, clindamycin and primaquine, dapsone.

OSTEOMYELITIS

Bone infection secondary to **direct spread** from a soft tissue infection (80% of cases) or **hematogenous seeding** (20% of cases). Direct spread is seen in patients with peripheral vascular disease, diabetes (chronic foot ulcers), and penetrating soft tissue injuries. Hematogenous osteomyelitis is most commonly found in children (affecting the metaphyses of the long bones) and IV drug users (affecting the vertebral bodies). Common pathogens are outlined in Table 2.10–5.

History/PE

Patients present with **fever** and **localized bone pain.** Localized warmth, tenderness, swelling, erythema, and limited motion of the adjacent joint.

TABLE 2.10–5. Common Pathogens in Osteomyelitis

If	Think
Most people	*S. aureus*
IVDU	*S. aureus* or *Pseudomonas*
Sickle cell disease	*Salmonella*
Hip replacement	*S. epidermidis*
Foot puncture wound	*Pseudomonas*
Chronic	*S. aureus, Pseudomonas,* Enterobacteriaceae

Differential

Cellulitis, soft tissue infection, septic arthritis, rheumatic fever, gout, Ewing's sarcoma, osteoarthritis.

Evaluation

Elevated **WBC** count, **ESR** (> 100), and **CRP** levels. Blood cultures may be positive. Radiographs are often negative on acute presentation; however, radiographic findings **(periosteal elevation)** may be seen 10–14 days later. **Bone scans** are sensitive for osteomyelitis but lack specificity; **indium-labeled leukocyte scanning** is more specific. **MRI** (test of choice) will show increased signal in the bone marrow consistent with bone marrow edema and may also reveal associated soft tissue infection. Definitive diagnosis is made by **bone aspiration** (Gram stain and culture).

Treatment

Treat with **IV antibiotics** for 4–6 weeks and with **surgical debridement** of necrotic, infected bone. Empiric antibiotic selection is based on the suspected organism and Gram stain. Consider oxacillin, nafcillin, a cephalosporin, vancomycin, or a quinolone plus rifampin if *S. aureus* is suspected. Empiric gram-negative coverage includes a third-generation cephalosporin and gentamicin or ciprofloxacin.

Complications

Chronic osteomyelitis, sepsis, soft tissue infection, septic arthritis. Long-standing chronic osteomyelitis with a draining sinus tract may eventually lead to **squamous cell carcinoma** (Marjolin's ulcer).

OTITIS EXTERNA

An inflammation of the skin lining the ear canal and surrounding soft tissue, also known as "swimmer's ear." *Pseudomonas* (from poorly chlorinated pools) and Enterobacteriaceae are the most common etiologic agents. Both grow in the presence of excess moisture.

History/PE

Presents with pain, pruritus, and a possible purulent discharge from the ear canal. Exam reveals pain with movement of the tragus/pinna (unlike otitis media) and an edematous and erythematous ear canal.

Otitis media should not cause pain with movement of the tragus/pinna.

Differential

Varicella zoster, foreign body, otitis media.

Evaluation

Clinical diagnosis. Gram stain and culture are helpful if a fungal etiology is suspected. CT scan if the patient is toxic appearing.

Treatment

Eardrops with polymyxin B, neomycin, and hydrocortisone usually suffice. Use **dicloxacillin** for acute disease. **Diabetics** are at risk for malignant otitis externa and osteomyelitis of the skull base and thus require hospitalization and **IV antibiotics.**

PNEUMONIA

An infection of the bronchoalveolar unit with an inflammatory exudate. Causes are often broadly categorized as **"typical,"** caused by bacteria from the nasopharynx, or **"atypical,"** caused by organisms (bacteria, viruses, fungi) inhaled from the environment. Atypical organisms are often difficult to visualize on Gram stain and are not susceptible to antibiotics that act on the cell wall (e.g., β-lactams). **Aspiration pneumonia** occurs secondary to inhalation of colonized oropharyngeal secretions into the larynx and lower respiratory tract. Aspiration pneumonia is distinct from **aspiration pneumonitis** (Mendelson's syndrome), which is secondary to inhalation of sterile gastric contents causing a chemical injury to the lungs.

History

Classic symptoms are **productive cough** (purulent yellow/green sputum or hemoptysis), dyspnea, fever/chills, night sweats, and **pleuritic chest pain.** Atypical organisms may present with a more gradual onset, dry cough, headaches, myalgias, sore throat, and pharyngitis.

PE

Decreased or bronchial breath sounds, crackles, wheezing, dullness to percussion, egophony, and tactile fremitus. Elderly patients as well as those with COPD or diabetes may have minimal signs on physical exam.

Differential

Lung abscess, aspiration pneumonitis, atelectasis, chronic bronchitis, COPD, lung cancer, TB, bronchiectasis.

Evaluation

- **CBC:** Leukocytosis and left shift (bands > 5% and/or immature WBCs).
- **Sputum Gram stain and culture:** Identifies the pathogenic organism and the organism's antibiotic susceptibilities (see Figures 2.10–2 through 2.10–4). A good sputum sample (i.e., one not contaminated by

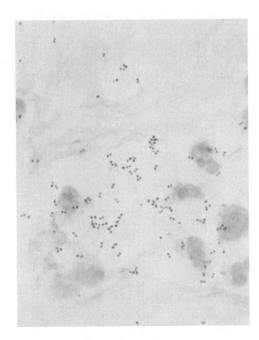

FIGURE 2.10–2. *Staphylococcus aureus.* These clusters of gram-positive cocci were isolated from the sputum of a patient who developed pneumonia while hospitalized.

oropharyngeal flora) has many PMNs (> 25 cells/hpf) and few epithelial cells (< 25 cells/hpf).

- **Blood culture:** If the patient appears very ill, suspect sepsis due to pneumonia.
- **ABGs:** Ill patients will have poor O_2 saturation and acid-base disturbances.
- **CXR:** Look for lobar consolidation or patchy or diffuse infiltrates.

For recurrent pneumonias, consider underlying disease processes, including obstruction, bronchogenic carcinoma, lymphoma, Wegener's, or unusual organisms (e.g., TB, *Nocardia*, *Coxiella burnetii*, *Aspergillus*).

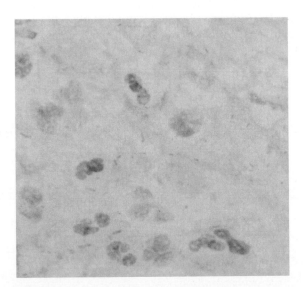

FIGURE 2.10–3. *Pseudomonas.* Sputum sample from a patient with pneumonia reveals gram-negative rods. The large number of neutrophils and relative paucity of epithelial cells indicate that this sample is not contaminated with oropharyngeal flora.

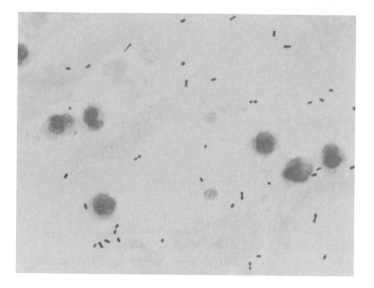

FIGURE 2.10–4. *Streptococcus pneumoniae.* Sputum sample from a patient with pneumonia. Note the characteristic lancet-shaped gram-positive diplococci.

Treatment

Empiric treatment is based on patient demographic and environmental information. Table 2.10–6 summarizes the recommended initial treatment for pneumonia.

- In uncomplicated cases, treat community-acquired pneumonia on an outpatient basis with oral antibiotics (e.g., macrolides).
- Patients > 65 years old as well as those with comorbidity (alcoholism, COPD, diabetes, malnutrition), immunosuppression, unstable vitals or signs of respiratory failure, altered mental status, and/or multilobar involvement require hospitalization with IV antibiotics.
- For patients with obstructive diseases (e.g., CF or bronchiectasis), consider adding pseudomonal coverage.
- Administer the **pneumococcal vaccine** in patients > 65 years old and those with chronic illnesses, immune compromise, asplenia, and sickle cell disease.

UCV *IM2.23,25*

TABLE 2.10–6. Treatment of Pneumonia

Patient Type	Suspected Pathogens	Initial Coverage
Outpatient community-acquired pneumonia, ≤ 65 years old, otherwise healthy.	*S. pneumoniae, M. pneumoniae, Chlamydia pneumoniae, H. flu,* viral.	Erythromycin, tetracycline. Consider clarithromycin or azithromycin in smokers to treat *H. flu.*
As above except ≥ 65 years old or with comorbidity (COPD, heart failure, renal failure, diabetes, liver disease, EtOH abuse).	*S. pneumoniae, H. flu,* aerobic gram-negative rods (GNRs—*E. coli, Enterobacter, Klebsiella*), *S. aureus, Legionella,* viruses.	Second-generation cephalosporin (cefuroxime), TMP-SMX, amoxicillin. Add erythromycin if atypicals (*Legionella, Mycoplasma, Chlamydia*) are suspected.
Community-acquired pneumonia requiring hospitalization.	*S. pneumoniae, H. flu,* anaerobes, aerobic GNRs, *Legionella, Chlamydia.*	Second- or third-generation cephalosporin (cefotaxime or ceftriaxone) or a β-lactam with β-lactamase inhibitor. Add erythromycin if atypicals are suspected.
Severe community-acquired pneumonia requiring hospitalization (generally needs ICU care).	*S. pneumoniae, H. flu,* anaerobes, aerobic GNRs, *Mycoplasma, Legionella, Pseudomonas.*	Erythromycin or other macrolide, a third-generation cephalosporin with anti-pseudomonal activity (or another anti-pseudomonal agent), and an aminoglycoside.
Nosocomial pneumonia—patient hospitalized > 48 hours or in a long-term care facility > 14 days.	GNRs, including *Pseudomonas, S. aureus, Legionella,* and mixed flora.	Third-generation cephalosporin with anti-pseudomonal activity and an aminoglycoside (gentamicin).

HIGH-YIELD FACTS

Infectious Disease

ROCKY MOUNTAIN SPOTTED FEVER (RMSF)

A tick-borne rickettsial disease caused by **Rickettsia rickettsii** and carried by the **Dermacentor** tick. The organism invades the endothelial lining of capillaries and leads to **small vessel vasculitis.**

History/PE

Headache, fever, malaise, and **rash.** The characteristic rash is initially macular (beginning on the **palms** and **soles**) but becomes **petechial/purpuric as it spreads centrally.** Altered mental status or DIC may develop in severe cases.

Differential

Meningococcemia, Lyme disease, measles, typhoid, endocarditis, hemorrhagic fevers (Ebola, Hanta), vasculitis, leptospirosis, other rickettsial diseases (e.g., ehrlichiosis).

RMSF starts on the palms and soles and then spreads centrally.

Evaluation

Clinical diagnosis is confirmed retrospectively with acute and convalescent antibody titers utilizing complement fixation or the **Weil-Felix test** (antigen cross-reactivity with *Proteus* antigens).

Treatment

Treat with **doxycycline;** use chloramphenicol in children and pregnant women. The condition can be rapidly fatal if left untreated.

SEPSIS

Systemic inflammatory response syndrome (SIRS) with a **documented infection.** Septic shock refers to sepsis-induced hypotension (systolic BP < 90). **Gram-positive shock** (e.g., staphylococci and streptococci) occurs secondary to fluid loss caused by **exotoxins. Gram-negative shock** (e.g., *E. coli, Klebsiella, Proteus,* and *Pseudomonas*) is caused by vasodilation due to **endotoxin** (lipopolysaccharide). Other etiologies are as follows:

- **Neonates:** Group B streptococci, *E. coli, Klebsiella.*
- **Children:** *H. influenzae,* pneumococcus, meningococcus.
- **Adults:** Gram-positive cocci, aerobic bacilli, anaerobes.
- **IV drug users:** *S. aureus.*
- **Asplenic patients:** Pneumococcus, *H. influenzae,* meningococcus (encapsulated organisms).

History

Presents with abrupt onset of fever and chills, often associated with hyperventilation and altered mental status.

PE

Exam reveals **fever** (15% present with hypothermia), **tachycardia,** and tachypnea. **Hypotension** and shock occur in severe cases. Septic shock may start as warm shock with **warm skin and extremities** (peripheral vasodilation) and may then progress to cold shock with **cool skin and extremities** (peripheral vasoconstriction). Petechiae or ecchymoses suggest DIC, which occurs in 2–3% of cases.

Differential

Cardiogenic shock, hypovolemic shock, DIC, acute renal failure, DKA, anaphylaxis.

Evaluation

Neutropenia or neutrophilia with **increased bands. Thrombocytopenia** occurs in 50% of cases. Blood, sputum, and urine cultures (in urosepsis) may be positive, and CXR may show an infiltrate. Obtain coagulation studies and consider a **DIC panel** (fibrinogen, fibrin split products, D-dimer).

Treatment

May require ICU admission. Treat aggressively with IV fluids, pressors, and antibiotics. Treat underlying factors (e.g., remove Foley catheter or lines that may be infected). Primary goal is to maintain BP.

SEXUALLY TRANSMITTED DISEASES

CHLAMYDIA

The most common bacterial STD in the United States. Caused by *Chlamydia trachomatis*, which can infect genital tract, urethra, anus, and eye. It often co-exists with or mimics *Neisseria gonorrhoeae* infection, so patients should be tested for both at the same time.

History/PE

Infection is often asymptomatic, but may present with symptoms of **urethritis** (dysuria, urgency), **mucopurulent cervicitis** (vaginal discharge or bleeding, dyspareunia), and **salpingitis** or **PID** (abdominal pain, fever). Chlamydia is a common cause of nongonococcal urethritis in men. Exam in women may reveal mucopurulent cervical discharge and cervical or adnexal tenderness. Males may have penile discharge and testicular tenderness. Vertical transmission causes ocular effects or pneumonia in the newborn.

Differential

Gonorrhea, endometriosis, PID, orchitis, vaginitis, UTI, conjunctivitis.

Evaluation

Diagnosis is usually clinical. Urine tests (enzyme immunoassay or PCR) are a rapid means of detection, while cultures are difficult and take 48–72 hours. Gram stain of urethral or genital discharge may show PMNs but no bacteria.

Treatment

Doxycycline or azithromycin. Use erythromycin in pregnant patients.

Complications

Chronic infection and pelvic pain, Reiter's syndrome (urethritis, conjunctivitis, arthritis), Fitz-Hugh–Curtis syndrome (perihepatic inflammation and fibrosis). Infertility can result from PID (in women) and epididymitis (in men).

Treat patient with chlamydia for presumptive gonorrhea coinfections.

GONORRHEA

This gram-negative diplococcus can infect almost any site in the female reproductive tract, including Bartholin's ducts as well as the urethra, vagina, cervix, ovaries, fallopian tubes, and anus. Infection in men tends to be limited to the urethra. Eighty to ninety percent of women who have a single encounter with an infected individual contract the disease, whereas males become infected only 20–25% of the time after sex with an infected female. Infection may be indistinguishable from chlamydial disease.

History/PE

Greenish-yellow discharge, pelvic or **adnexal pain,** swollen Bartholin's glands. Men experience **purulent urethral discharge,** dysuria, and erythema of the urethral meatus.

Differential

Chlamydia, endometriosis, pharyngitis, PID, vaginitis, UTI, salpingitis, tubo-ovarian abscess.

Evaluation

Swab the pharynx, cervix, urethra, or anus as appropriate for culture on Thayer-Martin medium (80–95% sensitivity). Gram stain of cervical discharge shows gram-negative intracellular diplococci.

Treatment

IM ceftriaxone. Also treat for presumptive chlamydia coinfection (doxycycline or macrolide). Condoms are effective prophylaxis.

Complications

Persistent infection with pain, infertility, tubo-ovarian abscess with rupture.

UCV *IM2.18*

SYPHILIS

Caused by *Treponema pallidum*, a spirochete.

History/PE

Syphilis is the "great imitator" because the rash resembles many other diseases.

- **Primary** (10–60 days after infection): A **painless ulcer (chancre)** is found on or near the area of contact (see Figure 2.10–5). The lesion often goes unnoticed and heals spontaneously in 3–9 weeks.
- **Secondary** (4–8 weeks after appearance of chancre): Patients present with low-grade **fever,** headache, malaise, anorexia, and generalized **lymphadenopathy** with a diffuse, symmetric, asymptomatic **maculopapular rash on the soles and palms.** Meningitis, hepatitis, and nephritis may also be seen. Highly infective secondary eruptions (mucous patches) can coalesce, forming **condylomata lata;** lesions heal spontaneously in 2–6 weeks.
- **Early latent:** No symptoms, positive serology, first year of infection.
- **Late latent:** No symptoms, positive or negative serology, > 1 year of infection. One-third will progress to tertiary syphilis.

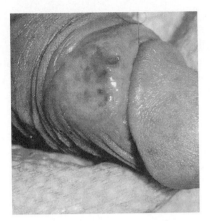

FIGURE 2.10–5. Primary syphilis. The chancre, which appears at the site of infection, is an ulcerated papule with a smooth, clean base; raised, indurated borders; and scant discharge. (Reproduced, with permission, from Bondi EE, *Dermatology: Diagnosis and Therapy*, 1st ed., Stamford, CT: Appleton & Lange, 1991: p. 394, Fig. 33.)

- **Tertiary** (1–20 years after initial infection): Destructive, granulomatous **gummas** can severely damage the skin, bones, and liver. Neurologic findings include **tabes dorsalis** (posterior column degeneration) and **Argyll Robertson pupil** (small, irregular pupil that accommodates but does not react to light). Cardiovascular findings include aortitis, aortic root aneurysms, and aortic regurgitation.

Differential

- **Primary:** Genital herpes, chancroid, lymphogranuloma venereum, lichen planus, psoriasis.
- **Secondary:** Hepatitis, infectious mononucleosis, drug eruptions, condylomata acuminata, viral exanthems, scabies.
- **Tertiary:** TB, sarcoid, lymphoma, CHF, HIV, stroke, seizures.

Evaluation

Evaluation (see Table 2.10–7) consists of **dark-field microscopy** (motile spirochetes) of primary or secondary lesions, **VDRL/RPR** (a rapid, nonspecific screening test), and **FTA-ABS/MHA-TP** (specific, diagnostic).

TABLE 2.10–7. Diagnostic Tests for Syphilis

Test	Comments
Dark-field microscopy	Identifies motile spirochetes (only primary and secondary lesions).
VDRL/RPR	Rapid and cheap, but sensitivity is only 60–75% in primary disease. Reverts to negative with successful treatment.
FTA-ABS	Sensitive, specific. Used as a secondary diagnostic test. Positive for life.

Treatment

Treat with IM **penicillin.** Tetracycline or doxycycline may be used in patients with penicillin allergies. **Neurosyphilis** should be treated with **IV penicillin;** penicillin-allergic patients should be desensitized prior to therapy.

UCV *IM2.27,28*

GENITAL LESIONS

See Table 2.10–8 for an outline of sexually transmitted genital lesions.

Infection of the sinuses due to an undrained collection of pus. Risk factors include barotrauma, allergic rhinitis, viral infection, asthma, smoking, and nasal decongestant overuse. The maxillary sinuses are most commonly infected.

- **Acute sinusitis** (symptoms lasting < 1 month) is most commonly associated with *S. pneumoniae, H. influenzae, Moraxella catarrhalis,* and viral infection.
- **Chronic sinusitis** (symptoms persisting > 3 months) is often due to obstruction of sinus drainage and ongoing low-grade anaerobic infections. In **diabetic** patients, **mucormycosis** infection may begin in the nose and maxillary sinuses.

History/PE

Always consider occult sinusitis in febrile ICU patients.

Fever, facial pain that can **radiate to the upper teeth,** nasal congestion, and **headache.** On exam, **tenderness,** erythema, swelling over the affected area, and **purulent discharge** may be noted. In chronic sinusitis, pain may be absent but nasal congestion, cough, and purulent drainage may continue. Febrile ICU patients may have **occult sinusitis,** especially if they are intubated or have NG tubes.

Differential

Migraine or cluster headache, dental abscess.

Evaluation

Sinusitis is a **clinical** diagnosis. Culture is generally not required. Clouding of sinuses may be observed on **transillumination,** but the test has low sensitivity. Maxillary sinus **radiographs** may be ordered if symptoms persist after therapy and may show air-fluid levels or opacification of the maxillary sinus (see Figure 2.10–6). Obtain a coronal CT if complications are suspected.

Treatment

- **Acute:** Amoxicillin or TMP-SMX for 10 days and symptomatic therapy (e.g., decongestants).

TABLE 2.10–8. Sexually Transmitted Genital Lesions

	Calymmato-bacterium granulomatis (granulona inguinale-donovanosis	*Haemophilus ducreyi (chancroid)*	**HSV-1 or -2[a]**	**HPV[b]**	*Treponema pallidum*
Lesion	Papule becomes beefy-red ulcer	Papule or pustule (Chancroid)	Vesicle	Papule (condylomata acuminata: warts)	Papule (chancre)
Appearance	Raised, red lesions	Irregular, deep, well demarcated	Regular, red, shallow	Irregular, pink or white, raised; cauliflower	Regular, red, round, raised
Number	1 or multiple	1–3	Multiple	Multiple	Single
Size	5–10 mm	10–20 mm	1–3 mm	1–5 mm	1 cm
Pain	No	Yes	Yes	No	No
Concurrent signs and symptoms	Granulomatous ulcers	Inguinal lymphadenopathy	Vulvar pain and pruritus	Pruritus	Regional adenopathy
Diagnosis	Clinical exam, visualize with smear	Difficult to culture; diagnosis made on clinical grounds	Tzanck smear or viral cultures	Clinical exam; biopsy for confirmation	Spirochetes seen under dark-field microscopy; *T. pallidum* identified by serum antibody test
Treatment	Doxycycline (100 mg bid × 3 weeks)	Ceftriaxone, erythromycin, or ciprofloxacin	Acyclovir for primary infection	Cryotherapy, topical agents such as podophyllin, trichloroacetic acid, or 5-FU cream	Penicillin

[a] 85% of genital herpes lesions are caused by HSV-2.
[b] HPV serotypes 6 and 11 are associated with genital warts; types 16, 18, and 31 are associated with cervical cancer.

- **Chronic:** 6–12 weeks of PO antibiotic treatment. If medical therapy does not work, treat with surgical drainage and correction of the cause of the obstruction.

Complications

Osteomyelitis of the frontal bone, meningitis, abscess of epidural or subdural spaces, orbital cellulitis, cavernous sinus thrombosis.

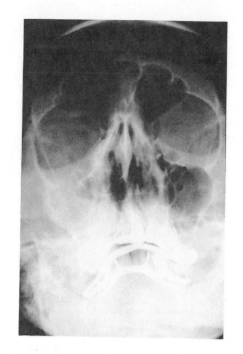

FIGURE 2.10–6. Sinusitis. Compare the opacified right maxillary sinus and normal air-filled left sinus on this sinus x-ray. (Reproduced, with permission, from Saunders CE. *Current Emergency Diagnosis & Treatment,* 4th ed. Stamford, CT: Appleton & Lange, 1992:443, Fig. 26–3.)

TUBERCULOSIS

Infection due to *Mycobacterium tuberculosis.* Most cases of symptomatic TB are due to reactivation of old infection rather than to primary disease and remain confined to the lung. Risk factors include **immunosuppression, alcoholism, preexisting lung disease,** diabetes, advancing age, homelessness, malnourishment, and crowded living conditions (e.g., prison). **Immigrants** from developing nations, health care workers, and other persons with "sick contacts" are also at high risk.

History/PE

TB is a common cause of FUO.

Cough, **hemoptysis,** dyspnea, **weight loss,** malaise, **night sweats,** fever, cachexia, hypoxia, tachycardia, lymphadenopathy, abnormal lung sounds. Pulmonary TB is a common cause of FUO, and the kidney is the most common site of extrapulmonary infection.

Differential

Pneumonia (bacterial, fungal, viral), other mycobacterial infections, HIV infection, UTI, lung abscess, lung cancer.

Evaluation

- Pulmonary TB is presumptively diagnosed by a **positive sputum acid-fast stain,** since culture may take several weeks (see Clinical Images).

PPD is injected intradermally on the volar surface of the arm. The transverse length of induration is measured at 48–72 hours. BCG vaccination typically renders a patient PPD positive for at least one year. The size of induration that indicates a positive test is as follows:

- Greater than **5 mm:** HIV or risk factors, close TB contacts, CXR evidence of TB.
- Greater than **10 mm:** Indigent/homeless, developing nations, IVDU, chronic illness, residents of health and correctional institutions.
- Greater than **15 mm:** Everyone else.

A **negative reaction** with negative controls implies anergy from immunosuppression, old age, or malnutrition and thus does not rule out TB.

FIGURE 2.10–7. PPD placement.

- **CXR** may show apical fibronodular infiltrates with or without cavitation.
- A positive PPD test (see Figure 2.10–7) indicates latent infection from previous exposure (not necessarily active infection) to M. *tuberculosis* and may not be present in immune-compromised individuals.

Treatment

- All cases should be reported to local and state health departments.
- Institute **respiratory isolation** (if TB is suspected) followed by directly observed multidrug therapy (usually **INH, pyrazinamide, rifampin, and ethambutol**). Therapy on at least rifampin and INH should continue for six months.
- Administer **vitamin B$_6$** (pyridoxine) with INH to prevent peripheral neuritis.
- Initiate prophylactic therapy (INH for nine months) for PPD conversion without active symptoms in patients with HIV or other causes of immunosuppression; IV drug users; those < 35 years of age; and those who have had close contact with an infected individual, a CXR suggestive of old TB infection, recent new conversion (< 2 years), poorly controlled diabetes, indigence and malnutrition, or institutional residence.
- Many physicians choose to forgo INH prophylaxis in patients < 35 years old because the risk of INH-induced liver toxicity increases with age.

UCV *IM2.29*

Rifampin turns body fluids orange. Ethambutol can cause optic neuritis.

Drugs for TB—

RESPIre
Rifampin
Ethambutol
Streptomycin
Pyrazinamide
INH

URINARY TRACT INFECTIONS

Include cystitis, pyelonephritis, and urosepsis. UTIs affect women more frequently than men, and positive *E. coli* cultures are obtained in 80% of cases. See the mnemonic **SEEKS PP** for other pathogens. Risk factors include use of a **Foley catheter** or other urologic instrumentation, anatomic abnormalities (e.g., BPH, vesicoureteral reflux), a history of previous UTIs or acute pyelonephritis, **diabetes mellitus,** recent antibiotic use, immunosuppression, and **pregnancy.**

UTI bugs—

SEEKS PP
S. *saprophyticus*
E. *coli*
Enterobacter
Klebsiella
Serratia
Proteus
Pseudomonas

History/PE

Patients complain of **urinary frequency, dysuria,** and **urgency.** Acute pyelonephritis may present with nausea, vomiting, **fever,** and **back/flank pain.** Children often present with **bedwetting,** and infants can present with poor feeding, recurrent febrile episodes, and foul-smelling urine.

Differential

Vaginitis, STDs, interstitial cystitis, prostatitis.

Evaluation

Urine dipstick may reveal **increased leukocyte esterase** (75% sensitive for WBCs), **elevated nitrites** (low sensitivity; false positives with bacterial contamination), elevated urine pH (characteristic of *Proteus* infections), or hematuria (seen with cystitis). Microscopic analysis may show **> 5 leukocytes/hpf** (indicative of GU infection) and a bacterial pathogen. WBC casts on UA indicate acute pyelonephritis. The gold standard is a clean-catch urine culture with **> 10^5 bacteria/mL** (diagnosis is often made on the basis of dipstick alone).

Treatment

Treat healthy young females on an outpatient basis with oral **TMP-SMX** or **ciprofloxacin** for three days. Elderly patients, those with comorbid diseases, or those with acute toxicity in the setting of acute pyelonephritis should be hospitalized and treated with **IV antibiotics** (ciprofloxacin or ampicillin and gentamicin to cover enterococcus). **Prophylactic antibiotics** may be given to those with recurrent UTIs.

UCV *IM2.31*

PYELONEPHRITIS

Infection of the renal parenchyma. Nearly 85% of community-acquired cases result from the same pathogens that cause UTIs. UTI and pyelonephritis share similar risk factors. Pyelonephritis is marked by **costovertebral angle tenderness,** mild abdominal tenderness, **fever,** nausea, vomiting, diarrhea, dysuria, frequency, and urgency. Unlike UTI, UA in pyelonephritis reveals WBC casts and CBC demonstrates leukocytosis. After obtaining a UA and culture, treat with a **fluoroquinolone** or other antibiotics with similar coverage. Fluids are recommended. Patients should be reevaluated in 72 hours and, if found to be appropriately improving, may continue outpatient treatment for 14–21 days.

Indications for radiographic evaluation include pregnancy, a history of urolithiasis, prior GU surgery, recurrent pyelonephritis, prepubescent age, fever for > 5–7 days without appropriate medical evaluation, and elderly patients. **IVP** is the initial study of choice in nonpregnant patients with adequate renal function. **U/S** is less invasive, is safe in pregnancy, and will not disturb renal function. **CT** is recommended for patients who do not respond to adequate therapy after three days of treatment or who have had nondiagnostic IVP and U/S evaluations.

Questions 1 and 2: Reproduced, with permission, from Reteguiz J, *PreTest: Physical Diagnosis*, 4th ed., New York: McGraw-Hill, 2001.
Questions 3 and 4: Reproduced, with permission, from Elkind MSV, *PreTest: Neurology*, 4th ed., New York: McGraw-Hill, 2001.
Questions 5 and 6: Reproduced, with permission, from Berk SL, *PreTest: Medicine*, 9th ed., New York: McGraw-Hill, 2001.

Questions

1. A 46-year-old woman with a history of sinusitis presents with a severe headache. She complains of neck stiffness and photophobia. On physical examination she has a temperature of 103.4°F. Blood pressure is normal and heart rate is 110/min. She has a normal funduscopic examination and no focal neurologic deficit. She has nuchal rigidity. Brudzinski and Kernig signs are positive. Which of the following is the most likely diagnosis?
   a. Migraine headache
   b. Cluster headache
   c. Torticollis
   d. Bacterial meningitis
   e. Cysticercosis
   f. Fever of unknown origin

2. A 41-year-old woman develops abdominal cramps and diarrhea two hours after eating fried rice. Physical examination is normal except for some mild abdominal tenderness with palpation. Examination of the stool reveals no fecal leukocytes. Which of the following is the most likely etiology for the symptoms?
   a. *Shigella*
   b. *Salmonella*
   c. *Vibrio cholerae*
   d. *Bacillus cereus*
   e. *Staphylococcus aureus*
   f. *Vibrio parahaemolyticus*

DIRECTIONS: The question below consists of lettered options followed by numbered items. For each numbered item, select the single most appropriate lettered option. Each lettered option may be used once, more than once, or not at all. **Choose exactly the number of options indicated following each item.**

Items 3–4

Select from the following list the condition that best fits each clinical scenario.
   a. Subacute HIV encephalomyelitis (AIDS encephalopathy)
   b. Subacute sclerosing panencephalitis (SSPE)
   c. Progressive multifocal leukoencephalitis (PML)
   d. Rabies encephalitis
   e. Guillain-Barré syndrome
   f. Tabes dorsalis
   g. Neurocysticercosis

3. A 27-year-old man developed recurrent episodes of involuntary movements. He had abused intravenous drugs for several years and had several admissions for recurrent infections, including subacute bacterial endocarditis. His invol-

untary movements were largely restricted to the right side of his body. Associated with this problem were hoarseness and difficulty swallowing. He had suffered a weight loss of 40 lb over the preceding four months. Examination revealed diffuse lymphadenopathy and right-sided hypertonia. His CSF was normal except for a slight increase in the protein content. Computed tomography revealed a large area of decreased density on the left side of the cerebrum. The EEG revealed diffuse slowing over the left side of the head. Biopsy of this lesion revealed oligodendrocytes with abnormally large nuclei that contained darkly staining inclusions. There was extensive demyelination and there were giant astrocytes in the lesion. Over the course of one month, this man exhibited increasing ataxia. Within two months, he had evidence of mild dementia and seizures. Within three months of presentation, his dementia was profound and he had bladder and bowel incontinence. Over the course of a few days he became obtunded and died. **(SELECT ONE CONDITION)**

4. A 50-year-old immigrant from eastern Europe developed problems with bladder control, an unsteady gait, and pain in his legs over the course of six months. On examination, it was determined that he had absent deep tendon reflexes in his legs, markedly impaired vibration sense in his feet, and a positive Romberg sign. Despite his complaint of unsteady gait, he had no problems with rapid alternating movement of the feet and no tremors were evident. He had normal leg strength. The pain in his legs was sharp, stabbing, and paroxysmal. His serum glucose and glycohemoglobin levels were normal. **(SELECT ONE CONDITION)**

Items 5–6

A 25-year-old male student presents with a chief complaint of rash. There is no headache, fever, or myalgia. A slightly pruritic maculopapular rash is noted over the abdomen, trunk, palms of hands, and soles of feet. Inguinal, occipital, and cervical lymphadenopathy is also noted. Hypertrophic, flat, wartlike lesions are noted around the anal area. Laboratory studies show the following:

    Hct: 40%
    Hgb: 14 g/dL
    WBC: 13,000/mm^3
    Differential:
      Segmented neutrophils 50%
      Lymphocytes 50%

5. The most useful laboratory test in this patient is
   a. Weil-Felix titer
   b. Venereal Disease Research Laboratory (VDRL) test
   c. *Chlamydia* titer
   d. Blood cultures

6. The treatment of choice for this patient would be
   a. Penicillin
   b. Ceftriaxone
   c. Tetracycline
   d. Interferon alpha
   e. Erythromycin

Answers

1. **The answer is d.** The patient is demonstrating signs of meningeal irritation. She has nuchal rigidity, a positive **Brudzinski sign** (involuntary flexion of the hips and knees when flexing the neck), and a positive **Kernig sign** (flexing the hip and knee when the patient is supine, then straightening out the leg, causes resistance and back pain). Other signs of meningitis include headache, photophobia, seizures, and altered mental status. Patients with meningitis (< 1%) rarely have papilledema secondary to increased intracranial pressure. Risk factors for meningitis include sinusitis, ear infection, and sick contacts. Fever of unknown origin **(FUO)** is defined as a fever of > 101°F for three weeks that remains undiagnosed after one week of aggressive investigation.

2. **The answer is d.** The incubation period for both *S. aureus* and *B. cereus* is 1–2 hours after eating. *B. cereus* toxicity is often due to eating fried (the toxin is heat-stable) or uncooked rice. *S. aureus* toxicity is usually due to eating ham, poultry, potato or egg salad, mayonnaise, or cream pastries. All the other organisms require an incubation period of > 16 hours. *V. cholerae* toxicity is due to eating shellfish and causes an inflammatory (presence of fecal leukocytes) diarrhea. *V. parahaemolyticus* toxicity is due to eating mollusks and crustaceans and causes dysentery (production of cytotoxins, bacterial invasion, and destruction of intestinal mucosal cells). *Salmonella* toxicity is due to eating beef, poultry, eggs, or dairy products and causes a watery diarrhea. *Shigella* causes dysentery and can be present in potato or egg salad, lettuce, or raw vegetables.

3. **The answer is c.** This patient probably had AIDS with PML as a complication of that disease. The inclusion bodies in the oligodendrocyte nuclei are JC virus, a papillomavirus. Primary infection with JC virus is universal and asymptomatic. Immunosuppression leads to reactivation of the virus. Diagnosis is typically made by MRI, which shows multiple, focal, well-defined white matter lesions that do not enhance or have mass effect. Cerebrospinal fluid PCR for JC virus is also available, obviating the need for brain biopsy in most cases. Treatment with cytarabine arabinoside has not been shown to be effective in clinical trials. Less than 10% of patients may experience spontaneous remission. PML may also develop with lymphomas, leukemias, or sarcoid, but the incidence of this disease in the U.S. population has expanded greatly since the dissemination of HIV in the population.

4. **The answer is f.** Tabes dorsalis is caused by *Treponema pallidum*, the agent responsible for all types of neurosyphilis, but it is a disease entity distinct from general paresis, the form of neurosyphilis in which personality changes and dementia do occur. With tabes dorsalis, the patient develops a leptomeningitis. The posterior columns of the spinal cord and the dorsal root ganglia are hit especially hard by degenerative changes associated with this form of neurosyphilis.

5–6. **The answers are 5-b, 6-a.** The diffuse rash involving palms and soles would in itself suggest the possibility of secondary syphilis. The hypertrophic, wartlike lesions around the anal area are called *condylomata lata*, which are specific for secondary syphilis. The VDRL slide test will be positive in all patients with secondary syphilis. The Weil-Felix titer has been used as a screening test for rickettsial infection. In this patient, who has condyloma and no systemic symptoms, Rocky Mountain spotted fever would be unlikely. No chlamydial infection would present in this way. Blood cultures might be drawn to rule out bacterial infection such as chronic meningococcemia; however, the clinical picture is not consistent with a systemic bacterial infection. Penicillin is the drug of choice for secondary syphilis. Ceftriaxone and tetracycline are usually considered to be alternative therapies. Interferon alpha has been used in the treatment of condyloma acuminatum, a lesion that can be mistaken for syphilitic condyloma.

Musculoskeletal

Brachial plexus

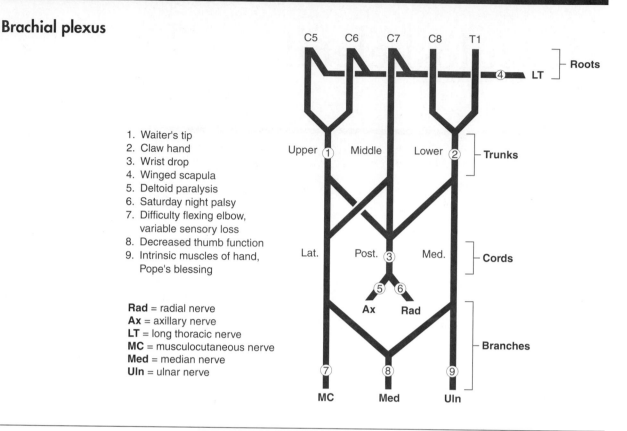

1. Waiter's tip
2. Claw hand
3. Wrist drop
4. Winged scapula
5. Deltoid paralysis
6. Saturday night palsy
7. Difficulty flexing elbow, variable sensory loss
8. Decreased thumb function
9. Intrinsic muscles of hand, Pope's blessing

Rad = radial nerve
Ax = axillary nerve
LT = long thoracic nerve
MC = musculocutaneous nerve
Med = median nerve
Uln = ulnar nerve

COX-2 inhibitors (celecoxib, rofecoxib)

Mechanism	Selectively inhibit cyclooxygenase (COX) isoform 2, which is found in inflammatory cells and mediates inflammation and pain; spares COX-1, which helps maintain the gastric mucosa. Thus, should not have the corrosive effects of other NSAIDs on the gastrointestinal lining.
Clinical use	Rheumatoid and osteoarthritis.
Toxicity	Similar to other NSAIDs; may have less toxicity to GI mucosa (i.e., lower incidence of ulcers, bleeding).

Elevated pressure within a confined space that compromises nerve, muscle, and soft tissue perfusion. Occurs most often in the lower leg (anterior compartment) or forearm. Etiologies include fractures, crush injuries, burns, and reperfusion following arterial repair in an ischemic extremity.

History/PE

Pain out of proportion to physical findings, **pain with passive motion** of the fingers and toes, **paresthesias,** a tense compartment on palpation, pallor, and poikilothermia are characteristic signs. **Pulselessness** and **paralysis** are late findings. **Volkmann's contracture** of the wrist and fingers can be secondary to vascular insufficiency due to supracondylar fractures.

Evaluation

This clinical diagnosis **must be recognized.** Measure compartment pressures (usually elevated to > 30 mmHg) if the diagnosis is uncertain. Delta pressures (the difference between diastolic and compartment pressures) are also used to evaluate compartment syndrome.

Treatment

This is a **surgical emergency** that requires **immediate fasciotomy of all compartments** to decrease compartmental pressures and restore tissue perfusion. Fasciotomies should be done in < 6 hours to reduce the risk of neurovascular and soft tissue compromise.

> **The 6 P's of compartment syndrome:**
>
> **P**ain
> **P**allor
> **P**oikilothermia
> **P**aresthesias
> **P**aralysis
> **P**ulselessness

An exceedingly common pain complex that may arise from paraspinous muscles, ligaments, facet joints, or disk or nerve roots. Strains are muscular injuries; sprains are ligamentous injuries.

History/PE

LBP is associated with the following manifestations and conditions:

- Paraspinous muscular pain/spasm suggests a back sprain or strain.
- Pain that worsens at night and is not relieved by rest or positional changes suggests malignancy.
- Point tenderness over a particular vertebral body suggests vertebral osteomyelitis, fracture, or malignancy.
- **Bowel or bladder dysfunction** and **saddle-area anesthesia** are consistent with **cauda equina syndrome.**
- See Table 2.9–1 for deficits associated with nerve pathology.

Cauda equina is a surgical emergency.

HIGH-YIELD FACTS

Musculoskeletal

251

TABLE 2.9–1. Motor and Sensory Deficits in Back Pain

Root	Associated Deficits
L4	Motor: Foot dorsiflexion (tibialis anterior). Reflex: Patellar. Sensory: Medial aspect of the leg.
L5	Motor: Big toe dorsiflexion (extensor hallucis longus). Reflex: None. Sensory: Medial forefoot and lateral aspect of the leg.
S1	Motor: Foot eversion (peroneus longus/brevis). Reflex: Achilles. Sensory: Lateral foot.

Differential

Herniation, strain, sprain, fracture, spondylolisthesis, OA, infection, cancer, cauda equina syndrome, ankylosing spondylitis (AS), aortic aneurysm.

Evaluation

Blastic lesions = prostate cancer.

Lytic lesions = breast or lung cancer.

Diagnosis is primarily **clinical.** X-rays may reveal evidence of osteomyelitis, cancer (e.g., pathologic vertebral fractures, punched-out lytic or sclerotic blastic lesions), fractures, or AS. Blastic lesions suggest prostate cancer; lytic lesions suggest breast or lung cancer. MRI scans and electrodiagnostic studies (e.g., nerve conduction velocity testing) can evaluate persistent radiculopathy or myelopathy.

Treatment

The majority of patients with lower back pain recover spontaneously within six weeks.

For sprains and strains, **NSAIDs,** physical therapy, and continuation of ordinary activities as tolerated are recommended. **Rest for > 1–3 days is considered unnecessary.** Ninety percent of patients recover spontaneously within six weeks. Surgery (e.g., laminectomy, diskectomy) is indicated for patients with correctable spinal disease. Cauda equina syndrome is a **surgical emergency** requiring immediate decompression with laminectomy.

UCV *Surg. 48*

HERNIATED DISK

A condition in which the nucleus pulposus herniates posteriorly, resulting in nerve root or cord compression with neck/back pain and sensory and motor deficits. Causes include degenerative changes, trauma, or neck/back strain or sprain. Disk herniations occur most frequently in middle-aged and older men and often follow strenuous activity. Herniation is most common in the lumbar region, especially at the **L4–L5 and L5–S1 levels.**

History/PE

Symptoms are usually preceded by several months of aching, "discogenic" pain, followed by the sudden onset of severe, electricity-like LBP. The pain is exacerbated by straining (e.g., coughing) and is characterized by **sciatica** (pain radiating down the leg in an L4–S3 distribution). Associated symptoms include tingling or numbness in a lower extremity, muscle weakness, atrophy, contractions, or spasms. **Passive straight leg** and sometimes **crossed straight leg raises** increase pain. Large midline herniations may result in **cauda equina syndrome** with bowel incontinence, bladder distention, impotence, and saddle anesthesia.

Evaluation

MRI can show disk herniation (see Figure 2.9–1).

Treatment

Bed rest, NSAIDs, physical therapy, and local heat lead to resolution within 2–3 weeks for the majority of cases. Persistent or disabling symptoms may require surgical removal of the disk (diskectomy).

SPINAL STENOSIS

A narrowing of the lumbar or cervical spinal canal that may cause compression of the nerve roots, most commonly due to degenerative joint disease. It is seen primarily in middle-aged or elderly patients.

History/PE

Patients may complain of neck pain, back pain that radiates to the buttocks and legs, or leg numbness and weakness. Leg cramping may occur **at rest, with standing, and with walking (pseudo- or neurogenic claudication); sitting of-**

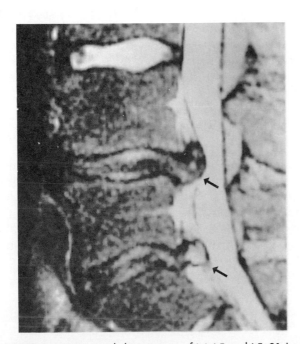

FIGURE 2.9–1. Disk herniation. MRI reveals herniations of L4–L5 and L5–S1 (arrows). (Reproduced, with permission, from Skinner HB. *Current Diagnosis & Treatment in Orthopedics,* 1st ed. Stamford, CT: Appleton & Lange, 1995:186, Fig. 5–10.)

ten provides relief. Patients can have pain while walking up hills and will flex at the hips to decrease their pain.

Evaluation

X-ray of the spine shows degenerative changes and a narrowed spinal canal. MRI or CT shows spinal stenosis. Unless comorbid vascular disease is present, the vascular exam is normal.

Treatment

Mild to moderate cases may be treated conservatively with NSAIDs and abdominal muscle strengthening. Epidural steroid injections can provide relief in advanced cases. When these measures fail, surgical laminectomy may achieve significant short-term success, although many patients will have a recurrence of symptoms.

ANKYLOSING SPONDYLITIS

AS is a chronic inflammatory disease of the spine and pelvis that causes sacroiliitis and, eventually, fusion of the affected joints. Age of onset is typically in the second and third decades. Like the other seronegative spondyloarthropathies (e.g., psoriatic, Reiter's, and enteropathic arthropathies), AS is strongly associated with **HLA-B27.** Additional risk factors include male gender and a positive family history.

History/PE

Patients present with intermittent hip and LBP that **worsens with inactivity and in the mornings** and that improves with activity over the course of the day. As the sacroiliitis progresses, there is decreased spine flexion (positive Schober test), a loss of lumbar lordosis, hip pain and stiffness, and limited chest expansion. Anterior uveitis and **third-degree heart block** may occur.

Differential

Remember for Reiter's: The patient "can't see, can't pee, and can't climb a tree."

Other seronegative spondyloarthropathies must be ruled out. These include:

- **Reiter's arthritis:** A disease of young men, the characteristic arthritis, uveitis, conjunctivitis, and urethritis usually follow an infection with *Campylobacter, Shigella, Salmonella, Chlamydia,* or *Ureaplasma.* Keratoderma blennorrhagicum and circinate balanitis may be present. (IM2.54)
- **Psoriatic arthritis:** An oligoarthritis of the **DIP joints.** Associated with psoriatic skin changes and **sausage-shaped digits** with **"mushroom caps."**

Evaluation

HLA-B27 will be positive. Spine and pelvic x-rays may demonstrate the characteristic late findings (fused **"bamboo spine"** and fused sacroiliac joints). ESR may be elevated; RF and ANA will both be negative.

Treatment

Minimize joint pain with NSAIDs and maximize exercise to improve posture and breathing.

UCV *IM2.50*

DUCHENNE MUSCULAR DYSTROPHY (DMD)

An **X-linked recessive disorder** that results from a deficiency of **dystrophin,** a subsarcolemmal cytoskeletal protein. DMD is the most common and most lethal muscular dystrophy with a usual onset between 2–6 years of age. Becker muscular dystrophy is a milder subtype that is also X-linked recessive and results from an abnormal-sized dystrophin.

History/PE

DMD affects the axial and proximal muscles before the distal muscles. Progressive **clumsiness, fatigability,** difficulty standing or walking, difficulty walking on toes (due to gastrocnemius shortening), and waddling gait may be present. **Gowers' maneuver** (pushing off with the hands when rising from the floor) is classic and indicates proximal muscle weakness. Exam will reveal **pseudohypertrophy of the gastrocnemius muscles** and possibly mental retardation.

Differential

Other muscular dystrophies (e.g., facioscapulohumeral, limb-girdle, myotonic, Becker), myasthenia gravis, metabolic myopathies.

Evaluation

CK is consistently elevated. Electromyogram (EMG) shows polyphasic potentials and increased recruitment. **Muscle biopsy** shows degeneration and variation in fiber size with fibrosis and basophilic fibers. Immunostaining for dystrophin expression (which is absent) is diagnostic. DNA analysis may reveal the dystrophin mutation, but this does not rule out Becker muscular dystrophy.

Treatment

As there is no cure for DMD, treatment is supportive. Patients are usually wheelchair bound by age 13; death generally occurs in the second decade. **Physical therapy** is necessary to maintain ambulation and prevent contractures. Perform Achilles tendon release if necessary.

UCV *Peds.49*

A common connective tissue disorder characterized by myalgias, weakness, and fatigability in the absence of inflammation. The etiology is unknown. Associated conditions include depression, anxiety, and irritable bowel syndrome. It is most common in **women > 50 years old.**

History/PE

Multiple (≥ 11 of 18), diffuse, tender areas and standard **"trigger points"** that, when palpated, reproduce the pain. Body aches, fatigue, and sleep disorders may also be present (see Figure 2.9–2).

Evaluation

This is a diagnosis of exclusion. The presence of < 11 of 18 tender points or non-fibromyalgia-associated tender points is known as myofascial pain syndrome.

Treatment

Treat with supportive measures such as stretching and heat application. Hydrotherapy as well as a transcutaneous electrical nerve stimulation (TENS) unit can also provide relief of symptoms. Reassurance about the benign nature of the disease, patient education, stress reduction, psychotherapy, and low-dose antidepressants may also help.

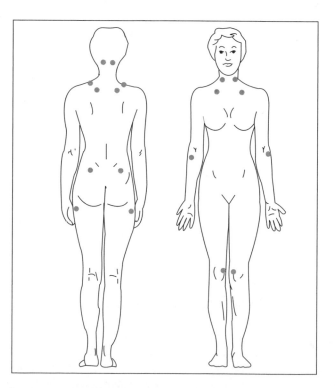

FIGURE 2.9–2.   (Reprinted, with permission, from Braunwald E. *Harrison's Principles of Internal Medicine,* 15th ed. New York: McGraw-Hill, 2001:2011, Fig. 325–2.)

A metabolic condition causing recurrent attacks of **acute monoarticular arthritis.** Results from the intra-articular deposition of **monosodium urate crystals** and is especially common among middle-aged, obese **men** (90%) and Pacific Islanders. Most patients have hyperuricemia secondary to uric acid underexcretion. Other causes include Lesch-Nyhan syndrome, diuretic use, cyclosporin use, malignancies, excessive ingestion of red meat or red wine, and hemoglobinopathies.

History/PE

Patients are typically awakened from sleep with the sudden onset of excruciating joint pain. Gout most commonly affects the **first metatarsophalangeal (MTP) joint** (podagra), midfoot, knees, ankles, and wrists; the hips and shoulders are generally spared. Joints are erythematous, swollen, and exquisitely tender. Patients with long-standing disease may develop **tophi,** deposits of urate crystals that lead to deformed joints.

Differential

Pseudogout (**positively birefringent rhomboid crystals** in aspirate; most commonly affects the **knee**), cellulitis, septic joint, trauma, foreign body synovitis, avascular necrosis (AVN), malignancy.

Pseudogout is often less severe.

Evaluation

Joint fluid aspiration may reveal **needle-shaped, negatively birefringent** (yeLLow when paraLLel to the condenser) **crystals** (see Clinical Images) and an elevated WBC. In many cases, serum uric acid is ≥ 7.5, but some patients have normal uric acid levels. Radiographs show no changes in early gout. Characteristic punched-out erosions with overhanging cortical bone (**"rat bite"**) are seen in more advanced gout.

The presence of crystals in the joint aspiration confirms the diagnosis of gout or pseudogout.

Gout = needle shaped, negatively birefringent. Pseudogout = rhomboid shaped, positively birefringent.

Treatment

For acute attacks, administer IV colchicine, high-dose **NSAIDs** (e.g., indomethacin), or **steroids.** For maintenance therapy, **allopurinol** (for overproducers) and **probenecid** (for undersecretors) can be given. Avoid thiazide/loop diuretics, red wine, red meat, and other triggers of hyperuricemia. The most frequent adverse effect of allopurinol is the precipitation of an acute gouty attack.

Avoid allopurinol during acute gout attacks.

UCV *IM2.52*

A chronic, noninflammatory arthritis of movable, weight-bearing joints that is also known as degenerative joint disease. OA has **no systemic manifestations** and is characterized by deterioration of the articular cartilage and osteophyte formation at joint surfaces. Risk factors include family history, **obesity,** and a **history of joint trauma** (particularly previous intra-articular fractures).

HIGH-YIELD FACTS

Musculoskeletal

History/PE

Crepitus, decreased range of motion, and insidious onset of joint stiffness and pain are usually present. Pain is generally **worsened by activity and weight bearing and relieved by rest.** Exam might show involvement of the **weight-bearing joints** (hip, knee, and lumbar spine) as well as the **DIP** joints **(Heberden's nodes), PIP** joints **(Bouchard's nodes),** MTP joint of the first toe, and cervical spine.

Evaluation

Lab values are normal. Radiographs show irregular **joint space narrowing,** osteophytes, subchondral sclerosis, and subchondral bone cysts. ESR is normal. Synovial fluid aspiration may reveal straw-colored fluid with a normal viscosity and a WBC count < 3000 cells/μL.

Treatment

Treat mild cases with physical therapy, **weight reduction,** and **NSAIDs.** Intra-articular corticosteroid injections may provide temporary relief of symptoms. **Elective joint replacement** (e.g., total hip/knee arthroplasty) may be necessary when symptoms significantly interfere with activities of daily living.

UCV *Surg. 44*

PAGET'S DISEASE (OSTEITIS DEFORMANS)

A poorly characterized disease with excessive bone turnover by osteoclasts. Paget's disease may be associated with paramyxovirus infection and is primarily a disease of the elderly.

History/PE

People with Paget's may complain that their hat size is increasing, that they are going deaf, and that their legs are starting to bow.

The condition is often asymptomatic, but patients may complain of deep bone pain. Bone softening results in tibial bowing, kyphosis, and frequent fractures. It is also associated with an increase in cranial diameter (frontal bossing) and with deafness (compression of CN VIII).

Evaluation

Alkaline phosphatase and urinary hydroxyproline are elevated. Serum Ca^{2+} and phosphate are normal. X-rays show a **markedly expanded bony cortex** with increased density, thickened bony trabeculae, bowing of the long bones, and a characteristic **jigsaw or mosaic** bone pattern (see Figure 2.9–3).

Treatment

Treatment of symptomatic patients includes NSAIDs, calcitonin, or most commonly, **alendronate.**

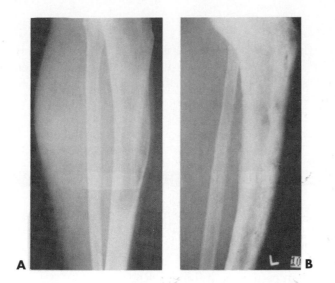

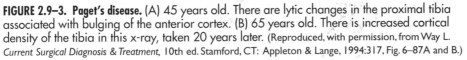

FIGURE 2.9–3. Paget's disease. (A) 45 years old. There are lytic changes in the proximal tibia associated with bulging of the anterior cortex. (B) 65 years old. There is increased cortical density of the tibia in this x-ray, taken 20 years later. (Reproduced, with permission, from Way L. *Current Surgical Diagnosis & Treatment,* 10th ed. Stamford, CT: Appleton & Lange, 1994:317, Fig. 6–87A and B.)

Complications

Fractures, vertebral collapse leading to spinal cord compression, high-output cardiac failure, arthritis, deafness, **secondary osteosarcoma.**

POLYMYOSITIS

A progressive, systemic connective tissue disease characterized by striated muscle inflammation. Thought to be an autoimmune disease, but its specific etiology is poorly understood. One-third of patients have **dermatomyositis** with coexisting cutaneous involvement. Patients may also develop myocarditis, cardiac conduction deficits, or malignancy. The condition may affect the young (5–15 years old) but is most commonly seen in older people (50–70 years old). Women are twice as likely as men to be affected.

History/PE

Symmetric, progressive, **proximal** muscle weakness and pain cause the classic complaint of difficulty rising from a chair. Patients may eventually have difficulty breathing or swallowing. Dermatomyositis may present with a **heliotrope rash** (violaceous periorbital rash) and **Grottron's papules** (papules located on the dorsum of the hands, over bony prominences).

Evaluation

Elevated serum creatine, aldolase, and CPK are generally present. EMG demonstrates fibrillations. Muscle biopsy shows inflammatory cells and muscle degeneration.

Treatment

High-dose corticosteroids generally result in improved muscle strength in 4–6 weeks and can be tapered to a lower dose for maintenance therapy. If the patient is unresponsive to initial treatment, immunosuppressive medication may be used. Monitor for malignancy.

UCV *IM2.51*

RHEUMATOID ARTHRITIS (RA)

A chronic, destructive, systemic inflammatory arthritis characterized by **symmetric** involvement of both large and small joints. RA causes synovial hypertrophy and pannus formation with resultant erosion of adjacent cartilage, bone, and tendons. It is most common in **females ≥ 35–50 years old.** There is a high incidence in patients with HLA-DR4.

History/PE

Unlike OA, the DIP joints in RA are spared.

Insidious onset of morning stiffness for ≥ 1 hour and painful, warm swelling of multiple symmetric joints for ≥ 6 weeks are characteristic complaints. Patients may also note fever, fatigue, malaise, anorexia, and weight loss. The most commonly involved joints are the **wrists, metacarpophalangeal (MCP)** and **PIP joints,** ankles, knees, shoulders, hips, elbows, and cervical spine. Ulnar deviation of the fingers with MCP joint hypertrophy is a common finding (see Figure 2.9–4). Extra-articular manifestations include ligament and tendon deformations (e.g., swan-neck and boutonnière deformities), **subcutaneous, painless Baker's cysts,** vasculitis, atlantoaxial subluxation, carpal tunnel syndrome, and Felty's syndrome.

Felty's triad = hepatosplenomegaly, thrombocytopenia, and RA.

Evaluation

Rheumatoid factor (anti-F_c IgG antibody) is elevated in ≥ 75% of cases but is not specific for RA. ESR can also be elevated. Synovial fluid aspiration reveals slightly turbid fluid with decreased viscosity and a WBC count of 3,000–50,000 cells/μL. Early in the course of the disease, radiographs show

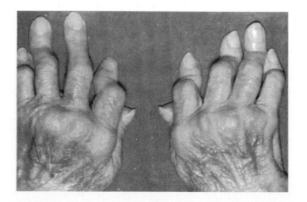

FIGURE 2.9–4. Rheumatoid arthritis. Note the boutonnière deformities of the digits, ulnar deviation of the fingers, MCP joint hypertrophy, and severe involvement of the PIP joints. (Reproduced, with permission, from Chandrasoma D. *Concise Pathology*, 3rd ed. Stamford, CT: Appleton & Lange, 1998:978, Fig. 68–2.)

soft tissue swelling and juxta-articular demineralization. Later findings include joint space narrowing and erosions.

Treatment

Treat with **NSAIDs,** including the COX-2 inhibitors. Severe cases are treated with corticosteroids, methotrexate, hydroxychloroquine sulfate, gold, or azathioprine. Operative therapy may be necessary in advanced cases.

UCV *IM2.55*

A nonmigratory, nonsuppurative mono- and poly-arthropathy with bony destruction that occurs in patients ≤ 16 years of age and lasts ≥ 6 weeks. In 95% of cases, the disease resolves by puberty.

History/PE

JRA can be classified into three subtypes:

- **Pauciarticular:** The **most common form** of JRA, this is a chronic arthritis frequently involving weight-bearing joints. Up to 30% will develop insidious **iridocyclitis,** which can cause blindness if left untreated.
  - **ANA type: Most common form;** results in asymmetric involvement of large joints with iridocyclitis.
  - **RF type:** Poor prognosis; most commonly found concurrently with AS in HLA-B27-positive men.
- **Polyarticular:** Resembles RA and involves multiple (≥ 5), symmetrically involved, inflamed small joints. Systemic features are less prominent; patients may develop iridocyclitis.
- **Systemic acute febrile:** The least common subtype, this form has characteristic arthritis with **daily high, spiking fevers** and an **evanescent, salmon-colored rash.** Hepatosplenomegaly and serositis may also be present.

All three patterns may be accompanied by **fever, nodules, erythematous rashes, pericarditis,** and **fatigue.**

Differential

Trauma, reactive arthritis, septic arthritis, systemic lupus erythematosus (SLE), Lyme disease, AS, OA, leukemia, acute rheumatic fever.

Evaluation

There is no diagnostic test for JRA. RF is positive in 15% of cases; ANA may be positive. ESR, WBCs, and platelets are commonly elevated; RBCs are generally decreased. A normal ESR does not exclude the diagnosis. Imaging may show soft tissue swelling and regional osteoporosis.

Treatment

Treat with **NSAIDs** or corticosteroids and range-of-motion and strengthening exercises. Methotrexate is used as a second-line agent. Monitor for iridocyclitis with routine ophthalmologic examinations.

UCV *Peds.55*

SCLERODERMA

Also called progressive systemic sclerosis, this is a multisystemic disease that most commonly manifests as the CREST syndrome and is most common in females aged 30–50 years old.

History/PE

Exam may reveal symmetric thickening of the skin of face and/or distal extremities. The **CREST syndrome** involves calcinosis, Raynaud's phenomenon, esophageal dysmotility, sclerodactyly, and telangiectasis. The more severe systemic form can result in pulmonary fibrosis, cor pulmonale, acute renal failure, and malignant HTN.

Evaluation

RF and ANA may be positive. **Anticentromere antibodies** are specific for CREST syndrome; **anti-Scl-70** (anti-topoisomerase 1) is specific for the systemic disease. CBC may reveal eosinophilia.

Treatment

Exacerbations may be treated with systemic glucocorticoids. Penicillamine can be used for skin changes, Ca^{2+} channel blockers for Raynaud's, and ACE inhibitors for renal disease and malignant HTN.

SYSTEMIC LUPUS ERYTHEMATOSUS

A multisystem autoimmune disorder that most frequently affects women (90%), especially **African-American women.** The pathogenesis of SLE is related to antibody-mediated cellular attack and to the deposition of antigen-antibody complexes. Drugs such as hydralazine, penicillamine, and procainamide may produce an SLE-like syndrome that resolves when the drug is discontinued.

History/PE

Nonspecific symptoms such as fever, anorexia, weight loss, and symmetric joint pain may be present. The mnemonic **DOPAMINE RASH** summarizes the criteria for diagnosing SLE (see Figure 2.9–5 and Clinical Images).

The symptoms of—

CREST syndrome
Calcinosis
Raynaud's phenomenon
Esophageal dysmotility
Sclerodactyly
Telangiectasias

Criteria for SLE—

DOPAMINE RASH
Discoid rash
Oral ulcers
Photosensitivity
Arthritis
Malar rash
Immunologic criteria
Neurologic symptoms (lupus cerebritis, seizures)
Elevated ESR
Renal disease
ANA +
Serositis
Hematologic abnormalities

HIGH-YIELD FACTS

Musculoskeletal

262

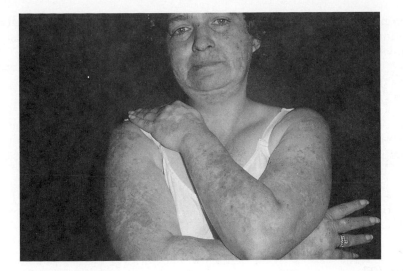

FIGURE 2.9–5. Systemic lupus erythematosus. Erythematous patches and plaques of SLE, predominantly in sun-exposed areas. Note the malar rash across the bridge of the nose. (Reproduced, with permission, from Hurwitz RM. *Pathology of the Skin: Atlas of Clinical-Pathological Correlation,* 2nd ed. Stamford, CT: Appleton & Lange, 1998:39, Fig. 2–41A.)

Evaluation

A positive ANA is sensitive but not specific. **Anti-dsDNA** and **anti-Sm antibodies** are highly specific but not as sensitive. During active attacks, there may be a decrease in C3 and C4. Drug-induced SLE has classic **antihistone antibodies.** Anti-Ro antibodies are associated with neonatal SLE. Antiphospholipid antibodies are associated with hypercoagulability, thromboembolic disease, and recurrent spontaneous abortions. Hematologically, anemia, leukopenia, and thrombocytopenia may be present.

Treatment

Treat with **NSAIDs** initially. **Steroids** are used for **acute exacerbations.** Steroids, hydroxychloroquine, cyclophosphamide, and azathioprine are used in progressive or refractory cases. Sun exposure and pregnancy exacerbate symptoms.

Complications

Opportunistic infections and progressive impairment of lung, heart, brain, or kidney function may occur. During pregnancy, there is an increased risk of spontaneous abortion; neonates have an increased risk of **congenital complete heart block.**

UCV *IM2.56*

TEMPORAL ARTERITIS (TA)

Generally not seen in patients < 50 years old. TA (or giant cell arteritis) affects twice as many women as men. Often due to subacute granulomatous inflammation of the large vessels, including the aorta, external carotid (especially the temporal branch), and vertebral arteries. The most feared complication of TA is **blindness** secondary to occlusion of the **central retinal artery** (a branch of the internal carotid artery). Half of all patients also have polymyalgia rheumatica (PMR).

History/PE

A new headache that is unilateral or bilateral and associated with scalp pain, **temporal tenderness, jaw claudication,** fever, and transient or permanent **monocular blindness** are classic. TA is also associated with weight loss, myalgias/arthralgias, and fever.

Differential

- **Large vessels:** Takayasu's arteritis
- **Medium vessels:** Churg-Strauss and polyarteritis nodosa (PAN, *IM2.53*)
- **Small vessels:** Wegener's granulomatosis and Henoch-Schönlein purpura (HSP *Peds.19*). HSP is an immune-mediated vasculitis affecting the GI tract, skin, joints, and kidneys. Average onset is 2–11 years old. It presents with **palpable purpura** on the buttocks and legs, **asymmetric migratory periarticular swelling,** and **abdominal pain.** Preceding URI is common (75%). Complications include GI bleeding, intussusception (check for stool occult blood), and glomerulonephritis (monitor for hematuria and proteinuria). The degree of renal involvement determines the prognosis. HSP is generally self-limited and treatment is supportive, but steroids might improve symptoms.

Evaluation

Obtain an **ESR** (> 50, usually > 100), an ophthalmologic evaluation, and a **temporal artery biopsy.** Biopsy will reveal thrombosis, necrosis of the media, and lymphocytes, plasma cells, and giant cells.

Treatment

If you suspect TA, start steroids before you biopsy.

Treat immediately with **high-dose prednisone** for 1–2 months before tapering. Unless biopsy is immediately available, do not delay treatment as blindness is permanent. Continue to follow the eye exam for improvements or changes.

UCV *Neuro.45*

POLYMYALGIA RHEUMATICA

A rheumatologic disorder most commonly seen in **elderly females.** PMR is considered part of the same disease spectrum as **TA** (same HLA haplotypes); the two frequently coexist.

History/PE

Pain and stiffness of the shoulder and pelvic girdle areas can be found in association with **fever,** malaise, weight loss, and minimal joint swelling. Patients classically have great difficulty getting out of a chair or lifting their arms above their heads. Weakness is generally not appreciated on exam.

Evaluation

Primarily clinical. **Anemia** and a markedly **elevated ESR** are almost always present.

Treatment

Low-dose prednisone (5–20 mg/day) works in almost all cases.

COMMON ADULT ORTHOPEDIC INJURIES

Table 2.9–2 summarizes the major adult orthopedic injuries.

COMMON PEDIATRIC ORTHOPEDIC INJURIES

Table 2.9–3 describes common pediatric orthopedic injuries.

DEVELOPMENTAL DYSPLASIA OF THE HIP (DDH)

Also called congenital hip dislocation (CHD), DDH is most commonly found in **first-born females** born in the **breech position**. DDH can result in subluxed, dislocatable, or dislocated femoral heads. Dislocations result from poor development of the acetabulum and hip due to lax musculature and **excessive uterine packing** in the flexed and adducted position (e.g., breech presentation), which leads to excessive stretching of the posterior hip capsule and adductor muscle contracture. The deformity will progress if it is not corrected.

History/PE

- **Barlow's maneuver:** Pressure is placed on the inner aspect of the abducted thigh and the hip is then adducted, causing posterior dislocation.
- **Ortolani's maneuver:** Like opening a book, the thighs are gently abducted from the midline with anterior pressure on the greater trochanter. A **soft click** signifies that the femoral head can be reduced into the acetabulum.
- **Allis' (Galeazzi's) sign:** The knees are at unequal heights when the hips and knees are flexed (the dislocated side is lower).

Additional signs include **asymmetric skin folds** and limited abduction of the affected hip secondary to adductor contracture.

Evaluation

Early detection is paramount to allow for proper hip development. Evaluation is clinical, although U/S may be helpful, especially after 10 weeks old. Because of the radiolucency of the neonatal femoral head, x-rays are unreliable until the patient is at least four months old.

TABLE 2.9–2. Common Adult Orthopedic Injuries

Injury	Mechanics	Treatment
Shoulder dislocation (*Surg.47*)	Most commonly an anterior dislocation with the **axillary artery and nerve** at risk. Posterior dislocations are associated with seizures and electrocutions and can injure the **radial artery.** Patients with anterior injuries hold the arm in external rotation; those with posterior injuries hold the arm in internal rotation.	Closed reduction followed by a sling and swath. Recurrent dislocations may need surgical repair.
Hip dislocation (*Surg.42*)	Most commonly a posterior dislocation via a posteriorly directed force **on an internally rotated, flexed,** adducted hip **("dashboard injury").** Anterior dislocations can injure the obturator nerve; posterior dislocations can injure the sciatic nerve and cause AVN.	Closed reduction followed by abduction pillow/bracing. Evaluate with CT scan after reduction.
Colles' fracture (*Surg.49*)	**The most common wrist fracture.** Involves the distal radius and commonly results from a **fall onto an outstretched hand,** resulting in a dorsally displaced, dorsally angulated fracture. Commonly seen in the **elderly** (osteoporosis) and in children.	Closed reduction followed by application of long arm cast. May need open reduction if fracture is intra-articular.
Scaphoid (carpal navicular) fracture	**Most commonly fractured carpal bone.** May take 1–2 weeks for radiographs to show the fracture; thus, a high index of suspicion is necessary. Assume a fracture if there is **tenderness in the anatomical snuff box.**	Thumb spica cast; if displacement or nonunion is present, treat with open reduction. With **proximal third** scaphoid fractures, **AVN** may result from disruption of blood flow.
Boxer's fracture	Fracture of the fifth metacarpal neck. Often results from forward trauma of a **closed fist** (e.g., punching a wall, an individual's jaw, or another fixed object).	Closed reduction and ulnar gutter splint; percutaneous pinning if fracture is excessively angulated. If skin is broken, assume infection by human oral pathogens **("fight bite")** and treat with surgical irrigation, debridement, and IV antibiotics to cover *Eikenella*.
Humerus fracture	Results from direct trauma and puts the **radial nerve** at risk (nerve travels in the spiral groove of the humerus). Signs of radial nerve palsy include **wrist drop** and loss of thumb abduction (see Figure 2.9–6).	Hanging arm cast versus coaptation splint and sling. Functional bracing.
"Nightstick fracture"	Ulna shaft fracture resulting from self-defense with arm against a blunt object.	Open reduction and internal fixation (ORIF) if significantly displaced.
Monteggia's fracture	Diaphyseal fracture of the proximal ulna with subluxation of the radial head.	ORIF of the shaft fracture (due to poor diaphyseal blood supply) and closed reduction of the radial head.

TABLE 2.9–2. Common Adult Orthopedic Injuries (continued)

Injury	Mechanics	Treatment
Galeazzi's fracture	Diaphyseal fracture of the radius with dislocation of the distal radioulnar joint. Results from a direct blow to the radius.	ORIF of the radius and casting of the forearm in supination to reduce the distal radioulnar joint.
Hip fracture *(Surg.43)*	**Most common in osteoporotic women** who sustain a fall. Patients present with a **shortened** and **externally rotated leg.** Displaced femoral neck fractures are associated with a high risk of AVN and fracture nonunion. Patients are at risk for subsequent DVTs.	ORIF with parallel pinning of the femoral neck. Displaced fractures in elderly patients (> 80 years old) may require a hip hemiarthroplasty. **Anticoagulation** is necessary for DVT prevention.
Femur fracture	Direct trauma (e.g., MVA). Beware of **fat emboli** (present with fever, scleral and axillary petechiae due to thrombocytopenia, confusion, dyspnea, and hypoxia).	Intramedullary nailing of the femur. Open fractures require thorough irrigation and debridement.
Tibial fracture	Direct trauma (car bumper + pedestrian injury). Watch for **compartment syndrome.**	Casting versus intramedullary nailing.
Open fractures	An **orthopedic emergency;** must be taken to the OR in < 6 hours owing to the risk of infection.	Must go to the OR **emergently** to repair fracture. Treat with antibiotics.
Achilles tendon rupture	Most commonly seen in unfit men who are participating in sports and hear a sudden **"pop" like a rifle shot.** Exam shows **limited plantar flexion** and a **positive Thompson test** (pressure on the gastrocnemius does not result in foot plantar flexion).	Treat with a long-leg cast for six weeks.
Knee injuries	Presents with knee instability, and possibly edema and hematoma. ■ **ACL:** Results from forced hyperflexion; positive anterior drawer and Lachman's tests. Rule out a meniscal or MCL injury. ■ **PCL:** Results from forced hyperextension; positive posterior drawer test. ■ **Meniscal tears: Clicking or locking** may be present. Exam shows **joint line tenderness** and a positive McMurray's test.	Treatment of MCL/LCL and meniscal tears is conservative unless tears are associated with symptoms or concurrent ligamentous injuries. Treatment of ACL injuries is generally surgical with graft from the patellar or hamstring tendons. Operative PCL repairs are reserved for highly competitive athletes.

HIGH-YIELD FACTS

Musculoskeletal

TABLE 2.9–3. Orthopedic Injuries in Children

Injury	Characteristics	Treatment
Clavicular fracture	**Most commonly fractured long bone in children.** May be birth-related (especially in large infants) and can be associated with **brachial nerve palsies.** Usually involve the **middle third of the clavicle,** with the proximal fracture end displaced superiorly due to the pull of the sternocleidomastoid muscle.	Figure-of-eight sling versus arm sling.
Greenstick fracture	Incomplete fracture involving the cortex of only one side of the bone.	Reduction with casting. Order films at 7–10 days.
Nursemaid's elbow	**Radial head subluxation** that typically occurs as a result of being **pulled or lifted by the hand.** The child complains of pain and **will not bend the elbow.**	Manual reduction by gentle supination of the elbow at 90° of flexion. No immobilization is necessary.
Torus fracture	Buckling of the cortex of a long bone secondary to trauma. Usually occurs in the distal radius or ulna.	Cast immobilization for 3–5 weeks, depending on age.
Supracondylar humerus fractures	Tends to occur at 5–8 years of age. Proximity to the **brachial artery** increases the risk of **Volkmann's contracture** (results from compartment syndrome of the forearm).	Cast immobilization; closed reduction with percutaneous pinning if fracture is significantly displaced.
Osgood-Schlatter disease	Overuse apophysitis of the tibial tubercle. Causes localized pain, especially with quadriceps contraction, in active young boys.	Decreased activity for 1–2 years. A neoprene brace may provide symptomatic relief.
Salter-Harris fractures	Fractures of the growth plate in children. Classified by fracture location: ■ **I:** Physis (growth plate). ■ **II:** Metaphysis and physis. ■ **III:** Epiphysis and physis. ■ **IV:** Epiphysis, metaphysis, and physis. ■ **V:** Crush injury of physis.	Types I and II can generally be treated nonoperatively. Others, including unstable fractures, must be treated operatively to prevent complications such as leg length inequality.

Treatment

Begin treatment early. Splint with a **Pavlik harness** (maintains hip flexed and abducted) if the child is < 6 months old. Older children can be treated with a spica cast (6–15 months old) or with open reduction (15–24 months old). If treatment is not instituted before two years of age, a significant defect is likely; various osteotomies can then be used to help correct deformities.

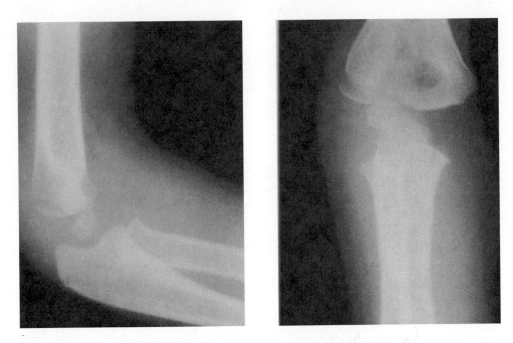

FIGURE 2.9–6. Lateral condyle fracture of the humerus. (Reproduced, with permission, from Skinner HB. *Current Diagnosis & Treatment in Orthopedics,* 2nd ed. Stamford, CT: Appleton & Lange, 2000:572, Fig. 11–45.)

Complications

Joint contractures and AVN of the femoral head can result.

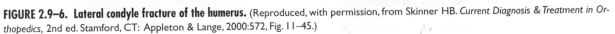 *Peds.51*

LIMP

One of the most common musculoskeletal disorders of childhood, limp has a number of etiologies. Trauma remains the most common etiologic factor.

History/PE

Parents may complain that the patient has a disruption in normal gait that may be associated with pain or fever. Inquire about a history of trauma, recent infection (especially when diagnosing septic joint, osteomyelitis, and toxic synovitis), or contact with TB-positive patients. Demographics are particularly important. Whereas young children and toddlers are more likely to have an infected joint, adolescents and teenagers are more likely to develop JRA, slipped capital femoral epiphyses (SCFE), and Legg-Calvé-Perthes (LCP). Exam may reveal a disruption in normal gait (e.g., Trendelenburg, antalgic gaits). Infection may cause erythema, edema, and limited range of motion. Point tenderness suggests trauma or tumor. Always evaluate for concurrent fever, signs of systemic infection, and neurologic involvement (e.g., reflexes, muscle atrophy, changes in sensation, bowel and bladder function).

Differential

The **STARTSS HOTT** mnemonic summarizes the differential for limp.

> **Differential diagnosis of limp—**
>
> **STARTSS HOTT**
> **S**eptic joint
> **T**umor
> **A**vascular necrosis (LCP)
> **R**heumatoid arthritis/JRA
> **T**uberculosis
> **S**ickle cell disease
> **S**CFE
> **H**SP
> **O**steomyelitis
> **T**rauma
> **T**oxic synovitis

Evaluation

A thorough history and physical exam are often the key. X-rays of the affected joint should include the joints above and below. A CBC, ESR, and C-reactive protein may be elevated, especially if an infection or a tumor is present. Additional tests might include a bone scan, nerve conduction studies, and for a suspected septic joint, joint aspiration and culture.

Treatment

Treatment is etiology-dependent. Immediately identify emergent causes, such as septic joint so that treatment may be initiated.

LEGG-CALVÉ-PERTHES DISEASE

Avascular necrosis (AVN) of the femoral head of unknown etiology, most commonly found in boys 4–10 years of age (see Figure 2.9–7). Can be bilateral.

History/PE

Hip pathology can present as referred knee pain.

Children are usually asymptomatic at first, but can develop a painless limp. If pain is present, it can be referred to the knee. Exam shows **limited abduction and internal rotation** as well as atrophy of the affected leg.

Treatment

The disease course is self-limited with the symptomatic interval generally lasting < 18 months. Children with limited femoral head involvement or with

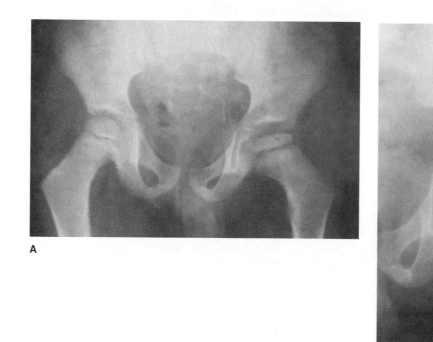

A

B

FIGURE 2.9–7. Legg-Calvé-Perthes. Avascular necrosis of the femoral head. (Reproduced, with permission, from Skinner HB. *Current Diagnosis & Treatment in Orthopedics,* 2nd ed. Stamford, CT: Appleton & Lange, 2000:543, Fig. 11–9)

full range of motion (ROM) can be treated conservatively with observation. If the disease is progressive or extensive or if ROM is impaired, treatment can include bracing, hip abduction with a Petrie cast, or an osteotomy. Prognosis depends on the patient's age (good if < 5 years of age), ROM, extent of femoral head involvement, and joint stability (good if there is little or no subluxation).

UCV *Peds.50*

SLIPPED CAPITAL FEMORAL EPIPHYSIS

Separation of the proximal femoral epiphysis through the growth plate such that the femoral head is displaced medially and posteriorly relative to the femoral neck. SCFE occurs most commonly in obese, African-American **adolescent (11- to 13-year-old) males.** Its etiology is unknown but may be due to an imbalance between growth hormone and sex hormones. The condition is bilateral in up to 30% of cases. SCFEs in younger individuals may be associated with hypothyroidism or other endocrinopathies.

History/PE

Presents with **thigh** or **knee pain** and a **painful limp.** Pain onset may be acute or insidious. In acute SCFE, there is restricted ROM and commonly, an **inability to bear weight.** Exam reveals limited internal rotation and abduction of the hip along with hip tenderness. Flexion of the hip leads to an **obligatory external rotation** secondary to physical displacement.

Evaluation

Radiographs of **both** hips in **AP and frog-leg lateral views** show **posterior and medial displacement** of the femoral head (see Figure 2.9–8). A TSH should be ordered to rule out hypothyroidism.

Treatment

The disease is progressive, and treatment should begin promptly. Patients **should not bear any weight** on the affected limb until the defect is promptly surgically stabilized with screws. **Gentle closed reduction** is warranted only in acute slips.

Complications

Can result in chondrolysis, AVN of the femoral head, and premature hip OA necessitating hip arthroplasty.

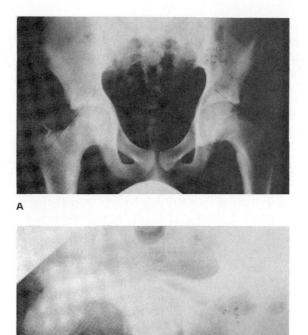

A

B

FIGURE 2.9–8. Slipped capital femoral epiphysis. (A) AP x-ray. The medial displacement of the left femoral epiphysis is best seen with a line drawn up the lateral femoral neck. The abnormal epiphysis does not protrude beyond this line. (B) Frog-leg lateral x-ray. Posterior displacement of the femoral epiphysis is characteristic. (Reproduced, with permission, from Skinner HB. *Current Diagnosis & Treatment in Orthopedics,* 2nd ed. Stamford, CT: Appleton & Lange, 2000:546, Fig. 11–13A and B.)

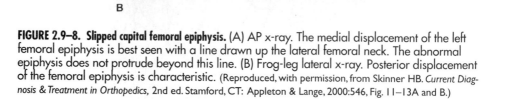

OSTEOSARCOMA

After multiple myeloma, osteosarcoma is the second common primary malignant tumor of bone. It tends to occur in the **metaphyseal** regions of the **distal femur, proximal tibia,** and proximal humerus and can metastasize to the lungs. It is most common in males during the second and third decades. Paget's disease can precede the development of secondary osteosarcoma.

History/PE

Patients generally present with progressive and eventually intractable pain that is worse at night. Constitutional symptoms such as fever, weight loss, and night sweats may be present. Exam may show a febrile patient with a zone of erythema and enlargement over the site of the tumor.

Differential

Ewing's sarcoma is also a common orthopedic tumor that presents most frequently in males aged 5–25 years old and is found in the **diaphyseal-metaphyseal** regions of the **pelvis, femur,** and tibia.

Evaluation

X-ray may show a classic **Codman's triangle** (periosteal new bone formation at the diaphyseal end of the lesion) or **"sunburst pattern"** of the osteosarcoma (see Figure 2.9–9); multilayered **"onion skinning"** is classic for Ewing's sarcoma. An MRI and CT should be performed to determine the extent of the tumor (soft tissue and bony invasion) and to plan for surgery.

Treatment

Treat osteosarcomas with limb-sparing surgical procedures and pre- and post-operative chemotherapy (e.g., methotrexate, doxorubicin, cisplatin, ifosfamide). Amputation may be necessary for large tumors. The five-year prognosis is 60%. Ewing's sarcoma may be treated with surgery (limb-sparing versus amputation), chemotherapy, and radiation; it carries a five-year survival rate of 70%.

UCV *Surg.45*

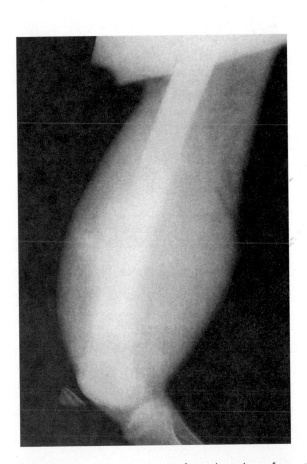

FIGURE 2.9–9. Osteosarcoma. "Sunburst" appearance of neoplastic bone formation in the femur of a 15-year-old girl. Amputation was required owing to the size of the tumor. (Reproduced, with permission, from Skinner HB. *Current Diagnosis & Treatment in Orthopedics,* 2nd ed. Stamford, CT: Appleton & Lange, 2000:272, Fig. 6–26.)

The following clinical questions and accompanying answers are reproduced, with permission, from Reteguiz J, *PreTest: Physical Diagnosis*, 4th ed., New York, McGraw-Hill, 2001.

Questions

For each patient in questions 1 and 2, choose among the following:
   a. Dermatomyositis
   b. Polymyositis
   c. Polymyalgia rheumatica
   d. Felty syndrome
   e. Scleroderma

1. A 75-year-old woman presents with malaise and myalgias for the last several months. She is chronically tired and has one hour of morning stiffness in the cervical, shoulder, and hip areas. She often has a low-grade temperature and has lost approximately 8 lb during this period. Neurologic exam reveals normal sensation, strength, and reflexes. **(CHOOSE ONE DIAGNOSIS)**

2. A 53-year-old woman presents with a two-month history of difficulty climbing stairs and rising from the seated position. On physical examination, she has a purplish discoloration of the skin over the forehead, eyelids, and cheeks. She has tenderness of the quadriceps muscles on palpation. **(CHOOSE ONE DIAGNOSIS)**

3. A 7-year-old boy presents with a one-year history of pain of the left anterior thigh. He has no history of trauma. On physical examination, he has limited hip motion, especially with abduction and internal rotation. A slight limp is noticeable with ambulation. Pain is brought on by activity and improves with rest. Which of the following is the most likely diagnosis?
   a. Legg-Calvé-Perthes disease
   b. Osgood-Schlatter's disease
   c. Muscular dystrophy
   d. Rickets
   e. Juvenile rheumatoid arthritis

4. An 81-year-old woman has recurrent back pain in her lumbar area. The pain radiates to her buttocks but is worse on the right side than the left side. Both sitting and walking aggravate the pain. She denies bladder dysfunction. On physical examination, the patient has diminished sensation and decreased reflexes of the right lower limb. Straight-leg raising and cross-leg raising tests are positive for reproduction of right lower limb symptoms. The patient has no spinal deformities. Which of the following is the most likely diagnosis?
   a. Sciatica
   b. Osteomyelitis
   c. Cauda equina syndrome
   d. Kyphosis
   e. Epidural abscess

Answers

1–2. The answers are 1-c, 2-a. **Polymyalgia rheumatica** affects older patients. They present with weight loss, profound fatigue, and pain and stiffness of the neck, shoulders, thighs, and hips. Physical examination is typically normal. **Temporal arteritis** may be seen in patients with polymyalgia rheumatica and must always be ruled out. **Dermatomyositis** is an autoimmune disease that causes proximal muscle weakness that involves the skin; **polymyositis** spares the skin. Patients with rheumatoid arthritis who develop splenomegaly and neutropenia are said to have **Felty syndrome.**

3. The answer is a. **Legg-Calvé-Perthes disease** (osteochondrosis) is an uncommon disorder that affects boys more than girls between the ages of 2 and 12. The hallmark is avascular necrosis of the capital femoral epiphysis, which has the potential to regenerate new bone. Consequently, children with Legg-Calvé-Perthes disease are of short stature and present with a "painless limp." **Osgood-Schlatter's disease** occurs in adolescence and is usually self-limiting. It is due to patellar tendon stress, which causes pain in the region of the tibial tuberosity especially when the patient extends the knee against resistance. **Rickets** is attributed to vitamin D deficiency and is manifested by bowing of the long bones, enlargement of the epiphyses of the long bones, delayed closure of the fontanelles, and enlargement of the costochondral junctions of the ribs (rachitic rosary). **Juvenile rheumatoid arthritis** is an inflammatory disorder that begins in childhood and may produce extraarticular symptoms, including iridocyclitis, fever, rash, anemia, and pericarditis. Muscular dystrophy is characterized by progressive weakness and muscle atrophy.

4. The answer is a. The sciatic nerve is located between the ischial tuberosity and the greater trochanter; tenderness over the nerve indicates irritation of the nerve roots forming the nerve. **The most common cause of sciatica is a herniated disk** usually occurring at the L4–L5 or L5–S1 levels. The **straight-leg raising test** is usually positive in sciatic nerve irritation (pain is produced with elevation of < 70° and worsened with dorsiflexion of foot or **Lasègue's sign**). A pulling or tight sensation in the hamstring is not a positive straight-leg raising test. **Cross-leg raising test** (elevation of unaffected leg causes pain in affected leg) may also be positive. Osteomyelitis and epidural abscesses are usually accompanied by systemic symptoms (i.e., fever) and are found in patients who are immunocompromised. The typical presentation for **cauda equina syndrome** is progressive weakness and numbness of the lower extremities bilaterally with urinary retention. There is perineal and perianal sensory loss (**"saddle anesthesia"**) and a lax anal sphincter. The cauda equina syndrome is a true surgical emergency. Kyphosis ("hunchback") is a smooth and rounded backward convexity of the thoracic region.

Neurology

Cerebral cortex functions

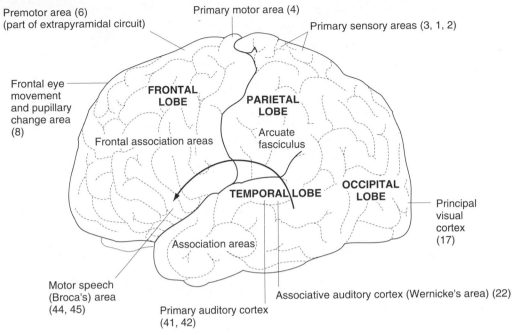

Premotor area (6)
(part of extrapyramidal circuit)

Primary motor area (4)

Primary sensory areas (3, 1, 2)

Frontal eye
movement
and pupillary
change area
(8)

FRONTAL LOBE

PARIETAL LOBE

Frontal association areas

Arcuate fasciculus

TEMPORAL LOBE

OCCIPITAL LOBE

Principal
visual
cortex
(17)

Association areas

Motor speech
(Broca's) area
(44, 45)

Primary auditory cortex
(41, 42)

Associative auditory cortex (Wernicke's area) (22)

Brain lesions

Area of lesion	Consequence	
Broca's area	Motor (expressive) aphasia with good comprehension	**BRO**ca's is **BRO**ken speech. Wernicke's is **W**ordy but makes no sense.
Wernicke's area	Sensory (fluent/receptive) aphasia with poor comprehension	
Arcuate fasciculus	Conduction aphasia; poor repetition with good comprehension, fluent speech	Connects Wernicke's to Broca's area.
Amygdala (bilateral)	Klüver-Bucy syndrome (hyperorality, hypersexuality, disinhibited behavior)	
Frontal lobe	Frontal release signs (e.g., personality changes and deficits in concentration, orientation, judgment)	
Right parietal lobe	Spatial neglect syndrome (agnosia of the contralateral side of the world)	
Reticular activating system	Coma	
Mammillary bodies (bilateral)	Wernicke-Korsakoff's encephalopathy (confabulations, anterograde amnesia)	

Lesions and deviations

CN XII lesion (LMN)—tongue deviates **toward** side of lesion (lick your wounds).

CN V motor lesion—jaw deviates **toward** side of lesion.

Unilateral lesion of cerebellum—patient tends to fall **toward** side of lesion.

CN X lesion—uvula deviates **away** from side of lesion.

CN XI lesion—head turns to ipsilateral side of lesion.

Visual field defects

Defect in visual field of

Lt. eye   Rt. eye

1. Right anopsia
2. Bitemporal hemianopsia
3. Left homonymous hemianopsia
4. Left upper quadrantic anopsia (right temporal lesion)
5. Left lower quadrantic anopsia (right parietal lesion)
6. Left hemianopsia with macular sparing

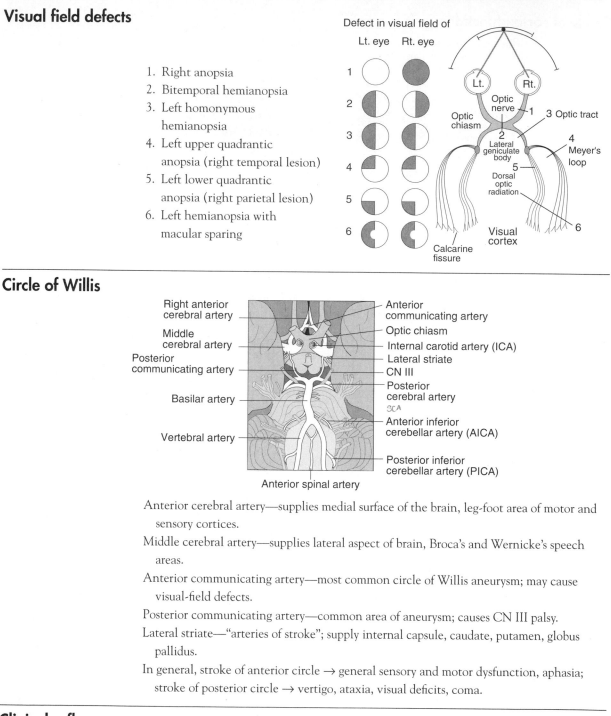

Circle of Willis

Anterior cerebral artery—supplies medial surface of the brain, leg-foot area of motor and sensory cortices.

Middle cerebral artery—supplies lateral aspect of brain, Broca's and Wernicke's speech areas.

Anterior communicating artery—most common circle of Willis aneurysm; may cause visual-field defects.

Posterior communicating artery—common area of aneurysm; causes CN III palsy.

Lateral striate—"arteries of stroke"; supply internal capsule, caudate, putamen, globus pallidus.

In general, stroke of anterior circle → general sensory and motor dysfunction, aphasia; stroke of posterior circle → vertigo, ataxia, visual deficits, coma.

Clinical reflexes

Biceps = C5 nerve root.

Triceps = C7 nerve root.

Patella = L4 nerve root.

Achilles = S1 nerve root.

Babinski—dorsiflexion of the big toe and fanning of other toes; sign of upper motor neuron lesion, but normal reflex in first year of life (upper motor neuron loss).

HIGH-YIELD FACTS

Neurology

Upper limb nerve injury

Nerve	Injury/deficit in motion	Deficit in sensation
Radial	Shaft of humerus—loss of triceps brachii (triceps reflex), brachioradialis (brachioradialis reflex), and extensor carpi radialis longus (→ wrist drop); often 2° to humerus fracture	Posterior brachial cutaneous Posterior antebrachial cutaneous
Median	Supracondyle of humerus—no loss of power in any of the arm muscles; loss of forearm pronation, wrist flexion, finger flexion, and several thumb movements; eventually, thenar atrophy	Loss of sensation over the lateral palm and thumb and the radial 2¹/₂ fingers
Ulnar	Medial epicondyle—impaired wrist flexion and adduction, and impaired adduction of thumb and the ulnar 2 fingers	Loss of sensation over the medial palm and ulnar 1¹/₂ fingers
Axillary	Surgical neck of humerus or anterior shoulder dislocation—loss of deltoid action	
Musculocutaneous	Loss of function of coracobrachialis, biceps, and brachialis muscles (biceps reflex)	

Spinal cord lesions

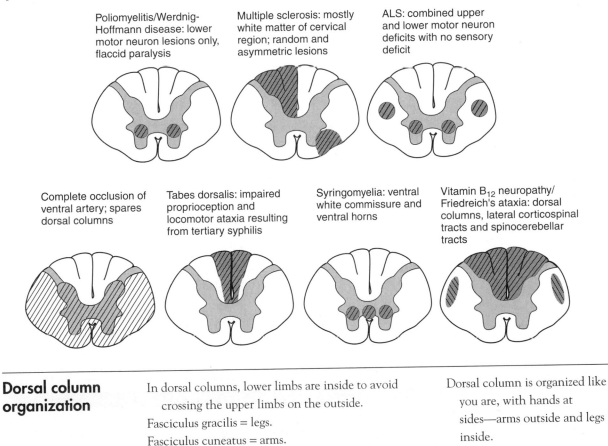

Poliomyelitis/Werdnig-Hoffmann disease: lower motor neuron lesions only, flaccid paralysis

Multiple sclerosis: mostly white matter of cervical region; random and asymmetric lesions

ALS: combined upper and lower motor neuron deficits with no sensory deficit

Complete occlusion of ventral artery; spares dorsal columns

Tabes dorsalis: impaired proprioception and locomotor ataxia resulting from tertiary syphilis

Syringomyelia: ventral white commissure and ventral horns

Vitamin B₁₂ neuropathy/Friedreich's ataxia: dorsal columns, lateral corticospinal tracts and spinocerebellar tracts

Dorsal column organization

In dorsal columns, lower limbs are inside to avoid crossing the upper limbs on the outside.
Fasciculus gracilis = legs.
Fasciculus cuneatus = arms.

Dorsal column is organized like you are, with hands at sides—arms outside and legs inside.

A general term for language disorders. The two principal aphasias are Broca's and Wernicke's. Aphasias generally result from insults (e.g., strokes, tumors, abscesses) to the "dominant hemisphere" (usually left hemisphere).

BROCA'S APHASIA

> Broca's is **B**roken speech.

A **disorder of language production** with **intact comprehension.** Due to an insult to Broca's area in the **posterior inferior frontal gyrus.** Also known as an expressive or nonfluent aphasia. Additional features include:

- Impaired repetition.
- Patients are aware of their deficits and are often **frustrated.**
- Associated with arm and face **hemiparesis,** hemisensory loss, and apraxia of oral muscles due to the proximity of Broca's area to the motor and sensory strips (the pre- and postcentral gyrus, respectively).
- Often secondary to a left superior **middle cerebral artery (MCA) stroke.**
- Treat with speech therapy.
- Wide range of outcomes with intermediate prognosis.

Insults to the basal ganglia that are associated with movement disorders may cause similar symptoms but are not considered Broca's aphasia.

UCV *Neuro.10*

WERNICKE'S APHASIA

> **W**ernicke's is **W**ordy but makes no sense.

A **disorder of language comprehension** with **intact yet nonsensical production.** Due to an insult to Wernicke's area in the left posterior superior temporal lobe (perisylvian). Also known as a fluent or receptive aphasia. Additional features include:

- Frequent use of **neologisms** (made-up words) and paraphasic errors (word substitutions).
- Patients are **unaware** of their deficit because they lack comprehension.
- No notable hemiparesis or dysarthria is present.
- Often secondary to left **inferior/posterior MCA** embolic stroke.
- Treat the underlying etiology and institute speech therapy.
- Poorer prognosis than with Broca's aphasia.

UCV *Neuro.16*

A profound suppression of responses to external and internal stimuli. Due to either catastrophic structural CNS injury or diffuse metabolic dysfunction. Causes include **hemorrhage, infarction,** abscesses, and tumors. Other causes include endogenous disturbances in electrolyte, endocrine, or metabolic function; **exogenous toxins** such as medications, EtOH, and other drugs; infectious or inflammatory disease; and generalized seizure activity or postictal states.

HIGH-YIELD FACTS

Neurology

Differential

Catatonic, hysterical, **"locked in,"** **persistent vegetative state.** Locked-in patients are awake and alert but are unable to move anything but their eyes and eyelids. Locked-in states are associated with central pontine myelinolysis, brain stem stroke, and advanced amyotrophic lateral sclerosis (ALS). A patient in a persistent vegetative state has normal wake-sleep cycles but is completely unaware of self or the environment. The most common causes are trauma with diffuse cortical injury or hypoxic ischemic injury.

Treatment

Initial treatment consists of the following measures:

1. **Stabilize the patient:** Attend to **ABCs**—**A**irway, **B**reathing, and **C**irculation.
2. **Reverse the reversible:** Administer **DONT**—**D**extrose, **O**xygen, **N**aloxone, and **T**hiamine.
3. **Identify and treat the underlying cause** and associated complications.
4. **Prevent further damage.**

DEMENTIA

A chronic, progressive, global decline in multiple cognitive areas (see **The 5 A's of dementia**). The most common etiology is Alzheimer's disease (AD), which accounts for 70–80% of cases. The differential diagnosis includes **DEMENTIAS.** Take care not to confuse delirium and dementia.

UCV *Neuro.17,36*

ALZHEIMER'S DISEASE

The **most common cause** of dementia. **Age** is the most important risk factor. Other risk factors include female gender, **family history, Down syndrome,** and low educational level. Pathology includes **neurofibrillary tangles, neuritic plaques** with **amyloid** deposition, amyloid angiopathy, and neuronal loss.

History/PE

Amnesia is usually the first presenting sign, followed by language deficits, acalculia, depression, agitation, and apraxia (inability to perform skilled movements).

Differential

Multi-infarct dementia, pseudodementia (due to depression), Pick's disease, normal pressure hydrocephalus, subdural hemorrhage, intracranial abscess, tumor.

Evaluation

AD is a **diagnosis of exclusion** that can be definitively **diagnosed only on autopsy.** MRI or CT may show atrophy and can rule out other causes. CBC,

---

The 5 A's of dementia:

Aphasia
Amnesia
Agnosia
Apraxia
Disturbances in
Abstract thought

DEMENTIAS:

Neuro**D**egenerative
diseases
Endocrine
Metabolic
Exogenous
Neoplasm
Trauma
Infection
Affective disorders
Stroke/**S**tructural

ESR, electrolytes, TSH, and serum B_{12} should all be within normal limits. Neuropsychological testing helps distinguish between dementia and depression.

Treatment

Institute supportive therapy. **Cholinesterase inhibitors** are first-line therapy and include donepezil, rivastigmine, and galantamine. Vitamin E (α-tocopherol) may also slow cognitive decline. Selegiline, other antioxidants, anti-inflammatories, and estrogen have not been shown unequivocally to affect disease course.

Complications

Survival is 5–10 years from the onset of symptoms. Death is usually secondary to **aspiration pneumonia** or other infections.

DYSEQUILIBRIUM

Peripheral causes of vertigo always produce horizontal nystagmus, whereas vertical nystagmus indicates a central lesion.

Refers to a number of phenomena, including **light-headedness** (as one might feel after standing up rapidly from a reclining position), **loss of balance,** or **vertigo** (a spinning sensation). Equilibrium is maintained through the input of **visual, vestibular,** and **proprioceptive** systems and through processing by the **cerebellum** and **brain stem.**

Differential

The most common causes are benign paroxysmal positional vertigo (BPPV) (~50%) and Ménière's disease. Other causes include hypothyroidism, aminoglycoside or furosemide toxicity, stroke, trauma, labyrinthitis, and acoustic neuroma.

Evaluation

Determine if the dysequilibrium is central or peripheral (see Table 2.10–1). A patient with a cerebellar lesion will have a positive **Romberg's sign** (inability

TABLE 2.10–1. Central vs. Peripheral Dysequilibrium

	Peripheral	Central
Vertigo	Often intermittent; severe.	Often constant; usually less severe.
Nystagmus	Always present; unidirectional; never vertical.	May be absent, uni- or bidirectional; may be vertical.
Associated findings		
Hearing loss or tinnitus	Often present.	Rarely present.
Intrinsic brain stem signs[a]	Absent.	Often present.

[a]Including ataxia, dysarthria, cranial nerve abnormalities, and motor system dysfunction.

to stand still with eyes closed). A patient with a vestibular lesion will often turn or fall to the ipsilateral direction. Other tests include assessment of thyroid function, B$_{12}$ level, and CSF for cells and oligoclonal bands (to rule out an infectious etiology and multiple sclerosis [MS], respectively). **Orthostasis** and **cardiac arrhythmias** should also be ruled out.

BENIGN PAROXYSMAL POSITIONAL VERTIGO

A common form of **peripheral vertigo** resulting from a **dislodged otolith** that causes disturbances in the semicircular canals.

History/PE

Transient, **episodic** vertigo (lasting < **1 minute**) and **nystagmus triggered by changes in head position** (classically while turning in bed or getting up in the morning), together with nausea and vomiting. Symptoms decrease with repetitive testing. **Recent trauma** is the most common identifiable etiology.

Evaluation

Evaluation should include the **Nylen-Bárány maneuver** (also known as the **Dix-Hallpike maneuver**)—i.e., having the patient go from a sitting to a supine position while quickly turning the head to the side. If vertigo and/or nystagmus is reproduced, BPPV is the likely diagnosis.

Treatment

Usually subsides spontaneously in weeks to months. Treat with repositioning exercises (e.g., the Epley maneuver).

MÉNIÈRE'S DISEASE (ENDOLYMPHATIC HYDROPS)

A form of **intermittent** peripheral vertigo that results from **distention of the endolymphatic compartment of the inner ear.** Causes include head trauma and syphilis; may also be **idiopathic.**

History/PE

Episodic vertigo associated with nausea, vomiting, **ear fullness, hearing loss, and tinnitus.** Episodes resolve within **hours to days.** Significant permanent hearing loss can occur over a period of years.

Evaluation

Audiometry shows low-frequency pure-tone hearing loss that fluctuates in severity.

Treatment

Treat with a **low-salt diet** and **acetazolamide.** Antihistamines, antiemetics, and benzodiazepines may be given for acute attacks. Surgical decompression may be necessary in refractory cases.

UCV *Neuro.25*

HEADACHE

Primary headache is generally classified into three categories: migraine, tension, and cluster. The causes of headache, however, are multiple and include the following:

- **Acute:** Subarachnoid hemorrhage (SAH), hemorrhagic stroke, meningitis, seizure, acutely elevated intracranial pressure (ICP), hypertensive encephalopathy, post-LP, ocular disease (glaucoma, iritis), new migraine headache.
- **Subacute:** Temporal arteritis (TA), intracranial tumor, subdural hematoma, pseudotumor cerebri, trigeminal/glossopharyngeal neuralgia, postherpetic neuralgia, HTN.
- **Chronic/episodic:** Migraine, cluster headache, tension headache, sinusitis, dental disease, neck pain.

Evaluation

Recent-onset headaches warrant immediate workup.

- **Is the headache new or old?** Recent or sudden-onset, severe headaches (such as headaches that awaken the patient) warrant immediate workup (e.g., for tumor, TA, and meningitis).
- **What are its characteristics?** Intensity, quality, location, and duration.
- **Are there associated symptoms?** Jaw claudication, fever, nausea, vomiting, and weight loss.
- **Are there neurologic symptoms?** Paresthesias, numbness, ataxia, visual disturbances, photophobia, and neck stiffness. Focal neurologic deficits and papilledema warrant immediate workup for more serious causes of headache.

CT without contrast is the preferred study for an acute hemorrhage.

- **If an SAH is suspected with a negative head CT, LP is mandatory.**
- Obtain a CBC, ESR, and CT/MRI in patients suspected of having SAH or elevated intracranial pressure (ICP) or if a patient has focal neurologic findings. Use **CT without contrast** to evaluate for an acute hemorrhage.

MIGRAINE HEADACHE

Most commonly affects **women** and those with a **family history.** Its etiology is unknown, but is likely related to **vascular** and brain neurotransmitter (**serotonin**) abnormalities. **Triggers** include certain foods (e.g., chocolate), fasting, stress, menses, OCPs, and bright light.

History/PE

Throbbing headache that lasts > **2 hours** but usually < 24 hours. Associated with **nausea and vomiting, photophobia,** and noise sensitivity. **"Classic mi-**

graines" are often **unilateral** and preceded by a visual **aura** in the form of either scintillating scotomas (bright light or flashing lights, often in a zigzag pattern, moving across the visual field) or field cuts (see Figure 2.10–1). By contrast, "**common migraines**" may be **bilateral** and periorbital and may present **without associated symptoms.**

Evaluation

Diagnosis is based on history. If headache is associated with focal neurologic deficits, rule out more serious etiologies with CT or MRI. Also rule out meningitis or SAH with an LP if symptoms are acute in onset.

Treatment

Avoid known triggers. Abortive therapy includes aspirin/NSAIDs and triptans (5-HT$_{1B/1D}$ agonists) (namely **sumatriptan**). **Prophylaxis** for patients with frequent/severe migraines includes β-blockers (propranolol), **tricyclic antidepressants** (TCAs) (amitriptyline), calcium channel blockers, and valproic acid. Narcotics should not be used prophylactically. *topiramate*

UCV *Neuro.28*

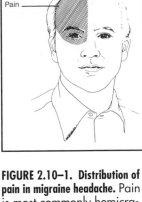

FIGURE 2.10–1. Distribution of pain in migraine headache. Pain is most commonly hemicranial but may be holocephalic, bifrontal, or unilateral frontal. (Reproduced, with permission, from Aminoff MJ. *Clinical Neurology*, 3rd ed. Stamford, CT: Appleton & Lange, 1996:91, Fig. 3–13.)

CLUSTER HEADACHE

Affects **men** more often than women, with an average age of onset of 25. Cluster headaches occur much less commonly than migraines.

History

A brief, severe, **unilateral periorbital headache** lasting 30 minutes to three hours (see Figure 2.10–2). Attacks tend to occur in **clusters,** affecting the same part of the head and taking place at the same time of day (usually at night) and at the same time of the year. Headaches may be precipitated by the use of alcohol or vasodilating drugs.

PE

Ipsilateral tearing of the eye, conjunctival injection, Horner's syndrome, and nasal stuffiness.

Evaluation

Classic presentations require no evaluation. Imaging may be necessary to rule out more catastrophic causes of extremely painful headache.

Treatment

Institute acute therapy with **high-flow O$_2$** (100% nonrebreather O$_2$), ergots, sumatriptan, intranasal lidocaine, and corticosteroids. Prophylactic therapy includes ergots, calcium channel blockers, prednisone, lithium, valproic acid, and topiramate.

UCV *Neuro.6*

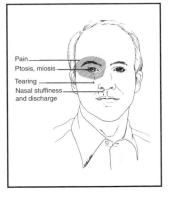

FIGURE 2.10–2. Distribution of pain in cluster headache. Pain is commonly associated with ipsilateral conjunctival injection, tearing, nasal stuffiness, and Horner's syndrome. (Reproduced, with permission, from Aminoff MJ. *Clinical Neurology*, 3rd ed. Stamford, CT: Appleton & Lange, 1996:92, Fig. 3–14.)

TENSION HEADACHE

The most common type of headache diagnosed in adults. Tension headaches are chronic headaches that do not share the specific symptomatology of migraine or cluster headaches yet respond to similar treatments.

History/PE

Patients complain of a **tight, bandlike pain** that is exacerbated by noise, bright lights, fatigue, and stress. Patients also report other nonspecific symptoms, such as anxiety, poor concentration, and difficulty sleeping. Headaches are generalized but may be most intense in the **occipital and neck region.** Surrounding musculature may also be tightly contracted. If a history of nausea and vomiting, photophobia, or family history is elicited, migraine headache is the more likely diagnosis.

Evaluation

A **diagnosis of exclusion.** There are no focal neurologic signs in tension headache.

Treatment

Relaxation, massage, hot baths, and **avoidance of exacerbating factors** may alleviate symptoms. **NSAIDs** are first-line abortive therapy, although triptans (e.g., sumatriptan) and ergots may be considered. Prophylactic treatment (calcium channel blockers, α-blockers, TCAs) can also be used.

UCV *Neuro.48*

HEMORRHAGE

SUBARACHNOID HEMORRHAGE

Commonly caused by a ruptured aneurysm (e.g., congenital berry), arteriovenous malformation (AVM), or trauma to the circle of Willis (often at the MCA). Trauma is the most common cause. Berry aneurysms are associated with polycystic kidney disease and coarctation of the aorta. SAH typically occurs at 50–60 years of age and has a high mortality rate (35%).

History/PE

A **sudden-onset, intensely painful headache,** often with **neck stiffness** and other signs of meningeal irritation, fever, nausea/vomiting, and a fluctuating level of consciousness. SAH may be preceded by milder **sentinel headaches** within weeks prior to its onset. Seizure may result from blood irritating the cerebral cortex. CN III palsy with pupil involvement is associated with berry aneurysms.

The three most common cerebral aneurysms are (1) anterior communicating (30%); (2) posterior communicating (25%); and (3) MCA (20%).

SAH will give the patient "the worst headache of my life."

Evaluation

Immediate head **CT without contrast** (see Figure 2.10–3) to look for blood in the subarachnoid space. Blood appears white on noncontrast CT (see Figure 2.10–3A). Obtain an immediate **LP if CT is negative** to look for RBCs, xanthochromia (yellowish CSF due to breakdown of RBCs), and elevated ICP. **Four-vessel angiography** should be performed once SAH is confirmed.

Treatment

Prevent rebleeding, which is most likely to occur in the first 48 hours after SAH. Prevent further neurologic deterioration due to vasospasm by administering **nimodipine** and IV fluids and keeping BP elevated. Administer **antiseizure medication** (phenytoin). Focus on **lowering ICP** by raising the head of the bed and possibly instituting hyperventilation. Surgical treatment involves open clipping or interventional radiologic coiling of vascular abnormalities. Treat pain, but not with NSAIDs.

Complications

Rebleeding (more common with aneurysm than with AVM), extension into the brain parenchyma (more common with AVM), arterial **vasospasm** (occurs in one-third of aneurysmal SAHs), and obstructive hydrocephalus. Ruptured aneurysms are reported to have a 50% one-month mortality rate.

UCV *Neuro.15*

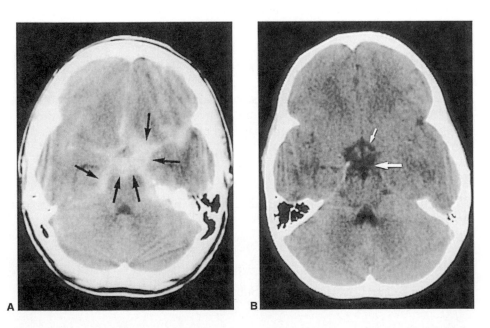

FIGURE 2.10–3. Subarachnoid hemorrhage. (A) CT scan without contrast reveals blood in the subarachnoid space at the base of the brain (arrows). (B) A normal CT scan without contrast shows no density in this region (arrows). (Reproduced, with permission, from Aminoff MJ. *Clinical Neurology*, 3rd ed. Stamford, CT: Appleton & Lange, 1996:78, Fig. 3–6A and B.)

EPIDURAL HEMATOMA

A traumatic intracranial hemorrhage of arterial origin that is commonly due to a **lateral skull fracture** (blunt trauma), with resultant tear of the **middle meningeal artery.**

History/PE

With an epidural hematoma, mental status changes occur within minutes to hours and have a classic "lucid" interval.

Patients present with a **lucid interval** ranging from several minutes to hours followed by the onset of headache, progressive obtundation, and hemiparesis. Ultimately epidural bleeding may lead to a **"blown pupil"** (fixed and dilated pupil).

Evaluation

CT shows a **lens-shaped, convex hyperdensity** that is limited by the sutures of the cranium where the dura inserts into the bone (see Figure 2.10–4B). Patients require **close observation** and **serial neurologic examinations** before surgery.

Treatment

Emergent **neurosurgical evacuation.**

SUBDURAL HEMATOMA

An intracranial hemorrhage that typically occurs after head trauma with resultant rupture of the **bridging veins** from the cortex to the dural sinuses (especially in the elderly and alcoholics).

History/PE

With a subdural hematoma, mental status changes can occur within days to weeks.

Headache, changes in mental status, contralateral hemiparesis, or other focal changes. Changes can be subacute or chronic and may present as dementia, especially in the elderly. There may be a remote history of a fall.

Evaluation

CT demonstrates a **crescent-shaped, concave hyperdensity** that does not cross the midline (see Figure 2.10–4A).

Treatment

Surgical evacuation if symptomatic. Subdural blood may regress spontaneously if it is chronic.

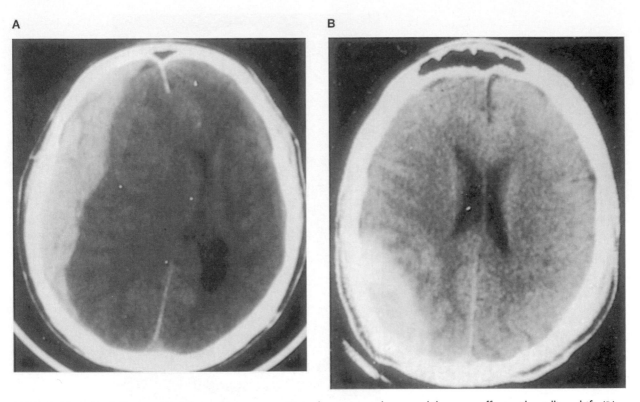

FIGURE 2.10–4. Head CT scans. (A) Subdural hematoma. Note the crescent shape and the mass effect with midline shift. (B) Epidural hematoma with classic biconvex lens shape. (Reproduced, with permission, from Aminoff MJ. *Clinical Neurology,* 3rd ed. Stamford, CT: Appleton & Lange, 1992:296.)

Parenchymal Hemorrhage

A hemorrhage within the brain parenchyma. Etiologies include HTN (usually in the basal ganglia), tumor, amyloid angiopathy (seen in the elderly), and vascular malformations (AVMs, cavernous hemangiomas). AVMs are more likely to produce an intraparenchymal hemorrhage than an SAH.

History/PE

Lethargy and headache; focal motor and sensory deficits. Patients may have some degree of obtundation.

Evaluation

Immediate non-contrast head **CT** reveals an intraparenchymal hemorrhage (see Figure 2.10–5). Look for mass effect or edema that may predict herniation.

Treatment

Treatment is similar to that for SAH: raise the head of the bed and institute antiseizure prophylaxis. Surgical evacuation may be necessary if mass effect is present, especially in the posterior fossa (threatening vital brain stem function).

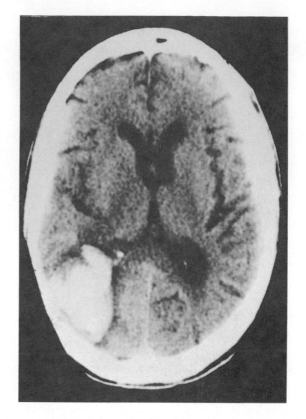

FIGURE 2.10–5. Intraparenchymal hematoma. Head CT without contrast reveals the irregularly shaped hyperdensity with midline shift of the choroid plexus. (Reproduced, with permission, from Saunders C. *Current Emergency Diagnosis & Treatment,* 4th ed. Stamford, CT: Appleton & Lange, 1992:248, Fig. 16–5.)

HERNIATION

Shifts in brain tissue through rigid, bony openings (see Figure 2.10–6). Several types exist, including central, **uncal,** subfalcine, and tonsillar. Can be secondary to any mass lesion, including **tumor, hemorrhage,** and abscess.

History/PE

Specific signs and symptoms depend on the type of herniation and the underlying mass lesion. The earliest symptoms of herniation are **altered mental status and/or consciousness.** Alterations in BP, HR, and respiratory patterns may also be a sign of increased ICP and impending herniation **(Cushing's triad).** A unilateral "blown pupil" is often a sign of **ipsilateral uncal herniation. Tonsillar herniation** is associated with **respiratory compromise.**

Evaluation

Noncontrast head CT to rule out mass lesion or hemorrhage.

Treatment

Treat the underlying cause. Signs of herniation can be managed by decreasing ICP with **hyperventilation,** IV **mannitol,** sedation, a ventriculostomy, and/or surgical decompression.

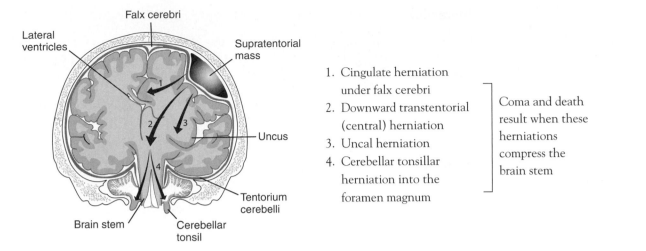

FIGURE 2.10–6. Herniation syndromes. (Adapted, with permission, from Simon RP et al. *Clinical Neurology*, 4th ed. Stamford, CT: Appleton & Lange, 1999:314.)

1. Cingulate herniation under falx cerebri
2. Downward transtentorial (central) herniation
3. Uncal herniation
4. Cerebellar tonsillar herniation into the foramen magnum

Coma and death result when these herniations compress the brain stem

MOVEMENT DISORDERS

PARKINSON'S DISEASE

An **idiopathic hypokinetic** disorder that occurs in all ethnic groups and usually begins after 50–60 years of age. Parkinson's is due to **dopamine depletion in the substantia nigra.** Life expectancy from the time of diagnosis is approximately nine years. Although most cases are idiopathic, other insults can decrease dopaminergic activity and lead to "parkinsonism," including **postencephalitic, toxic** (e.g., carbon disulfide, manganese, "designer drugs" such as **MPTP**), bihemispheric ischemic, traumatic, and iatrogenic (especially neuroleptic) insults.

History/PE

The **"Parkinson's tetrad"** consists of:

1. **Resting tremor** (e.g., "pill rolling") (see Figure 2.10–7).
2. **Rigidity:** Note that "cogwheeling" is due to the combined effects of rigidity and tremor.
3. **Bradykinesia:** Slowed movements and difficulty initiating movements. Also festinating gait (wide leg stance with short accelerating steps) without arm swing.
4. **Postural instability:** Stooped posture, impaired righting reflexes, freezing, and falls (see Figure 2.10–7).

Other common manifestations include masked facies, memory loss, and micrographia.

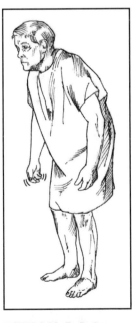

FIGURE 2.10–7. Patient with parkinsonism in typical flexed posture. Note the masked facies and resting hand tremor. (Reproduced, with permission, from Aminoff MJ. *Clinical Neurology*, 3rd ed. Stamford, CT: Appleton & Lange, 1996:220.)

Differential

Depression, normal pressure hydrocephalus, Wilson's disease, Creutzfeldt-Jakob disease, Shy-Drager syndrome, and Huntington's disease. Clues to **nonidiopathic Parkinson's** are **younger age of onset, lack of response to levodopa,** and **rapid progression of disease.** Consider Parkinson's-plus syndromes, which include additional prominent neurologic abnormalities (e.g., progressive supranuclear palsy [PSP]).

Treatment

Dopamine agonists (**bromocriptine**) are first line for early Parkinson's disease. **Levodopa/carbidopa** is the mainstay of therapy. Selegiline, an MAO-B inhibitor, may be neuroprotective and reduce the need for levodopa. Catechol-O-methyl-tranferase (COMT) inhibitors (entacapone) increase levodopa's availability to the brain and may decrease motor fluctuations. Amantadine and anticholinergics have limited efficacy. If medical therapy fails, attempt **surgical pallidotomy** (of the globus pallidus interna) or chronic **deep brain stimulation** of the globus pallidus interna and subthalamic nucleus.

UCV *Neuro.34*

HUNTINGTON'S DISEASE

A rare, **hyperkinetic, autosomal-dominant** disease involving multiple **abnormal CAG triplet repeats** on **chromosome 4p.** The number of repeats can expand from generation to generation, causing earlier expression and more severe disease in subsequent generations through a process known as **anticipation.** Fewer than 29 CAG repeats are considered normal, while mutant genes generally have > **39 repeats** (there is a gray area in between). Life expectancy is 20 years from time of diagnosis.

History/PE

Presents in patients 30–50 years of age with a gradual onset of **chorea, altered behavior,** and **dementia.** Dementia begins as irritability, moodiness, and antisocial behavior. This can develop into schizophreniform illness and depression.

Differential

Gilles de la Tourette's syndrome, senile chorea, hemiballismus, Wilson's disease, Parkinson's disease.

Evaluation

Clinical diagnosis. CT scans and MRI show cerebral atrophy (especially of the caudate and putamen). Molecular genetic testing to determine the number of CAG repeats.

Treatment

There is no cure, and the disease cannot be halted. Symptomatic treatment. Haloperidol for psychosis; reserpine to minimize unwanted movements. Genetic counseling should be offered to offspring.

UCV *Neuro.23*

NEOPLASMS

Intracranial neoplasms may be primary (30%) or **metastatic (70%).** The most common primary tumors include **meningiomas and glioblastoma multiforme (GBM) in adults** and **medulloblastomas and astrocytomas in children.** While **two-thirds of primary brain tumors in adults are supratentorial,** only **one-third are supratentorial in children.** Of all primary brain tumors, 40% are benign. Men are more likely to have GBM and women are more likely than men to have meningiomas. In general, benign disease affects those > 65 years old. Primary tumors rarely spread beyond the CNS.

Metastatic tumors (more common) are most often from primary **lung, breast, kidney, and GI tract neoplasms** and **melanoma.** Metastatic tumors most often occur supratentorially at the **gray-white junction** and are characterized by rapid growth, invasiveness, necrosis, and neovascularization. When **multiple discrete neoplastic** nodules appear in the brain simultaneously, metastatic disease should be suspected and a primary source should be sought.

The most common CNS tumor is metastatic disease.

The most common primary CNS tumors in adults are glioblastoma multiforme and meningioma.

The most common primary CNS tumors in children are medulloblastomas and astrocytomas.

History/PE

Symptoms depend on tumor type and location (see Table 2.10–2). Symptomatology is due to local growth and **resulting mass effect,** cerebral edema, increased ICP, and ventricular obstruction. Symptoms develop gradually and include nausea and vomiting, headache, and focal neurologic deficit. Other common symptoms include personality changes, lethargy, intellectual decline, aphasias, seizures, and mood swings.

Evaluation

CT with contrast and MRI with gadolinium to localize and determine the extent of the lesion. Histologic diagnosis may be obtained via CT-guided biopsy or during surgical tumor debulking. LP is rarely indicated.

Treatment

Resection (if possible), **radiation,** and **chemotherapy.** The type of therapy is highly dependent on the type of tumor and its histology, progression, and site (see Table 2.10–2). **Corticosteroids** can be used to reduce vasogenic edema. Management is often palliative.

UCV *Neuro.2,7,19,24,32,44*

Table 2.10–2. Most Common Primary Neoplasms

Tumor	Presentation	Treatment
Astrocytoma	Presents with headache and increased ICP. May cause unilateral paralysis in CN V–VII and CN X. Slow, **protracted course.** Prognosis much better than that of GBM.	Resection if possible. Radiation.
GBM (grade IV astrocytoma)	Most common primary brain tumor. Often presents with headache and increased ICP. Progresses rapidly. **Poor prognosis** (< 1 year from the time of prognosis).	Surgical removal/resection. Radiation and chemotherapy have variable results.
Meningioma	Originates from **dura mater or arachnoid.** Good prognosis. Incidence increases with age.	Surgical resection. Radiation for unresectable tumors.
Acoustic neuroma (schwannoma)	Presents with ipsilateral hearing loss, tinnitus, vertigo, and signs of cerebellar dysfunction. Derived from **Schwann cells.**	Surgical removal.
Medulloblastoma	**Common in children.** Arises from fourth ventricle and leads to increased ICP. Highly malignant; may seed subarachnoid space.	Surgical resection coupled with radiation and chemotherapy.
Ependymoma	Common in children. May arise from ependyma of a ventricle (commonly the fourth) or the spinal cord; may lead to hydrocephalus.	Surgical resection. Radiation.

NEUROCUTANEOUS SYNDROMES

NEUROFIBROMATOSES

*NF2 is associated with **bilateral** acoustic neuromas and a gene defect on chromosome **22.***

The most common of the neurocutaneous disorders. There are two major types: Neurofibromatosis 1 (NF1, or von Recklinghausen's syndrome) and neurofibromatosis 2 (NF2). NF1 is more common and is associated with the NFT-1 gene on chromosome 17q. NF2 is associated with a defective gene on chromosome 22.

History/PE

NF1 diagnostic criteria include two or more of the following: (1) **six café-au-lait spots** (each ≥ 5 mm in children or ≥ 15 mm in adults); (2) two neurofibromas of any type; (3) **freckling** in the axillary or inguinal area; (4) **optic glioma;** (5) **two Lisch nodules (pigmented iris hamartomas);** (6) osseous abnormality; and (7) a first-degree relative with NF1.

Numerous café-au-lait spots should make you think of NF1.

NF2 diagnostic criteria include **bilateral acoustic neuromas** or a first-degree relative with NF2 and either unilateral acoustic neuromas or two of any of the following: neurofibromas, meningiomas, gliomas, or schwannoma. Other NF2 features include seizures, skin nodules, and café-au-lait spots.

Evaluation

MRI of the brain, brain stem, and spine. Perform complete dermatologic exam, ophthalmologic exams, and family history. Consider testing hearing.

Treatment

No cure. Symptomatic treatment. Acoustic neuromas can be treated by surgery or radiosurgery.

TUBEROUS SCLEROSIS

Exhibits an extremely variable clinical course and is characterized by seizures (beginning in the first year of life), mental retardation (MR) (greater likelihood with earlier age of onset), and skin and eye lesions. Symptoms are secondary to small benign tumors that grow on the face, eyes, brain, kidney, and other organs.

History/PE

Patients usually present with **infantile spasms** and **"ash-leaf" hypopigmented lesions** on the trunk and extremities. Other skin manifestations include **sebaceous adenomas,** which are small red nodules over the nose and cheeks (may be confused with acne), and a **shagreen patch,** which is a rough papule in the lumbosacral region with an orange-peel consistency. Two retinal lesions are recognized: (1) mulberry tumors, which arise from the nerve head; and (2) phakomas, which are round, flat gray lesions near the disk.

Evaluation

Head CT shows calcified tubers in the periventricular area. These lesions may rarely transform into malignant astrocytomas. Skin lesions are enhanced by a Wood's UV lamp. ECG can evaluate for rhabdomyoma of the heart, especially in the apex of the left ventricle (~50% of tuberous sclerosis patients). Rhabdomyomas may cause CHF, although they usually resolve spontaneously. Renal U/S may reveal renal hamartomas or polycystic disease. Pulmonary manifestations include angiomyolipomas that may cause generalized cystic or fibrous pulmonary changes.

Treatment

Treatment is symptomatic. Maintain seizure control with clonazepam or valproic acid (as in infantile spasms). Signs of increased ICP may indicate a tuber obstructing the foramen of Munro. Surgical intervention may be indicated.

NUTRITIONAL DEFICIENCIES

Several nutritional deficiencies are associated with specific neurologic syndromes. The important syndromes are described in Table 2.10–3.

SEIZURES

Evaluate patients after their first seizure (e.g., for mass lesions) before initiating treatment for epilepsy.

Due to **excessive or hypersynchronous discharge by neurons,** resulting in focal and/or general neurologic symptoms. Patients with a first seizure should be evaluated prior to the initiation of treatment. An **aura,** which is a subjective sensation/feeling preceding the onset of a seizure, is experienced by 50–60% of patients with epilepsy. The EEG is the most important diagnostic test. Common etiologies of seizures according to age are listed in Table 2.10–4.

TABLE 2.10–3. Neurologic Syndromes Associated with Nutritional Deficiencies

Vitamin	Syndrome	Signs/Symptoms	Classic Patients	Treatment
Thiamine (vitamin B_1)	Wernicke's encephalopathy	Classic triad: **encephalopathy, ophthalmoplegia** (nystagmus, lateral rectus palsy, conjugate-gaze palsy), **ataxia** (polyneuropathy, cerebellar and vestibular dysfunction).	**Alcoholics,** hyperemesis, starvation, renal dialysis, AIDS. **Can be elicited by large-dose glucose administration.**	Reversible, almost immediately, with thiamine administration.
	Korsakoff's dementia	Above, plus **amnesia,** horizontal nystagmus.	Same as above.	Irreversible.
Cyanocobalamin (vitamin B_{12})[a]	Combined system disease (CSD) *or* subacute combined degeneration	Gradual, progressive onset. Symmetric paresthesias, leg stiffness, spasticity, paraplegia, bowel and bladder dysfunction. Dementia.	Patients with pernicious anemia.	B_{12} injections or large oral doses.
Folate[a]	Folate deficiency	Irritability, memory loss, personality changes without the neurologic systems of CSD.	**Alcoholics,** patients with pernicious anemia.	Reversible if corrected early.

[a]Associated with elevated homocysteine and increased risk of vascular events.

TABLE 2.10–4. Causes of Seizures

Infant	Child (2–10)	Adolescent	Adult (18–35)	Adult (35+)
Perinatal injury	Idiopathic	Idiopathic	Trauma	Trauma
Infection	Infection	Trauma	Alcoholism	Stroke
Metabolic	Trauma	Drug withdrawal	Brain tumor	Metabolic disorder
Congenital	Febrile seizure	AVM		Alcoholism
				Brain tumor

Evaluation

- **Was the seizure epileptic?** Use the history to differentiate. Elevated prolactin levels are consistent with an epileptic seizure.
- **Was the seizure provoked by a systemic process?** If there is a clear, treatable, non-neurologic cause, further neurologic investigation may be unnecessary. Such disorders include **hypoglycemia, hyponatremia, hypocalcemia, hyperosmolar states, hepatic encephalopathy,** uremia, porphyria, **drug overdose** (especially cocaine, antidepressants, neuroleptics, methylxanthines, and lidocaine), **drug withdrawal** (especially alcohol and other sedatives), eclampsia, hyperthermia, hypertensive encephalopathy, and cerebral hypoperfusion.
- **Was the seizure caused by an underlying neurologic disorder?** Seizures with focal onset (or focal postictal deficit) suggest focal CNS pathology. Seizures may be the presenting sign of a tumor, stroke, AVM, infection, or hemorrhage, or they may represent the delayed presentation of a developmental abnormality.
- **Is anticonvulsant therapy indicated?** First seizures are frequently not treated when the underlying cause is unknown.

> *Workup should focus on reversible causes of seizure first.*

FOCAL (PARTIAL) SEIZURES

Arise from a **discrete region** in one cerebral hemisphere and **do not lead to loss of consciousness (LOC)** unless they secondarily generalize. Can be simple or complex.

History/PE

Simple partial seizures may include motor (e.g., jacksonian march, the progressive jerking of successive body regions), sensory (parietal lobe), autonomic (BP, HR, PVR), or psychic features (fear, déjà vu) without alteration of consciousness. Postictally, there may be a focal neurologic deficit (Todd's paralysis) that resolves within 1–2 days. It is often confused with acute stroke and can be differentiated with MRI. **Complex partial seizures** typically involve the temporal lobe (70–80%) and are characterized by **impaired level of consciousness,** auditory or visual hallucinations, déjà vu, automatisms (e.g., lip smacking, chewing, or even walking), and postictal confusion/disorientation and amnesia. Symptoms may mimic schizophrenia or acute psychosis. Both simple partial and complex partial seizures may evolve into secondary generalized tonic-clonic (grand mal) seizures.

Workup

Obtain an **EEG.** Rule out systemic causes with CBC, electrolytes, calcium, fasting glucose, LFTs, renal panel, RPR, ESR, and toxicology screen. A focal seizure implies a focal brain lesion. Rule out a mass by MRI or CT with contrast.

Treatment

Treat the underlying cause. For recurrent partial seizures, phenytoin, oxcarbazepine, tegretol, phenobarbital, and valproic acid can be administered as monotherapy. In children, phenobarbital is the first-line anticonvulsant. For intractable temporal lobe seizures, surgical options include **anterior temporal lobectomy.** Prior to surgery, patients undergo **Wada testing,** in which sodium amytal, a brain-numbing agent, is injected into the anterior temporal lobe (via the MCA) to determine if resection would cause a functional deficit.

UCV *Neuro.41*

PRIMARY (IDIOPATHIC) GENERALIZED SEIZURES

Involve **both cerebral hemispheres** and lead to **sudden LOC,** usually without aura, followed by a period of **postictal confusion.** The two most common types are tonic-clonic (grand mal) and absence (petit mal).

TONIC-CLONIC (GRAND MAL) SEIZURES

History/PE

Primary (idiopathic) tonic-clonic seizures begin suddenly with tonic extension of the back and extremities, continuing with 1–2 minutes of repetitive, symmetric clonic movements. Marked by **incontinence** and **tongue biting.** Patients may appear **cyanotic** during the ictal period. Consciousness is slowly regained in the postictal period. Postictally, the patient may complain of muscle aches and headaches. Partial seizures can evolve into secondarily generalized tonic-clonic seizures as well.

Differential

Syncope, cardiac dysrhythmias, brain stem ischemia, and pseudoseizures. Refer to Table 2.10–5 to differentiate between syncope and seizures.

Treatment

Treat the underlying cause. Valproate is first-line therapy for primary (idiopathic) generalized tonic-clonic seizures. Lamotrigine or topiramate may be used as adjunctive therapy. For secondarily generalized tonic-clonic seizures, use the same therapy as would be used for focal (partial) seizures.

UCV *Neuro.43*

ABSENCE (PETIT MAL) SEIZURES

Begin in **childhood,** subside before adulthood, and are often **familial.**

TABLE 2.10–5. Seizure vs. Syncope

	Seizure	Syncope
Onset	Sudden onset without prodrome. Focal sensory or motor phenomena. Sensation of fear, smell, memory.	Progressive light-headedness. Dimming of vision, faintness.
Course	Sudden LOC with tonic-clonic activity. May last 1–2 minutes. May see tongue laceration, head trauma, and bowel/urinary incontinence.	Gradual LOC, limp or with jerking. Rarely lasts longer than 15 seconds. Less commonly injured.
Postspell	Postictal confusion and disorientation.	Typically immediate return to lucidity.

History/PE

Present with brief, often unnoticeable episodes of **impaired consciousness** lasting **only 5–10 seconds** and occurring up to hundreds of times per day. Patients are **amnestic** during and immediately after seizures. Classically, a teacher may observe a child **"daydreaming"** or **"staring"** in class. No loss of muscle tone. Eye fluttering or lip smacking during absence seizures is common.

Children with absence seizures often get into trouble for daydreaming in class.

Evaluation

EEG shows classic three-per-second spike-and-wave discharges.

Treatment

Ethosuximide is the first-line agent. Valproic acid or zonisamide may also be used.

UCV *Neuro.40*

INFANTILE SPASMS (WEST SYNDROME)

A syndrome characterized by (1) **infantile spasms** (generalized seizures), (2) an **abnormal interictal EEG** (very high amplitude slow waves), and (3) **arrest of psychomotor development** at the age of seizure onset. It generally starts between 3 and 12 months of age, exhibiting a male predominance and a family history in a small percentage of cases. Seizures are tonic, bilateral, and symmetric and tend to occur in clusters of 5–10 individual spasms. Seizures tend to occur while drowsy or immediately upon awakening. MR is found in the majority of patients. Treatment includes hormonal therapy with **ACTH**, prednisone, and antiepileptic medications (clonazepam and valproic acid).

STATUS EPILEPTICUS

Status epilepticus is a medical emergency with a 20% mortality!

A **medical emergency** consisting of prolonged (> **30 minutes**) or repetitive seizures without a return to baseline consciousness. Common causes include anticonvulsant withdrawal/noncompliance, anoxic brain injury, EtOH/sedative withdrawal or other drug intoxication, metabolic disturbances (e.g., hyponatremia), trauma, and infection. Status epilepticus is associated with a 20% mortality rate.

Evaluation

First, **protect the airway.** Determine the underlying cause with pulse oximetry, CBC, electrolytes, calcium, glucose, ABGs, LFTs, BUN/Cr, ESR, and toxicology screen. **Defer EEG and brain imaging until the patient is stabilized.** Perform LP in the setting of fever or meningeal signs (only after having done a CT scan to ensure the safety of the LP).

Treatment

Maintain **ABCs.** Consider rapid intubation for airway protection. Administer an **IV benzodiazepine** such as lorazepam or diazepam and a loading dose of **phenytoin.** If seizures continue, intubate and load with **phenobarbital.** Consider an IV sedative such as midazolam or pentobarbital if seizures continue. **Glucose, thiamine, and naloxone** may also be given to presumptively treat other potential etiologies.

STROKE

Hemorrhagic strokes are far less common than ischemic strokes.

Acute onset of focal neurologic deficits resulting from diminished blood flow (**ischemic stroke, 85%**) or hemorrhage (**hemorrhagic stroke, 15%**). Nonmodifiable risk factors are **age, male** gender, genetics, and **race** (African-Americans, Hispanics, Asians). Modifiable risk factors include **HTN, diabetes mellitus, obesity, smoking, hypercholesterolemia,** carotid stenosis, heavy alcohol intake, cocaine, IVDU, and **atrial fibrillation (AF).** The most common etiology is atherosclerosis of the extracranial vessels (internal and common carotids, basilar, and vertebral arteries). Lacunar infarcts occur in regions supplied by small perforating vessels and result from atherosclerosis, HTN, or diabetes. Other causes include **fibromuscular dysplasia** (especially in young females), inflammatory diseases, arterial dissection, migraine, and venous thrombosis.

Cardiac causes of stroke include AF (the most common cause of cardioembolic stroke) as well as embolism of mural thrombi, thrombi from diseased or prosthetic valves, other arrhythmias, endocarditis (septic, fungal, or marantic emboli), and paradoxic (venous) emboli in patients with right-to-left shunt in the heart (from atrial septal defect or patent foramen ovale). Patients with AF have a five- to sixfold greater risk of stroke than the general population.

History/PE

- **Middle cerebral artery:** Aphasia (dominant hemisphere), neglect (nondominant hemisphere), contralateral hemiparesis, gaze preference, and homonymous hemianopsia (Neuro.13,14).

- **Anterior cerebral artery:** Leg paresis, amnesia, personality changes, foot drop, gait dysfunction, and cognitive changes.
- **Posterior cerebral artery:** Homonymous hemianopsia, memory deficits, and dyslexia/alexia.
- **Basilar artery:** Coma, cranial nerve palsies, apnea, visual symptoms, drop attacks, and dysphagia.
- **Lacunar stroke:** Pure motor or sensory stroke, dysarthria–clumsy hand syndrome, ataxic hemiparesis *(Neuro.12)*.
- **TIA:** Transient neurologic deficit that lasts < 24 hours (although most last < 1 hour).

Differential

Todd's paralysis (postictal), brain tumor, subdural or epidural hematoma, brain abscess, endocarditis, MS, metabolic abnormalities (hypoglycemia), neurosyphilis.

Evaluation

- **CT without contrast** (to differentiate ischemic from hemorrhagic stroke) (see Figure 2.10–8).
- **MRI** (to identify early ischemic changes and neoplasms and to adequately image the brain stem/posterior fossa).
- **ECG** and an echocardiogram if embolic stroke is suspected (transesophageal echo is most sensitive for mural thrombus).
- **Vascular studies** for extracranial disease (carotid U/S, magnetic resonance angiography [MRA] or traditional angiography) and for intracranial disease (transcranial Doppler or MRA) (see Figure 2.10–9A).
- **Screen for hypercoagulable states** (if history of bleeding, first stroke, or < 50 years of age).
- Physical exam may reveal the source of an embolic stroke. Look for clues of cardiac arrhythmias (especially AF) and atherosclerotic disease (bruits).

Treatment

- Maintain vigilance for signs and symptoms of brain swelling, increased ICP, and herniation, which occur in large hemispheric strokes.
- **tPA** (tissue plasminogen activator) is indicated for ischemic stroke if administered **within three hours** of onset of symptoms. **Contraindications** to tPA therapy include systolic blood pressure (SBP) > 185 or diastolic blood pressure (DBP) > 110 despite aggressive antihypertensive therapy, prior intracranial hemorrhage, stroke or head trauma in the last three months, a recent MI, current anticoagulant therapy with INR > 1.7, use of heparin in the last 48 hours with prolonged PTT, a platelet count < 100,000/mm^3, major surgery in the past 14 days, GI or urinary bleeding in the past 21 days, seizures present at the onset of stroke, blood glucose < 50 or > 400 mg/dL, and age < 18.
- **ASA** reduces morbidity and mortality in acute ischemic stroke presenting within 48 hours (assuming no ASA allergy, no GI bleeding, and no tPA use).

Allow BP to rise up to 200/100 to maintain cerebral perfusion.

A

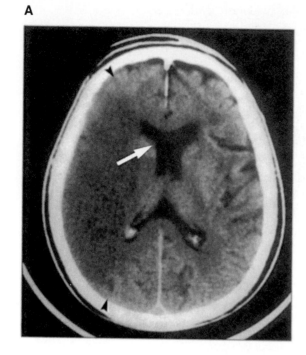

B

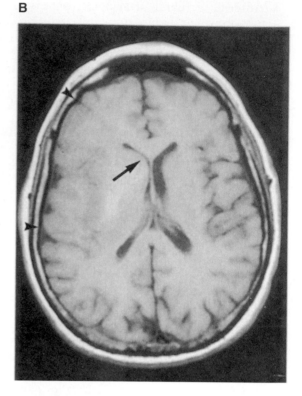

C

FIGURE 2.10–8. CT-MRI findings in ischemic stroke in the right MCA territory. (A) CT shows low density and effacement of cortical sulci (between arrowheads) and compression of the anterior horn of the lateral ventricle (arrow). (B) T1-weighted MRI shows loss of sulcal markings (between arrowheads) and compression of the anterior horn of the lateral ventricle (arrow). (C) T2-weighted MRI scan shows increased signal intensity (between arrowheads) and ventricular compression (arrow). (Reprinted, with permission, from Aminoff MJ. *Clinical Neurology*, 3rd ed. Stamford, CT: Appleton & Lange, 1996:275.)

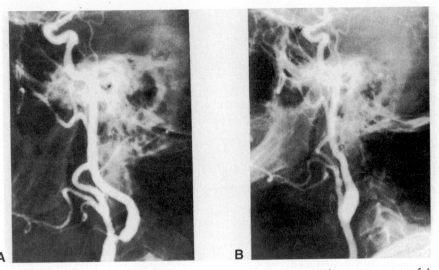

FIGURE 2.10–9. Pre- and post-endarterectomy. (A) Carotid arteriogram showing stenosis of the proximal internal carotid artery. (B) Postoperative arteriogram with restoration of the normal luminal size following endarterectomy. (Reproduced, with permission, from Way LW. *Current Diagnosis & Treatment,* 10th ed. Stamford, CT: Appleton & Lange, 1994:763, Fig. 35–11.)

- **Avoid hypotension, hypoxemia, and hypoglycemia.** SBP should generally be maintained approximately 20 mmHg above the patient's normal SBP.
- Treat aspiration pneumonia, UTI, or DVT, the main causes of morbidity and mortality following stroke.

Preventive and long-term treatment should consist of the following:

- **ASA,** clopidogrel, or dipyridamole/ASA if stroke is secondary to small vessel disease or thrombosis or if anticoagulation is contraindicated.
- **Carotid endarterectomy** if stenosis is > 70% in symptomatic patients or > 60% in asymptomatic patients (endarterectomy is contraindicated in vessels that are 100% occluded). See Figure 2.10–9.
- **Anticoagulation** (heparin initially, then warfarin) in cases of cardiac emboli, new AF, or hypercoagulable states. Target INR is 2–3.
- **Management of HTN** (including isolated systolic HTN), **hypercholesterolemia,** and **diabetes.**

Rule out hemorrhage before administering heparin.

VASCULAR SYNDROMES

VON HIPPEL–LINDAU DISEASE

An autosomal-dominant disorder characterized by **multiple vascular neoplasms,** including retinal angiomas, hemangioblastomas of the brain and spinal cord (especially the cerebellum), renal cell carcinoma, and pheochromocytoma.

Cerebellar hemangioblastoma and retinal angioma should make you think of von Hippel–Lindau.

History/PE

Similar to any posterior fossa mass, including nausea, vomiting, headache, and cerebellar symptoms. Retinal angiomas are usually peripheral and may cause retinal detachment.

Evaluation

CT reveals an isodense posterior fossa mass, sometimes cystic. MRI may reveal serpentine signal voids. Angiography reveals intense vascularity. CBC reveals polycythemia. Further evaluation should rule out the presence of a retinal angioma as well as catecholamine production from pheochromocytoma.

Treatment

Surgical resection or radiation.

UCV *Neuro.50*

OSLER-WEBER-RENDU SYNDROME

Remember the triad of Osler-Weber-Rendu:

(1) telangiectasia,

(2) recurrent epistaxis,

(3) family history.

Stroke in a young person should prompt an inspection for manifestations of HHT.

Cerebral abscess should always be suspected in patients with HHT and neurologic symptoms.

Also known as hereditary hemorrhagic telangiectasia (HHT), this disorder is an autosomal-dominant fibrovascular dysplasia in which telangiectasias, AVMs, and aneurysms are widely distributed throughout the body, especially the lungs, GI system, and brain.

History/PE

Recurrent epistaxis. The cardinal GI manifestation is painless bleeding from AVMs and telangiectasia in the upper and lower bowel. Hepatic AV fistulas may cause **hepatomegaly and RUQ pain,** a pulsatile mass, a palpable thrill or audible bruit, and/or liver failure. Left-to-right shunting through the fistula may cause a hyperdynamic circulatory state and high-output CHF. Portosystemic shunting may result in hepatic encephalopathy. Right-to-left shunting may cause cyanosis, hypoxemia and secondary polycythemia, exertional dyspnea, and clubbing. Neurologic complications result from (1) pulmonary AV fistula, (2) vascular malformation of the brain and spinal cord, and (3) portosystemic encephalopathy. Asymptomatic pulmonary AV fistulas may present initially as cerebral embolism or brain abscess. Because of the random distribution of vascular malformations, affected persons may be asymptomatic or may present at any age with a wide range of clinical manifestations.

Treatment

Iron and folate supplementation because of bleeding. Symptomatic treatment of epistaxis. ASA and other medications that impair hemostasis are contraindicated. Embolization, surgical excision, or ligation is indicated for enlarging or symptomatic fistulas.

WEAKNESS

Think anatomically! Pathology can occur in several locations, and all should be considered. First seek to differentiate upper motor neuron (UMN) from lower motor neuron (LMN) disease (see Table 2.10–6). Four commonly tested causes of weakness—carpal tunnel syndrome, Guillain-Barré syndrome (GBS), ALS, and myasthenia gravis—are described in further detail below. Table 2.10–7 reviews the results of different studies for different etiologies of weakness.

TABLE 2.10–6. Anatomic

Clinical Features	UMN	LMN
Pattern of weakness	Pyramidal (arm extensors, leg flexors)	Variable
Tone	Spastic (increased: initially flaccid)	Flaccid (decreased)
DTRs	Increased (initially decreased)	Normal, decreased, absent
Miscellaneous signs	Babinski's, other CNS signs	Atrophy, fasciculations

GUILLAIN-BARRÉ SYNDROME

An **acute, rapidly progressive,** acquired demyelinating autoimmune disorder of the peripheral nerves resulting in weakness (see **the 5 A's of GBS**). GBS is associated with recent *Campylobacter jejuni* infection, preceding viral infection, and recent vaccination. Approximately 85% of patients make a complete or near-complete recovery. The mortality rate is roughly 5%.

History/PE

Rapidly progressive **ascending paralysis** that begins distally and progresses proximally to involve the trunk, diaphragm, and cranial nerves **(ascending paralysis).** Autonomic symptoms and a reflexion may be present as well. **Areflexia is seen.** Dysesthesias may also be present.

Differential

Myasthenia gravis, MS, ALS, poliomyelitis, porphyria, heavy metal poisoning, botulism, transverse myelitis.

Evaluation

Evidence of diffuse demyelination on **EMG** and **nerve conduction studies.** Diagnosis is supported by a **CSF protein level > 55 mg/dL** with little or no pleocytosis (albuminocytologic dissociation).

Treatment

Admit to the ICU for close monitoring because of the risk of **respiratory failure. Plasmapheresis** and **IVIG** are first-line treatments. Most patients will regain premorbid function, but this may take up to a year. Aggressive rehabilitation is imperative.

UCV *Neuro.20*

> **The 5 A's of GBS:**
>
> **A**cute inflammatory demyelinating polyradiculopathy
> **A**scending paralysis
> **A**utonomic neuropathy
> **A**rrythmias
> **A**lbuminocytologic dissociation

Closely monitor respiratory function in patients with GBS.

TABLE 2.10–7. Investigation of a Patient with Weakness

Test	Spinal Cord	Anterior Horn Cell Disorders	Peripheral Nerve or Plexus	Neuro-muscular Junction	Myopathy
Serum enzymes	Normal.	Normal.	Normal.	Normal.	Normal or increased.
Electromyography	Reduced number of motor units under voluntary control. With lesions causing axonal degeneration, may be abnormal spontaneous activity (e.g., fasciculations, fibrillations) if sufficient time has elapsed after onset; with reinnervation, motor units may be large, long, and polyphasic. Variability in size.			Often normal, but individual motor units may show abnormal variability in size.	Small, short, abundant polyphasic motor unit potentials. Abnormal spontaneous activity may be conspicuous in myositis.
Nerve conduction velocity	Normal.	Normal.	Slowed, especially in demyelinative neuropathies. May be normal in axonal neuropathies.	Normal.	Normal.
Muscle response to repetitive motor nerve stimulation	Normal.	Normal except in active stage of disease.	Normal.	Abnormal decrement or increment depending on stimulus frequency and disease.	Normal.
Muscle biopsy	May be normal in acute stage but subsequently suggestive of denervation.			Normal.	Changes suggestive of myopathy.
Myelography or spinal MRI	May be helpful.	Helpful in excluding other disorders.	Not helpful.	Not helpful.	Not helpful.

Reproduced, with permission, from Aminoff MJ. *Clinical Neurology*, 3rd ed. Stamford, CT: Appleton & Lange, 1996:156.

Myasthenia Gravis

An **autoimmune disease** caused by antibodies that bind to **postsynaptic ACh receptors** (as opposed to Lambert-Eaton syndrome, which is characterized by autoantibodies to presynaptic Ca^{2+} channels). Occurs most often in young adult women and can be associated with **thyrotoxicosis, thymoma,** and autoimmune disorders (e.g., rheumatoid arthritis [RA] or SLE).

History/PE

Fluctuating **fatigable ptosis or double vision.** Difficulty swallowing and proximal muscle weakness. **Symptoms typically worsen throughout the day.** Respiratory compromise and aspiration are rare but potentially lethal complications and are termed "myasthenic crisis."

Differential

Lambert-Eaton myasthenic syndrome (associated with small cell carcinoma of the lung), botulism, drug-induced myasthenic syndrome (aminoglycosides).

Evaluation

Edrophonium testing is diagnostic, leading to rapid amelioration of clinical symptoms. Abnormal **single-fiber EMG** and/or a **decremental response to repetitive nerve stimulation** can give additional confirmation. ACh antibodies are positive in 85–90% of patients with myasthenia gravis, and antistriational (striated muscle) antibodies are positive in 85% of patients with thymoma. CT of the chest is used to evaluate for thymoma.

Treatment

- Anticholinesterase drugs (**neostigmine** and pyridostigmine) are symptomatic therapies.
- **Prednisone** and other immunosuppressants are mainstays of treatment.
- In severe cases, plasmapheresis or IVIG may provide temporary relief (days to weeks).
- **Resection of thymoma** can be curative.

UCV *Neuro.30*

Amyotrophic Lateral Sclerosis

A **chronic, progressive degenerative disease** of unknown etiology characterized by loss of **motor neurons within the spinal cord,** brain stem, and motor cortex. ALS almost always progresses to respiratory failure and death.

History/PE

Asymmetric, slowly progressive weakness affecting the arms, legs, and cranial nerves. Some patients initially complain of fasciculations. Presents with **UMN signs** (spasticity, increased DTRs, upward-going toes) and/or **LMN signs** (flaccid paralysis, loss of DTRs, fasciculations, downward-going toes, tongue fasciculations).

A combination of upper and lower motor neuron signs in three or more extremities is diagnostic of ALS.

Differential

Spondylitic cervical myopathy, syringomyelia, neoplasms, demyelinating diseases, benign fasciculations, polio, hypothyroidism, hyperparathyroidism, dysproteinemia, lymphoma, heavy metal poisoning, postradiation effects, GBS.

Evaluation

Clinical presentation is most often diagnostic. **EMG/nerve conduction studies** reveal widespread denervation and fibrillation potentials. Obtain CT/MRI of the cervical spine to exclude structural lesions. Rule out systemic causes with CBC, TSH, SPEP, UPEP, Ca^{2+}, PTH, urine for heavy metals (if history of exposure), and PFTs.

Treatment

Supportive measures, patient education, and aggressive pulmonary toilet. Riluzole (reduces presynaptic glutamate release), may slow disease progression.

UCV *Neuro.1*

CARPAL TUNNEL SYNDROME

Results from **median nerve** compression at the wrist where it passes through the carpal tunnel. Most common in women 30–55 years of age. Risk factors include **repetitive use injury, pregnancy, diabetes, hypothyroidism, acromegaly,** RA, and obesity.

History/PE

Symtoms include wrist pain; numbness and tingling of the thumb, index finger, middle finger, and lateral half of the ring finger; weak grip; and decreased thumb opposition. Symptoms may awaken patients at night and are relieved by **shaking out the wrists.** Patients often complain of **nocturnal pain** and paresthesias. **Thenar atrophy** may occur in severe cases.

Workup

Tinel's sign is produced by Tapping on the wrist.

Tinel's sign involves tapping on the palmaris longus tendon at the wrist over the median nerve to elicit a tingling sensation in the thumb and affected fingers. **Phalen's sign** requires that the patient appose the dorsal aspects of the hands with the wrists flexed at 90 degrees for at least 30 seconds. The onset of paresthesias confirms the diagnosis. **EMG** and **NCV** are confirmatory and assess degree of compromise. Evaluate for risk factors, including diabetes and hypothyroidism.

Treatment

Neutral wrist splints; activity modification. Create a more **ergonomic work environment. NSAIDs** to control inflammation. Direct injection of corticosteroid into the carpal space may also provide temporary relief. If symptoms persist, surgical **carpal tunnel release** is indicated.

MULTIPLE SCLEROSIS

An acquired **demyelinating** disease of the CNS that may have a **T-cell-mediated autoimmune** pathogenesis (involving both environmental and genetic components). MS has a female-to-male ratio of 2:1, shows a peak incidence at 20–40 years of age, and is thought to have a genetic component. The incidence of MS increases with **increased distance from the equator;** those who move before the age of 15 inherit the susceptibility of the new geographic location. Subtypes are relapsing, remitting, secondary progressive, and primary progressive.

The classic triad in MS is scanning speech, intranuclear ophthalmoplegia, and nystagmus.

History/PE

Multiple neurologic complaints that are separated in time and space and cannot be explained by a single lesion. The most common presenting complaints include limb weakness, optic neuritis, paresthesias, diplopia, urinary retention, and vertigo. Neurologic symptoms can wax and wane or be progressive. Exacerbating factors include infection, heat, trauma, pregnancy, and vigorous activity. Pregnancy, by contrast, is often associated with a decreased frequency of exacerbations.

Differential

CNS tumors or trauma, **multiple CVAs,** [*cerebral vascular accident*] vasculitis, vitamin B$_{12}$ deficiency, CNS infections (Lyme disease, neurosyphilis), sarcoidosis, atypical presentations of other autoimmune diseases (e.g., SLE and Sjögren's syndrome).

Evaluation

MRI reveals **multiple, asymmetric,** often **periventricular** lesions in white matter. **Corpus callosum lesions are virtually pathognomonic.** Active lesions enhance with gadolinium on MRI. CSF analysis may show mononuclear pleocytosis (> 5 cells/µL) in 25% of cases, elevated CSF IgG in 80% of cases, and/or oligoclonal bands (nonspecific)-**albuminocytologic dissociation.** Abnormal somatosensory, or visual evoked potentials may also be present.

Treatment

Steroids should be given during acute exacerbations. Immunomodulators alter relapse rates in relapsing/remitting MS and are as easy as **ABC: A**vonex/Rebif (interferon-β-1a), **B**etascron (interferon-β-1b), and **C**opaxone (copolymer-1). For worsening relapsing/remitting MS or progressive MS, the chemotherapeutic agent **mitozantrone** can be used. Remember, symptomatic treatment of spasticity, pain, fatigue, and depression.

> **MS treatment is as easy as ABC:**
> **A**vonex/Rebif
> **B**etaseron
> **C**opaxone

OPHTHALMOLOGIC TOPICS

CLOSED-ANGLE GLAUCOMA

This medical emergency occurs most often in older patients and in Asians. The cause is an **acute** closure of a narrow anterior chamber angle (usually unilateral). This type of injury generally occurs with **pupillary dilation** (prolonged time in a darkened area, stress, medications), anterior uveitis, or dislocation of the lens.

History/PE

Do not dilate the pupil in suspected closed-angle glaucoma.

Patients present with extreme **pain** and blurred vision. The eye is hard and red, and the pupil is dilated and nonreactive to light. Nausea and vomiting are not uncommon. Intraocular pressure is elevated.

Differential

Conjunctivitis, uveitis, corneal trauma, infectious processes.

Treatment

- **Lower intraocular pressure** with acetazolamide.
- Once pressure drops, use pilocarpine.
- **Laser iridotomy** is curative.

OPEN-ANGLE GLAUCOMA

The most common form of glaucoma; almost always bilateral. It occurs most often in individuals > 40 years of age and in those with a **family history. African-Americans,** diabetics, and those with myopia are also at increased risk. In open-angle glaucoma, intraocular pressure becomes elevated secondary to a diseased trabecular meshwork that obstructs proper drainage of the eye. The pressure rises **gradually,** causing progressive vision loss. The eye appears structurally normal. Vision loss begins **peripherally** and moves centrally, ultimately resulting in blindness.

History/PE

Initially asymptomatic. However, glaucoma should be suspected in patients > 35 years of age who need **frequent lens changes** and have mild headaches, visual disturbances, and impaired adaptation to darkness. The earliest visual defect is seen in the peripheral nasal fields. **Cupping** of the optic disk may be seen on funduscopic examination.

Evaluation

Tonometry, ophthalmoscopic visualization of the optic nerve, and central field testing are the most important examinations in evaluating glaucoma. All examinations must be evaluated on a **long-term basis** owing to wide variations in intraocular pressure. Because of its insidious nature, glaucoma can be difficult to diagnose until its advanced stages.

Treatment

Prevention is the most important treatment available. All people > 40 years of age should visit an ophthalmologist every 3–5 years. Annual examinations are recommended for individuals with increased risk factors. Most cases can be controlled with topical α-blockers (timolol, betaxolol), which decrease aqueous humor production, or pilocarpine, which increases aqueous outflow. Carbonic anhydrase inhibitors are used when eye drops do not adequately control intraocular pressure. If medication fails, laser trabeculoplasty can be performed to improve aqueous drainage.

MACULAR DEGENERATION

In the United States, macular degeneration is the leading cause of **permanent, bilateral visual loss** in the elderly. There is a higher incidence of macular degeneration in Caucasians, females, smokers, and those with a family history. Vision loss occurs centrally; patients do not lose their peripheral vision and ability to move around safely. Types include:

- **Atrophic macular degeneration:** Causes gradual vision loss.
- **Exudative macular degeneration:** Causes more rapid and severe vision damage.

History/PE

Painless loss of central vision. Funduscopy reveals pigmentary or hemorrhagic disturbance in the macular region.

Treatment

Treatment is greatly limited. **Laser photocoagulation** may delay loss of central vision in exudative macular disease.

RETINAL OCCLUSION

Retinal occlusion can be arterial or venous.

History/PE

- **Central retinal artery occlusion:** Sudden, painless, **unilateral blindness.** The pupil accommodates but is sluggishly reactive to direct light. On funduscopic exam, there may be a **cherry-red spot** on the fovea (see Clinical Images); arteries may appear bloodless, and retinal swelling may be present.
- **Central retinal vein occlusion:** Rapid, painless vision loss. Retinal hemorrhage, cotton wool spots, and edema of the fundus may be seen on funduscopic exam. Occurs in **elderly patients** and is often idiopathic. Results in macular disease and glaucoma.

Treatment

- **Central retinal artery occlusion: Thrombolysis** of the ophthalmic artery within eight hours of onset of symptoms. Reduction of intraocular pressure through drainage of the anterior chamber, IV acetazolamide may also improve perfusion of the retina. If treatment is not instituted immediately, retinal infarction and permanent blindness may result.
- **Central retinal vein occlusion:** Laser photocoagulation has variable results.

The following clinical questions and accompanying answers are reproduced, with permission, from Elkind MSV, *PreTest: Neurology*, 9th ed., New York: McGraw-Hill, 2001.

Questions

A 73-year-old man with a history of hypertension complains of a ten-minute episode of left-sided weakness and slurred speech. On further questioning, he relates three brief episodes in the last month of sudden impairment of vision affecting the right eye. His examination now is normal.

1. Which of the following would be the most appropriate next diagnostic test?
   a. Creatine phosphokinase (CPK)
   b. Holter monitor
   c. Visual evoked responses
   d. Carotid artery Doppler ultrasound
   e. Conventional cerebral angiography

2. The episodes of visual loss are most likely related to
   a. Retinal vein thrombosis
   b. Central retinal artery ischemia
   c. Posterior cerebral artery ischemia
   d. Middle cerebral artery ischemia
   e. Posterior ciliary artery ischemia

3. A 23-year-old woman complained of two days of visual loss associated with discomfort in the right eye. She appeared otherwise healthy, but her family reported recurrent problems with bladder control over the prior two years, which the patient was reluctant to discuss. On neurologic examination, this young woman exhibited dysmetria in her right arm, a plantar extensor response of the left foot, and slurred speech. The most informative ancillary test would be expected to be
   a. Visual evoked response (VER) testing
   b. Sural nerve biopsy
   c. Electroencephalography (EEG)
   d. Magnetic resonance imaging (MRI)
   e. Computed tomography (CT)

4. For the following clinical scenario, pick the most likely diagnosis.
   a. Hepatolenticular degeneration
   b. Hyperparathyroidism
   c. Central pontine myelinolysis
   d. Akinetic mutism
   e. MPTP poisoning
   f. Locked-in syndrome
   g. Postencephalitic parkinsonism
   h. Neuroleptic effect
   i. Essential tremor
   j. Vegetative state
   k. Hypermagnesemia
   l. Rhombencephalitis

A 19-year-old woman developed auditory hallucinations and persecutory delusions over the course of three days. She was hospitalized and started on haloperidol (Haldol), 2 mg three times daily. Within a week of treatment, she developed stooped posture and a shuffling gait. Her head was slightly tremulous and her movements were generally slowed. Her medication was changed to thioridazine (Mellaril), and trihexyphenidyl (Artane) was added. Over the next two weeks, she became much more animated and reported no recurrence of her hallucinations. **(SELECT ONE DIAGNOSIS)**

1. **The answer is d.** This patient is experiencing the classical symptoms of extracranial internal carotid artery disease, which include episodes of ipsilateral transient monocular blindness, or amaurosis fugax, and contralateral transient ischemic attacks consisting of motor weakness. Patients with symptomatic extracranial carotid artery disease have a high likelihood of going on to develop strokes (approximately 26% over two years on medical therapy). The appropriate test to confirm the suspicion of carotid stenosis is a Doppler ultrasound test of the carotid arteries. This test utilizes the fact that sound waves will bounce back from particles moving in the bloodstream, primarily red blood cells, at a different frequency, depending upon the velocity and direction of the blood flow. A great deal of important information about the structure of the blood vessel can be obtained in this way. Although angiography can also provide this information, it is invasive, carries a risk of causing a stroke, and is more expensive.

2. **The answer is b.** The presumed mechanism of transient monocular blindness in carotid artery disease is embolism to the central retinal artery or one of its branches. Although classic teaching has emphasized the role that cholesterol emboli play in causing this blindness, it has been noted that cholesterol emboli (Hollenhorst plaques) may be seen on funduscopic examination even of asymptomatic individuals. Retinal vein thrombosis may produce a rapidly progressive loss of vision, with hemorrhages in the retina, but would not be associated with the transient ischemic attacks (TIAs) described here. Although both posterior and middle cerebral artery ischemia can cause visual loss, they would not be expected to cause the monocular blindness described here. Posterior ciliary artery ischemia can cause ischemic optic neuropathy, but this is usually acute, painless, and not associated with preceding transient monocular blindness or TIAs.

3. **The answer is d.** This young woman almost certainly has MS. Her visual loss can be explained by optic neuritis. Her bladder problems may be from demyelination of corticospinal tract fibers. Many patients are reluctant to discuss minor problems with bladder, bowel, or sexual function with a physician of the opposite sex. The positive Babinski sign, focal dysmetria, and apparent dysarthria all support the diagnosis of a multifocal CNS lesion. Multiple lesions disseminated in time and space are typical of MS. With MRI, the multifocal areas of demyelination should be apparent. Many more lesions may be evident on MRI than are suggested by the physical examination.

4. **The answer is h.** Butyrophenones, the most commonly prescribed of which is haloperidol, routinely produce some signs of parkinsonism if they are used at high doses for more than a few days. This psychotic young woman proved to be less sensitive to the parkinsonian effects of the phenothiazine thioridazine than she was to haloperidol. Adding the anticholinergic trihexyphenidyl may also have helped to reduce the patient's parkinsonism. Another commonly used medication that can cause parkinsonism, in addition to tardive dyskinesia, is metoclopramide hydrochloride (Reglan).

Obstetrics

Estrogen

Source   Ovary (estradiol), placenta (estriol), blood (aromatization), testes.

Function
1. Growth of follicle
2. Endometrial proliferation, myometrial excitability
3. Development of genitalia
4. Stromal development of breast
5. Female fat distribution
6. Hepatic synthesis of transport proteins
7. Feedback inhibition of FSH
8. LH surge (estrogen feedback on LH secretion switches to positive from negative just before LH surge)
9. ↑ myometrial excitability

Potency—estradiol > estrone > estriol.

Estrogen hormone replacement therapy after menopause → ↓ hot flashes and ↓ postmenopausal bone loss.

Unopposed estrogen therapy— ↑ risk of endometrial cancer; use of progesterone with estrogen ↓ this risk.

Progesterone

Source   Corpus luteum, placenta, adrenal cortex, testes.

Function
1. Stimulation of endometrial glandular secretions and spiral artery development
2. Maintenance of pregnancy
3. ↓ myometrial excitability
4. Production of thick cervical mucus, which inhibits sperm entry into the uterus
5. ↑ body temperature
6. Inhibition of gonadotropins (LH, FSH)
7. Uterine smooth muscle relaxation

Elevation of progesterone is indicative of ovulation.

hCG

Source   Syncytiotrophoblast of placenta.

Function
1. Maintains the corpus luteum for the 1st trimester by acting like LH. In the 2nd and 3rd trimester, the placenta synthesizes its own estrogen and progesterone and the corpus luteum degenerates.
2. Used to detect pregnancy because it appears in the urine 8 days after successful fertilization (blood and urine tests available).
3. Elevated hCG in women with hydatidiform moles or choriocarcinoma.

Menstrual cycle

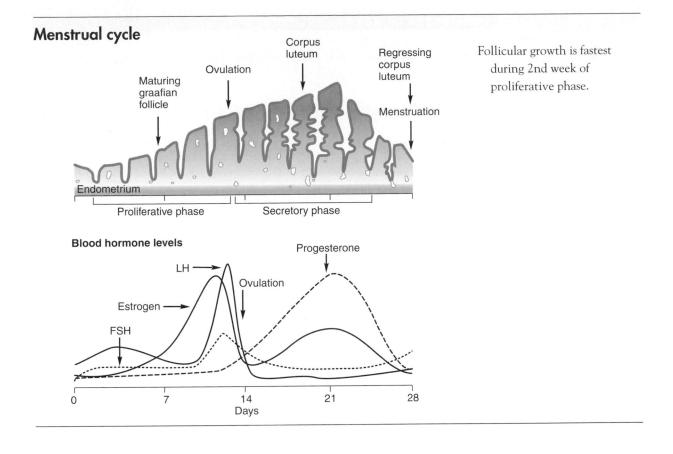

Follicular growth is fastest during 2nd week of proliferative phase.

Table 2.11–1 summarizes normal physiologic changes during pregnancy.

TABLE 2.11–1. Normal Physiologic Changes During Pregnancy

Organ/System	Physiologic Change
Cardiovascular	**Increase in cardiac output (30–50%), HR** (10–15 bpm), and **stroke volume.** Systolic murmur and audible S3 are normal; **new diastolic murmurs are not normal.** Decrease in systemic vascular resistance (progesterone causes smooth muscle relaxation). **BP decreases** in the first trimester, reaches nadir at 24 weeks, and normalizes by 40 weeks. Growing uterus displaces heart upward and to the left. This results in the appearance of cardiomegaly on CXR.
Cervix	Softening and cyanosis ~ 4 weeks. Thick mucus clot in cervical os is expelled at or near labor **("bloody show"),** and progesterone causes cervical mucus to look granular when spread on a glass slide.
Endocrine	High estrogen levels lead to increased thyroid-binding globulin. Total and bound T_3 and T_4 increase, but active unbound hormone is unchanged. Human placental lactogen (HPL) acts as an insulin antagonist to maintain fetal glucose levels. This results in prolonged postprandial **hyperglycemia,** fasting **hyperinsulinemia/ hypertriglyceridemia,** and exaggerated starvation **ketosis** response. Changes can worsen diabetes or cause gestational diabetes. Increase in total and free cortisol (produced by fetal adrenal gland and placenta).
GI	**Nausea and vomiting** (in up to 70% of pregnancies) resolves by 14–16 weeks. **Increased acid reflux** from lowered gastroesophageal junction sphincter tone. **Constipation** from decreased large bowel motility and increased water resorption. Increased biliary cholesterol saturation predisposes to gallstone formation.
Hematologic (OB.35, 36)	Increase in **plasma volume (50%)** and RBC mass (30%) leads to decrease in Hb and HCT **("physiologic anemia"). Hb < 11.0 mg/dL is never normal** and is likely due to iron deficiency. WBC count increases throughout pregnancy to a mean of 10.5 million/mL but can rise during labor to > 20 million/mL. Pregnancy is a **hypercoagulable** state. DVT risk is highest in the puerperium. The **number one nonobstetric cause of postpartum death is thromboembolic disease.**
Musculoskeletal	Increased motility of sacroiliac, sacrococcygeal, and pubic joints.
Pulmonary	Increase in **tidal volume** (40%). Decrease in total lung capacity, residual volume, and expiratory reserve volume. **RR is unchanged.** Increased minute ventilation (VT × RR) results in increased alveolar and arterial P_{O_2} and decreased alveolar and arterial P_{CO_2}. **"Dyspnea of pregnancy"** is common and likely caused by increased VT and decreased P_{CO_2}.
Renal	Kidneys dilate. **GFR increases by 50%.** Renal plasma flow increases by 30%. **Dilation of the collecting system may be mistaken for hydronephrosis.** Elevated estrogen and progesterone stimulate the renin-angiotensin system. **Increased aldosterone** contributes to water retention and increased plasma volume.

Organ/System	Physiologic Change
Skin	Increased estrogen may cause changes that resemble cirrhotic disease, such as **striae** (on abdomen, breasts, thighs), **spider angiomas,** and **palmar erythema.** **Hyperpigmentation** over the midline **(linea nigra),** face **(chloasma),** and perineum is due to increased α-melanocyte-stimulating hormone and steroids. Rectus muscles may separate in the midline (diastasis recti), leaving part of the anterior uterus covered only by skin, fascia, and peritoneum.
Uterus	**At 12 weeks,** uterus contacts anterior abdominal wall, displaces intestines, and is felt above the symphysis pubis. Irregular painless **(Braxton Hicks)** contractions occur throughout pregnancy and may become frequent and rhythmic late in the third trimester **("false labor").**
Vagina	Thick, acidic secretions. Violet coloration **(Chadwick's sign)** from increased blood flow.

UCV OB.40

PRENATAL CARE AND NUTRITION

The goal is to prevent, diagnose, and treat conditions that cause adverse outcomes in pregnancy. In women with regular menstrual cycles, calculate the estimated date of delivery (EDD) using **Nägele's rule:** add nine months plus seven days to the first day of the last menstrual period (LMP). Gestational age (GA) can be determined by uterine size, quickening (at 17–18 weeks), fetal heart tones (at 10 weeks via Doppler), or U/S (fetal crown–rump length at 5–12 weeks; biparietal diameter at 20–30 weeks).

Nägele's rule: due date = LMP + nine months + seven days.

- **Weight gain:** The recommended gain for an average-size woman is **25–35 lbs.** Obese women should gain less (15–25 lbs) and thin women more. Average caloric requirements are 2,000–2,500 kcal/day. An **additional 300 kcal/day** is needed during pregnancy and 500 kcal/day during breast-feeding.
- **Nutrition:** Requirements for protein, iron, folate, calcium, and other vitamins and minerals are increased in pregnancy. Most can be met through diet, but all patients are advised to take prenatal vitamins. Folate and iron are particularly important:
  - Folate is required by dividing cells. All women should receive **1 mg of folate daily,** via diet or supplementation, to decrease the risk of neural tube defects.
  - Iron demand is increased by fetal needs and by the expanding maternal blood supply. Supplement with **30–60 mg/day of elemental iron** in the latter half of pregnancy to prevent anemia.
- **Prenatal labs:** See Table 2.11–2 for a recommended schedule.

Leg cramps are the classic symptom of calcium deficiency in a pregnant woman.

HIGH-YIELD FACTS

Obstetrics

TABLE 2.11–2. Standard Prenatal Labs and Studies

Gestation	Labs to Be Obtained
Initial visit	CBC; UA and culture; Pap smear; blood type, Rh, and Ab screen; rubella Ab titer; HBV surface Ag test, syphilis screen (RPR, VDRL); cervical gonorrhea and chlamydia cultures. PPD, glucose testing, sickle prep, and HIV (in high-risk groups).
15–19 wks	Maternal serum α-fetoprotein (MSAFP) OR **triple screen (MSAFP, estriol, β-hCG).** Offer amniocentesis to patients of advanced maternal age (> 35 years at delivery).
18–20 wks	U/S to determine GA (if unknown or uncertain) and to survey fetal anatomy, amniotic fluid volume, and placental location.
26–28 wks	Glucose loading test (GLT). Repeat HCT.
28 wks	RhoGAM given to patients who are Rh-antibody negative.
32–36 wks	Cervical chlamydia and gonorrhea cultures in high-risk patients. Repeat HCT. **Screen for group B strep (GBS). If positive, give penicillin during labor** to prevent transmission to the infant.

PRENATAL DIAGNOSTIC TESTING

ALPHA-FETOPROTEIN (AFP)

AFP is produced by the fetus and found primarily in amniotic fluid. Small amounts cross the placenta and enter maternal circulation. **Measure MSAFP at 15–20 weeks' gestation.** Results are reported as multiples of the median (MoMs) and depend on accurate gestational dating. The causes of elevated MSAFP (> 2.5 MoMs) include open neural tube defects (anencephaly, spina bifida), abdominal wall defects (gastroschisis, omphalocele), multiple gestation, incorrect gestational dating, fetal death, and placental abnormalities (e.g., placental abruption). Abnormally low MSAFP levels (< 0.5 MoM) warrant amniocentesis and karyotyping to rule out chromosomal abnormalities. Sensitivity for detecting chromosomal abnormalities is increased by adding estriol and β-hCG (triple screen). In trisomy 18, all three are low. In trisomy 21, AFP and estriol are low and β-hCG is high.

AMNIOCENTESIS

Transabdominal removal of amniotic fluid using a U/S-guided needle and evaluation of fetal cells for chromosomal abnormalities. There is ample fluid in **weeks 15–17** to perform the test. Risks are fetal-maternal hemorrhage (1–2%) and fetal loss (0.5%). Amniocentesis is used:

The triple screen is more sensitive than MSAFP alone for detecting trisomies.

- In women who will be **> 35 years old at the time of delivery.**
- In conjunction with an abnormal triple screen (together they detect 65% of fetuses with trisomy 21).
- In Rh-sensitized pregnancy to obtain fetal blood type or to detect fetal hemolysis.
- For the evaluation of fetal lung maturity via a lecithin-sphingomyelin ratio ≥ 2.5 or to detect the presence of phosphatidyl glycerol.

CHORIONIC VILLUS SAMPLING (CVS)

Transvaginal or transabdominal aspiration of chorionic villus tissue (the precursor to the placenta). Advantages include diagnostic accuracy comparable to that of amniocentesis and availability earlier in pregnancy, at **10–12 weeks' gestation.** Disadvantages include a **1% risk of fetal loss and inability to diagnose neural tube defects.** Limb defects have been associated with CVS performed at ≤ 9 weeks.

PERCUTANEOUS UMBILICAL BLOOD SAMPLING (PUBS)

Performed in the second and third trimesters when umbilical cord vessels are large enough to puncture safely. PUBS is used for:

- Assessment and treatment of Rh isoimmunization/erythroblastosis fetalis.
- Fetal karyotyping.
- Fetal infection (e.g., CMV, toxoplasmosis, rubella).
- Evaluation of genetic diseases (e.g., sickle cell disease, thalassemia).
- Evaluation of fetal acid-base status.

NORMAL LABOR AND DELIVERY

STAGES OF LABOR

Table 2.11–3 and Figure 2.11–1 depict the normal stages of labor.

> **Factors affecting active phase—3 P's:**
>
> **P**ower
> **P**assenger
> **P**elvis

TABLE 2.11–3. Stages of Labor

Stage	Starts/Ends	Duration		Comments
First		Primi[a]	Multi[b]	
Latent	Onset of labor to 3–4 cm dilation	6–11 hrs	4–8 hrs	Prolongation seen with excessive sedation and hypertonic uterine contractions.
Active	4 cm to complete cervical dilation (10 cm)	4–6 hrs (1.2 cm/hr)	2–3 hrs (1.5 cm/hr)	Prolongation seen with **cephalopelvic disproportion.**
Second	Complete cervical dilation to delivery of infant	0.5–3.0 hrs	5–30 min	Baby goes through all cardinal movements of labor.
Third	Delivery of infant to delivery of placenta	0–0.5 hr	0–0.5 hr	Placenta separates and uterus contracts to establish hemostasis.

[a]Primiparous (first-time mother).
[b]Multiparous (prior pregnancy and delivery).

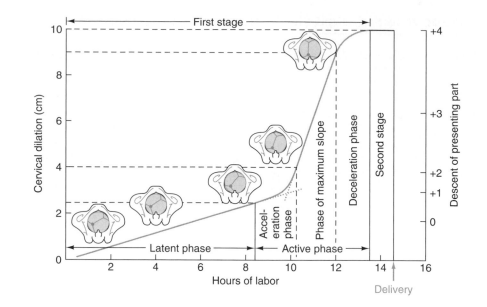

FIGURE 2.11–1. Stages of labor. Cervical dilation, level of descent, and orientation of occipitoanterior presentation during various stages of labor. (Reproduced, with permission, from DeCherney AH. *Current Obstetric & Gynecologic Diagnosis & Treatment,* 8th ed. Stamford, CT: Appleton & Lange, 1994:211, Fig. 10–5.)

TESTS OF FETAL WELL-BEING

- **Nonstress test (NST):** Performed with the mother resting in the left lateral supine position (to prevent supine hypotension). Fetal heart rate (FHR) is monitored externally by Doppler and correlated with spontaneous fetal movements as reported by the mother (see Table 2.11–4). A normal response is acceleration of **≥ 15 bpm above baseline for at least 15 seconds.** A normal "reactive" test includes two such accelerations in a 20-minute period. If the test is "nonreactive," perform further tests (e.g., a biophysical profile). Lack of FHR accelerations may occur with any of the following: GA < 30 weeks, fetal sleeping, fetal CNS anomalies, maternal sedative or narcotic administration, and fetal hypoxia (rare).

- **Contraction stress test (CST):** Used in high-risk pregnancies to assess uteroplacental dysfunction. FHR is monitored during spontaneous or induced (via nipple stimulation or oxytocin) contractions. Reactivity is determined as in the NST. A "positive" CST, defined by repetitive late decelerations **during at least three contractions in ten minutes,** raises concerns about fetal jeopardy. A "negative" CST (no late decelerations) is highly predictive of fetal well-being when seen with a reactive NST (see Table 2.11–4 and Figure 2.11–2).

- **Biophysical profile (BPP):** Real-time U/S is used to assess five parameters (see mnemonic). A score of 2 (normal) or 0 (abnormal) is given to each. A "negative" test (score of 8–10) is reassuring of fetal well-being. A "positive" test (score of 0–2) is worrisome for fetal compromise. Immediate delivery should ensue if no nonhypoxic explanation is found.

When performing a BPP, remember to—

Test the **B**aby, **MAN!**
Fetal **T**one
Fetal **B**reathing
Fetal **M**ovement
Amniotic fluid volume
Nonstress test

TABLE 2.11–4. Fetal Heart Decelerations

Type	Description	Most Common Cause
Early	Decelerations begin and end at approximately the same time as the maternal contraction.	Cephalic compression (no fetal distress).
Variable	Decelerations occur at any time during the maternal contraction.	Umbilical cord compression. Change mother's position (e.g., back to side).
Late	Decelerations begin at the peak of the contraction and persist until after the contraction has finished.	Uteroplacental insufficiency and fetal hypoxemia, possibly due to abruption or hypotension. Further testing for reassurance is necessary. If late decelerations are repetitive and severe, deliver the baby ASAP.

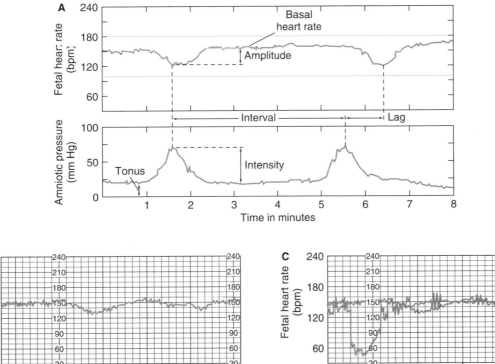

FIGURE 2.11–2. Fetal heart tracings. (A) Schematic tracing. (B) Late deceleration. (C) Variable deceleration. (Reproduced, with permission, from DeCherney AH. *Current Obstetric & Gynecologic Diagnosis & Treatment,* 8th ed. Stamford, CT: Appleton & Lange, 1994:301, Fig. 13–13A, C, and D.)

HYPEREMESIS GRAVIDARUM

Intractable nausea and vomiting that typically **persists beyond 14–16 weeks' gestation** and results in dehydration, electrolyte abnormalities, and **poor weight gain or weight loss.** More common in nulliparas and **molar pregnancies** (with elevated β-hCG). Differentiate from "morning sickness," acid reflux, and gastroenteritis. Evaluate for ketonemia, ketonuria, hyponatremia, and hypokalemic-hypochloremic metabolic alkalosis. Treatment includes frequent small meals, antiemetics, and IV hydration.

UCV *OB.42*

GESTATIONAL DIABETES MELLITUS

Hyperglycemia in the first trimester usually suggests preexisting diabetes.

Occurs in **3–5% of all pregnancies.** Typically a disorder of **late pregnancy.** Hyperglycemia in the first trimester usually suggests preexisting diabetes. Its etiology is unknown but may result from insulin-antagonist hormones from the placenta (e.g., HPL, cortisol). Risk factors include obesity, a family or personal history of diabetes, recurrent abortions, stillbirths, maternal age > 25 years, a prior macrosomic (4,000–4,500 g) or congenitally deformed infant, or prior polyhydramnios.

History/PE

A fetus that is large for GA may indicate occult diabetes.

Typically asymptomatic. Edema, polyhydramnios, or a **large-for-GA infant (> 90th percentile) may be warning signs.**

Differential

Preexisting diabetes, volume or glucose overload, urinary tract abnormalities.

Evaluation

UA reveals glycosuria. Diagnosis requires two abnormal glucose tests, including **fasting serum glucose > 126 mg/dL,** random glucose > 200 mg/dL, or an **abnormal glucose tolerance test (GTT),** routinely performed at 24–28 weeks' gestation. A one-hour (50-g) GTT with serum glucose > 140 mg/dL is suggestive. Confirm with a three-hour (100 g) GTT showing any two of the following: fasting ≥ 95; one hour ≥ 180; two hours ≥ 155; three hours ≥ 140.

Management

Tight maternal glucose control (e.g., average of 90 mg/dL) improves outcomes. Start with the **ADA diet** and regular exercise. **Add insulin** if dietary control is insufficient. **Avoid oral hypoglycemics** (can cause fetal hypoglycemia). Obtain periodic U/S and NSTs to assess fetal growth and well-being. Give intrapartum insulin and dextrose to maintain tight control during delivery. May need to induce labor with oxytocin at 38–40 weeks.

Complications

More than 50% of patients go on to **develop glucose intolerance and/or type 2 diabetes mellitus (DM).**

UCV *OB.39*

PREGESTATIONAL DIABETES AND PREGNANCY

Poorly controlled DM (HbA$_{1C}$ > 10%) is associated with an increased **risk of congenital malformations** and greater maternal/fetal morbidity during labor and delivery.

Management

Mother:
- Routine prenatal screening/care and nutritional counseling.
- Renal, ophthalmologic, and cardiac evaluation to assess end-organ damage.
- Strict glucose control to minimize fetal defects. Type 1 DM patients should receive insulin with the goal of maintaining the following blood glucose levels:
  - Fasting morning: 60–90 mg/dL.
  - Pre-lunch: 60–105 mg/dL.
  - Two-hour postprandial: < 120 mg/dL.

Fetus:
- **16–20 weeks:** U/S to determine fetal age and growth and to detect macrosomia, polyhydramnios, and intrauterine growth retardation (IUGR); AFP to screen for developmental anomalies.
- **20–22 weeks:** Echocardiogram to detect cardiac anomalies.
- **Third trimester:** Close fetal surveillance (e.g., NST, CST, BPP). Admit at 32–36 weeks if maternal DM has been poorly controlled or fetal parameters are a concern.

Delivery and postpartum:
- Maintain normoglycemia (80–100 mg/dL) during labor.
- Consider early delivery if there is poor maternal glucose control, preeclampsia, macrosomia, or evidence of fetal lung maturity.
- Cesarean delivery is indicated for fetal macrosomia.
- Continue glucose monitoring postpartum. Insulin needs rapidly decrease after delivery.

Complications

See Table 2.11–5 for complications.

GESTATIONAL AND CHRONIC HYPERTENSION

Pregnancy-induced HTN is idiopathic HTN without significant proteinuria (< 300 mg/L) that begins in the second half of pregnancy, during labor, or within 48 hours of delivery. It is a retrospective diagnosis (made at least one week after delivery). **Chronic HTN** is present before conception, at < 20 weeks' gestation, or persists for > 6 weeks postpartum. One-third of patients

TABLE 2.11–5. Complications of Pregestational Diabetes Mellitus

Maternal Complications	Fetal Complications
DKA (type 1) or HHNK (type 2)	Macrosomia
Preeclampsia/eclampsia	Cardiac and renal defects
Cephalopelvic disproportion (from macrosomia) and need for C-section	Neural tube defects (e.g., sacral agenesis)
	Hypocalcemia
Preterm labor	Polycythemia
Infection	Hyperbilirubinemia
Polyhydramnios	IUGR
Postpartum hemorrhage	Hypoglycemia from hyperinsulinemia
Maternal mortality	Respiratory distress syndrome (RDS)
	Birth injury (e.g., shoulder dystocia)
	Perinatal mortality

develop superimposed preeclampsia. Monitor BP closely and treat with appropriate antihypertensives (e.g., methyldopa, β-blockers, hydralazine). **Do not give ACE inhibitors (ACEIs) or diuretics.** Complications are similar to those of preeclampsia.

PREECLAMPSIA AND ECLAMPSIA

> **HELLP syndrome—**
>
> **H**emolysis
> **E**levated **L**FTs
> **L**ow **P**latelets
> (thrombocytopenia)

Preeclampsia is defined as **new-onset HTN, proteinuria,** and/or **nondependent (hand and face) edema** occurring at **> 20 weeks' gestation. Eclampsia** is defined as **seizures** in a patient with preeclampsia. Risk factors include nulliparity, black race, extremes of age (< 20 or > 35), multiple gestation, molar pregnancy, renal disease (due to systemic lupus erythematosus or type 1 DM), a family history of preeclampsia, and chronic HTN. **HELLP syndrome** is a variant of preeclampsia with a poor prognosis (see mnemonic). The etiology is unknown, but clinical manifestations are explained by vasospasm causing hemorrhage and organ necrosis.

History/PE

See Table 2.11–6 for signs and symptoms of preeclampsia and eclampsia.

Differential

Molar pregnancy, primary HTN, renal disease, renovascular HTN, Conn's or Cushing's syndromes, pheochromocytoma, primary seizure disorder, thrombotic thrombocytopenic purpura.

Evaluation

UA, 24-hour urine protein, CBC, electrolytes, BUN/Cr, uric acid, precise measurement of fetal age, **amniocentesis** (to assess **fetal lung maturity**), LFTs, PT/PTT, fibrinogen and fibrin split products (for DIC), urine toxicology screen, U/S, NST/CST/BPP (as indicated).

UCV OB.51

Treatment

The only cure for preeclampsia/eclampsia is delivery. See Table 2.11–6 for management.

TABLE 2.11–6. Signs, Symptoms, and Management of Preeclampsia and Eclampsia

	Mild Preeclampsia	Severe Preeclampsia	Eclampsia
Signs and symptoms	BP > **140/90** on two occasions > 6 hours apart. Rapid weight gain and nondependent edema. Proteinuria (> 300 mg/24 hrs or 1–2+ urine dipstick). Often asymptomatic, so routine prenatal screening is essential for early detection.	BP > **160/110** on two occasions > 6 hours apart. Proteinuria (> 5 g/24 hrs or 3–4+ urine dipstick). HELLP syndrome. Oliguria (< 500 mL/24 hrs). Oligohydramnios or IUGR. Pulmonary edema/cyanosis. RUQ/epigastric pain. **Cerebral changes** (headache, somnolence). **Visual changes** (blurred vision, scotomata). **Hyperactive reflexes**/clonus.	The three most common symptoms preceding an eclamptic attack are **headache, visual changes, and RUQ/epigastric pain.** **Seizures** are severe if not controlled with anticonvulsant therapy.
Management	If close to term, fetal lungs are mature, or preeclampsia worsens, induce delivery with IV oxytocin, prostaglandins, or amniotomy. If far from term, modified bed rest and **expectant management.**	**Control BP** with hydralazine ± labetalol (goal BP < 160/110, with diastolic BP ~ 90–100 to maintain fetal blood flow). **Prevent seizures with MgSO$_4$.** When patient stabilizes, deliver fetus by C-section or induction of labor. **Postpartum,** continue seizure prophylaxis with MgSO$_4$ for the first 24 hours. Monitor for signs of **Mg^{2+} toxicity (loss of DTRs, respiratory paralysis, coma).** Treat Mg$^+$ toxicity with IV calcium gluconate.	Monitor ABCs closely. Give supplemental O$_2$. Seizure control/prophylaxis with MgSO$_4$. If seizures recur, consider IV diazepam. Control BP (hydralazine ± labetalol). Limit fluids, Foley catheter to check I/Os, monitor blood Mg$^+$ level, watch for Mg$^+$ toxicity, monitor fetal status. Initiate delivery once patient is stable and convulsions are controlled. Postpartum: same as preeclampsia. Seizures may occur antepartum (25%), intrapartum (50%), and postpartum (25%; most within 48 hours after delivery).

Complications

- **Preeclampsia:** Prematurity, fetal distress, stillbirth, placental abruption, seizure, DIC, cerebral hemorrhage, serous retinal detachment, fetal/maternal death.
- **Eclampsia:** Cerebral hemorrhage, aspiration pneumonia, hypoxic encephalopathy, thromboembolic events, fetal/maternal death.

TERATOGENIC DRUGS

Table 2.11–7 summarizes the effects of common teratogens.

TABLE 2.11–7. Common Teratogenic Drugs

Teratogen[a]	Effect
Alcohol	Fetal alcohol syndrome (microcephaly, midfacial hypoplasia, mental retardation [MR], IUGR, cardiac defects).
Cocaine	Bowel atresias, IUGR, microcephaly.
Streptomycin	CN VIII damage/ototoxicity.
Tetracycline	Tooth discoloration, inhibition of bone growth, small limbs, syndactyly.
Sulfonamides	Kernicterus.
Quinolones	Cartilage damage.
Isotretinoin	Heart and great vessel defects, craniofacial dysmorphism, deafness.
Iodide	Congenital goiter, hypothyroidism, MR.
Methotrexate	CNS malformations, craniofacial dysmorphism, IUGR.
Diethylstilbestrol (DES)	Clear cell adenocarcinoma of the vagina/cervix, genital tract abnormalities (cervical hood, T-shaped uterus, hypoplastic uterus), cervical incompetence.
Thalidomide	Limb reduction (phocomelia), ear and nasal anomalies, cardiac and lung defects, pyloric or duodenal stenosis, GI atresia.
Coumadin	Stippling of bone epiphyses, IUGR, nasal hypoplasia, MR.
ACEIs	Oligohydramnios, fetal renal damage.
Lithium	Ebstein's anomaly, other cardiac diseases.
Carbamazepine	Fingernail hypoplasia, IUGR, microcephaly, neural tube defects.
Phenytoin	Nail hypoplasia, IUGR, MR, craniofacial dysmorphism, microcephaly.
Valproic acid	Neural tube defects, craniofacial and skeletal defects.

[a]The fetus is most susceptible during gestational weeks 3–8 (organogenesis).

INTRAUTERINE GROWTH RETARDATION

Defined by fetal weight < 10th percentile for GA. Suspect IUGR if there is a discrepancy of > 4 between fundal height (in centimeters) and GA (in weeks) on exam. Occurs in 3–7% of pregnancies. See Table 2.11–8 for differences between symmetric and asymmetric IUGR.

Evaluation/Treatment

- **Serial exams** with U/S evaluation every 3–4 weeks.
- Fetal monitoring with NST, CST, BPP; Doppler flow studies to evaluate uterine/umbilical artery flow.
- **Steroids** to accelerate fetal lung maturity.
- Consider early delivery, particularly with asymmetric IUGR, since uterine environment later in pregnancy is critical.
- Continuous FHR monitoring during labor; C-section if decelerations persist.

OLIGOHYDRAMNIOS

A deficiency of amniotic fluid volume defined by an **amniotic fluid index (AFI)** < 5 on U/S. Without rupture of membranes (ROM), it is associated with a 40-fold increase in perinatal mortality. It is usually asymptomatic, but IUGR or fetal distress may be present. Common etiologies are **fetal urinary tract abnormalities** (e.g., renal agenesis, polycystic kidney disease, GU obstruction), **chronic uteroplacental insufficiency** (associated with small-for-GA fetus), or **ROM.** Rule out inaccurate gestational dates. Treat the underlying cause if possible. Patients with ROM may benefit from amnio infusion. Complications include musculoskeletal abnormalities (e.g., club foot, facial distortion), **pulmonary hypoplasia,** fetal hypoxia due to umbilical cord compression, and IUGR.

Oligohydramnios almost always indicates the presence of a fetal abnormality.

TABLE 2.11–8. Types of Intrauterine Growth Retardation

	Symmetric	**Asymmetric**
Prevalence	20% of cases	80% of cases
Ultrasonic parameters		
Biparietal diameter	↓	Normal
Head circumference	↓	Normal
Abdominal circumference	↓	↓
Femur length	↓	Normal
Time of insult	Early in pregnancy	Late in pregnancy
Etiology	Fetal problem:	Placenta mediated:
	Cytogenetic	HTN
	Infection	Poor nutrition
	Anomalies	Maternal smoking
		(OB.50)

POLYHYDRAMNIOS

An excess of amniotic fluid volume defined by an **AFI > 20** on U/S. It may be present in normal pregnancies, but fetal chromosomal or developmental abnormalities are common. Although usually asymptomatic, exam may reveal fundal height greater than expected. Etiologies include **maternal DM, multiple gestation** *(OB.52)*, isoimmunization, pulmonary abnormalities (e.g., cystic lung malformations), fetal anomalies (e.g., duodenal atresia, tracheoesophageal fistula, or **anencephaly**), and twin-twin transfusion syndrome. Evaluation includes U/S for fetal anomalies, glucose testing for DM, and Rh screen. Treatment depends on the cause. Complications include preterm labor, fetal malpresentation, and cord prolapse.

UCV *OB.45*

RHESUS ISOIMMUNIZATION

Rhesus (Rh) factor is an antigenic protein located on RBCs in Rh-positive individuals. Transmission is autosomal dominant, so an Rh-positive father and an Rh-negative mother can have an Rh-positive fetus. When fetal RBCs leak into maternal circulation, maternal anti-Rh IgG antibodies can form. These antibodies can cross the placenta, react with Rh-positive RBCs, and cause fetal hemolysis (**erythroblastosis fetalis;** *Peds.40*; see Figure 2.11–3). Hemolytic disease usually occurs during the second pregnancy owing to rapid production of anti-Rh IgG antibodies by memory plasma cells.

History/PE

Inquire about prior events that may have exposed the mother to Rh-positive blood, including ectopic pregnancy, **abortion,** blood transfusions, **prior delivery of an Rh-positive child,** amniocentesis, or other traumatic procedures during pregnancy.

Evaluation

- **Maternal:** On initial visit, test for ABO and Rh blood groups and perform antibody screening (indirect Coombs' test). If negative, repeat Coombs' test at 26–28 weeks. If positive, test serially for high titers of maternal anti-Rh IgG (> 1:16).

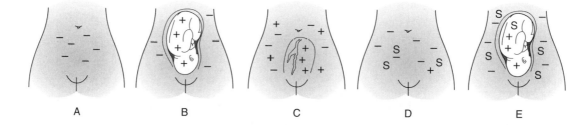

FIGURE 2.11–3. Rh disease. (A) Rh-negative woman before pregnancy. (B) Pregnancy occurs. The fetus is Rh-positive. (C) Separation of the placenta. (D) Following delivery, Rh isoimmunization occurs in the mother, and she develops antibodies (S = antibodies). (E) The next pregnancy with an Rh-positive fetus. Maternal antibodies cross the placenta, enter the bloodstream, and attach to Rh-positive cells, causing hemolysis. RhoGAM (Rh IgG) is given to the Rh-negative mother to prevent sensitization. (Adapted, with permission, from DeCherney AH. *Current Obstetric & Gynecologic Diagnosis & Treatment*, 8th ed. Stamford, CT: Appleton & Lange, 1994:339, Fig. 15–1.)

- **Fetal:** Assess during pregnancy using amniocentesis or U/S-guided umbilical blood sampling for fetal blood type, Coombs' titer, bilirubin levels, HCT, and reticulocytes, or determine Rh status and HCT postnatally using fetal cord blood.

Treatment

- **Prevention:** If the mother is Rh negative at 28 weeks and (1) the father is Rh positive, (2) father's Rh status is unknown, or (3) paternity is uncertain, **give RhoGAM** (RhIgG). If the baby is Rh positive, give RhoGAM postpartum as well. Give RhoGAM to Rh-negative mothers who undergo abortion (therapeutic or spontaneous) or who have had an ectopic pregnancy, amniocentesis, vaginal bleeding, or placenta previa/placental abruption.
- Sensitized Rh-negative mothers with titers > 1:16 should be closely monitored (for evidence of fetal hemolysis) with serial U/S and amniocentesis.
- In severe cases, initiate preterm delivery when fetal lungs are mature (enhance lung maturity with betamethasone). Prior to delivery, intrauterine blood transfusions may be given to correct a low fetal HCT.

RhoGAM (anti-RhIgG) destroys Rh-positive cells in maternal circulation and prevents Rh sensitization.

Complications

Fetal hypoxia and acidosis, kernicterus, prematurity, or death. **Hydrops fetalis** (decreased protein and oncotic pressure, edema, jaundice, high-output cardiac failure) occurs when Hb drops to > 7 g/dL below normal.

GESTATIONAL TROPHOBLASTIC DISEASE (GTD)

A range of proliferative trophoblastic abnormalities that can be benign (e.g., hydatidiform mole) or malignant (e.g., choriocarcinoma). **Hydatidiform mole (or molar pregnancy) accounts for approximately 80% of cases. Complete moles** usually result from sperm fertilization of an empty ovum, have a chromosomal pattern of **46,XX,** and are paternally derived. **Incomplete (partial) moles** result when a normal ovum is fertilized by two sperm (or a haploid sperm that duplicates its chromosomes), usually have a chromosomal pattern of **69,XXY, and contain fetal tissue.** Risk factors for GTD include extremes of age (< 20 or > 40), a diet deficient in folate or β-carotene, and blood group (type A woman impregnated by type O man). Molar pregnancy may progress to malignant GTD, including invasive moles (10–15%) and choriocarcinoma (2–5%).

Partial moles can contain fetal parts.

History/PE

First-trimester **uterine bleeding** (most common), **hyperemesis gravidarum, preeclampsia-eclampsia** at < 24 weeks, **uterine size greater than dates,** and hyperthyroidism (HTN, tachycardia, tachypnea). No fetal heartbeat is detected. Pelvic exam may reveal enlarged ovaries with bilateral theca-lutein cysts and possible **expulsion of grapelike molar clusters** into the vagina or blood in the cervical os.

Preeclampsia in the first trimester is pathognomonic for hydatidiform mole.

Complete hydatidiform mole has a "snow-storm" appearance on pelvic U/S.

Differential

Normal pregnancy, spontaneous abortion, ectopic pregnancy, preeclampsia, placenta previa, placental abruption, multiple gestation.

Evaluation

Look for **markedly elevated serum β-hCG** (usually > 100,000 mIU/mL) and a **"snowstorm" appearance on pelvic U/S** with no gestational sac or fetus present. CXR may show lung metastases.

Treatment

Dilation and curettage (D&C) reveals "cluster-of-grapes" tissue (see Figure 2.11–4). **Follow β-hCG** closely and **prevent pregnancy** for **one year** to ensure accurate monitoring. Treat malignant disease with **chemotherapy** (methotrexate or dactinomycin) and **residual uterine disease with hysterectomy.** Chemotherapy and irradiation are highly successful for metastases (90%).

Complications

Malignant GTD, pulmonary or CNS metastases, trophoblastic pulmonary emboli, acute respiratory insufficiency.

THIRD-TRIMESTER BLEEDING

Describes any bleeding **after 20 weeks' gestation.** Prior to 20 weeks, bleeding is referred to as threatened abortion. Complicates ~3–5% of pregnancies. The **most common causes are placental abruption and placenta previa** (see Figure 2.11–5) (OB.43,44), which are compared in Table 2.11–9. Other causes include bloody show, ruptured vasa previa, early labor, ruptured uterus, marginal placental separation, genital tract lesions and trauma, and placenta accreta (placental adherence to myometrium).

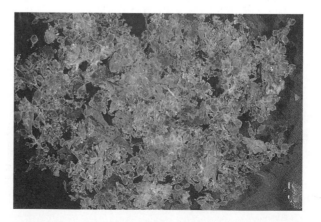

FIGURE 2.11–4. Hydatidiform mole. Note the characteristic "bunch-of-grapes" appearance on this gross specimen. (Reproduced courtesy of Dr. Raoul Fresco, Loyola University.)

TABLE 2.11–9. Placental Abruption vs. Placenta Previa

	Placental Abruption	Placenta Previa
Pathophysiology	**Premature** (before onset of labor) **separation** of normally implanted placenta.	Abnormal placental implantation: ■ **Total:** placenta covers cervical os. ■ **Marginal:** placenta extends to margin of os. ■ **Low-lying** placenta in close proximity to os.
Incidence	1 in 100.	1 in 200.
Risk factors	HTN, abdominal/pelvic trauma, tobacco or cocaine use, previous abruption, rapid decompression of overdistended uterus.	Prior C-sections, grand multiparous, advanced maternal age, multiple gestation, prior placenta previa.
Symptoms	**Painful, dark** vaginal bleeding that does not spontaneously cease. Abdominal pain, uterine hypertonicity. Fetal distress.	**Painless, bright red** bleeding that often ceases in 1–2 hours with or without uterine contractions. First bleeding episode at 29–30 weeks. Usually no fetal distress.
Diagnosis	**Primarily clinical.** Transabdominal/transvaginal U/S sensitivity is only 50%; look for retroplacental clot; most useful for ruling out previa.	**Transabdominal/transvaginal U/S sensitivity is > 95%;** look for abnormally positioned placenta.
Management	Stabilize patient with mild abruption and premature fetus; **manage expectantly** (hospitalize, start IV and fetal monitoring, type and cross blood, bed rest). **Moderate to severe abruption:** immediate delivery (vaginal delivery with amniotomy if mother and fetus are stable, C-section for maternal or fetal distress).	**NO vaginal exam!** **Stabilize patient with premature fetus;** manage expectantly. Give tocolytics (MgSO₄). Serial U/S to assess fetal growth, resolution of partial previa. Assess fetal lung maturity with amniocentesis and augment with betamethasone. **Deliver by C-section. Indications for delivery: persistent labor, life-threatening bleeding, fetal distress, documented fetal lung maturity, 36 weeks' GA.**
Complications	Hemorrhagic shock. Coagulopathy: **DIC** in 10%. Recurrence risk is 5–16%; rises to 25% after two previous abruptions. Fetal hypoxia.	Increased risk of placenta accreta. Vasa previa (fetal vessels crossing the internal os). Preterm delivery, PROM, IUGR, congenital anomalies. Recurrence risk is 4–8%.

HIGH-YIELD FACTS

Obstetrics

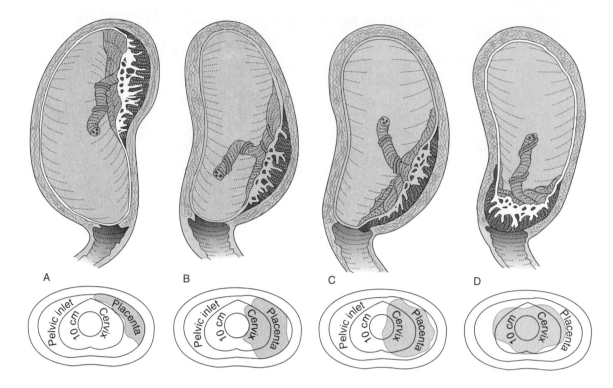

FIGURE 2.11–5. Placental implantation. (A) Normal placenta. (B) Low implantation. (C) Partial placenta previa. (D) Complete placenta previa. (Adapted, with permission, from DeCherney AH. *Current Obstetric & Gynecologic Diagnosis & Treatment,* 8th ed. Stamford, CT: Appleton & Lange, 1994:404, Fig. 20–2.)

ABNORMAL LABOR AND DELIVERY

PREMATURE RUPTURE OF MEMBRANES (PROM)

Spontaneous ROM before onset of labor. May be precipitated by vaginal or cervical infections, abnormal membrane physiology, and cervical incompetence. Preterm PROM (PPROM) occurs at < 37 weeks' gestation. Risk factors include low socioeconomic status, young maternal age, smoking, and STDs. Prolonged ROM is defined as rupture > 18 hours prior to delivery.

History/PE

Patients often report a **"gush" of clear or blood-tinged vaginal fluid.** Uterine contractions may be present.

Differential

Urinary leakage, excess vaginal discharge, bloody show.

Evaluation

Sterile speculum exam reveals **pooling** of amniotic fluid in vaginal vault, **positive nitrazine paper test** (paper turns blue in alkaline amniotic fluid), and **positive fern test** (ferning pattern seen under a microscope after amniotic fluid dries on a glass slide). U/S to assess amniotic fluid volume. Cultures or smears to rule out infections. To minimize infection risk, **do not** perform digital vaginal exams. Check fetal heart tracing, maternal temperature, WBC count, and uterine tenderness for evidence of chorioamnionitis.

UCV OB.38

Do not perform digital vaginal exams in women with PROM to minimize risk of infection.

Treatment

Depends on GA and fetal lung maturity. In general, if there is no sign of infection, delivery is delayed with **tocolytics:** β-agonists (i.e., ritodrine or terbutaline), magnesium, NSAIDs (e.g., indomethacin), or Ca^{2+} channel blockers (e.g., nifedipine). **Prophylactic antibiotics** are given to prevent infection. **Corticosteroids** (e.g., betamethasone or dexamethasone × 48 hours) can be given to promote fetal lung maturity. If signs of infection or fetal distress develop, give antibiotics (ampicillin ± erythromycin) and induce labor.

Complications

Preterm labor and delivery, chorioamnionitis, placental abruption, cord prolapse.

PRETERM LABOR

Onset of labor between **20–37 weeks' gestation.** Occurs in ~10% of all U.S. pregnancies and is the primary cause of neonatal morbidity and mortality. Risk factors include multiple gestation, infection, PROM, uterine anomalies, previous preterm labor or delivery, polyhydramnios, placental abruption, poor maternal nutrition, and low socioeconomic status. However, **most patients have no identifiable risk factors.**

History/PE

Patients may have menstrual-like cramps, onset of low back pain, pelvic pressure, and new vaginal discharge or bleeding.

Differential

Cervical incompetence (treated with cerclage), preterm uterine contractions (self-limited).

Evaluation

Diagnosis requires **regular uterine contractions** (≥ 3 contractions of 30 seconds each over a 30-minute period) and **concurrent cervical change** at < 37 weeks' gestation. **Assess for contraindications to tocolysis** (e.g., infection, nonreassuring fetal testing, placental abruption). Perform a **sterile speculum exam** to rule out PROM. Obtain **U/S** to rule out fetal or uterine anomalies, verify GA, and assess fetal presentation and amniotic fluid volume. Obtain cultures for chlamydia, gonorrhea, and GBS. Obtain a UA/urine culture.

HIGH-YIELD FACTS

Obstetrics

Treatment

Begin with hydration and bed rest. Unless contraindicated, begin **tocolytic therapy** and **steroids** to accelerate fetal lung maturation. Give **penicillin or ampicillin for GBS prophylaxis** if preterm delivery is likely.

Complications

RDS, intraventricular hemorrhage, patent ductus arteriosus (PDA), necrotizing enterocolitis *(Ped.43)*, retinopathy of prematurity, bronchopulmonary dysplasia, death.

FETAL MALPRESENTATION

Breech presentation is the most common fetal malpresentation.

Defined as any presentation other than vertex (i.e., head closest to birth canal, chin to chest, occiput anterior). Risk factors include **prematurity,** prior breech delivery, uterine anomalies, poly- or oligohydramnios, multiple gestations, PPROM, hydrocephalus, anencephaly, and placenta previa. **Breech presentations** are the most common (3% of all deliveries) and involve presentation of fetal lower extremities or buttocks into the maternal pelvis (see Figure 2.11–6). Subtypes include:

- **Frank breech** (50–75%): Thighs flexed and knees extended.
- **Footling breech** (20%): One or both legs extended below the buttocks.
- **Complete breech** (5–10%): Thighs and knees flexed.

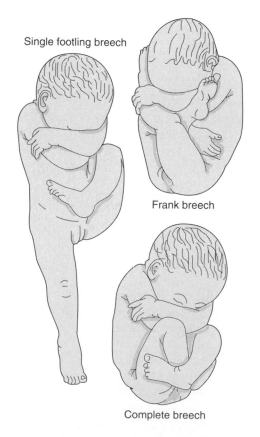

FIGURE 2.11–6. Types of breech presentations. (Reproduced, with permission, from DeCherney AH. *Current Obstetric & Gynecologic Diagnosis & Treatment,* 8th ed. Stamford, CT: Appleton & Lange, 1994:411, Fig. 21–1.)

TABLE 2.11–10. Indications for Cesarean Section

Maternal Factors	Fetal and Maternal Factors	Fetal Factors
Prior classical C-section (vertical incision predisposes to uterine rupture with vaginal delivery)	Cephalopelvic disproportion (most common cause of primary C-section)	Fetal malposition (e.g., posterior chin, transverse lie, shoulder presentation)
Active genital herpes infection	Placenta previa/placental abruption	Fetal distress
Cervical carcinoma	Failed operative vaginal delivery	Cord compression
Maternal trauma/demise	Post-term pregnancy (relative indication)	Erythroblastosis fetalis (Rh incompatibility)

Evaluation

Use Leopold maneuvers to identify fetal lie (transverse or vertical) and presentation (vertex or breech).

Treatment

- **Follow:** Up to 75% spontaneously change to vertex by week 38.
- **External version:** If the fetus has not reverted spontaneously, apply pressure to the maternal abdomen to turn the infant to vertex. Success rate is ~75%. Risks are placental abruption and cord compression, so be prepared for an emergency C-section.
- **Elective C-section:** The standard of care in many hospitals, but it has **not** been shown to improve outcome.
- **Trial of breech vaginal delivery:** Attempt **only if delivery is imminent.** Otherwise contraindicated. Complications include cord prolapse and/or head entrapment.

INDICATIONS FOR CESAREAN SECTION

See Table 2.11–10 for indications.

PUERPERIUM

POSTPARTUM HEMORRHAGE

Defined as a loss of **> 500 mL of blood for vaginal delivery** or **> 1000 mL for C-section** occurring before, during, or after delivery of the placenta. Table 2.11–11 summarizes common causes. Complications include acute blood loss (potentially fatal), anemia due to chronic blood loss (predisposes to puerperal infection), and **Sheehan's syndrome** (see below).

POSTPARTUM INFECTIONS

Genital tract infection with a temperature $\geq 38°C$ for **at least two of the first ten postpartum days (not including the first 24 hours).** Endometrial infection is most common. Incidence is increased after C-section. Other risk factors include emergent C-section, PROM, prolonged labor, multiple intra-

TABLE 2.11–11. Common Causes of Postpartum Hemorrhage

	Uterine Atony	Genital Tract Trauma	Retained Placental Tissue
Risk factors	Uterine overdistention (multiple gestation, macrosomia, polyhydramnios). Exhausted myometrium (rapid or prolonged labor, oxytocin stimulation). Uterine infection. Conditions interfering with contractions (anesthesia, myomas, $MgSO_4$).	Precipitous labor. Operative vaginal delivery (forceps, vacuum extraction). Large infant. Inadequate episiotomy repair.	Placenta accreta/increta/ percreta. Placenta previa. Uterine leiomyomas. Preterm delivery. Previous C-section/curettage.
Diagnosis	Palpation of soft, enlarged, "boggy" uterus. **Most common cause of postpartum hemorrhage (90%).**	Manual and visual inspection of lower genital tract for any laceration > 2 cm long.	Manual and visual inspection of placenta and uterine cavity for missing cotyledons. U/S may also be used to inspect uterus.
Treatment[a]	Bimanual **uterine massage** (usually successful). **Oxytocin** infusion. **Methergine** (methylergonovine) if not hypertensive. **Prostin** ($PGF_{2\alpha}$) if not asthmatic.	Surgical repair of the physical defect.	Manual removal of remaining placental tissue. Curettage with suctioning (take care not to perforate the uterine fundus).

[a]For all uterine causes, when bleeding persists after conventional therapy, uterine/internal iliac artery ligation or hysterectomy can be lifesaving.

The 7 W's of postpartum fever:

Womb (endomyometritis)
Wind (atelectasis, pneumonia)
Water (UTI)
Walk (DVT, PE)
Wound (incision, episiotomy)
Weaning (breast engorgement, abscess, mastitis)
Wonder drugs (drug fever)

partum vaginal exams, and intrauterine manipulations. Causes are outlined in the **7 W's.** Perform a pelvic exam to rule out hematoma or lochial block. Consider UA/culture (for UTI) and blood cultures (for sepsis [OB.47]). Hospitalize and give **broad-spectrum IV antibiotics** (e.g., clindamycin and gentamicin) **until patients have been afebrile for 48 hours.** Add ampicillin for complicated cases. Consider other diagnoses (e.g., pelvic abscess, **septic pelvic thrombophlebitis**) if the three-drug regimen is not effective after 48 hours.

SHEEHAN'S SYNDROME (POSTPARTUM PITUITARY NECROSIS)

Pituitary ischemia and necrosis resulting in anterior pituitary insufficiency secondary to massive obstetric hemorrhage and shock. The primary cause of anterior pituitary insufficiency in adult females. The **most common presenting syndrome is failure to lactate** (due to decreased prolactin levels). Other symptoms include weakness, lethargy, cold insensitivity, genital atrophy, and menstrual disorders.

UCV *OB.49*

- **Physiology:** During pregnancy, elevated estrogen and progesterone induce breast hypertrophy and inhibit prolactin release. After delivery of the placenta, hormone levels drop markedly and prolactin is released, stimulating milk production. Periodic infant suckling causes further release of **prolactin** and **oxytocin,** which stimulates myoepithelial cell contraction and milk ejection ("let-down reflex").

- **Breast-feeding:** Colostrum ("early breast milk") contains protein, fat, **secretory IgA,** and minerals. Within one week postpartum, mature milk with protein, fat, lactose, and water is produced. High IgA levels in colostrum provide **passive immunity** for the infant and protect against enteric bacteria. High leukocyte levels in breast milk provide **active immunity.** Other benefits include decreased incidence of allergies, mother-child bonding, and maternal weight loss. Breast-feeding contraindications are HIV infection, active hepatitis, and use of certain medications (e.g., tetracycline, chloramphenicol, warfarin).

Breast-feeding is contraindicated in maternal HIV infection, active hepatitis, and use of certain medications.

MASTITIS

Cellulitis of the periglandular tissue caused by nipple trauma from breast-feeding coupled with introduction of *Staphylococcus aureus* from the infant's nostrils into the nipple ducts. Symptoms often begin 2–4 weeks postpartum, are **usually unilateral,** and include focal breast tenderness, erythema, edema, warmth, and possible purulent nipple drainage. Differentiate from simple breast engorgement. Infection is suggested by focal symptoms, positive breast milk culture, elevated WBC count, and fever. Treatment includes **continued breast-feeding** and PO antibiotics (e.g., penicillin, dicloxacillin, erythromycin). Incision and drainage of breast abscess if present.

Treatment of mastitis includes antibiotics and continued breast-feeding.

HIGH-YIELD FACTS

Obstetrics

The following clinical questions and accompanying answers are reproduced, with permission, from Evans MI, *PreTest: Obstetrics & Gynecology*, 9th ed., New York: McGraw-Hill, 2001.

Questions

1. In terms of birth defect potential, the safest of the following drugs is
   a. Alcohol
   b. Isotretinoin (Accutane)
   c. Tetracyclines
   d. Progesterones
   e. Phenytoin (Dilantin)

2. A 24-year-old woman appears at eight weeks of pregnancy and reveals a history of pulmonary embolism seven years ago during her first pregnancy. She was treated with intravenous heparin followed by several months of oral warfarin (Coumadin) and has had no further evidence of thromboembolic disease for over six years. Which of the following statements about her current condition is true?
   a. Having no evidence of disease for over five years means that the risk of thromboembolism is not greater than normal
   b. Impedance plethysmography is not a useful study to evaluate her for deep venous thrombosis in pregnancy
   c. Doppler ultrasonography is not a useful technique to evaluate her for deep venous thrombosis in pregnancy
   d. The patient should be placed on low-dose heparin therapy throughout pregnancy and puerperium
   e. The patient is at highest risk for recurrent thromboembolism during the second trimester of pregnancy

3. A 29-year-old, gravida 3, para 2 black woman in the 33rd week of gestation is admitted to the emergency room because of acute abdominal pain that developed and is increasing during the past 24 hours. The pain is severe and is radiating from the epigastrium to the back. The patient has vomited a few times and has not eaten or had a bowel movement since the pain started. On examination you observe an acutely ill patient lying on the bed with her knees drawn up. Her blood pressure is 150/100 mmHg, her pulse is 110 beats/min, and her temperature is 38.18°C (100.68°F). On palpation the abdomen is somewhat distended and tender, mainly in the epigastric area, and the uterine fundus reaches 31 cm above the symphysis. Hypotonic bowel sounds are noted. Fetal monitoring reveals a normal pattern of fetal heart rate (FHR) without uterine contractions. On ultrasonography the fetus is in vertex presentation and appropriate in size for gestational age; fetal breathing and trunk movements are noted and the volume of amniotic fluid is normal. The placenta is located on the anterior uterine wall and of grade 2 to 3. Laboratory values show mild leukocytosis (12,000 cells/μL); a hematocrit of 43; mildly elevated serum glutamic-oxaloacetic transaminase (SGOT), serum glutamic-pyruvic transaminase (SGPT), and bilirubin; and serum amylase of 180 U/dL. Urinalysis is normal.

The most probable diagnosis in this patient is
   a. Acute degeneration of uterine leiomyoma
   b. Acute cholecystitis
   c. Acute pancreatitis
   d. Acute appendicitis
   e. Severe preeclamptic toxemia

4. When treating urinary tract infection (UTI) in the third trimester, the antibiotic of choice should be
   a. Cephalosporin
   b. Tetracycline
   c. Sulfonamide
   d. Nitrofurantoin

1. **The answer is d.** Alcohol is an enormous contributor to otherwise preventable birth defects. Sequelae include retardation of intrauterine growth, craniofacial abnormalities, and mental retardation. The occasional drink in pregnancy has not been proved to be deleterious. Isotretinoin (Accutane) is a powerful drug for acne that has enormous potential for producing congenital anomalies when ingested in early pregnancy; it should never be used in pregnancy. Tetracyclines interfere with development of bone and can lead to stained teeth in children. Progesterones have been implicated in multiple birth defects but controlled studies have failed to demonstrate a significant association with increased risk. Patients who have inadvertently become pregnant while on birth control pills should be reassured that the incidence of birth defects is no higher for them than for the general population. Phenytoin (Dilantin) is used for epilepsy and can be associated with a spectrum of abnormalities, including digital hypoplasia and facial abnormalities.

2. **The answer is d.** Patients with a history of thromboembolic disease in pregnancy are at high risk to develop it in subsequent pregnancies. Impedance plethysmography and doppler ultrasonography are useful techniques even in pregnancy and should be done as baseline studies. Patients should be treated prophylactically with low-dose heparin therapy through the postpartum period as this is the time of highest risk of this disease. Coumadin is contraindicated in pregnancy.

3. **The answer is c.** The most probable diagnosis in this case is acute pancreatitis. The pain caused by a myoma in degeneration is more localized to the uterine wall. Low-grade fever and mild leukocytosis may appear with a degenerating myoma, but liver function tests are usually normal. The other obstetric cause of epigastric pain, severe preeclamptic toxemia (PET), may exhibit disturbed liver function (sometimes associated with the HELLP syndrome [hemolysis, elevated liver enzymes, low platelets]), but this patient has only mild elevation of blood pressure and no proteinuria. Acute appendicitis in pregnancy is one of the more common nonobstetric causes of abdominal pain. In pregnancy, symptoms of acute appendicitis are similar to those in nonpregnant patients, but the pain is more vague and poorly localized and the point of maximal tenderness moves with advancing gestation to the right upper quadrant. Liver function tests are normal with acute appendicitis. Acute cholecystitis may cause fever, leukocytosis, and pain of the right upper quadrant with abnormal liver function tests, but amylase levels would be elevated only mildly, if at all, and pain would be less severe than described in this patient. The diagnosis that fits the clinical description and the laboratory findings is acute pancreatitis. This disorder may be more common during pregnancy, with an incidence of 1:100 to 1:10,000 pregnancies. Cholelithiasis, chronic alcoholism, infection, abdominal trauma, some medications, and pregnancy-induced hypertension are known predisposing factors. Patients with pancreatitis are usually in acute distress—the classic finding is a person who is rocking with knees drawn up and trunk flexed in agony. Fever, tachypnea, hypotension, ascites, and pleural effusion may be observed. Hypotonic bowel sounds, epigastric tenderness, and signs of peritonitis may be demonstrated on examination.

Leukocytosis, hemoconcentration, and abnormal liver function tests are common laboratory findings in acute pancreatitis. The most important laboratory finding is, however, an elevation of serum amylase levels, which appears 12–24 hours after onset of clinical disease. Values may exceed 200

U/dL (normal values are 50 to 160 U/dL). A useful diagnostic tool in the pregnant patient with only modest elevation of amylase values is the amylase/creatinine ratio. In patients with acute pancreatitis, the ratio of amylase clearance to creatinine clearance is always greater than 5–6%.

Treatment considerations for the pregnant patient with acute pancreatitis are similar to those in nonpregnant patients. Intravenous hydration, nasogastric suction, enteric rest, and correction of electrolyte imbalance and of hyperglycemia are the mainstays of therapy. Careful attention to tissue perfusion, volume expansion, and transfusions to maintain a stable cardiovascular performance are critical. Gradual recovery occurs over 5–6 days.

4. **The answer is a.** Although quite effective, sulfonamides should be avoided during the last few weeks of pregnancy because they competitively inhibit the binding of bilirubin to albumin, which increases the risk of neonatal hyperbilirubinemia. Nitrofurantoin may not be tolerated in pregnancy because of the effect of nausea. It should also be avoided in late pregnancy because of the risk of hemolysis due to the deficiency of erythrocyte phosphate dehydrogenase in the newborn. Tetracyclines are contraindicated during pregnancy because of dental staining in the fetus. Thus, the drugs of choice for treatment of UTI in pregnancy are ampicillin and the cephalosporins.

HIGH-YIELD FACTS

Obstetrics

Gynecology

Characterized by abnormalities in frequency, duration, volume, and/or timing of menstrual bleeding (see Table 2.12–1).

Evaluation

To distinguish ovulatory from anovulatory disorders, take a thorough menstrual history and characterize bleeding frequency, volume, and duration. Complete a bimanual exam and screen for cervical cancer with a Pap smear. If cycles appear **ovulatory,** diagnostic tools include transvaginal U/S, sonohysterogram, or dilation and curettage (D&C; gold standard) with hysteroscopy. If cycles appear **anovulatory,** perform β-hCG, CBC, coagulation profile, and endocrine tests (FSH, LH, TSH, and prolactin). Perform an **endometrial biopsy** (EMB) to screen for endometrial hyperplasia and cancer in **all women** with postmenopausal or chronic anovulatory bleeding.

TABLE 2.12–1. Abnormal Uterine Bleeding

Name	Definition	Causes
Menorrhagia	Excessive bleeding (> 80 mL blood loss/cycle) or prolonged bleeding (flow lasting > 8 days).	Leiomyoma, adenomyosis, endometrial hyperplasia or polyps, endometrial or cervical cancer, primary bleeding disorders, pregnancy complications.
Metrorrhagia	Bleeding between periods.	Endometrial polyps, endometrial or cervical cancer, pregnancy complications, exogenous estrogen.
Menometrorrhagia	Heavy bleeding between and during menstrual periods.	Same as above.
Polymenorrhea	Frequent menstruation (< 21-day cycle).	Anovulation.
Oligomenorrhea	Infrequent menstruation (> 35-day cycle).	Pregnancy (most common), hypothalamic-pituitary-gonadal-axis disruption, systemic disease.
Hypomenorrhea	Unusually low menstrual volume and duration; regular frequency.	Hypogonadotropic hypogonadism (common in anorexics and athletes), OCPs, Asherman's syndrome (uterine scarring due to surgery or infection), outlet obstruction.
Dysfunctional uterine bleeding (DUB) *(OB.8)*	A diagnosis of exclusion. Describes abnormal menstrual bleeding when no pathologic cause is found.	Anovulation (90%).
Postmenopausal bleeding	Uterine bleeding > 1 year after menopause.	Vaginal atrophy, exogenous hormones, cancer.

Treatment

Treat the underlying disorder. Treat anovulatory bleeding with **OCPs** or cyclic progestin therapy (**medroxyprogesterone** 10 mg/day for 10 days/month). Control profuse bleeding with **high-dose IV estrogen, D&C,** endometrial ablation, or hysterectomy (a last resort). Treat ovulatory DUB with NSAIDs +/– OCPs.

AMENORRHEA

Primary amenorrhea is the absence of menses and the lack of secondary sexual characteristics by age 14 or the absence of menses by age 16 with or without secondary sexual characteristics. **Secondary amenorrhea** is the absence of menses for three cycles or for six months with prior normal menses.

Differential

Table 2.12–2 summarizes the causes of amenorrhea.

Evaluation

Physical exam to assess for outflow tract abnormalities and β-hCG to rule out pregnancy (the most common cause). The workup of primary amenorrhea is based on the presence or absence of a uterus and breasts (see Figure 2.12–1). The workup of secondary amenorrhea includes serum prolactin and TSH. Further studies may include progestin challenge, serum FSH and estradiol, and CT or MRI (see Figure 2.12–2).

- **Prolactin:** Elevated prolactin inhibits the release of FSH and LH. It can be caused by a pituitary tumor, hypothyroidism, and dopamine antagonists (e.g., phenothiazines). Check TSH and obtain a CT or MRI to visualize the pituitary. If negative, perform a progestin challenge.

Always rule out pregnancy in a patient with amenorrhea.

TABLE 2.12–2. Causes of Amenorrhea

	Primary	Secondary
Anatomic abnormalities	Müllerian anomalies Vaginal agenesis Imperforate hymen Testicular feminization	Asherman's syndrome Cervical stenosis (scarring of os)
Ovarian or uterine dysfunction	Ovarian failure Gonadal dysgenesis (e.g., Turner's) Steroidogenic enzyme defects Constitutional developmental delay	Ovarian failure **Pregnancy** Polycystic ovarian syndrome (PCOS)
Central regulatory disorders	Hypothalamic dysfunction (Kallmann's syndrome, anorexia, excess exercise, weight loss, stress, tumor, infection) Primary pituitary dysfunction (rare)	Hypothalamic dysfunction (anorexia, excess exercise, weight loss, stress) Pituitary dysfunction (**Sheehan's syndrome,** panhypopituitarism) Hyperprolactinemia

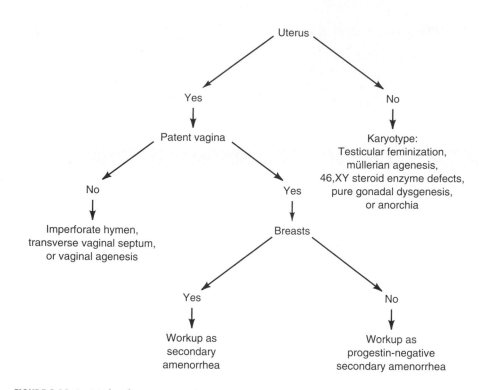

FIGURE 2.12–1. Workup for patients with primary amenorrhea. (Reproduced, with permission, from DeCherney AH. *Current Obstetric & Gynecologic Diagnosis & Treatment,* 8th ed. Stamford, CT: Appleton & Lange, 1994:1010, Fig. 54–2.)

- ■ **Progestin challenge:** If withdrawal bleeding occurs after a five-day course of progesterone (positive test), this means that estrogen is present, the outflow tract is patent, and the problem is anovulation. Causes include hypothalamic dysfunction, polycystic ovarian syndrome (PCOS), Cushing's syndrome; or ovarian or adrenal tumor. If no bleeding occurs, perform an estrogen-progesterone challenge.

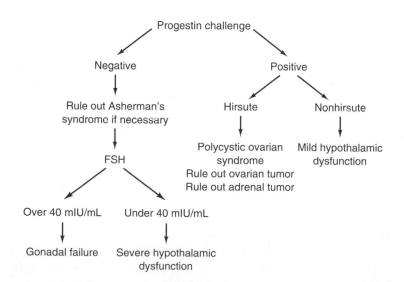

FIGURE 2.12–2. Workup for patients with secondary amenorrhea without hyperprolactinemia. (Reproduced, with permission, from DeCherney AH. *Current Obstetric & Gynecologic Diagnosis & Treatment,* 8th ed. Stamford, CT: Appleton & Lange, 1994:1012, Fig. 54–4.)

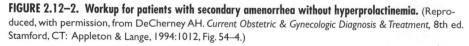

- **Estrogen-progesterone challenge:** Bleeding suggests a functional uterus with inadequate estrogen stimulation (a problem with the follicle or hypothalamic-pituitary axis [HPA]). Absence of bleeding indicates **Asherman's syndrome.**
- **Gonadotropins (FSH/LH):** Hypogonadotropism suggests HPA dysfunction (e.g., Sheehan's syndrome). Hypergonadotropism suggests gonadal failure (e.g., 17-hydroxylase deficiency, gonadal agenesis).

Treatment

Treat the underlying cause. Patients with low estrogen should receive HRT and elemental calcium supplementation.

UCV OB.22,23,26

BENIGN BREAST DISORDERS

Include fibrocystic change (most common), fibroadenoma, intraductal papilloma (common cause of bloody nipple discharge; OB.2), duct ectasia, galactoceles, fat necrosis, and breast abscess.

Intraductal papilloma is a common cause of bloody nipple discharge.

FIBROCYSTIC CHANGE

A spectrum of clinical findings (e.g., cystic change, nodularity, stromal proliferation, epithelial hyperplasia) commonly seen in **premenopausal women** (up to 50%). Caused by exaggerated stromal response to hormones and growth factors. Symptoms include cyclic, often premenstrual, bilateral breast pain, tenderness, and swelling. Exam reveals excessive tissue nodularity. Diagnose with fine-needle aspiration and cytologic examination of the dominant lesion. Management may include decreased caffeine and nicotine, vitamin E supplementation, hormonal therapy (e.g., progestins, danazol, tamoxifen), and diuretics for premenstrual mastalgia. Breast cancer risk is increased only if cellular atypia is present.

FIBROADENOMA

A benign, slow-growing breast tumor with epithelial and stromal components. The **most common breast lesion in women < 30 years of age.** Usually presents as a round, firm, discrete, mobile, nontender, solitary mass. Surgical excision provides tissue for diagnosis and is the treatment of choice. Recurrence is common. **Phyllodes tumor** is a rapidly growing, often large type of fibroadenoma that is rarely malignant (cystosarcoma phyllodes).

Fibroadenoma is the most common breast lesion in women < 30 years old.

BREAST CANCER

The most common cancer and the second most common cause of cancer death in women (next to lung cancer). Risk factors include female gender, older age, breast cancer in first-degree relatives, personal history of breast cancer, history of fibrocystic change with cellular atypia, nulliparity, early menar

Increased exposure to estrogen (early menarche, late menopause, nulliparity) increases the risk of breast cancer.

che, late menopause, and first full-term pregnancy after age 35. Late menarche is associated with decreased risk. BRCA-1 and BRCA-2 mutations are associated with early-onset, often familial breast and ovarian cancer.

History/PE

Patients often present with a **hard, irregular, immobile, painless breast lump** and possibly nipple discharge. **Skin changes** (dimpling, redness, ulceration, edema) and **axillary adenopathy** indicate more advanced disease. Cancers may be asymptomatic and nonpalpable and may thus be detected on **mammogram only.** The most common location is the **upper outer quadrant.** Metastatic sites include **lymph nodes, bones, brain, lung,** and **liver.**

Differential

Mammary dysplasia, fibroadenoma, intraductal papilloma, mastitis, fat necrosis.

Evaluation

Diagnosis is suggested by a palpable mass or **mammogram abnormalities** (e.g., microcalcifications, hyperdense regions). **U/S** may also be used. If cystic, perform FNA; if cyst doesn't resolve, fluid is bloody, or cyst recurs, excise. If solid, biopsy. **Biopsy** techniques include direct needle core biopsy (of a palpable lump), stereotactic core biopsy (of a nonpalpable lesion), or open surgical biopsy (with needle localization if the mass is not palpable). Test for prognostic factors, including estrogen/progesterone receptors (ER/PR) and herzneu amplification. Special forms of breast cancer include:

Positive estrogen receptor status is a good prognostic indicator.

- **Inflammatory breast cancer:** A highly aggressive, rapidly growing cancer; invades lymphatics and causes skin inflammation; poor prognosis.
- **Paget's disease:** Ductal carcinoma in situ (DCIS) of the nipple with itching, burning, and nipple erosion (may be mistaken for infection). Associated with a focus of invasive carcinoma.
- **Bilateral breast cancer:** More common in young women and with lobular carcinoma.

Treatment

Treatment depends on the type and **stage:**

Lobular carcinoma in situ increases risk of invasive carcinoma in both breasts.

- **Carcinoma in situ (CIS):** Classified as lobular (LCIS) or ductal (DCIS). LCIS increases the risk of subsequent invasive carcinoma in both breasts, so patients should have close follow-up or bilateral mastectomy (in high-risk patients). DCIS treatment depends on size; treat small tumors with local excision and close follow-up and larger tumors with wide local excision plus radiation or simple mastectomy (no node dissection necessary).
- **Invasive cancer:** Can be lobular or ductal (most common type). Staging is based on size, node status, and metastases (perform a bone scan, CBC, serum calcium, and CXR). Treat localized disease with **lumpectomy plus axillary node dissection and radiation** or with **modified radical mastectomy** (simple mastectomy plus axillary node dissection). Use chemotherapy in all premenopausal women with positive nodes (regardless of hormone receptor status) and in postmenopausal women with positive nodes and negative hormone receptors.

- Tumors with a positive **estrogen receptor status** can be treated with hormone therapy (e.g., tamoxifen). Treat metastatic or recurrent disease with chemotherapy.
- Patients with herzneu amplification and metastatic disease can receive Herceptin.

UCV OB.3

Stage is a key prognostic factor for breast cancer.

CONTRACEPTION

Table 2.12–3 describes the various methods of contraception.

DYSMENORRHEA

Characterized by marked pain with menstrual periods that requires medication and prevents normal activity. **Primary dysmenorrhea** has no obvious organic cause, usually occurs before age 20, and may result from high levels of PGs and leukotrienes or from psychological factors. Treat with NSAIDs and OCPs. **Secondary dysmenorrhea** is associated with a specific pelvic pathology, including **endometriosis** (most common), adenomyosis (endometrial glands and stroma within the myometrium), myomas, pelvic congestion, PID, ovarian cysts, cervical stenosis, and pelvic adhesions.

ENDOMETRIOSIS

Defined as the presence of endometrial glands and stroma outside the uterus. Common sites include the **ovaries,** cul-de-sac, and uterosacral ligaments. Proposed etiologies include endometrial cell implantation via retrograde menstruation; vascular and lymphatic dissemination of endometrial cells; and metaplasia within the peritoneal cavity. Typically found in women of reproductive age. Risk factors include positive family history, nulliparity, and infertility.

Endometrial implants are commonly found in the ovaries, cul-de-sac, and uterosacral ligaments.

History/PE

Premenstrual pain (resolves at onset of menstruation), **dyschezia** (painful defecation), **chronic pelvic pain, dyspareunia** (painful intercourse), abnormal bleeding, and/or **infertility.** Pelvic exam may reveal tender **nodularity along the uterosacral ligament;** a **fixed, retroverted uterus;** and tender, fixed adnexal masses.

Differential

PID, pelvic adhesions, ectopic pregnancy, appendicitis, adnexal torsion, ruptured corpus luteum cyst, tumors.

Evaluation

Definitive diagnosis can be made with direct visualization of endometrial tissue via **laparoscopy** or laparotomy. Implants often appear as rust-colored to dark brown **"powder burns"** or as raised blue **"raspberry lesions."** In severe disease, implants may be surrounded by extensive adhesions. The ovary may contain endometriomas or **"chocolate cysts"** (large cystic collections of en-

TABLE 2.12–3. Contraceptive Methods

Type	Description	Side Effects
Behavioral methods		
Rhythm	Uses body temperature and cervical mucus consistency to predict time of fertility.	Unreliable compared to other methods.
Coitus interruptus	Withdrawal of the penis before ejaculation.	High failure rate.
Barrier methods		
Diaphragm and cervical caps	Domed sheet of rubber or latex placed over cervix. Must be fitted by physician and remain in vagina 6–8 hours after intercourse.	Possible allergy to latex or spermicides. Risk of UTI, toxic shock syndrome (TSS).
Condoms	Latex sheaths cover penis during intercourse.	Possible allergy to latex or spermicides.
IUD	Plastic and/or metal device placed in uterus. Causes local sterile inflammatory reaction within uterine wall such that sperm are engulfed and destroyed.	Increased vaginal bleeding,[a] uterine perforation, IUD migration, infection, increased risk of PID and ectopic pregnancy.[b]
Hormonal methods		
OCPs	Suppress ovulation by inhibiting FSH/LH; change consistency of cervical mucus, making the endometrium unsuitable for implantation.	Nausea, breast tenderness, acne, mood changes, HTN, hepatic adenoma, weight gain, increased risk of thromboembolism (e.g., PE, DVT; OB.15).
Levonorgestrel (Norplant)[c]	Progestin-only subdermal implant. Suppresses ovulation, thickens cervical mucus, and makes endometrium unsuitable for implantation. Effect lasts five years.	Irregular vaginal bleeding, weight gain, galactorrhea, acne, breast tenderness, headache. Difficult removal.
Postcoital "morning-after pill"	Progesterone ± estrogen taken within 72 hours of unprotected sex to suppress ovulation or discourage implantation.	Nausea, vomiting, fatigue, headache, dizziness, breast tenderness.
Medroxyprogesterone (Depo-Provera)	IM injection given every three months. Suppresses ovulation, thickens cervical mucus, and makes endometrium unsuitable for implantation.	Irregular vaginal bleeding, depression, weight gain, breast tenderness, delayed restoration of ovulation after discontinuation.
Surgical sterilization (tubal litigation, vasectomy)	Tubes are ligated, cauterized, or mechanically occluded.	Essentially irreversible (OB.25); bleeding, infection, failure, ectopic pregnancy.

[a] Seen with copper IUDs but not with progesterone IUDs.
[b] Overall rate of pregnancy is much lower with IUD use, but if pregnancy does occur, there is a higher risk that it will be ectopic.
[c] Product was taken off the market in 2002.

UCV

dometriosis filled with thick, dark, old blood). **Pain severity does not always correlate with extent of disease.**

Treatment

Depends on the extent and location of disease, symptom severity, and the desire for future fertility. **Medical options** include **OCPs** or progestin (to suppress ovulation and menstruation) and **danazol** or GnRH agonists (to suppress estrogen production). **Surgical options** include **laparoscopic ablation** of visible implants or **total abdominal hysterectomy and bilateral salpingo-oophorectomy (TAH-BSO)** with lysis of adhesions for severe, recurrent disease.

UCV OB.10

ECTOPIC PREGNANCY

Any pregnancy that implants outside the uterine cavity (see Figure 2.12–3). The most common location is the ampulla of the oviduct (95%). Risk factors include a **history of PID** (most common), prior ectopic pregnancy, tubal/pelvic surgery, diethylstilbestrol (DES) exposure in utero, and IUD use. Incidence is ~ 1 in 100 pregnancies.

The ampulla of the oviduct is the most common location for an ectopic pregnancy.

History/PE

The classic symptom triad is **amenorrhea, light vaginal bleeding, and lower abdominal or pelvic pain.** A tender **pelvic or adnexal mass** may be palpable. A ruptured ectopic pregnancy may present with sudden, sharp abdominal pain accompanied by **orthostatic hypotension,** tachycardia, generalized abdominal and adnexal tenderness with rebound tenderness, shoulder pain, and **shock.**

Any woman with abdominal pain needs a urine pregnancy test.

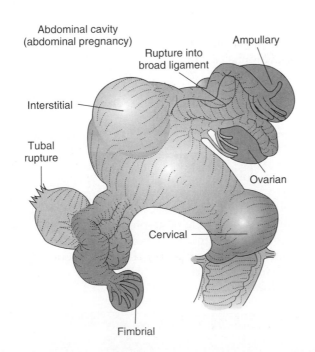

FIGURE 2.12–3. Sites of ectopic pregnancy. (Adapted from Benson RC. *Handbook of Obstetrics & Gynecology,* 8th ed. Stamford, CT: Appleton & Lange, 1983.)

Differential

Spontaneous abortion (SAB), molar pregnancy, ruptured corpus luteum cyst, PID, adnexal torsion, appendicitis, pyelonephritis, pancreatitis, diverticulitis, regional ileitis, ulcerative colitis.

Evaluation

Elevated β-hCG in the absence of an intrauterine pregnancy on U/S is suspicious for an ectopic pregnancy.

Measure β-hCG and follow the rate of rise. Levels are lower than expected for normal pregnancies of the same duration and have prolonged doubling times (normal is two days). Serum progesterone is often below normal (usually < 15 ng/mL) but this is nonspecific. Use transabdominal U/S (at β-hCG levels of 5000 mIU/mL) or transvaginal U/S (at β-hCG levels of 1,500 mIU/mL) to look for an intrauterine pregnancy and rule out an ectopic. **Elevated β-hCG in the absence of an intrauterine pregnancy on U/S** is highly suspicious. The return of > 5 cc of nonclotting blood on culdocentesis identifies hemoperitoneum but is not sensitive or specific. Definitive diagnosis is made by laparoscopy, laparotomy, or U/S visualization.

Treatment

- Follow patients closely with serial β-hCG and U/S studies.
- Use expectant management for asymptomatic patients with decreasing β-hCG, fallopian tube pregnancy, no U/S evidence of intra-abdominal bleeding, and a < 3.5-cm ectopic mass.
- Use **methotrexate** for early, stable, unruptured ectopic pregnancies.
- All others require stabilization and **surgery** with salpingostomy, salpingectomy, or salpingo-oophorectomy.
- Give a **RhoGAM** shot if appropriate based on blood type and antibody screen.

Complications

Inevitable loss of fetus, hemorrhagic shock, **future ectopic pregnancy,** infertility, maternal death, Rh sensitization.

UCV *OB.41*

GYNECOLOGIC INFECTIONS

VAGINITIS

The vagina normally contains mixed bacterial flora in an acidic environment (pH 3.5–4.5) maintained by lactic acid–producing lactobacilli. A change in this environment (e.g., due to medications, illness, frequent intercourse) can lead to overgrowth of other bacteria and clinical infection. Vaginitis may be bacterial (often polymicrobial, including *Gardnerella vaginalis*), fungal (*Candida*), or protozoal (*Trichomonas*).

History/PE

Presents with an **increased vaginal discharge** and **vulvovaginal pruritus** with or without a burning sensation or odor. Exam may reveal vulvar edema/erythema and white or colored discharge.

Differential

UTIs, STDs (other than *Trichomonas*), normal physiologic secretions, malignancy.

Evaluation/Treatment

Determine **vaginal pH** with nitrazine paper. **Microscopic examination of vaginal discharge** in saline **(wet prep)** and **KOH** (see Figure 2.12–4). Rule out STDs with a Gram stain of vaginal discharge and *Chlamydia* antigen tests. Rule out UTI with a clean-catch urine culture and UA. See Table 2.12–4 for findings and treatment.

Complications

Increased risk of PID (with bacterial vaginosis) and preterm labor or rupture of membranes (if infection occurs during pregnancy).

UCV *OB.1,30,31*

	Bacterial Vaginosis (usually polymicrobial)	***Trichomonas***	**Yeast (usually *Candida*)**
Relative frequency	50%.	25% (may coexist with bacterial vaginitis).	25%.
Main symptom	Stale odor.	Discharge.	Pruritus.
Exam	Mild vulvar irritation.	Strawberry petechiae in upper vagina/cervix.	Erythematous, excoriated vulva/vagina.
Discharge	Homogenous, **grayish-white, fishy**/stale odor.	Profuse, malodorous, **yellow-green, frothy.**	Thick, white, **cottage-cheese texture.**
Vaginal pH	> 4.5.	> 4.5.	Normal vaginal pH (3.5–4.5).
Saline smear[a]	**Clue cells** (epithelial cells coated with bacteria; see Figure 2.12–4).	**Motile trichomonads** (flagellated organisms just larger than WBCs).	Nothing.
KOH prep	Positive whiff test (fishy smell).	Nothing.	**Pseudohyphae** (see Figure 2.12–4).
Treatment	PO metronidazole.[b]	PO metronidazole.[b] **This is an STD;** treat partner and test for other STDs.	Topical antifungals (e.g., miconazole) or PO fluconazole.

TABLE 2.12–4. Causes of Vaginitis

[a]If there are many WBCs and no organisms on saline smear, suspect *Chlamydia*.
[b]Patients taking metronidazole should not drink alcohol (can lead to disulfiram-like reaction). Not recommended during the first trimester of pregnancy owing to teratogenic effects.

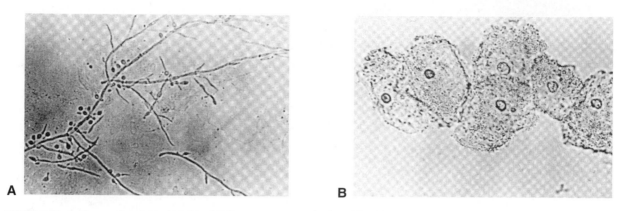

FIGURE 2.12–4. Causes of vaginitis. (A) Candidal vaginitis. Branched and budding *Candida albicans* are evident on KOH preparation of vaginal discharge. (B) *Gardnerella vaginalis.* Saline wet mount of vaginal fluid reveals granulations on vaginal epithelial cells ("clue cells") due to adherence of *G. vaginalis* organisms to the cell surface. (Reproduced, with permission, from DeCherney AH. *Current Obstetric & Gynecologic Diagnosis & Treatment,* 8th ed. Stamford, CT: Appleton & Lange, 1994:692, Figs. 34–2 and 34–4.)

CERVICITIS

Neisseria gonorrhoeae and *Chlamydia trachomatis* are STDs that can infect the cervical glandular epithelium and cause a yellowish-green, mucopurulent discharge. Coinfection is common (50% of patients with gonorrhea also have chlamydia). Diagnose when **cervical motion tenderness (CMT) is present in the absence of other signs of PID** (see below). For a complete discussion, see "Sexually Transmitted Disease," pp. 237–240.

PELVIC INFLAMMATORY DISEASE (PID)

Use of OCPs and barrier contraception decreases the risk of PID.

A variety of acute, subacute, and chronic infections of the ascending genital tract, including the endometrium **(endometritis),** oviducts **(salpingitis),** ovary **(oophoritis),** uterine wall **(myometritis),** and portions of the parietal peritoneum **(peritonitis).** Most cases are bacterial. Risk factors include multiple sexual partners, unprotected or frequent intercourse, young age at first intercourse, mucopurulent cervicitis, prior PID, and IUD use. The incidence of PID decreases with use of OCPs and barrier contraception.

History/PE

A one- to three-day history of **lower abdominal pain** with or without fever, nausea, and vomiting. A **history of recent menses** and an **abnormal cervical/ vaginal discharge** is common. On exam, look for uni- or bilateral lower abdominal, uterine, adnexal, and cervical motion tenderness and/or purulent cervical discharge.

Differential

Ectopic pregnancy, endometriosis, ovarian tumors or hemorrhagic cysts, adnexal torsion, UTI/pyelonephritis, appendicitis, diverticulitis, regional ileitis, ulcerative colitis.

Evaluation

Minimal diagnostic criteria include **lower abdominal, adnexal,** and **cervical motion tenderness** (e.g., chandelier sign). Other supportive data include fever (> 38°C), elevated ESR, elevated CRP, WBC > 10,000, a cervical swab positive for chlamydia or gonorrhea, and pelvic abscess on U/S. **For definitive diagnosis,** use **laparoscopy** (will reveal pus in the peritoneal cavity). Obtain a β-hCG (for pregnancy status). Consider RPR/VDRL, HIV test, and LFTs.

"Chandelier sign": severe CMT on exam that makes the patient "jump for the chandelier."

Treatment

Antibiotics should target common pathogens (e.g., *N. gonorrhoeae, C. trachomatis,* anaerobes).

- **Inpatient IV antibiotic regimen:** Cefoxitin (or cefotetan) and doxycycline **or** clindamycin and gentamicin until the patient is asymptomatic for 48 hours. Follow with doxycycline PO for a total of 14 days.
- **Outpatient antibiotic regimen:** Ceftriaxone plus doxycycline **or** ofloxacin plus clindamycin or metronidazole for 14 days.
- Hospitalize for pelvic/tubo-ovarian abscess (TOA), peritonitis, noncompliance, nausea/emesis preventing PO meds, high fever, or high WBC count. Also hospitalize teenage or nulliparous patients or patients who do not improve after 48–72 hours of outpatient treatment.

Complications

- Suspect **TOA** in patients with severe pain, high fever, nausea/emesis, signs of sepsis, peritoneal signs, or adnexal mass (if exam is even possible). Hospitalize patients for IV antibiotics, hydration, and possible surgical intervention (drainage or TAH-BSO).
- **Ectopic pregnancy,** chronic pelvic pain, **infertility,** Fitz-Hugh–Curtis syndrome (perihepatitis with RUQ pain; occurs in 5–10% of PID patients).

UCV *OB.18*

Toxic Shock Syndrome

Acute illness caused by a **preformed *Staphylococcus aureus* toxin (TSST-1).** Patients have sudden onset of **fever, diffuse sunburn-like rash,** diarrhea, vomiting, sore throat, headache, and/or myalgia that can rapidly progress to **hypotensive shock. Desquamation (especially palms and soles)** occurs within 1–2 weeks. Menses and tampon use are associated in 50% of cases. Hospitalize and support with fluids, pressors, transfusion, and ventilation as needed. Treat infection with IV anti-staph antibiotics (e.g., nafcillin, oxacillin). Steroids can decrease symptom severity.

UCV *OB.27*

VULVAR CANCER

The fourth most common gynecologic malignancy. Usually occurs **after menopause** (peak incidence in the 60s). The vast majority (90%) are **squamous cell carcinoma (SCC).** Risk factors include diabetes, obesity, HTN, vulvar dystrophies, and HPV-16/18 infection *(OB.11)*. May present with **vulvar pruritus (most common),** but early stages are often asymptomatic. On exam, look for an erythematous or ulcerated **vulvar lesion and/or a palpable vulvar mass. Biopsy is necessary for diagnosis.** Staging is surgical and is based on tumor size, invasiveness, nodal involvement, and distant metastases. Treat primary disease with **wide local excision and regional lymph node dissection.** Radiation is used to reduce tumor burden and for metastatic or recurrent disease.

UCV *Ob/Gyn.32*

CERVICAL CANCER

Infection with HPV-16, 18, and 31 increases risk of cervical cancer.

Although incidence and mortality rates have decreased since the introduction of the **screening Pap smear,** cervical cancer remains the third most common gynecologic malignancy. Cervical dysplasia is thought to be the precursor. Risk factors include early onset of sexual activity, multiple sexual partners, immune-compromised status (e.g., HIV), **tobacco use, STDs,** and **HPV (types 16, 18, and 31).**

History/PE

Asymptomatic patients are usually diagnosed by Pap smear, colposcopy, and biopsy. Symptomatic patients may have meno- and/or metrorrhagia, **postcoital bleeding,** pelvic pain, and vaginal discharge. Exam may reveal **cervical discharge/ulceration,** pelvic mass, or fistulas.

Differential

Cervicitis, vaginitis, STDs, actinomycosis.

Evaluation

Biopsy all lesions. Patients with abnormal Pap smears showing dysplasia, squamous intraepithelial neoplasia, or two consecutive findings of atypical squamous cells of undetermined significance (ASCUS) should undergo colposcopy and endocervical curettage (ECC). Cancers are categorized as **invasive cervical carcinoma** (depth > 3 mm, width > 7 mm) or **cervical intraepithelial neoplasia (CIN).** CIN I (mild dysplasia) is also known as low-grade squamous intraepithelial lesion (LSIL). CIN II (moderate) and III (severe) are known as high-grade squamous intraepithelial lesions (HSIL). **Staging is clinical** and based on invasion into adjacent structures and metastases (perform pelvic exam under anesthesia; obtain CXR and IVP). **CT/MRI cannot be used for staging.**

Treatment

- **CIN I:** Most regress spontaneously. Reliable patients can be **observed** (Pap smears and colposcopy every three months for one year).
- **CIN II/III:** Treat with **cryosurgery,** laser, or **LEEP (loop electro-cautery excision procedure). Cold knife conization** of the cervix (performed under anesthesia in the OR) has a higher complication rate and is used for lesions that cannot be fully visualized, discrepancies between high-grade cytology and biopsy, adenocarcinoma in situ, a positive ECC, or microinvasive SCC.
- **Invasive cancer:** Early stages may be treated with **radical hysterectomy and lymph node dissection.** All stages can be treated with **radiation and chemotherapy** or less radical surgeries. Use radiation +/– chemotherapy with bulky tumors or advanced disease to improve survival.

UCV *OB.4*

Uterine Leiomyoma (Fibroids)

The most common **benign** gynecologic lesion. More common in black women and patients > 35 years old. These smooth muscle cell tumors are **hormonally responsive,** often **increase in size with pregnancy,** and usually **regress after menopause.** Malignant transformation to **leiomyosarcoma is very rare** (0.1–0.5%).

History/PE

Usually **asymptomatic,** but may present with **abnormal uterine bleeding,** anemia, pelvic pressure, dysmenorrhea, urinary frequency, pain (due to vascular compromise), or infertility (uncommon). Pelvic exam often reveals a firm, nontender, irregularly enlarged **("lumpy-bumpy")** uterus.

Differential

Carcinoma (cervical, endometrial, or ovarian), pregnancy, endometriosis, or adenomyosis.

If a uterine mass continues to grow after menopause, it is not a leiomyoma.

Evaluation/Treatment

- **U/S** can be used to confirm the diagnosis.
- Definitively diagnosed asymptomatic fibroids can be managed **expectantly** with serial exams and U/S to monitor growth.
- Fibroids that cause severe symptoms or exhibit postmenopausal growth can be managed with **hysterectomy or myomectomy (to preserve fertility).**
- **Medical therapies** (e.g., medroxyprogesterone, danazol, GnRH agonists) are effective for shrinking tumors, but growth usually continues when medications are stopped. They may be useful in perimenopausal women while awaiting decline of endogenous estrogen levels.

UCV *OB.28*

ENDOMETRIAL CANCER

The most common gynecologic malignancy. Strongly associated with exposure to **high levels of unopposed estrogen,** as seen in estrogen replacement therapy, chronic anovulation, early menarche, late menopause, ovarian granulosa cell tumors, obesity, and tamoxifen use. Other risk factors include diabetes, HTN, nulliparity, and a positive family history. Peak onset is between ages 50 and 70. Most tumors are adenocarcinomas. Metastasis occurs through **direct extension** (cervix), **intraperitoneal seeding,** and **lymphatic** (aortic and pelvic nodes) or **hematogenous** (lungs and vagina) spread.

History/PE

Postmenopausal bleeding should never be attributed to atrophic vaginitis until endometrial sampling has ruled out carcinoma.

Common symptoms are **postmenopausal bleeding, menorrhagia, metrorrhagia,** lower abdominal pain, and cramping. The uterus may be fixed and immobile if cancer has spread to the adnexa and peritoneum. Signs of metastatic disease include hepatosplenomegaly, general lymphadenopathy, and abdominal masses.

Differential

Uterine/cervical polyps, fibroids, endometrial hyperplasia, exogenous estrogen use, atrophic vaginitis, hemorrhoids.

Evaluation/Treatment

Grade is a key prognostic factor for endometrial cancer.

- **Pap smear** may detect asymptomatic disease **but is not very sensitive.**
- Use **U/S** to rule out fibroids, polyps, and endometrial hyperplasia.
- **ECC and EMB** show glandular cell hyperplasia and anaplasia with invasion of stroma, myometrium, or blood vessels. Use D&C if sample is inadequate.
- **Surgical staging** based on abdominal exploration, peritoneal washings, TAH-BSO, and selective pelvic/periaortic node sampling is used to determine the extent of spread. **Grade** is a key prognostic factor.
- Adjuvant radiation in patients with cervical/extrauterine spread.
- **Hormone therapy** (high-dose progestins) for stage I disease. **Chemotherapy** (doxorubicin and cisplatin) for advanced and recurrent disease.

UCV *OB.9*

OVARIAN CANCER

The **leading cause of U.S. gynecologic cancer deaths.** Most common in postmenopausal and prepubescent females. Risk factors include **family history** of breast or ovarian cancer and chronic uninterrupted ovulation (e.g., **nulliparity,** delayed childbearing, **infertility,** late menopause). **OCPs have a protective effect** through suppression of ovulation. Primary ovarian tumors are categorized by site of origin and include epithelial cell (e.g., serous cystadenocarcinoma), germ cell (e.g., dysgerminoma), and sex cord-stromal tumors (e.g., functional tumors). Epithelial tumors **(most common)** occur most often in women > 20 years of age.

History/PE

Usually **asymptomatic** until late in the course of disease. Patients may have abdominal pain, bloating, pelvic pressure, urinary frequency, early satiety, constipation, vaginal bleeding, and systemic symptoms (fatigue, malaise, weight loss). Exam findings may include a palpable **solid, fixed, nodular pelvic mass, ascites, and pleural effusion.**

Differential

Uterine leiomyomas (should not enlarge after menopause), ectopic pregnancy, pelvic kidney, retroperitoneal fibrosis/tumor, colorectal cancer, PID, ovarian cyst, metastasis (e.g., Krukenberg tumor), endometriosis.

Evaluation/Treatment

- Evaluate an adnexal mass with **pelvic U/S** and possibly CT or MRI.
- Serum tumor markers (**CA-125,** α-fetoprotein, LDH, and hCG) are used to monitor tumor progression but are **not useful screening tests** owing to low specificity.
- Staging is surgical and includes **TAH-BSO, omentectomy, and tumor debulking.**
- Radiation therapy is effective for dysgerminomas.
- Postsurgical **chemotherapy** (carboplatin and paclitaxel) is used for epithelial cell tumors, which have a high recurrence rate and a **poor prognosis.**

CA-125 levels may be elevated in ovarian cancer.

Dysgerminomas are sensitive to radiation therapy.

Prevention

Women with a strong family history ($\geq$ 2 first-degree relatives) should have annual screening with **CA-125** and **transvaginal U/S.** After childbearing, **prophylactic oophorectomy** may be recommended. OCPs may help decrease risk.

UCV *OB.16*

HIRSUTISM AND VIRILIZATION

Hirsutism (increased male-pattern hair growth on a female) and virilization (male-pattern balding, increased muscle mass, clitoromegaly, deepening voice, and male body habitus) are **clinical manifestations of increased androgens.** Causes in women include congenital adrenal hyperplasia *(Ped.5)*, medications, Cushing's syndrome, PCOS, Sertoli-Leydig cell ovarian tumors, luteoma of pregnancy, and adrenal neoplasms.

POLYCYSTIC OVARIAN SYNDROME

Defined as oligomenorrhea with signs and symptoms of increased circulating androgens. Characterized by bilateral polycystic ovaries (see Figure 2.12–5), chronic anovulation, and infertility. PCOS affects **women aged 15–30** who are often **obese and hirsute.** The cause is unknown, but symptoms are secondary to excess LH and androgen overproduction. **Insulin resistance** and **diabetes** are associated, and endometrial cancer risk is increased as a result of unopposed estrogen.

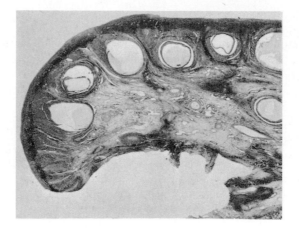

FIGURE 2.12–5. Polycystic ovary with prominent multiple cysts. (Reproduced, with permission, from DeCherney AH. *Current Obstetric & Gynecologic Diagnosis & Treatment,* 8th ed. Stamford, CT: Appleton & Lange, 1994:747, Fig. 37–3.)

History/PE

Patients usually seek treatment for **hirsutism, amenorrhea, or infertility.** Virilization, **obesity,** acne, diabetes, HTN, and acanthosis nigricans may be present. Enlarged cystic ovaries are found on bimanual exam.

Evaluation

Findings include a **serum LH/FSH ratio > 3** and **increased serum androstenedione and DHEA.** U/S shows enlarged ovaries with numerous large subcapsular cysts.

Treatment

PCOS is treated with OCPs.

Weight reduction improves insulin resistance. Infertility usually responds to **clomiphene citrate or metformin. OCPs** (which suppress LH secretion) are used to treat hirsutism, amenorrhea, and acne.

UCV OB.20

INFERTILITY

Endometriosis is the most common cause of female infertility, followed by PID.

Inability of a couple to conceive **after one year** of regular intercourse without contraception. Etiologies include male dysfunction (30–40%) and female dysfunction (60–70%), which includes ovulatory problems (15–20%); peritoneal factors (40%); uterine-tubal factors (30%); and cervical factors (5%). Multiple factors are present in ~20% of cases, and the cause is unknown in 5–20% of cases. Endometriosis is the number one cause of female infertility.

Differential

Ovulatory dysfunction (ovarian failure, prolactinoma), genital tract anomalies/damage (myomas, endometriosis, PID), defects in spermatogenesis, varicoceles (interfere with normal sperm development), endocrine dysfunction (thyroid/adrenal disease, PCOS).

Evaluation

Includes semen analysis (to rule out male factor), serum FSH/LH/TSH/prolactin (to rule out endocrine dysfunction), and hysterosalpingography (to rule out tubal and uterine cavity abnormalities).

Treatment

Treat the underlying cause. Fertility rates in endometriosis may be improved by laparoscopic removal of implants. Ovulation may be induced with clomiphene citrate or Pergonal (purified human FSH and LH), but this can cause ovarian hyperstimulation and multiple gestation. Advanced reproductive technologies (e.g., GIFT, IVF) can be used for refractory cases.

UCV *OB.13*

MENOPAUSE

The permanent cessation of menstruation due to end-organ ovarian resistance to gonadotropins. The median age of onset in U.S. women is 50–52. Premature menopause occurs **before age 40** and is often due to idiopathic premature ovarian failure. Early menopause is associated with **cigarette smoking.** Artificial menopause occurs after removal or irradiation of the ovaries. Postmenopausal women lose the protective effects of estrogen and are at increased risk for **osteoporosis** and **heart disease.**

History/PE

See the mnemonic **HAVOC.** Patients may have menstrual irregularities, **sweating,** sleep disturbances, **mood changes,** decreased libido, dyspareunia (from decreased vaginal wall lubrication), cystocele, urinary frequency/incontinence, and **dysuria.** Exam may reveal vaginal dryness, decreased breast size, and genital tract atrophy.

> **Menopause wreaks HAVOC:**
>
> **H**ot flashes (vasomotor instability)
> **A**trophy of the
> **V**agina
> **O**steoporosis
> **C**oronary artery disease

Evaluation

Elevated serum FSH is suggestive. Diagnosis requires one year without menses.

Treatment

- **HRT** can relieve symptoms and help prevent osteoporosis. Contraindications include undiagnosed vaginal bleeding, liver disease, acute vascular thrombosis, and a history of endometrial or breast cancer.
- Use combined progesterone/estrogen if the patient still has her uterus. Estrogen can be used alone in women who have undergone a TAH-BSO.
- Alternatives to HRT include clonidine (for vasomotor instability); topical estrogens (for vaginal atrophy); and calcium, vitamin D, calcitonin, and bisphosphonates (to prevent osteoporosis).

UCV *OB.14*

Defined as nonelective termination of a pregnancy at < **20 weeks' gestational age** (GA). SAB or "miscarriage" occurs in 15–25% of recognized pregnancies and is a **common cause of first-trimester bleeding.** Most first-trimester SABs are caused by fetal factors (e.g., **chromosomal abnormalities**). Most second-trimester SABs are caused by maternal factors (e.g., cervical incompetence, infection, hypercoagulable states). Risk factors include advanced maternal/paternal age, increased gravidity, minority status, and history of prior SAB. See Table 2.12–5 for types of SAB.

History/PE

Ask about history of abortions, infections, and familial genetic abnormalities. On pelvic exam, note vaginal bleeding, passage of tissue (products of conception [POC]), and open or closed cervical os.

Differential

Postcoital bleeding, ectopic pregnancy, vaginal or cervical lesions, extrusion of molar pregnancy.

TABLE 2.12–5. Types of Spontaneous Abortion

Type	Symptoms	PE /Ultrasound	Treatment[a]
Threatened abortion	**Minimal bleeding.** Possible abdominal pain. **No POC expelled.**	**Closed** internal cervical os. **Normal U/S.**	Avoid heavy activity; pelvic and bed rest.
Inevitable abortion	**Profuse bleeding.** Severe **cramping**.	**Open** internal cervical os.	Emergent D&C.
Incomplete abortion	**Some POC expelled.**	**Open** internal cervical os. Retained fetal tissue on U/S.	Emergent D&C.
Complete abortion	Minimal bleeding/cramping. **All POC expelled.**	**Closed** internal cervical os. Empty uterus on U/S.	
Missed abortion	No uterine bleeding. **No POC expelled.**	**Closed** internal cervical os. **No fetal cardiac activity.** Retained fetal tissue on U/S.	Evacuate uterus; D&C.
Septic abortion	Fever/chills, peritoneal signs. Often recent history of therapeutic abortion (maternal mortality 10–50%).	Hypotension, hypothermia, oliguria, respiratory distress if in shock. Elevated WBC count.	Evacuate uterus, D&C, and IV antibiotics.
Intrauterine fetal demise	Mother may report absence of fetal movements.	Uterus small for GA. No fetal heart tones or movement on U/S.	Induce labor and evacuate uterus to avoid DIC.

[a]All patients should receive RhoGAM if appropriate.

Evaluation/Treatment

Ensure hemodynamic stability if there has been significant bleeding. Check β-hCG (qualitative/quantitative) to confirm pregnancy, establish GA, or check for remaining tissue after completed abortion. Use transvaginal U/S to assess fetal viability. Check CBC, blood type, and antibody screen and **give RhoGAM if appropriate.** Typical management includes **uterine evacuation** and prevention of infection.

UCV OB.33

Give RhoGAM to an Rh-negative woman after an SAB.

URINARY INCONTINENCE

Involuntary loss of urine is a problem that affects nearly 50% of all women occasionally and 20% of older women on a regular basis. Risk factors include **older age** and **pelvic relaxation,** which can be caused by **obstructed labor, traumatic delivery, menopause** (hormonal changes cause decreased tissue resiliency), chronic cough, straining, ascites, and large pelvic tumors. See Table 2.12–6 for types of urinary incontinence.

TABLE 2.12–6. Urinary Incontinence

	Stress Incontinence	Urge Incontinence
History/PE	Urine loss **(small amounts)** with exertion or straining (coughing, laughing). **No symptoms when supine or asleep.** Exam may show cystocele or urethrocele (OB.29)	Unpredictable urine loss **(large volumes).** Day and nighttime urgency/frequency. Exam often normal.
Mechanism	Change in urethrovesical angle causes intra-abdominal pressure increases to be transmitted to bladder more than urethra.	Involuntary, uninhibited detrusor muscle contractions.
Risk factors	Pelvic relaxation, chronically increased intra-abdominal pressure, weakened urethral closing mechanisms (e.g., estrogen deficiency, medications).	UTIs, bladder stones, bladder cancer, neurologic disease (e.g., Alzheimer's, Parkinson's), diabetes.
Diagnosis	Normal UA/urine culture, neurologic exam, and cystometrogram. Demonstrable leakage with stress. Positive "Q-tip test" (angle of cotton swab shows > 30° change when patient strains).	Cystometrogram reveals involuntary bladder contractions associated with urinary leakage, normal residual volume and sensation.
Treatment	Pelvic (Kegel) exercises, estrogen, pessaries, and/or surgery.	Anticholinergics (e.g., oxybutynin), β-adrenergics (e.g., metaproterenol), behavior modification, and/or surgical denervation.

The following clinical questions and accompanying answers are reproduced, with permission, from Evans MI, *PreTest: Ob/Gyn*, 9th ed., New York: McGraw-Hill, 2001.

Questions

1. A 62-year-old woman presents for annual examination. Her last spontaneous menstrual period was nine years ago, and she has been reluctant to use postmenopausal hormone replacement because of a strong family history of breast cancer. She now complains of diminished interest in sexual activity. Which of the following is the most likely cause of her complaint?
   a. Decreased vaginal length
   b. Decreased ovarian function
   c. Alienation from her partner
   d. Untreatable sexual dysfunction
   e. Physiologic anorgasmia

2. Which of the following contraceptives appear to increase the risk for development of pelvic inflammatory disease?
   a. Condoms without spermicide
   b. Oral contraceptives
   c. Intrauterine device
   d. Diaphragm
   e. Vasectomy

3. A patient is diagnosed with carcinoma of the breast. The most important prognostic factor in the treatment of this disease is
   a. Age at diagnosis
   b. Size of tumor
   c. Axillary metastases
   d. Estrogen receptors on the tumor
   e. Progesterone receptors on the tumor

4. Women who have ovarian carcinoma most commonly present with which of the following symptoms?
   a. Vaginal bleeding and anorexia
   b. Weight loss and dyspareunia
   c. Nausea and vaginal discharge
   d. Constipation and frequent urination
   e. Abdominal distention and pain

5. Women who have endometrial carcinoma most frequently present with which of the following symptoms?
   a. Bloating
   b. Weight loss
   c. Postmenopausal bleeding
   d. Vaginal discharge
   e. Hemoptysis

Answers

1. **The answer is b.** Sexuality continues despite aging. However, there are physiologic changes that must be recognized. Diminished ovarian function may lower libido, but estrogen replacement therapy (ERT) may help. Sexual dysfunction can be physiologic, e.g., from lowered libido. As with younger patients, however, lowered libido is in most cases treatable. Because aging does not alter the capacity for orgasm or produce vaginismus, a further evaluation should be initiated if these symptoms persist after a postmenopausal woman is placed on ERT.

2. **The answer is c.** Acute salpingitis, or pelvic inflammatory disease (PID), is a disease predominantly of nulliparous young women. The intrauterine device (IUD) increases the risk of developing salpingitis three- to fivefold; the number of sexual partners and the incidence of sexually transmitted disease in a population also influence the development of PID in IUD users. Oral contraceptives are felt to have a protective effect on developing infections; the risk is 30–90% that of nonusers. Condoms, diaphragms, and chemical barriers also provide protection from disease. Vasectomy does not appear to influence the risk for development of PID.

3. **The answer is c.** Recognition of the high risk associated with axillary metastases for early death and poor five-year survival have led to the use of postsurgical adjuvant chemotherapy in these patients. Patients who have estrogen- or progesterone-receptive tumors (i.e., receptor present or receptor positive) are particular candidates for this adjuvant therapy, as 60% of estrogen-positive tumors will respond to hormonal therapy. Age and size of the tumor are certainly factors of importance, but they are secondary in importance to the presence or absence of axillary metastases.

4. **The answer is e.** Approximately 50% of women who have ovarian cancer present with abdominal distention, and 50% present with abdominal pain. Gastrointestinal symptoms, which occur in about 20% of affected women, are often secondary to the development of ascites or partial bowel obstruction from the tumor. Urinary tract symptoms, caused by the pressure exerted by a rapidly growing mass, and abnormal vaginal bleeding are the initial symptoms of ovarian cancer in only 15% of affected women.

5. **The answer is c.** Postmenopausal bleeding is the most common presenting symptom of women who have endometrial carcinoma. Because this warning signal is present even in the earliest stages of disease, early diagnosis and treatment are possible and likely.

HIGH-YIELD FACTS

Gynecology

Pediatrics

Autosomal trisomies

Down syndrome (trisomy 21), 1:700	Most common chromosomal disorder and cause of congenital mental retardation. Findings: mental retardation, flat facial profile, prominent epicanthal folds, simian crease, duodenal atresia, congenital heart disease (most common malformation is septum primum–type ASD due to endocardial cushion defects), Alzheimer's disease in affected individuals > 35 years old, ↑ risk of ALL. 95% of cases due to meiotic nondisjunction of homologous chromosomes; associated with advanced maternal age (from 1:1500 in women < 20 to 1:25 in women > 45). 4% of cases due to robertsonian translocation, and 1% of cases due to Down mosaicism (no maternal association).	**Drinking** age (21). ↓ levels of AFP.
Edwards' syndrome (trisomy 18), 1:8000	Findings: severe mental retardation, rocker bottom feet, low-set ears, micrognathia, congenital heart disease, clenched hands (flexion of fingers), prominent occiput. Death usually occurs within 1 year of birth.	**Election** age (18).
Patau's syndrome (trisomy 13), 1:6000	Findings: severe mental retardation, microphthalmia, microcephaly, cleft lip/palate, abnormal forebrain structures, polydactyly, congenital heart disease. Death usually occurs within 1 year of birth.	**Puberty** (13).

Genetic gender disorders

Klinefelter's syndrome [male] (XXY), 1:850	Testicular atrophy, eunuchoid body shape, tall, long extremities, gynecomastia, female hair distribution. Presence of inactivated X chromosome (Barr body).	One of the most common causes of hypogonadism in males.
Turner's syndrome [female] **(XO)**, 1:3000	Short stature, ovarian dysgenesis, webbing of neck, coarctation of the aorta, most common cause of primary amenorrhea. No Barr body.	"Hugs and kisses" **(XO)** from Tina **Turner** (female).
Double Y males [male] (XYY), 1:1000	Phenotypically normal, very tall, severe acne, antisocial behavior (seen in 1–2% of XYY males).	Observed with ↑ frequency among inmates of penal institutions.

Phenylketonuria

	Normally, phenylalanine is converted into tyrosine (nonessential aa). In PKU, there is ↓ phenylalanine hydroxylase or ↓ tetrahydrobiopterin cofactor. Tyrosine becomes essential and phenylalanine builds up, leading to excess phenylketones.	Screened for at birth. Phenylketones—phenylacetate, phenyllactate, and phenylpyruvate in urine.
	Findings: mental retardation, fair skin, eczema, musty body odor.	
	Treatment: ↓ phenylalanine (contained in Nutrasweet) and ↑ tyrosine in diet.	

Lysosomal storage diseases	Each is caused by a deficiency in one of the many lysosomal enzymes.	
Fabry's disease	Caused by deficiency of α-galactosidase A, resulting in accumulation of ceramide trihexoside. Finding: renal failure.	X-linked recessive.
Krabbe's disease	Absence of galactosylceramide β-galactosidase leads to the accumulation of galactocerebroside in the brain. Optic atrophy, spasticity, early death. *Bio.61*	Autosomal recessive.
Gaucher's disease	Caused by deficiency of β-glucocerebrosidase, leading to glucocerebroside accumulation in brain, liver, spleen, and bone marrow (Gaucher's cells with characteristic "crinkled paper" enlarged cytoplasm). Type I, the more common form, is compatible with a normal life span.	Autosomal recessive.
Niemann-Pick disease	Deficiency of sphingomyelinase causes buildup of **sphingo**myelin and cholesterol in reticuloendothelial and parenchymal cells and tissues. Patients die by age 3.	Autosomal recessive. No **man PICK**s (Niemann-**PICK**) his nose with his **sphing**er.
Tay-Sachs disease	Absence of hexosaminidase A results in GM$_2$ ganglioside accumulation. Death occurs by age 3. Cherry-red spot visible on macula. Carrier rate is 1 in 30 in Jews of European descent (1 in 300 for others).	Autosomal recessive. **Tay-saX** lacks he**X**osaminidase.
Metachromatic leukodystrophy	Deficiency of arylsulfatase A results in the accumulation of sulfatide in the brain, kidney, liver, and peripheral nerves.	Autosomal recessive.
Hurler's syndrome	Deficiency of α-L-iduronidase results in corneal clouding and mental retardation.	Autosomal recessive.
Hunter's syndrome	Deficiency of iduronate sulfatase. Mild form of Hurler's with no corneal clouding and mild mental retardation.	**X**-linked recessive. Hunters aim for the **X**.

Fragile X syndrome	X-linked defect affecting the methylation and expression of the *FMR1* gene. The 2nd most common cause of genetic mental retardation (the most common cause is Down syndrome). Associated with macro-orchidism (enlarged testes), long face with a large jaw, large everted ears, and autism.	Triplet repeat disorder (CGG$_n$) that may show genetic anticipation. Fragile **X** = e**X**tra large testes, jaw, ears.

373

Red flags are raised if the caretaker's story does not match the child's injury.

Includes neglect and physical, sexual, and emotional abuse. Suspect abuse if the **history is discordant with physical findings** and there is a **delay in obtaining appropriate medical care.**

History/PE

Pain, swelling, and bruises. Infants may have apnea, seizures, or failure to thrive (FTT). Neglect may result in poor hygiene and behavioral abnormalities. Exam findings include:

Spiral fractures suggest child abuse.

- **Cutaneous:** Oddly situated (e.g., face, thighs) **ecchymoses of varying ages** or **patterned injuries** (e.g., immersion burns, cigarette burns, belt marks).
- **Skeletal: Spiral fractures** of the humerus and femur in children < 3 years of age suggest abuse until proven otherwise; **epiphyseal/metaphyseal injuries** can occur in infants from pulling or twisting of the limbs. Look for **rib injuries** in children < 2 years of age.
- **Sexual abuse:** STDs or genital trauma.

Differential/Evaluation

Rule out conditions that mimic abuse, such as bleeding disorders, mongolian spots (bruises), osteogenesis imperfecta (fractures), bullous impetigo (blisters may mimic cigarette burns), and "coining" (alternative therapy used in certain cultures). **Skeletal survey and bone scan can show fractures in various stages of healing.** Test for gonorrhea, chlamydia, and HIV if sexual abuse is suspected. To rule out shaken baby syndrome, perform an ophthalmologic exam for **retinal hemorrhages** (see Clinical Images), CT for **bilateral subdural hemorrhages,** and MRI for white matter changes.

Treatment

Document injuries. Notify child protective services for evaluation and possible removal from the home. Hospitalize if necessary to stabilize injuries or to protect the child.

UCV *Ped.53*

Left-to-right shunts—

The 3 D's:
VS**D**
AS**D**
P**D**A

Generally classified by the presence or absence of cyanosis. Cyanotic conditions have right-to-left shunts, in which deoxygenated blood is shunted into systemic circulation. Noncyanotic conditions have left-to-right shunts, in which oxygenated blood from the lungs is shunted back into pulmonary circulation. Intrauterine risk factors include maternal alcohol and drug use, exogenous hormones (e.g., OCPs), lithium, and congenital infection.

ATRIAL SEPTAL DEFECT (ASD)

An opening in the atrial septum allows blood to flow between the atria. **Left-to-right shunting** occurs as a result of lower right-sided pressures, and **blood flow to the lungs is increased.**

History/PE

Usually presents in late childhood or early adulthood. Symptom onset and severity depend on the size of the defect. Large defects can lead to CHF, which may cause cyanosis. Other symptoms include easy fatigability, frequent respiratory infections, and FTT. Exam reveals an RV heave, wide and **fixed, split S2,** and systolic ejection murmur (SEM) at the upper left sternal border (from increased flow across the pulmonary valve).

ASD has a fixed, split S2.

Evaluation

Echocardiogram with color flow Doppler shows blood flow between the atria (diagnostic), paradoxic ventricular wall motion, and a dilated RV. ECG shows **right-axis deviation;** CXR shows cardiomegaly and **increased pulmonary vascular markings.**

Treatment

- Small defects may close spontaneously and do not require treatment.
- **Antibiotic prophylaxis** before dental procedures is required for ostium primum defects to prevent bacterial endocarditis.
- Perform surgical closure in infants with CHF and patients with > 2:1 ratio of pulmonary to systemic blood flow. Early correction improves prognosis by preventing complications such as **arrhythmias,** RV dysfunction, and **Eisenmenger's syndrome** (left-to-right shunt causes pulmonary vascular hyperplasia, irreversible pulmonary HTN, and shunt reversal).

Eisenmenger's syndrome: left-to-right shunt causes pulmonary HTN and shunt reversal.

UCV *Surg.1*

VENTRICULAR SEPTAL DEFECT (VSD)

A "hole" in the ventricular septum allows blood to flow between ventricles. Symptoms depend on the degree of **left-to-right** shunting. VSDs are the **most common congenital heart defect** and are more common in patients with Apert's syndrome (cranial deformities with fusion of fingers and toes), Down syndrome, cri-du-chat syndrome, and trisomies 13 and 18.

VSD is the most common congenital heart defect.

History/PE

Small defects are usually **asymptomatic** at birth. Large defects can present with frequent respiratory infections, FTT, and CHF. Exam reveals a **pansystolic murmur at the lower left sternal border** and a **loud pulmonic S2.** In severe defects, systolic thrill, cardiomegaly, and crackles may be present.

Evaluation

Echocardiogram is diagnostic. ECG may show RVH or LVH but is normal with small VSDs.

Treatment

- Treat existing CHF (with diuretics and inotropes) and respiratory infections.
- Most small VSDs will close spontaneously.
- Large VSDs (or VSDs in Down syndrome patients) require early surgical repair to prevent complications (e.g., Eisenmenger's syndrome).
- Endocarditis and septic emboli prophylaxis (e.g., amoxicillin) before dental or pulmonary procedures.

UCV *Ped.3*

PATENT DUCTUS ARTERIOSUS (PDA)

Failure of the ductus arteriosus to close in the first few days of life results in a **left-to-right shunt** from the aorta to the pulmonary artery. Risk factors include high altitude (low O_2 tension) and maternal first-trimester **rubella** infection. More common in **premature infants** and **females.**

History/PE

Typically asymptomatic, but may present with slowed growth, recurrent lower respiratory tract infections, lower extremity clubbing, and symptoms of CHF. Exam reveals a **wide pulse pressure, continuous "machinery murmur"** at the second left intercostal space at the sternal border, **loud S2,** and **bounding peripheral pulses.**

Evaluation

With larger PDAs, echocardiography shows LA and LV enlargement; ECG may show LVH, and CXR may show cardiomegaly. Small PDAs often have no signs of cardiomegaly. A color flow Doppler demonstrating blood flow from the aorta into the pulmonary artery is diagnostic.

Treatment

- Give **indomethacin** unless the PDA is needed for survival (e.g., transposition of the great vessels).
- If indomethacin fails or the child is > 6–8 months old, surgical closure is preferred.

UCV *Peds.1*

COARCTATION OF THE AORTA

Coarctation is a cause of secondary HTN.

Constriction of a portion of the aorta leads to increased flow above and decreased flow below the coarctation. More common in males. **Turner's syndrome** is a risk factor. One-fourth of patients have a bicuspid aortic valve.

History/PE

Often presents in childhood with **asymptomatic HTN.** Dyspnea on exertion, syncope, claudication, epistaxis, and headache may be present. On exam, **sys-**

tolic BP is higher in the upper extremities and may be **greater in the right arm.** Femoral pulses are weak or delayed, a late systolic murmur is heard in the left axilla, and apical impulse is forceful. Advanced cases may have **lower extremity wasting** from decreased blood flow.

In advanced cases of coarctation, patients may have a well-developed upper body and lower-extremity wasting.

Differential

Primary HTN, pheochromocytoma, aortic stenosis, renal artery stenosis, renal disease, Cushing's syndrome, hyperaldosteronism.

Evaluation

Perform ECG (showing LVH), echocardiography, and color flow Doppler. Cardiac catheterization (aortography) is diagnostic. CXR may reveal a **"reverse 3" sign** due to pre- and post-dilatation of the coarct segment and **"rib notching"** due to collateral circulation through intercostal arteries.

Treatment

- **Surgical correction** or **balloon angioplasty** (controversial).
- Continue **endocarditis prophylaxis** even after treatment.

UCV *Surg.2*

TRANSPOSITION OF THE GREAT VESSELS

A condition in which pulmonary and systemic circulations exist in **parallel.** The aorta is connected to the RV and the pulmonary artery to the LV. Without a septal defect or a PDA, it is incompatible with life. Risk factors include Apert's syndrome, Down syndrome, cri-du-chat syndrome, and trisomies 13 and 18.

> **Right-to-left shunts—**
>
> **The 5 T's:**
> **T**etralogy
> **T**ransposition
> **T**runcus arteriosus
> **T**ricuspid atresia
> **T**otal anomalous pulmonary venous return

History/PE

Critical illness and cyanosis typically occur immediately after birth. Exam reveals tachypnea and progressive respiratory failure. Some have signs of CHF.

Evaluation

Echocardiography. CXR may show narrow heart base and absence of main pulmonary artery segment (**"egg-shaped silhouette"**).

In transposition of the great vessels, a PDA or septal defect is required for mixing of pulmonary and systemic blood flow.

Treatment

- Keep the PDA open with **prostaglandin E$_1$ (PGE$_1$).**
- **Balloon atrial septostomy** if immediate surgery is not feasible.
- **Surgical correction** (arterial or atrial switch)

TETRALOGY OF FALLOT

Consists of VSD, RV outflow obstruction, RVH, and overriding aorta. Early cyanosis results from right-to-left shunting across the VSD. Risk factors include Down syndrome, cri-du-chat syndrome, and trisomies 13 and 18.

> **Tetralogy of Fallot—**
>
> **PROVe**
> **P**ulmonary stenosis
> **R**VH
> **O**verriding aorta
> **V**SD

History/PE

Presents during infancy with **cyanosis, dyspnea,** and fatigability. Children often **squat for relief** during hypoxemic episodes (**"tet spells"**). Hypoxemia may cause FTT or mental status changes. Exam reveals an **SEM** at the left sternal border (due to RV outflow obstruction), **RV lift,** single S2, and possibly signs of CHF.

Evaluation

Echocardiography and catheterization. CXR shows a **"boot-shaped" heart** with decreased pulmonary vascular markings. ECG shows right-axis deviation and RVH.

Treatment

- Administer PGE_1 to keep the PDA open.
- Treat cyanotic spells with O_2, propranolol, knee-chest position, fluids, and morphine.
- Temporary palliation can be achieved through creation of an artificial shunt (e.g., balloon atrial septostomy) before surgical correction.

UCV *Surg.3*

DEVELOPMENT

CHILDHOOD VACCINATIONS

Table 2.13–1 summarizes the recommended childhood immunizations. **Contraindications** to vaccination are as follows:

- Current moderate to severe illness (with or without fever).
- Severe allergy to a vaccine component or prior dose of vaccine.
- Encephalopathy within seven days of prior pertussis vaccination.
- Anaphylactic egg allergy for influenza vaccine (do prior skin testing).
- Recent administration of antibody-containing blood products (for live injected vaccines).
- Avoid live vaccines (OPV, varicella, MMR) in immune-compromised and pregnant patients (exception: HIV patients without immune compromise may receive MMR and varicella).

The following are **not contraindications** to vaccination:

- Mild illness and/or low-grade fever; current antibiotic therapy; prematurity.

Precautions to vaccination include the following:

- Progressive neurologic disorders.
- Prior reactions to pertussis vaccine (i.e., fever > 40.5°C, shocklike state, persistent crying for > 3 hours within 48 hours of vaccination, or seizure within three days of vaccination).

TABLE 2.13–1. Immunization Schedule

Vaccine[a-c]	Birth	2 Months	4 Months	6 Months	12–15 Months	15–18 Months	2 Years	4–6 Years
HBV	x	x		x				
DTaP		x	x	x		x		x
Hib		x	x	x	x			
IPV		x	x	x				x
PPV		x	x	x	x			
MMR					x			x
Varicella					x			
HAV							x	

[a]Influenza vaccine is indicated in patients > 6 months old with asthma *(Ped.54)*, CF *(Ped.11.)*, diabetes, HIV, bronchopulmonary dysplasia, sickle cell disease *(Ped.21)*, and chronic heart disease.
[b]HAV vaccine is recommended at age two in certain regions and high-risk groups.
[c]PPV is recommended for all children aged 2–23 months and certain children > 24 months, but fewer doses are needed.

DEVELOPMENTAL MILESTONES

Table 2.13–2 highlights major developmental milestones.

FAILURE TO THRIVE

Defined as persistent weight below the third to fifth percentile for age or falling off the growth curve (i.e., crossing two major percentile lines on a growth chart). Identified as **organic** when an underlying medical condition is present and **nonorganic (most cases)** when psychosocial factors are thought to be the cause. Risk factors include chronic illness, poverty, low maternal age, chaotic environment, genetic disease (e.g., CF), inborn errors of metabolism, and HIV.

History/PE

Patients are of **low weight for age and height** with minimal weight gain or weight loss. Plot height, weight, and head circumference on a growth chart and compare to population norms. Look for signs of systemic disease. Take a diet history and observe caregiver-child interaction.

Differential

Often no organic cause is found. The vast differential includes inadequate or improper feeding; mechanical GI dysfunction; structural abnormalities (e.g., pyloric stenosis); infection; and endocrine, cardiac, pulmonary, or neurologic diseases.

TABLE 2.13–2. Developmental Milestones

Age	Gross Motor	Fine Motor	Language	Social/Cognitive
2 months	Lifts head/chest when prone	Tracks past midline	Alerts to sound, coos	Recognizes parent, social smile
4–5 months	Rolls front to back, back to front (5 mos)	Grasps rattle	Orients to voice, "ah-goo," razzes	Enjoys looking around, laughs
6 months	**Sits unassisted**	**Transfers objects,** raking grasp	Babbles	**Stranger anxiety**
9–10 months	Crawls, pulls to stand	Uses three-finger pincer grasp	Says mama/dada (nonspecific)	Waves bye-bye, plays pat-a-cake
12 months	Cruises (11 mos), walks alone	Uses two-finger pincer grasp	Says mama/dada (specific)	Imitates actions
15 months	Walks backward	Uses cup	Uses 4–6 words	Temper tantrums
18 months	Runs, kicks a ball	Builds tower of 2–4 cubes	Names common objects	Copies parent in tasks (e.g., sweeping)
2 years	Walks up/down steps with help, jumps	Builds tower of six cubes	Uses **two-word** phrases	Follows **two-step** commands, removes clothes
3 years	Rides **tricycle,** climbs stairs with alternating feet (3–4 years)	Copies a circle, uses utensils	Uses **three-word** sentences	Brushes teeth with help, washes/dries hands
4 years	Hops	Copies a cross	Counts to ten	Cooperative play

Evaluation/Treatment

Start a calorie count. Tests include CBC, electrolytes, Cr, albumin, and total protein. Consider a sweat chloride test (for CF), UA/culture, stool culture/ova and parasites, and assessment of bone age. Treatment will depend on the cause. **Supplement nutrition** if breast-feeding is inadequate. **Hospitalize** if there is neglect or severe malnourishment.

GASTROENTEROLOGY

INTUSSUSCEPTION

One portion of the bowel telescopes into an adjacent segment, usually proximal to the ileocecal valve (see Figure 2.13–1). The **most common cause of bowel obstruction in the first two years of life.** Affects more males than females. The cause is often unknown, but risk factors include Meckel's diverticulum, intestinal lymphoma (> 6 years of age), **Henoch-Schönlein purpura,** parasites, polyps, adenovirus or rotavirus infection, celiac disease, and CF.

History/PE

Abrupt-onset colicky abdominal pain in apparently healthy children, often with drawing up of the legs and vomiting. Young infants may have pallor and sweating. Advanced signs include bloody mucus in stools (**red "currant jelly" stool),** lethargy, and fever. On exam, look for abdominal tenderness, positive stool guaiac, and a palpable **"sausage-shaped" RUQ abdominal mass.**

Differential

Rule out above risk factors, constipation, and meconium ileus (neonates).

Evaluation/Treatment

- Correct any volume or electrolyte abnormalities and check CBC (for leukocytosis).
- Abdominal plain films and U/S may be helpful.
- **Air contrast barium enema** is diagnostic and often curative. If child is unstable or enema reduction is unsuccessful, perform **surgical reduction** and resection of gangrenous bowel.

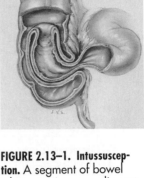

FIGURE 2.13–1. Intussusception. A segment of bowel telescopes into an adjacent segment, causing obstruction. (Reproduced, with permission, from Way L. *Current Surgical Diagnosis & Treatment,* 10th ed. Stamford, CT: Appleton & Lange, 1994:1222, Fig. 46–13.)

PYLORIC STENOSIS

Hypertrophy of the pyloric sphincter causes gastric outlet obstruction. **First-born males** are more often affected. Incidence is 1 in 500 births.

History/PE

Nonbilious emesis progresses to projectile emesis after every feeding in the first two weeks to four months of life. Babies feed well initially but eventually suffer from malnutrition and dehydration. Exam may reveal a palpable **olive-shaped, mobile, nontender epigastric mass** and visible gastric peristaltic waves.

Differential

Hiatal hernia, duodenal atresia ("double-bubble" sign on x-ray), malrotation/volvulus, meconium ileus, GERD, gastroenteritis, pylorospasm, overfeeding.

Evaluation/Treatment

- **Abdominal U/S** showing a hypertrophic pylorus is diagnostic. Barium studies reveal a narrow pyloric channel (**"string sign"**) or a **pyloric beak.**
- Check for **hypochloremic-hypokalemic metabolic alkalosis** due to persistent emesis and correct existing dehydration and acid-base/electrolyte abnormalities. NG tube placement may be necessary.
- **Surgical correction** with **pyloromyotomy** after correction of metabolic abnormalities.

First correct metabolic abnormalities; then perform pyloromyotomy for pyloric stenosis.

IMMUNODEFICIENCY DISORDERS

Congenital immunodeficiencies are rare and often present with **chronic or recurrent infections** (e.g., chronic thrush), unusual or opportunistic organisms, incomplete treatment response, or FTT. Categorization is based on the primary immune system component that is abnormal (see Table 2.13–3):

> **DiGeorge syndrome is a—**
>
> **CATCH-22**
> **C**ongenital heart disease
> **A**bnormal facies
> **T**hymic aplasia
> **C**left palate
> **H**ypocalcemia
> **22**q deletion

- **B-cell deficiencies:** Most common (50%). Typically present **after six months of age** (when transplacentally acquired maternal antibodies decline) with recurrent sinopulmonary, GI, and urinary tract infections with encapsulated organisms (*Haemophilus influenzae, Streptococcus pneumoniae, Neisseria meningitidis*).
- **T-cell deficiencies:** Tend to present earlier (1–3 months) with opportunistic and low-grade fungal, viral, and intracellular bacterial infections (e.g., mycobacteria). May have secondary B-cell dysfunction.
- **Phagocyte deficiencies:** Characterized by **mucous membrane infections, abscesses,** and **poor wound healing.** Catalase-positive (e.g., *Staphylococcus aureus*) and gram-negative enteric organisms are common. Delayed umbilical cord separation may be an early sign.
- **Complement deficiencies:** Characterized by recurrent bacterial infections with encapsulated organisms.

KAWASAKI DISEASE

Multisystem acute vasculitis mainly affecting young children (80% are < 5 years of age), particularly those of Asian ancestry. Acute phase manifestations include:

> **Kawasaki disease symptoms—**
>
> **"CRASH and burn"**
> **C**onjunctivitis
> **R**ash
> **A**denopathy
> **S**trawberry tongue
> **H**ands and feet (red, swollen, flaky skin)
> **AND**
> **Burn** = fever > 40°C for ≥ 5 days

- Fever (usually > 40°C) for at least five days.
- Bilateral nonexudative painless conjunctivitis.
- Polymorphous rash (primarily truncal).
- Cervical lymphadenopathy (often unilateral, at least one node ≥ 1 cm).
- Diffuse mucous membrane erythema (e.g., strawberry tongue).
- Erythema of palms and soles; indurative edema of hands and feet; and late desquamation of fingertips.
- Fever plus ≥ 4 of the remaining criteria are required for diagnosis.

The subacute phase is characterized by **thrombocytosis and increased ESR.** During convalescence, untreated patients are at risk for **coronary artery aneurysms** (40%) and MI. Prognosis is tied to the severity of cardiac involvement. **Acute-phase treatment** includes **high-dose aspirin** (for inflammation and fever) and **IVIG** (to prevent aneurysms). **Corticosteroids** may increase aneurysm formation and are currently **contraindicated.**

INFECTIOUS DISEASE

BRONCHIOLITIS

Acute inflammatory illness of the small airways that **primarily affects infants and children < 2 years of age. RSV is the most common cause.** Progression to

TABLE 2.13–3. Pediatric Immunodeficiency Disorders

Disorder	Description	Diagnosis/Treatment
B-cell		
X-linked (Bruton's) agammaglob-ulinemia *(Ped.36)*	Profound **B**-cell deficiency in **B**oys only. May present at < 6 months of age. At risk for life-threatening *Pseudomonas* infections.	Diagnose with **quantitative Ig levels** (subclasses) and specific Ab responses. Treat with prophylactic antibiotics and IVIG.
Common variable immunodeficiency	Ig levels drop in the second to third decade of life. Increased risk of lymphoma and autoimmune disease.	
IgA deficiency	Most common immunodeficiency. Usually asymptomatic, but recurrent infections may occur.	
T-cell		
Thymic aplasia (DiGeorge syndrome)	See the mnemonic **CATCH-22.** Presents with **tetany** (due to hypocalcemia) in the first days of life.	Diagnose with absolute lymphocyte count, mitogen stimulation response, and delayed hypersensitivity skin testing.
Ataxia-telangiectasia	Oculocutaneous telangiectasias and progressive cerebellar ataxia. This is a DNA repair defect.	Treat with **bone marrow transplant (BMT)** for severe disease and **IVIG** for Ab deficiency. Can do thymus transplant instead of BMT for DiGeorge. No therapy to limit progression of ataxia-telangiectasia.
Combined		
Severe combined immunodeficiency (SCID) *Ped.37*	Severe lack of B and T cells. Patients present with frequent, severe bacterial infections, chronic candidiasis, and opportunistic organisms.	Treat SCID with **BMT** or **stem cell** transplant and IVIG for Ab deficiency. *Pneumocystis carinii* **pneumonia (PCP) prophylaxis** until **BMT.** Gene therapy may be a future option.
Wiskott-Aldrich syndrome *Ped.23*	X-linked disorder with less severe B- and T-cell dysfunction. Patients have **eczema,** elevated IgE and IgA, decreased IgM, and **thrombocytopenia.**	Treatment for Wiskott-Aldrich is supportive (IVIG and aggressive antibiotic treatment of infection). Patients rarely survive to adulthood.
Phagocytic		
Chronic granulo-matous disease (CGD)	X-linked or autosomal-recessive disorder with deficient superoxide production by PMNs and macrophages. Results in chronic pulmonary, GI, and urinary tract infections, osteomyelitis, and hepatitis. Anemia, lymphadenopathy, and hypergammaglobulinemia may be present.	Diagnose with absolute neutrophil count and adhesion, chemotaxic, phagocytic, and bactericidal assays. **Nitroblue tetrazolium test is diagnostic for CGD.** Treat with **daily trimethoprim-sulfamethoxazole (TMP-SMX).** Judicious antibiotic use during infections. γ-interferon therapy can reduce the incidence of serious infection.
Chédiak-Higashi syndrome	Autosomal-recessive disorder causing a defect in neutrophil chemotaxis. Syndrome includes oculocutaneous albinism, neuropathy, and neutropenia.	

TABLE 2.13–3. Pediatric Immunodeficiency Disorders (continued)

Disorder	Description	Diagnosis/Treatment
Complement		
C1 esterase deficiency (hereditary angioneurotic edema)	Autosomal-dominant disorder with recurrent episodes of angioedema lasting 2–72 hours and provoked by stress or trauma. Can result in life-threatening airway edema.	Diagnose with **total hemolytic complement (CH_{50});** assess quantity and function of individual classical and alternative pathway components.
Terminal complement deficiency (C5–C9)	Patients are susceptible to recurrent meningococcal or gonococcal infections and, rarely, systemic lupus erythematosus or glomerulonephritis.	**Treat** C1 esterase deficiency with daily prophylactic danazol. Purified C1 esterase and FFP can be used prior to surgery. Treat terminal complement deficiency with meningococcal vaccine and appropriate antibiotics.

respiratory failure is a potentially fatal complication. Risk factors for severe RSV include age < 6 months, prematurity, heart or lung disease, and immunodeficiency.

History/PE

Often presents with low-grade **fever, rhinorrhea, cough,** and **apnea** (in young infants). Exam reveals **tachypnea, wheezing,** crackles, prolonged expiration, and **hyperresonance to percussion.**

Differential

Reactive airway disease, pneumonia, CHF, foreign body aspiration.

Evaluation

The most common cause of bronchiolitis is RSV.

CXR reveals hyperinflation of the lungs, interstitial infiltrates, and atelectasis. **ELISA** of nasal washings for RSV is highly sensitive and specific.

Treatment

- Mild disease: Outpatient management with fluids, nebulizers, and O_2 (if needed).
- Hospitalize for marked respiratory distress, O_2 saturation < 95%, toxic appearance, dehydration/poor oral feeding, history of **prematurity** (< 34 weeks), **age < 3 months,** underlying **cardiopulmonary disease,** or unreliable parents.

- Treat inpatients with contact isolation, hydration, O₂. **Ribavirin** aerosol may shorten symptom course and decrease viral shedding in infants at risk for severe RSV infection.
- **RSV prophylaxis** with injectable poly- or monoclonal antibodies (i.e., **RespiGam or Synagis**) is recommended in winter for high-risk patients.

UCV *Ped.24*

CROUP (LARYNGOTRACHEOBRONCHITIS)

Acute inflammatory disease of the larynx, primarily within the **subglottic** space. Pathogens include parainfluenza virus-1 **(PIV-1) (most common),** PIV-2 and -3, RSV, influenza, rubeola, adenovirus, and *Mycoplasma pneumoniae*.

History/PE

Typically prodromal URI symptoms are followed by low-grade fever, mild dyspnea, inspiratory stridor that worsens with agitation, hoarse voice, and a characteristic **barking cough** (usually at night).

Differential

See Table 2.13–4. Also foreign body aspiration, angioedema, and retropharyngeal abscess.

TABLE 2.13–4. Characteristics of Croup, Epiglottitis, and Tracheitis

	Croup	Epiglottitis	Tracheitis
Age group	3 months to 3 years	3–7 years	3 months to 2 years
Incidence in children presenting with stridor	88%	8%	2%
Pathogen	PIV	*H. influenzae*	Often *S. aureus*
Onset	Prodrome (1–7 days)	Rapid (4–12 hrs)	Prodrome (3 days) → acute decompensation (10 hrs)
Fever severity	Low grade	High grade	Intermediate grade
Associated symptoms	Barking cough, hoarseness	Muffled voice, drooling	Variable respiratory distress
Position preference	None	Seated, neck extended	None
Response to racemic epinephrine	Stridor improves	None	None
CXR findings	"Steeple sign" on AP film	"Thumbprint sign" on lateral film	Subglottic narrowing

Evaluation

Diagnosis is primarily **clinical.** AP neck film may show subglottic narrowing (**"steeple sign"**; see Figure 2.13–2).

Treatment

- **Mild cases:** Outpatient management with **cool mist therapy** and fluids.
- **Moderate cases:** May require addition of oral **corticosteroids.**
- **Severe cases** (i.e., respiratory distress at rest): Hospitalize and give **nebulized racemic epinephrine.**

UCV *Ped.28*

EPIGLOTTITIS

Epiglottitis may cause life-threatening airway obstruction.

A serious and rapidly progressive infection of **supraglottic structures** (e.g., epiglottis, arytenoids). Prior to immunization, **H. influenzae type B** was the primary pathogen. Common causes now include *Streptococcus* species, nontypable *H. flu,* and viral agents. Incidence has decreased with widespread use of the Hib vaccine.

History/PE

Sudden-onset high **fever** (39–40°C), **dysphagia, drooling, muffled voice,** inspiratory retractions, cyanosis, and **soft stridor.** Patients sit with the neck hyperextended and chin protruding (**"sniffing dog"** position) and lean forward in a **"tripod"** position. Untreated infection can lead to life-threatening airway obstruction and respiratory arrest.

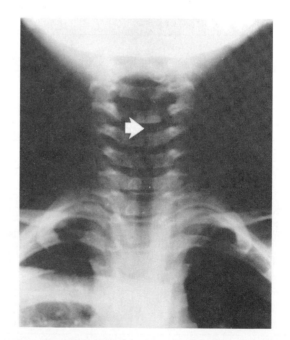

FIGURE 2.13–2. Croup. The x-ray shows marked subglottic narrowing of the airway (arrow). (Reproduced, with permission, from Saunders C. *Current Emergency Diagnosis & Treatment,* 4th ed. Stamford, CT: Appleton & Lange, 1992:448, Fig. 26–9.)

Differential

See Table 2.13–4. Also foreign body aspiration, angioedema, and retropharyngeal abscess.

Evaluation

Diagnosis is primarily clinical. **Do not examine the throat** unless an anesthesiologist is present. Definitive diagnosis is made via direct fiberoptic visualization of cherry-red, swollen epiglottis and arytenoids. Lateral x-ray shows a swollen epiglottis obliterating the valleculae (**"thumbprint sign"**; see Figure 2.13–3).

Throat examination may precipitate laryngospasm and airway obstruction.

Treatment

- This disease is a true emergency. Keep the patient (and parents) calm, call anesthesia, and **transfer the patient to the OR.**
- Treat with **endotracheal intubation or tracheostomy** and **IV antibiotics** (ceftriaxone or cefuroxime).

OTITIS MEDIA (OM)

A middle ear infection commonly caused by **S. pneumoniae, H. flu,** or **Moraxella catarrhalis.** Children are predisposed owing to a shorter, more horizontal eustachian tube. Risk factors include viral URIs, trisomy 21, CF, immunodeficiencies, smoke exposure, day-care attendance, bottle-feeding, cleft palate, and prior OM.

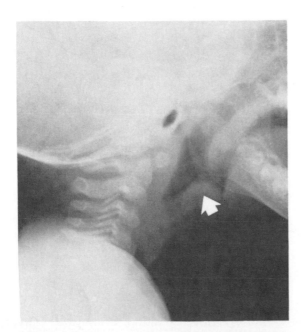

FIGURE 2.13–3. Epiglottitis. The classic swollen epiglottis ("thumbprint sign"; arrow) and obstructed airway are seen on lateral neck x-ray. (Reproduced, with permission, from Saunders C. *Current Emergency Diagnosis & Treatment,* 4th ed. Stamford, CT: Appleton & Lange, 1992: 447, Fig. 26–8B.)

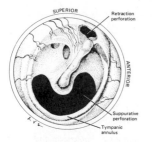

FIGURE 2.13–4. Perforated TM. Common sites of TM perforation. (Reproduced, with permission, from Saunders C. *Current Emergency Diagnosis & Treatment*, 4th ed. Stamford, CT: Appleton & Lange, 1992:433, Fig. 26–2.)

History/PE

Parents may report **fever, ear tugging, hearing loss, irritability,** crying, feeding difficulties, and vomiting. Classic exam findings are **erythema,** opacity, **bulging,** and **decreased mobility** (with insufflation) of the **tympanic membrane** (TM) with **loss of the light reflex and bony landmarks.** The TM may be perforated (see Figure 2.13–4).

Differential

Otitis externa, toothache, trauma, foreign body, ear canal furuncle, hard cerumen.

Evaluation/Treatment

Diagnosis is clinical. Erythema alone is insufficient (it may be caused by vigorous crying). Treat with **amoxicillin for ten days.** Patients with treatment failure (i.e., persistent ear pain, fever, or bulging TM) after three days can be switched to amoxicillin–clavulanic acid, ceftriaxone, or cefuroxime.

Complications

Mastoiditis, meningitis, hearing loss, cholesteatoma, tympanosclerosis, chronic suppurative OM.

VIRAL EXANTHEMS

Table 2.13–5 discusses common viral exanthems.

NEONATOLOGY

APGAR SCORING

A rapid scoring system that helps evaluate the need for neonatal resuscitation. Each of five parameters (see the mnemonic **APGAR**) is assigned a score of 0–2 at one and five minutes after birth. Scores of 8–10 typically reflect good cardiopulmonary adaptation. Scores of 4–7 indicate the possible need for resuscitation—infants should be observed, stimulated, and possibly given ventilatory support. Scores of 0–3 indicate the need for immediate resuscitation.

CONGENITAL MALFORMATIONS

Table 2.13–6 describes selected congenital malformations.

NEONATAL JAUNDICE

Elevated serum bilirubin concentration (> 5 mg/dL) due to increased production (e.g., hemolysis) or decreased excretion. **Conjugated (direct) hyperbilirubinemia is always pathologic. Unconjugated** (indirect) hyperbilirubinemia may be physiologic or pathologic. See Table 2.13–7 for differentiating characteristics. **Kernicterus** is a feared complication of unconjugated hyperbilirubinemia and results from irreversible bilirubin deposition in the basal ganglia, pons,

> **APGAR:**
>
> **A**ppearance (color)
> **P**ulse (heart rate)
> **G**rimace (reflex irritability)
> **A**ctivity (muscle tone)
> **R**espiratory effort

Direct hyperbilirubinemia is always pathologic.

TABLE 2.13–5. Viral Exanthems

Disease	Cause	Characteristics	Complications
Erythema infectiosum (fifth disease)	Parvovirus B19	Prodrome: none; fever often absent or low grade. Rash: **"slapped cheek"** erythematous rash; erythematous, pruritic, maculopapular rash starts on arms and spreads to trunk and legs; **worse with fever and sun exposure.**	Arthritis, hemolytic anemia, encephalopathy. Congenital infection associated with fetal hydrops and death.
Measles *Ped.30*	Paramyxovirus	Prodrome: low-grade fever with cough, coryza, conjunctivitis (the "**three C's**"); Koplik's spots (small irregular red spots with central gray specks) on buccal mucosa after 1–2 days. Rash: erythematous, maculopapular rash spreads from head toward feet.	Common: otitis media, pneumonia, laryngotracheitis. Rare: subacute sclerosing panencephalitis *(Neuro.46)*.
Rubella	Rubella virus	Prodrome: asymptomatic or tender, generalized, lymphadenopathy. Rash: erythematous, tender, maculopapular rash and slight fever. Polyarthritis may be seen in adolescents.	Encephalitis, thrombocytopenia (rare complication of postnatal infection). Congenital infection associated with congenital anomalies.
Roseola infantum	HHV-6	Prodrome: acute onset of high fever (> 40°C); no other symptoms for 3–4 days. Rash: **maculopapular rash appears as fever breaks** (begins on trunk, quickly spreads to face and extremities) and often lasts < 24 hours.	**Febrile seizures** may occur as a result of rapid fever onset.
Varicella *Ped.35*	Varicella-zoster virus (VZV)	Prodrome: mild fever, anorexia, and malaise precede rash by 24 hours. Rash: generalized, pruritic, **"teardrop" vesicular rash** begins on trunk, spreads to periphery; **lesions often at different stages of healing.** Infectious from 24 hours before eruption until lesions crust over.	Progressive varicella with meningoencephalitis and hepatitis occurs in immune-compromised children. Congenital infection associated with congenital anomalies.
Varicella zoster	VZV	Prodrome: reactivation of varicella infection, starts as pain along an affected sensory nerve. Rash: pruritic "teardrop" vesicular rash in a **dermatomal distribution.** Uncommon unless immunocompromised.	Encephalopathy, aseptic meningitis, pneumonitis, thrombotic thrombocytopenic purpura, Guillain-Barré syndrome, cellulitis, arthritis.
Hand-foot-and-mouth disease	Coxsackie A	Prodrome: fever, anorexia, oral pain. Rash: **oral ulcers;** maculopapular **vesicular rash** on hands, feet, and sometimes buttocks.	None (self-limited).

TABLE 2.13–6. Selected Congenital Malformations

Malformation	Presentation/Diagnosis/Treatment
Tracheoesophageal fistula	Tract between trachea and esophagus. Associated with defects such as esophageal atresia and **VACTERL** anomalies (**V**ertebral, **A**nal, **C**ardiac, **T**racheal, **E**sophageal, **R**enal, **L**imb). Presentation: polyhydramnios in utero, increased oral secretions, inability to feed, gagging, respiratory distress. Diagnosis: CXR after NG tube placement identifies esophageal atresia. The presence of air in the GI tract is suggestive; confirm with bronchoscopy. Treatment: surgical repair.
Congenital diaphragmatic hernia *Ped.38*	GI tract segments protrude through diaphragm into thorax; **90% are posterior left (Bochdalek).** Presentation: respiratory distress (from **pulmonary hypoplasia and pulmonary HTN**), **sunken abdomen, bowel sounds over left hemithorax.** Diagnosis: U/S in utero; confirmed by postnatal CXR. Treatment: high-frequency ventilation or extracorporeal membrane oxygenation (ECMO) to manage pulmonary HTN; surgical repair.
Gastroschisis	Herniation of intestine through the abdominal wall next to umbilicus (usually on right) with **no sac.** Presentation: polyhydramnios in utero, often premature, associated with GI stenoses or atresia. Treatment: **a surgical emergency!** Single-stage closure is possible in only 10%.
Omphalocele	Herniation of abdominal viscera through the abdominal wall at umbilicus **into a sac covered by peritoneum and amniotic membrane.** Presentation: polyhydramnios in utero, often premature, associated with other GI and cardiac defects. Treatment: C-section can prevent sac rupture; **if sac is intact, postpone surgical correction** until patient is fully resuscitated. Keep sac covered/stable with petroleum and gauze. Intermittent NG suction to prevent abdominal distention.
Duodenal atresia *Ped.39*	Complete or partial failure of duodenal lumen to recanalize during gestational weeks 8–10. Presentation: polyhydramnios in utero; **bilious emesis** within hours **after first feeding, associated with Down syndrome** and other cardiac/GI anomalies (e.g., annular pancreas, malrotation, imperforate anus). Diagnosis: abdominal radiographs show **"double-bubble" sign** (air bubbles in the stomach and duodenum) proximal to the site of atresia. Treatment: surgical repair.
Meckel's diverticulum *Ped.10*	Vestigial remnant of omphalomesenteric duct (**most common congenital GI tract anomaly**). **Rule of 2's:** 2 times as many males affected; 2 feet from the ileocecal valve (most common); 2 types of mucosa (gastric, pancreatic); 2% of people affected. Presentation: **painless rectal bleeding** (most common), intestinal obstruction from intussusception or volvulus, painful diverticulitis (often mistaken for appendicitis). Diagnosis: Meckel's scan (for ectopic gastric mucosa; uses IV **technetium pertechnetate,** which is preferentially taken up by gastric mucosa).
Hirschsprung's disease (congenital aganglionic megacolon)	Absence of autonomic innervation of bowel wall; inadequate relaxation and peristalsis lead to intestinal obstruction. Presentation: abdominal distention, bilious vomiting, **failure to pass meconium** in the first 24 hours of life. Diagnosis: **barium enema** reveals dilated proximal segment and narrowed distal segment. **Rectal biopsy** with lack of ganglion cells is confirmatory. Treatment: colostomy prior to corrective surgery allows for pelvic growth and normalization of dilated bowel.

TABLE 2.13–6. Selected Congenital Malformations (continued)

Malformation	Presentation/Diagnosis/Treatment
Hypospadias	Abnormal urethral opening on ventral surface of penis due to incomplete development of distal urethra. Presentation: curved penis (**chordee**); associated with hernias and cryptorchidism. Treatment: **circumcision is contraindicated;** surgical repair uses preputial tissue.

and cerebellum. It typically occurs at levels of > 20 mg/dL and can be fatal. Risk factors for kernicterus include prematurity, asphyxia, and sepsis.

History/PE

Ask if child is **breast or formula fed.** Note intrauterine drug exposure and family history of hemoglobinopathies, enzyme deficiencies, or RBC defects. Symptoms include abdominal distention, delayed passage of meconium, **light-colored stools, dark urine,** low Apgar scores, weight loss, and vomiting. Kernicterus presents with lethargy, poor feeding, high-pitched cry, hypertonicity, and seizures. Jaundice may follow a **cephalopedal progression** as concentration increases. Look for signs of infection, congenital malformations, cephalohematomas, bruising, pallor, petechiae, and hepatomegaly.

Differential

- **Conjugated:** Extrahepatic cholestasis (biliary atresia, choledochal cysts), intrahepatic cholestasis (neonatal hepatitis, inborn errors of metabolism, TPN cholestasis), ToRCHeS infections.
- **Unconjugated:** Physiologic jaundice, hemolysis, breast milk jaundice, increased enterohepatic circulation (e.g., GI obstruction), disorders of bilirubin metabolism, sepsis.

Evaluation

CBC with peripheral blood smear, blood typing of mother and infant (for **ABO or Rh incompatibility**), Coombs' test, and bilirubin levels. For direct hyperbilirubinemia, check LFTs, bile acids, blood cultures, sweat test, and tests for aminoacidopathies and α_1-antitrypsin deficiency. A jaundiced

A jaundiced neonate with abnormal vital signs requires a full workup for sepsis.

TABLE 2.13–7. Differentiating Physiologic and Pathologic Jaundice

Physiologic Jaundice	Pathologic Jaundice
Not present until 72 hours after birth.	Present in the first 24 hours of life.
Bilirubin increases < 5 mg/dL/day.	Bilirubin increases > 0.5 mg/dL/hour.
Bilirubin peaks at < 14–15 mg/dL.	Bilirubin rises to > 15 mg/dL.
Direct bilirubin is < 10% of total.	Direct bilirubin is > 10% of total.
Resolves by one week in term infants and two weeks in preterm infants.	Persists beyond one week in term infants and two weeks in preterm infants.

HIGH-YIELD FACTS

Pediatrics

neonate who is febrile, hypotensive, and/or tachypneic needs a full sepsis workup and ICU monitoring.

Treatment

- Treat underlying causes (e.g., infection).
- Treat unconjugated hyperbilirubinemia with **phototherapy** (mild elevations) or **exchange transfusion** (severe elevations). Start phototherapy earlier (10–15 mg/dL) for preterm infants. Phototherapy with conjugated hyperbilirubinemia can cause skin-bronzing.

UCV *Ped.45*

RESPIRATORY DISTRESS SYNDROME (RDS)

The most common cause of respiratory failure in **preterm infants** (affects > 70 % of infants born at 28–30 weeks' gestation). **Surfactant deficiency** results in poor lung compliance and atelectasis. Risk factors include maternal diabetes mellitus, male sex, and the second born of twins.

History/PE

Presents in the **first 48–72 hours of life** with **RR > 60/min,** progressive **hypoxemia,** cyanosis, **nasal flaring, intercostal retractions,** and **expiratory grunting.**

Differential

Transient tachypnea of the newborn (TTN), meconium aspiration, congenital pneumonia, spontaneous pneumothorax, diaphragmatic hernia, cyanotic heart disease.

Evaluation

Check ABGs, CBC, and blood cultures to rule out infection. Diagnosis is based mainly on characteristic CXR findings:

- **RDS:** Bilateral diffuse atelectasis causes **"ground-glass"** appearance and air bronchograms.
- **TTN:** Retained amniotic fluid causes prominent perihilar streaking in interlobular fissures.
- **Meconium aspiration:** Coarse, irregular infiltrates, hyperexpansion, and pneumothoraces.
- **Congenital pneumonia:** Nonspecific patchy infiltrates; neutropenia, tracheal aspirate, and Gram stain suggest the diagnosis.

Treatment

- **Continuous positive airway pressure (CPAP)** or intubation and mechanical **ventilation.**
- **Artificial surfactant** administration decreases mortality.
- To prevent, pretreat mothers at risk for preterm delivery with **corticosteroids** and monitor fetal lung maturity via **lecithin-sphingomyelin ratio** and phosphatidylglycerol.

Complications

Persistent PDA and bronchopulmonary dysplasia. Retinopathy of prematurity, intraventricular hemorrhage, and necrotizing enterocolitis are complications of treatment.

CEREBRAL PALSY (CP)

A range of **nonprogressive,** nonhereditary disorders of movement and posture. The most common movement disorder in children. The cause in most cases is unknown, but it often results from perinatal neurologic insult. Risk factors include prematurity, perinatal asphyxia, intrauterine growth retardation, early infection or trauma, brain malformation, and neonatal cerebral hemorrhage. Categories include:

- **Pyramidal (spastic):** Spastic paresis of any or all limbs. Accounts for 75% of cases. Mental retardation is present in up to 90%.
- **Extrapyramidal (nonspastic):** Result of damage to extrapyramidal tracts. Subtypes are **ataxic** (difficulty coordinating purposeful movements), **choreoathetoid,** and **dystonic** (uncontrollable jerking, writhing, or posturing). Abnormal movements worsen with stress and disappear during sleep.

History/PE

May be associated with **seizure** disorder, behavioral disorder, hearing or vision impairment, **learning disabilities,** and **speech deficits.** Affected limbs may show **hyperreflexia,** pathologic reflexes (e.g., Babinski), **increased tone/contractures,** weakness, and/or underdevelopment. Toe walking and scissor gait are common. Hip dislocations and scoliosis may occur.

Differential/Evaluation

Rule out metabolic disorders, cerebellar dysgenesis, and spinocerebellar degeneration. Diagnosis is largely clinical. EEG may be useful in patients with seizures.

Treatment

Special education, physical therapy, braces, and surgical release of contractures may help. Treat spasticity with **diazepam, dantrolene, or baclofen.** Baclofen pumps and posterior rhizotomy may alleviate severe contractures.

UCV *Neuro.5*

FEBRILE SEIZURES

Usually occur in children between **six months and six years** of age who have **no evidence of intracranial infection or other cause.** Risk factors include a **rapid rise in temperature** and a history of febrile seizures in a close relative.

History/PE

Seizures usually **occur during onset of fever** and may be the first sign of an underlying illness (e.g., OM, **roseola**). They are classified as simple or complex:

- **Simple:** Short-duration (< 15 minutes), **generalized seizure** with one in a 24-hour period. High fever (> 39°C) and fever onset within hours of the seizure are typical.
- **Complex:** Long-duration (> 15 minutes), **focal seizure** with > 1 seizure in a 24-hour period. Low-grade fever and fever for several days before seizure onset may be present.

Differential

Infection, dehydration, electrolyte imbalance, CNS malformations, trauma, tumors, intoxication.

Evaluation

Focus on finding a source of infection. **LP is indicated if there are clinical signs of CNS infection** (e.g., altered consciousness, meningismus, tense/bulging anterior fontanelle—after ruling out increased ICP). No lab studies are needed if presentation is consistent with febrile seizures. For atypical presentations, obtain electrolytes, serum glucose, blood cultures, UA, and CBC with differential. The utility of **EEG and MRI** in evaluating **complex febrile seizures** is controversial.

Treatment

For simple seizures, use aggressive **antipyretic therapy** (avoid aspirin owing to the risk of Reye's syndrome) and treat any underlying illness. For complex seizures, perform a thorough neurologic evaluation. Chronic anticonvulsant therapy (e.g., diazepam or phenobarbital) may be necessary.

Complications

Febrile seizure will recur in 30% of children, but there is **no increased risk of epilepsy** or developmental, intellectual, or growth abnormalities. Patients with complex seizures have a 10% risk of developing epilepsy.

UCV *Neuro.42*

ONCOLOGY

NEUROBLASTOMA

This **embryonal tumor of neural crest cell origin.** More than half of patients are < 2 years old. Associations include neurofibromatosis and Hirschsprung's disease, and the N-myc oncogene.

History/PE

Lesions may occur anywhere in the body (e.g., abdomen, mediastinum). Symptoms vary with location and may include a **nontender abdominal mass** (may cross midline), **Horner's syndrome, HTN,** or cord compression (from a paraspinal tumor). Patients may have anemia, FTT, and fever. Site-specific metastases may cause **proptosis** and **periorbital bruising ("raccoon eyes"), subcutaneous tumor nodules,** bone pain with pancytopenia (from bone marrow infiltration), and **opsoclonus/myoclonus ("dancing eyes, dancing feet").**

Differential

Wilms' tumor, rhabdomyosarcoma, peripheral neuroepithelioma, lymphoma, renal cell carcinoma (RCC), ovarian tumors, hydronephrosis, polycystic kidney disease (PCKD).

Evaluation

Check abdominal CT and 24-hour urinary catecholamines (for **elevated VMA** and **HVA**). Assess disease extent with CXR, bone scan, CBC, LFTs, BUN/Cr, and coagulation panel.

Treatment

Localized tumors are usually cured with **excision.** Chemotherapy includes **cyclophosphamide and doxorubicin;** adjunctive radiation may be used for tumor spread beyond the organ of origin. Prognosis is improved in a subtype that occurs in infants < 1 year of age.

UCV *Neuro.32*

WILMS' TUMOR

This **renal tumor of embryonal origin** is the most common renal tumor in children. Usually seen between two and four years of age. Associated with a family history, Beckwith-Wiedemann syndrome (hemihypertrophy, macroglossia, visceromegaly), neurofibromatosis, and **WAGR** syndrome (**W**ilms', **A**niridia, **G**enitourinary abnormalities, mental **R**etardation).

History/PE

Patients may have nausea, emesis, bone pain, dysuria, polyuria, weight loss, **hematuria** (usually microscopic), **fever,** and **HTN.** Most common finding is a **painless abdominal/flank mass** (does not cross midline).

Wilms' tumor is associated with aniridia and hemihypertrophy.

Differential

Neuroblastoma, RCC, lymphoma, ovarian tumors, hydronephrosis, PCKD, splenomegaly.

Evaluation

Abdominal **CT or U/S** shows a solid **intrarenal mass.** Assess for metastases with CXR, chest CT, CBC, LFTs, and BUN/Cr.

Treatment

- **Transabdominal nephrectomy** and **postsurgical chemotherapy** with **vincristine and dactinomycin.**
- Flank irradiation is used in some cases.
- Prognosis is generally good but depends on staging and histology.

UCV *Ped.48*

Questions 1, 2, and 3: Reproduced, with permission, from Yetmar KJ, *PreTest: Pediatrics*, 9th ed., New York: McGraw-Hill, 2001.
Question 4: Reproduced, with permission, from Ratelle S, *PreTest: Preventive Medicine and Public Health*, 9th ed., New York: McGraw-Hill, 2001.

Questions

1. You are called to the nursery to see a baby who was noted to be jaundiced and has a serum bilirubin concentration of 13 mg/dL at 18 hours of age. The baby is a 3500-g boy who was born at term to a 27-year-old primigravida 16 hours after membranes ruptured. There were no prenatal complications. Breast-feeding has been well tolerated. Of the following, which is LEAST likely to be responsible for the jaundice in this baby?
   a. Rh or ABO hemolytic disease
   b. physiologic jaundice
   c. sepsis
   d. congenital spherocytic anemia
   e. glucose-6-phosphate dehydrogenase (G6PD) deficiency

2. During a regular checkup on an 8-year-old child, you note a loud first heart sound with a fixed and widely split second heart sound at the upper left sternal border that does not change with respirations. The patient is otherwise active and healthy. The most likely heart lesion to explain these findings is
   a. atrial septal defect
   b. ventricular septal defect
   c. isolated tricuspid regurgitation
   d. tetralogy of Fallot
   e. mitral valve prolapse

3. A 4-year-old boy presents with a history of constipation since the age of 6 months. His stools, produced every 3–4 days, are described as large and hard. Physical examination is normal; rectal examination reveals a large ampulla, poor sphincter tone, and stool in the rectal vault. The next step in the management of this infant would be
   a. lower GI barium study
   b. parental reassurance and counseling
   c. serum electrolyte measurement
   d. upper GI barium study
   e. initiation of synthroid

4. A 20-month-old child presents to your office with a mild viral infection. The results of examination are normal except for a temperature of 37.2°C (99°F) and clear nasal discharge. Review of her vaccination records reveals that she received only two doses of polio vaccine and diphtheria-tetanus-pertussis (DTaP) vaccine, and that she did not receive the measles-mumps-rubella (MMR) vaccine. The mother is 20 weeks pregnant. Her brother is undergoing chemotherapy for leukemia. Which of the following is the most appropriate intervention?
   a. Schedule a visit in two weeks for DTaP
   b. Administer inactivated polio vaccine (IPV) and DTaP
   c. Administer DTaP, oral polio vaccine (OPV), and MMR
   d. Administer DTaP, IPV, and MMR
   e. Administer DTaP and OPV and schedule a visit in three months for MMR

HIGH-YIELD FACTS

Pediatrics

Answers

1. **The answer is b.** The development of jaundice in a healthy full-term baby may be considered the result of a normal physiologic process if the time of onset and duration of the jaundice and the pattern of serially determined serum concentrations of bilirubin are in conformity with currently accepted safe criteria. Physiologic jaundice becomes apparent on the second or third day of life, peaks to levels no higher than about 12 mg/dL on the fourth or fifth day, and disappears by the end of the week. The rate of rise is less than 5 mg/dL per 24 h and levels of conjugated bilirubin do not exceed about 1 mg/dL. Concern about neonatal jaundice relates to the risk of the neurotoxic effects of unconjugated bilirubin. The precise level and duration of exposure necessary to produce toxic effects are not known, but bilirubin encephalopathy, or kernicterus, is rare in term infants whose bilirubin level is kept below 18 to 20 mg/dL. Certain risk factors affecting premature or sick newborns increase their susceptibility to kernicterus at much lower levels of bilirubin. The diagnosis of physiologic jaundice is made by excluding other causes of hyperbilirubinemia by means of history, physical examination, and laboratory determinations. Jaundice appearing in the first 24 hours is usually a feature of hemolytic states and is accompanied by an indirect hyperbilirubinemia, reticulocytosis, and evidence of red-cell destruction on smear. In the absence of blood group or Rh incompatibility, congenital hemolytic states (e.g., spherocytic anemia) or G6PD deficiency should be considered. With infection, hemolytic and hepatotoxic factors are reflected in the increased levels of both direct and indirect bilirubin.

   Studies should include maternal and infant Rh types and blood groups and Coombs' tests to detect blood group or Rh incompatibility and sensitization. Measurements of total and direct bilirubin concentrations help to determine the level of production of bilirubin and the presence of conjugated hyperbilirubinemia. Hematocrit and reticulocyte count provide information as to the degree of hemolysis and anemia, and a complete blood count screens for the possibility of sepsis and the need for cultures. Examination of the blood smear is useful in differentiating common hemolytic disorders. Except for determinations of total and direct bilirubin, tests of liver function are not particularly helpful in establishing the cause of early-onset jaundice. Transient elevations of transaminases (AST and ALT) related to the trauma of delivery and to hypoxia have been noted. Biliary atresia and neonatal hepatitis can be accompanied by elevated levels of transaminase but characteristically present as chronic cholestatic jaundice with mixed hyperbilirubinemia after the first week of life.

2. **The answer is a.** Most commonly, children with an atrial septal defect (ASD) are asymptomatic with the lesion found during a routine examination. In older children, exercise intolerance can be noted if the lesion is of significant size. On examination, the pulses are normal, a right ventricular systolic lift at the left sternal border is palpable, and a fixed splitting of the second heart sound is audible. For lesser degrees of ASD, surgical treatment is more controversial. Ventricular septal defects commonly present as a harsh or blowing holosystolic murmur best heard along the left lower sternum, often with radiation throughout the precordium. Tricuspid regurgitation is a mid-diastolic rumble at the lower left sternal border. Often, a history of birth asphyxia or findings of other cardiac lesions are present. Tetralogy of Fallot is a very common form of congenital heart disease. The four abnormalities include right ventricular outflow obstruction, ventricular septal defect, dextroposition of the aorta, and right ventricular hyper-

trophy. The cyanosis presents in infants and in young children. Mitral valve prolapse occurs with the billowing into the atria of one or both mitral valve leaflets at the end of systole. It is a congenital abnormality that frequently only manifests during adolescence or later. It is more common in girls than in boys and seems to be inherited in an autosomal dominant fashion. On clinical examination, an apical murmur is noted late in systole, which can be preceded by a mid systolic click. The diagnosis is confirmed with an echocardiogram that shows prolapse of the mitral leaflets during mid to late systole. Antibiotic prophylaxis is recommended for dental work (especially if a murmur is present) as the incidence of endocarditis can be higher in these patients.

3. **The answer is b.** Hirschsprung's disease is usually suspected in the chronically constipated child despite the fact that 98% of such children have functional constipation. Finding a dilated, stool-filled anal canal with poor tone on the physical examination of a well-grown child supports the diagnosis of functional constipation. The difficulty in treating functional constipation once it has been established emphasizes the need for prompt identification and treatment of problems with defecation and for counseling of parents regarding proper toileting behavior. The extensive workup of this patient would likely be negative and expensive and is not indicated.

4. **The answer is d.** Children who are late in their immunization schedule should be vaccinated when the opportunity arises. Mild acute illness or antibiotic use is not a contraindication to immunization. MMR is not contraindicated in children of pregnant women. OPV, but not MMR, is contraindicated in any household contact of a severely immunocompromised person. In fact, in an effort to reduce vaccine-associated paralytic polio (VAPP), OPV is no longer recommended for the first two doses of polio immunizations in infants since 1997, and effective January 2000, the CDC recommendations are to give four doses of IPV at 2 months, 4 months, 6–18 months, and then at 6–8 years. OPV can be considered only under a few specific circumstances. If the parents refuse the schedule, OPV could be given only for the third or fourth dose and parents should be counseled about the possible occurrence of VAPP. In this scenario, however, OPV would not be acceptable given the sibling situation. Live and inactivated vaccines can be given at the same time.

Psychiatry

HIGH-YIELD FACTS

Psychiatry

Sleep stages

Stage (% of total sleep time in young adults)	Description	Waveform
	Awake (eyes open), alert, active mental concentration	Beta (highest frequency, lowest amplitude)
	Awake (eyes closed)	Alpha
1 (5%)	Light sleep	Theta
2 (45%)	Deeper sleep	Sleep spindles and K-complexes
3–4 (25%)	Deepest, non-REM sleep; sleepwalking; night terrors, bed-wetting (slow-wave sleep)	Delta (lowest frequency, highest amplitude)
REM (25%)	Dreaming, loss of motor tone, possibly a memory processing function, erections, ↑ brain O_2 use	Beta
		At night, **BATS** Drink **B**lood.

1. Serotonergic predominance of raphe nucleus key to initiating sleep
2. Norepinephrine reduces REM sleep
3. Extraocular movements during REM due to activity of PPRF (paramedian pontine reticular formation/conjugate gaze center)
4. REM sleep having the same EEG pattern as while awake and alert has spawned the terms "paradoxical sleep" and "desynchronized sleep"
5. Benzodiazepines shorten stage 4 sleep; thus useful for night terrors and sleepwalking
   BehSci.39, 87
6. Imipramine is used to treat enuresis since it decreases stage 4 sleep   *BehSci.36*

REM sleep

↑ and variable pulse, rapid eye movements (REM), ↑ and variable blood pressure, penile/clitoral tumescence. 25% of total sleep. Occurs every 90 minutes; duration ↑ through the night. REM sleep ↓ with age. Acetylcholine is the principal neurotransmitter involved in REM sleep.

REM sleep is like sex:
↑ pulse, penile/ clitoral tumescence, ↓ with age.

Narcolepsy

Person falls asleep suddenly. May include hypnagogic (just before sleep) or hypnopompic (just before awakening) hallucinations. The person's nocturnal and narcoleptic sleep episodes start off with REM sleep. **Cataplexy** (sudden collapse while awake) in some patients. Strong genetic component. Treat with stimulants (e.g., amphetamines).

Sleep patterns of depressed patients

Patients with depression typically have the following changes in their sleep stages:
1. ↓ slow-wave sleep
2. ↓ REM latency
3. Early-morning awakening (important screening question)

GENERALIZED ANXIETY DISORDER (GAD)

Characterized by **chronic, excessive anxiety or worry** about a **broad spectrum of activities or life events** that causes significant impairment or distress. Lifetime prevalence is 5%. The male-to-female ratio is 1:2, and clinical onset is usually in the early 20s.

Anxiety disorders are the most prevalent psychiatric disorders.

History/PE

Patients have anxiety/worry on most days for ≥ **6 months and ≥ 3 somatic symptoms,** including restlessness, fatigue, difficulty concentrating, irritability, muscle tension, and sleep disturbance.

Differential

Substance-related or medical disorders (e.g., hyperthyroidism), depression, other anxiety disorders, somatoform disorders.

Treatment

Pharmacologic therapy with selective serotonin reuptake inhibitors (SSRIs), venlafaxine, and buspirone. Benzodiazepines with longer half-lives (e.g., clonazepam) may be used for immediate symptom relief. Relaxation training and psychotherapy may be useful.

UCV *Psych.6*

OBSESSIVE-COMPULSIVE DISORDER (OCD)

Characterized by obsessions and/or compulsions that patients try to suppress, that they **recognize as excessive and irrational products of their own minds,** and that cause significant distress or impairment (e.g., take > 1 hour/day). Lifetime prevalence is 2–3%. Typically presents in late adolescence or early adulthood.

History/PE

Obsessions are **persistent, intrusive ideas, thoughts, impulses, or images** that cause marked anxiety or distress. Common themes are contamination and fear of harm to oneself or loved ones. Compulsions are **conscious, repeated mental acts** (e.g., counting) **or behaviors** (e.g., checking) that neutralize anxiety from obsessions. Common compulsions include hand washing (e.g., look for chafed hands from frequent/caustic washing), elaborate rituals for ordinary tasks (e.g., walking through a doorway), or excessive checking (e.g., returning home repeatedly to check that the door is locked). Adults recognize that thoughts or behaviors are excessive or unreasonable (although children may not) but are unable to control them.

Differential

Tourette's disorder, other anxiety disorders, depression (with obsessive rumination), obsessive-compulsive personality disorder (recurrent obsessions/compulsions are not present), schizophrenia, organic causes (e.g., stroke, temporal lobe epilepsy).

Treatment

Pharmacotherapy (i.e., clomipramine or SSRIs) and **cognitive-behavioral therapy** (CBT) using exposure and response prevention and desensitization.
UCV *Psych.7*

PANIC DISORDER

Patients with panic disorder often have agoraphobia.

Characterized by recurrent, unexpected panic attacks. Common in females in their 20s. Patients have an increased incidence of mitral valve prolapse and thyroid problems. **Agoraphobia** is present in 30–50% of cases. *(Psych.7)*

History/PE

- Panic attacks—discrete periods of intense fear or discomfort in which four (or more) of the following symptoms develop abruptly and peak within 10 minutes: chest pain, palpitations, diaphoresis, nausea, tachypnea, trembling, dizziness, fear of dying or "going crazy," and depersonalization.
- At least **one month** of concern about having additional attacks or implications of the attacks (e.g., having a heart attack), or significant behavior change (e.g., avoiding public places).

Differential

Medical conditions (e.g., angina, hyperthyroidism, hypoglycemia), substance-induced anxiety disorder, other anxiety disorders.

Treatment

CBT, respiratory training, and antidepressants (e.g., SSRIs, tricyclic antidepressants [TCAs]). Benzodiazepines (e.g., clonazepam) may be used for immediate relief, but avoid long-term use owing to their addictive potential.
UCV *Psych.5,8*

PHOBIAS (SOCIAL AND SPECIFIC)

Social phobia is characterized by marked anxiety provoked by **social or performance situations** in which embarrassment may occur. It may be specific (e.g., public speaking) or general (e.g., social interaction) and often begins in adolescence. In **specific phobia,** anxiety is provoked by exposure to a **feared object or situation** (e.g., animals, heights). Most begin in childhood, and although common, most are not severe enough to warrant diagnosis.

History/PE

Persistent excessive or unreasonable fear and/or avoidance of an object or situation results in significant distress or impairment. Related history of traumatic events or panic attacks may be present.

Differential

Appropriate anxiety, avoidant or schizoid personality disorder, depression, psychosis, panic disorder with agoraphobia, post-traumatic stress disorder (PTSD), OCD.

Treatment

Therapy employs desensitization through incremental exposure to the feared object or situation. Other options include relaxation and breathing techniques; hypnosis; and supportive, family, and insight-oriented psychotherapy. SSRIs, low-dose benzodiazepines, or β-blockers (for performance anxiety) may be used for social phobia.

UCV *Psych.10*

POST-TRAUMATIC STRESS DISORDER

Characteristic symptoms develop following exposure to an extreme traumatic stressor (e.g., assault, combat, witnessing a violent crime) that evoked intense fear, helplessness, or horror. Lifetime prevalence is 8% for U.S. adults but is higher in traumatized individuals.

History/PE

Symptoms must persist for **> 1 month** and must include **reexperiencing of the event** (e.g., nightmares), avoidance of stimuli associated with the trauma, numbed responsiveness (e.g., detachment, anhedonia), and increased arousal (e.g., hypervigilance, exaggerated startle). Watch for survivor guilt, irritability, poor concentration, amnesia, personality change, sleep disturbance, substance abuse, depression, and suicidality.

Acute stress disorder: symptoms last < 1 month. Post-traumatic stress disorder: symptoms last > 1 month.

Differential

Acute stress disorder (within one month of a trauma; **lasts < 1 month**), adjustment disorder with anxious features (within three months of a stressor, lasts < 6 months), depression, OCD, borderline personality disorder.

Treatment

First-line agents include **SSRIs, buspirone,** and **mood stabilizers** (e.g., lithium). Agents **targeting anxiety** include β-blockers, benzodiazepines, and α_2-agonists (e.g., clonidine). **CBT** and **support groups** are also effective.

UCV *Psych.9*

ANXIOLYTIC MEDICATIONS

Unlike benzodiazepines, buspirone does not cause tolerance, dependence, or withdrawal.

- **Benzodiazepines:** Used for anxiety, insomnia, anesthesia, alcohol withdrawal, seizures, and muscle spasm. Effective, safe, and well tolerated. **Rapid onset of action.** Cons are risk of abuse, tolerance, dependence (often with high-potency agents such as alprazolam and clonazepam), and withdrawal (often with shorter-acting agents such as triazolam and midazolam). They **augment sedation and respiratory depression** from other CNS depressants (e.g., alcohol). P450 inhibitors (e.g., cimetidine, fluoxetine) increase levels; carbamazepine and rifampin decrease levels.
- **Buspirone:** A 5-HT$_{1A}$ partial agonist. Used for GAD and to augment depression/OCD treatment. **Not used for panic disorder. Few side effects** and **no tolerance, dependence,** or **withdrawal.** Slow onset of action and lower efficacy than with benzodiazepines. Do not use with monoamine oxidase inhibitors (MAOIs).
- **Zolpidem:** Non-benzodiazepine for insomnia. Rapid onset. Rare withdrawal.

CHILDHOOD AND ADOLESCENT DISORDERS

ATTENTION-DEFICIT HYPERACTIVITY DISORDER (ADHD)

A persistent pattern of excessive inattention and/or hyperactivity-impulsivity with a prevalence of 3–7%. It is more common in males, typically presents between ages 3 and 13, and often shows a familial pattern.

History/PE

Children must exhibit ADHD symptoms in two or more settings (e.g., home and school).

Diagnosis requires ≥ **6 symptoms** from each category for ≥ **6 months** in **at least two settings** (e.g., school, home) causing significant social and academic impairment. Some symptoms must be present in patients **before age seven.**

- **Inattention: Poor attention span** for schoolwork/play; poor attention to detail or careless mistakes; does not listen when spoken to; has **difficulty following instructions or finishing tasks;** loses items needed to complete tasks; forgetful and **easily distracted.**
- **Hyperactivity/impulsivity: Fidgets;** leaves seat in classroom; runs around inappropriately; cannot play quietly; appears "driven by a motor"; talks excessively; blurts out answers; **does not wait turn; interrupts others.**

Differential

Normal active child, medication side effects, learning disabilities, mood or anxiety disorders, head trauma, Tourette's disorder, conduct or oppositional defiant disorder (common comorbidity).

Treatment

Initial treatment may be nonpharmacologic (e.g., behavior modification). Sugar and food additives are not considered etiologic factors. Pharmacologic treatment includes:

- **Psychostimulants: Methylphenidate** (beware of abuse potential), dextroamphetamine. Adverse effects include insomnia, irritability, decreased appetite, tic exacerbation, and reduced growth velocity (should normalize when medication stops).
- **Antidepressants** (e.g., nortriptyline, bupropion) and α_2-**agonists** (e.g., clonidine).

Reduced growth velocity from psychostimulants should normalize when medication stops.

UCV *Psych.11*

AUTISTIC DISORDER

Characterized by abnormal or **impaired social interaction and communication** and **restricted activities and interests** evident **before age three.** More common in males. May be associated with **tuberous sclerosis and fragile X syndrome.** Symptom severity and IQ vary widely.

History/PE

Patients fail to develop normal social behaviors (e.g., social smile, eye contact) and lack interest in relationships. Language development is delayed or absent. Children show **stereotyped speech and behavior** (e.g., hand flapping) and restricted interests (e.g., preoccupation with objects) and activities (e.g., inflexible rituals).

Differential

Includes other pervasive developmental disorders:

- **Asperger's syndrome:** Autistic-like disorder without marked language or cognitive delays.
- **Rett's disorder:** Genetic neurodegenerative disorder of **females** with progressive impairment (e.g., language, coordination) after five months of normal development.
- **Childhood disintegrative disorder:** Severe developmental regression after ≥ 2 years of normal development.

Treatment

Intensive special education, **behavioral management,** and symptom-targeted medications. Family support and counseling are crucial.

UCV *Psych.12*

CONDUCT AND OPPOSITIONAL DEFIANT DISORDERS

Conduct disorder is a repetitive, persistent pattern of **violating the basic rights of others** or age-appropriate **societal norms or rules** for ≥ 1 year. Behaviors may be **aggressive** (e.g., rape, robbery) or **nonaggressive** (e.g., stealing, lying). More common in males and patients with a history of abuse. Some progress to antisocial personality disorder (diagnosed after age 18). **Oppositional defiant disorder** is a pattern of **negativistic, defiant, disobedient, and hostile behavior** toward authority figures (e.g., losing temper, arguing) for ≥ 6 months. Patients do not seriously violate social norms or the rights of others. Treat with individual and family therapy.

Children with oppositional defiant disorder are argumentative and defiant, but do not violate the rights of others.

UCV *Psych.14*

LEARNING DISORDERS

Characterized by **academic functioning substantially below expected for age, intelligence, and education** as measured by standardized test achievement in reading, mathematics, or written expression. Learning problems interfere significantly with academic functioning and/or daily activities. More males are affected, and there is often a familial pattern. Rule out physical (e.g., deafness) or social factors (e.g., non–English speakers). Interventions include remedial classes or individualized learning strategies.

MENTAL RETARDATION (MR)

Defined as significantly subaverage intellectual functioning **(an IQ of ≤ 70)** with **deficits in adaptive functioning** (e.g., hygiene, social skills) and onset before age 18. Prevalence is ~1%. More males are affected. Causes include chromosomal abnormalities, congenital infections, teratogens, and inborn errors of metabolism. Levels of severity are **mild (IQ 50–70; 85% of cases)**, moderate (IQ 35–49), severe (IQ 20–34), and profound (IQ < 20).

TOURETTE'S DISORDER

Stimulants can precipitate or exacerbate tics.

Characterized by **multiple motor** (e.g., blinking, grimacing) and **vocal** (e.g., grunting, coprolalia) **tics** occurring many times per day, recurrently, for > 1 year. It is more common in males, has a genetic predisposition, and begins prior to age 18. Stimulants (dopamine [DA] agonists) can worsen or precipitate tics. **Associated with ADHD, learning disorders, and OCD.** Treatment is pharmacologic (i.e., haloperidol, pimozide, or clonidine). Counseling can aid social adjustment and coping.

COGNITIVE DISORDERS

DELIRIUM

DeMENtia = MEMory impairment. DeliRIUM = change in sensoRIUM.

A **transient disturbance of consciousness** with **altered cognition** not attributable to dementia. Develops over a short period of time (usually hours to days). Children, the elderly, and hospitalized patients **(e.g., ICU psychosis)** are particularly susceptible. Major causes are outlined in the mnemonic **HIDE.** Other causes are seizure, CVA, endocrine and autoimmune diseases, **uremia,** hepatic encephalopathy, Wilson's disease, heavy metal poisoning, and drugs (e.g., alcohol, **corticosteroids,** TCAs, antihistamines, **anticholinergics,** phenytoin, β-blockers, digitalis, lithium, barbiturates, benzodiazepines).

History/PE

Major causes of delirium—

HIDE
Hypoxia
Infection (especially UTI)
Drugs (especially anticholinergics)
Electrolyte disturbances

Acute onset of **waxing and waning consciousness** and **perceptual disturbances** (hallucinations, illusions). Patients may be anxious, paranoid, or combative. They may have decreased attention span and short-term memory, reversed sleep-wake cycle, autonomic disturbances (e.g., tachycardia), and increased symptoms at night **("sundowning").**

Differential

Dementia, schizophrenia, mania, dissociative disorders, psychotic depression.

Evaluation

Check vitals, pulse oximetry, and glucose; perform physical and neurologic exams. Note recently started medications, substance use, prior episodes, medical problems, signs of organ failure, and infection (**occult UTI is common in the elderly; check UA**). Studies may include CBC, chem 7, tox screen, ABG, CXR, ECG, LP, and head CT.

Always check the medication list of delirious patients.

Treatment

Treat underlying causes (delirium is often reversible); normalize fluids and electrolytes; and **optimize the sensory environment.** Use low-dose **antipsychotics** (e.g., haloperidol) or **benzodiazepines** (e.g., lorazepam) for agitation. Use **physical restraints** if necessary to prevent harm to the patient or others.

UCV *Psych.1*

DEMENTIA

Characterized by the development of **multiple cognitive deficits with memory impairment.** Prevalence is highest in people > 85 years old. Course is typically chronic and progressive, and < 15% of cases are reversible (e.g., normal pressure hydrocephalus [NPH] *[Neuro.33]*). The most common causes are **Alzheimer's disease** *(Psych.2)* and **vascular dementia** *(Neuro.17)*. Other causes are outlined in the mnemonic **DEMENTIAS.**

History/PE

Patients have **memory impairment and ≥ 1 of the following: aphasia, apraxia, agnosia,** or **impaired executive function** (e.g., planning) in the presence of a **clear sensorium.** Symptoms may worsen at night (**"sundowning"**). Personality, mood, and behavior changes are common.

Differential

Delirium, depression (pseudodementia), age-related cognitive decline, schizophrenia, amnestic disorder, MR, substance intoxication, traumatic brain injury.

Evaluation/Treatment

Work up for reversible causes and treat appropriately. Provide **environmental cues.** Low-dose **antipsychotics** may be used for agitation. **Avoid benzodiazepines,** which may worsen disinhibition and confusion.

Avoid benzodiazepines in demented patients.

DEMENTIAS:

Degenerative diseases (Parkinson's, Huntington's)
Endocrine (thyroid, parathyroid, pituitary, adrenal)
Metabolic (alcohol, electrolytes, B$_{12}$ deficiency, glucose, hepatic, renal, Wilson's disease)
Exogenous (heavy metals, carbon monoxide, drugs)
Neoplasia
Trauma (subdural hematoma)
Infection (meningitis, encephalitis, endocarditis, syphilis, HIV, prion diseases, Lyme disease)
Affective disorders (pseudodementia)
Stroke/**S**tructure (vascular dementia, ischemia, vasculitis, NPH)

HIGH-YIELD FACTS

Psychiatry

ANOREXIA NERVOSA

Characterized by **refusal to maintain normal body weight** (> 85% ideal weight), intense **fear of weight gain,** distorted body image **(patients perceive themselves as fat),** and **amenorrhea** in postmenarchal females (missing three consecutive cycles). Females account for 90% of cases. Peak onset is between ages 10 and 30. Patients may recover (40%), improve (30%), or become chronic (30%). Mortality from suicide or medical complications is > 10%.

History/PE

Patients **restrict** (e.g., **fasting, excessive exercise**) or **binge and purge (i.e., vomiting, laxatives, and diuretics). Appetite is normal.** Patients are often preoccupied with food rituals, base self-image on weight, and deny the medical consequences of their behaviors. Signs/symptoms include **lanugo,** dry skin, lethargy, bradycardia, hypotension, cold intolerance, hypothermia, and hypercarotenemia.

Evaluation

Measure height and weight. Check CBC, electrolytes, endocrine tests, and ECG. Perform a psychiatric evaluation.

Treatment

- **Early treatment:** Monitor caloric intake to stabilize weight and then focus on **weight gain;** hospitalize if necessary to restore nutritional status and correct electrolyte imbalances.
- **Later treatment:** Individual, family, and group **psychotherapy;** SSRIs to treat comorbid depression and anxiety.

UCV *Psych.27*

BULIMIA NERVOSA

Characterized by **binge eating, compensatory methods to prevent weight gain,** and **dependence of self-evaluation on weight.** Patients usually maintain normal body weight. Prevalence is 1–3%. Peak onset is in late adolescence, and course is usually chronic or intermittent.

History/PE

At least twice a week for three months patients have episodes of **binge eating** (with a sense of **being out of control**) and **compensatory behaviors,** which include vomiting, laxatives, and diuretics **(purging type)** or fasting and exercise **(nonpurging type).** Patients are usually **ashamed** and conceal their behaviors. **Signs** include **dental enamel erosion, enlarged parotid glands,** and **scars on the dorsal hand surfaces** (from inducing vomiting).

Evaluation/Treatment

Assess and correct fluid and electrolyte abnormalities. **Psychotherapy** focuses on behavior modification and body image. **Antidepressants** are effective for depressed and nondepressed patients.

UCV *Psych.28*

MOOD DISORDERS

MAJOR DEPRESSIVE DISORDER (MDD)

A unipolar mood disorder characterized by ≥ 1 major depressive episode (MDE). The **male-to-female ratio is 1:2.** Lifetime prevalence is 10–25% for females and 5–12% for males. Onset may occur at any age, but average is in the mid-20s. In the elderly, prevalence increases with age. **Chronic illness and stress** increase risk, but socioeconomic status and race do not appear to do so. **Untreated MDEs typically last ≥ 4 months,** and recurrence risk is 60% after one MDE. Up to 15% die by suicide.

History/PE

Diagnosis requires **depressed mood or loss of interest/pleasure AND ≥ 5 SIG E CAPS signs/symptoms** nearly every day **for a two-week period** causing significant distress or impairment. Selected depression subtypes include:

- **Psychotic features** (typically mood-congruent delusions/hallucinations).
- **Postpartum** (within one month postpartum; 10% incidence; high recurrence risk).
- **Atypical** (weight gain, hypersomnia, rejection sensitivity).
- **Seasonal** (recurrent fall and winter depression; treat with bright light therapy).
- **Double depression** (MDE in a dysthymic patient).

Differential

- **Mood disorder due to a medical condition** (e.g., hypothyroidism, Parkinson's) *(Psych.41)*.
- **Substance-induced mood disorder** (e.g., illicit drugs, β-blockers).
- Adjustment disorder with depressed mood (milder, within three months of stressor, lasts < 6 months).
- Normal bereavement (no severe impairment/suicidality; usually resolves in one year but varies with cultural norms) *(Psych.39)*.
- **Dysthymia (milder, chronic depression for ≥ 2 years;** often treatment resistant)*(Psych.43)*.
- Dementia (rule out pseudodementia in the elderly), bipolar disorder, schizophrenia, schizoaffective disorder.

> **Symptoms of a depressive episode—**
>
> **SIG E CAPS**
> **S**leep (hypersomnia or insomnia)
> **I**nterest (loss of interest or pleasure in activities)
> **G**uilt (feelings of worthlessness or inappropriate guilt)
> **E**nergy (decreased)
> **C**oncentration (decreased)
> **A**ppetite (increased or decreased)
> **P**sychomotor agitation or retardation
> **S**uicidal ideation

Always assess suicide risk in patients with depression.

Treatment

Psychotherapy plus antidepressants is more effective than either treatment alone.

- **Pharmacotherapy:** Effective in 50–70% of patients, but requires 3–4 weeks for effect. Treat for at least six months. Specific antidepressants are discussed below.
- **Electroconvulsive therapy (ECT):** Safe, highly effective, potentially lifesaving therapy reserved for refractory or catatonic depression. May also be used for acute mania and acute psychosis. Usually requires 6–12 treatments. Adverse effects include postictal confusion, arrhythmias, headache, and **retrograde amnesia.** Contraindications include recent MI/stroke, intracranial mass, seizure disorder, and high anesthetic risk (relative contraindication).
- **Psychotherapy:** **Psychotherapy plus antidepressants is more effective than either treatment alone.** Cognitive, behavioral, and interpersonal therapies are among the techniques with proven efficacy.

UCV *Psych.42*

ANTIDEPRESSANT MEDICATIONS

TCAs can be lethal in overdose.

- **SSRIs:** Fluoxetine, sertraline, paroxetine, citalopram, fluvoxamine. First-line therapy for depression and anxiety. Well tolerated, effective, and relatively safe in overdose. Side effects include **sexual dysfunction,** anxiety, tremor, insomnia, nausea, anorexia, and headache. Beware drug interactions via P450 inhibition, particularly with fluoxetine. **Serotonin syndrome** (fever, myoclonus, mental status changes, cardiovascular collapse) can occur if used with other serotonergic agents (e.g., MAOIs).
- **TCAs:** Nortriptyline, desipramine, imipramine, amitriptyline, clomipramine, doxepin. Block reuptake of norepinephrine (NE) and 5-HT. Used for depression, bedwetting (imipramine), OCD, chronic pain, and migraine. Cheap and effective, but have drug interactions and side effects including anticholinergic symptoms, α-blocking effects (orthostasis), sedation, sexual dysfunction, and arrhythmias **(check ECG before therapy).** See the mnemonic **Tri-C's** for serious toxicity. **Tertiary TCAs (imipramine, amitriptyline) have more anticholinergic effects.** Desipramine is the least sedating. Watch for confusion and hallucinations in the elderly. **TCAs can be lethal in overdose,** so use with caution in suicidal patients.

> **TCA toxicity—**
> **Tri-C's:**
> **C**onvulsions
> **C**oma
> **C**ardiac arrhythmias

- **Heterocyclic antidepressants:**
  - **Bupropion:** May act via DA reuptake inhibition. First-line therapy for depression and smoking cessation. May cause stimulant effects and aggravation of psychosis (uncommon).
  - **Venlafaxine:** Main action is 5-HT and NE reuptake inhibition. Used for MDD and GAD. Rapid onset of action (1–2 weeks). Can cause nausea, sedation, anticholinergic effects, sexual inhibition, dizziness, and **diastolic HTN (monitor BP).** Avoid cimetidine and MAOIs.
  - **Mirtazapine:** An α_2-antagonist (increases NE and 5-HT transmission) and 5-HT$_2$ receptor antagonist. Efficacy is comparable to that of TCAs. Few sexual side effects. Causes marked sedation, increased cholesterol, and weight gain.
  - **Nefazodone and trazodone:** Primarily inhibit 5-HT reuptake. Efficacy is comparable to that of SSRIs. Improves sleep, but can cause nausea, orthostasis, sedation (mainly trazadone), and **priapism (trazodone).**

Cheese and red wine can precipitate a hypertensive crisis when taking an MAOI.

- **MAOIs:** Phenelzine, tranylcypromine, isocarboxazid. Nonselective MAOIs effective for treatment-resistant and atypical depressions. Common side effects include orthostasis, headache, weight gain, insomnia, and sexual dysfunction. May cause **hypertensive crisis with tyramine ingestion** (e.g., in cheese) or pressor medication. **Serotonin syndrome** can occur when used with other serotoninergic drugs (e.g., **SSRIs, meperidine,** TCAs, and indirect sympathomimetics [in many **OTC cold remedies**]).

MAOIs used with meperidine or SSRIs can precipitate serotonin syndrome.

UCV *Psych.23*

BIPOLAR DISORDERS

Prevalence is ~1%, and the male-to-female ratio is 1:1. A family history of bipolar illness significantly increases risk. Average age of onset is 20, and the frequency of mood episodes tends to increase with age. Up to 10–15% die by suicide. Bipolar disorders are divided into the following categories:

- **Bipolar I: At least one manic or mixed episode** (usually requiring hospitalization) that may alternate with MDE or hypomanic episodes.
- **Bipolar II: At least one MDE and one hypomanic episode** (less intense than mania). Patients do not meet criteria for full manic or mixed episodes.
- **Rapid cycling:** Four or more episodes (MDE, manic, mixed, or hypomanic) in one year.
- **Cyclothymic:** Chronic and less severe, with periods of hypomania and moderate depression.

History/PE

The mnemonic **DIG FAST** outlines the clinical presentation of mania. Patients may report excessive spending or sexual activity, speeding tickets, and/or psychotic features. **Antidepressants may trigger manic episodes.**

Differential

Schizophrenia, schizoaffective disorder, MDD, substance-induced mood disorder, borderline personality disorder, ADHD. Medical conditions (e.g., temporal lobe epilepsy, CNS infections) may mimic bipolar disorder.

Evaluation

A manic episode is $\geq$ **1 week** (less if patient is hospitalized) of **persistently elevated, expansive, or irritable mood** and **three DIG FAST symptoms.** Symptoms are not due to a substance or medical condition and cause significant functional impairment. Hypomania is similar but does not cause marked functional impairment and is of shorter duration.

Treatment

- **Acute mania:** Control mood with mood stabilizers (discussed below). Manage psychosis with antipsychotics (e.g., risperidone) and agitation with benzodiazepines.
- **Bipolar depression:** Mood stabilizers +/– antidepressant. **Start mood stabilizers first** to avoid inducing mania. ECT may be used to treat refractory cases.

UCV *Psych.40*

Symptoms of mania—

DIG FAST
Distractibility
Insomnia (decreased need for sleep)
Grandiosity (increased self-esteem)
Flight of ideas (or racing thoughts)
Increase in goal-directed **A**ctivities/ Psychomotor **A**gitation
Pressured **S**peech
Thoughtlessness (poor judgment)

HIGH-YIELD FACTS

Psychiatry

Chronic lithium use can cause hypothyroidism and nephrotoxicity.

- **Lithium:** First-line agent for acute and chronic treatment of bipolar disorders (highly effective for mania) and to augment depression treatment (mild antidepressant effect). Has a **narrow therapeutic index** requiring regular serum level monitoring (0.6–1.2 mEq is therapeutic; 1.5–2.0 mEq is toxic). May be less effective for rapid cyclers. Side effects include **fine tremor, polyuria** (ADH antagonism causes nephrogenic diabetes insipidus), GI distress, cognitive dulling, acne, and weight gain. Toxicity includes **coarse tremor, ataxia,** confusion, seizures, coma, and teratogenesis *(Psych.21)*. Chronic effects include **hypothyroidism** and **nephrotoxicity** (monitor TFTs and BUN/Cr). A change in renal function (e.g., acute renal failure, diuretics) can increase levels.
- **Valproic acid:** First-line agent that augments CNS GABA function. Effective in rapid cyclers (patients may need additional antidepressant). Side effects include sedation, tremor, ataxia, and GI distress. Pancreatitis, thrombocytopenia, fatal hepatotoxicity, and agranulocytosis are uncommon. Monitor drug levels, platelets, and LFTs.
- **Carbamazepine:** Second-line agent that may cause nausea, skin rash, and leukopenia. Toxic reactions are atrioventricular (AV) block, respiratory depression, and coma; rare associations are aplastic anemia and Stevens-Johnson syndrome. Monitor CBC.
- **Lamotrigine and gabapentin:** May be used for treatment-refractory patients (gabapentin is an adjunctive treatment only). **Lamotrigine** may cause ataxia, blurred vision, GI distress, and potentially **life-threatening skin rash.**

Lamotrigine can cause a life-threatening skin rash.

PERSONALITY DISORDERS

Enduring patterns of inner experience and behavior that deviate markedly from cultural expectations, are pervasive and inflexible, begin in adolescence or early adulthood, are stable over time, and lead to distress or impairment (see the mnemonic **MEDIC**). Prevalence is 10% in the general population, 30% among psychiatric outpatients, and 40% among psychiatric inpatients. For specific disorders, see Table 2.14–1.

> **Personality disorders—**
>
> **MEDIC**
> **M**aladaptive
> **E**nduring
> **D**eviates from cultural norms
> **I**nflexible
> **C**auses impairment in social functioning

Evaluation

Rule out Axis I disorders. Ask about attitudes, moral/religious views, mood variability, activities, fantasies, and reaction to stress. Patients may have transient psychotic symptoms under stress, but reality testing is typically intact. Consider psychological testing (e.g., Minnesota Multiphasic Personality Inventory [MMPI]).

Treatment

Psychotherapy and symptom-targeted **pharmacotherapy.** Treat comorbid disorders.

UCV *Psych.44,45,46*

TABLE 2.14–1. Signs and Symptoms of Personality Disorders

Cluster	Disorders	Characteristics	Clinical Dilemma/Strategy
Cluster A: "weird"	Paranoid	Distrustful, suspicious; interpret others' motives as malevolent.	Patients are suspicious and distrustful of doctors and rarely seek medical attention.
	Schizoid	Isolated, detached "loners." Restricted emotional expression.	Be clear, honest, noncontrolling, and nondefensive. Avoid humor.
	Schizotypal	Odd behavior, perceptions, appearance. Magical thinking, ideas of reference.	Maintain emotional distance.
Cluster B: "wild"	Borderline	Unstable mood/relationships, feelings of emptiness. Impulsive.	Patients change the rules, demand attention, and feel they are special. Will manipulate staff and doctor ("splitting").
	Histrionic	Excessively emotional and attention seeking. Sexually provocative.	Be firm: Stick to treatment plan.
	Narcissistic	Grandiose, need admiration, sense of entitlement. Lack empathy.	Be fair: Do not be punitive or derogatory.
	Antisocial	Violate rights of others, social norms, laws. Impulsive. Lack remorse.	Be consistent: Do not change rules.
Cluster C: "worried and wimpy"	Obsessive-compulsive	Preoccupied with perfectionism, order, control. Inflexible morals, values.	Patients are controlling and may sabotage their treatment. Words may be inconsistent with actions.
	Avoidant	Socially inhibited, rejection sensitive. Fear being disliked or ridiculed.	Avoid power struggles. Give clear recommendations, but do not push patients into decisions.
	Dependent	Submissive, clingy, need to be taken care of. Difficulty making decisions.	

PSYCHOTIC DISORDERS

SCHIZOPHRENIA

Characterized by impairment in thought content and form, perception, affect, and general function. Its prevalence is 0.5–1.5%, and the male-to-female ratio is 1:1. **Peak onset is earlier in males (ages 18–25)** than in **females (ages 25–35).** Schizophrenia in first-degree relatives increases risk. Etiologic theories focus on neurotransmitter abnormalities such as DA dysregulation (frontal hypoactivity, limbic hyperactivity) and brain abnormalities on CT and MRI. Course is often chronic. **Ten percent commit suicide** and 20–40% make an attempt. See Table 2.14–2 for schizophrenia subtypes.

Schizophrenics are at high risk for suicide.

History/PE

Two or more of the following are present for ≥ 1 month with some signs present for ≥ 6 months and marked **social or occupational dysfunction:**

- **Positive symptoms:** Hallucinations (usually auditory), delusions, disorganized speech and behavior.
- **Negative symptoms:** Affective flattening, alogia (poverty of speech), avolition.

TABLE 2.14–2. Subtypes of Schizophrenia

Subtype	Description
Paranoid	Delusions and/or hallucinations present. Cognitive function and affect are relatively preserved. Best overall prognosis.
Disorganized	Disorganized speech and behavior with flat or inappropriate affect. Worst prognosis.
Catatonic	Psychomotor disturbance with two of the following: excessive motor activity, immobility, extreme negativism, mutism, waxy flexibility, echolalia, or echopraxia.
Undifferentiated	Characteristics of > 1 subtype present.
Residual	Met criteria in the past, but now lacks prominent positive symptoms.

Differential

> **Bleuler's symptoms of schizophrenia—**
>
> **The 4 A's:**
> **A**ssociations (loose)
> **A**ffect (flat)
> **A**utism (self-preoccupation, noncommunication)
> **A**mbivalence (uncertainty)

- Substance-induced psychosis (e.g., amphetamines), drug withdrawal (e.g., alcoholic hallucinosis), or psychosis due to a medical condition (e.g., CNS tumor, Cushing's syndrome).
- **Schizophreniform disorder** (symptoms **last < 6 months;** better prognosis).
- **Brief psychotic disorder** (≥ 1 symptoms for < **1 month;** often after a psychosocial stressor; better prognosis) *(Psych.47)*.
- **Delusional disorder** (nonbizarre delusions for ≥ **1 month** without hallucinations, disorganized speech/behavior, or negative symptoms; typical onset in 40s, often chronic; treat with psychotherapy)
- **Schizoaffective disorder** (**meets criteria for schizophrenia AND major mood episode;** psychotic symptoms also present for two weeks without significant mood symptoms).
- Mood disorder with psychotic features.

Treatment

Antipsychotics (see below) and hospitalization during psychotic episodes. Supportive psychotherapy and social skills training may help. Negative symptoms may be more difficult to treat.

UCV *Psych.49*

ANTIPSYCHOTIC MEDICATIONS

Typical Antipsychotics

> *High-potency antipsychotics cause more EPS. Low-potency antipsychotics cause more anticholinergic effects.*

Act through DA receptor blockade (mostly D_2 and D_4 subtypes). Used for psychotic disorders and acute agitation. Cheap and effective, particularly for positive symptoms. High-potency agents (haloperidol, droperidol, fluphenazine, thiothixene) cause more extrapyramidal symptoms (EPS). Low-potency agents (thioridazine, chlorpromazine) cause more sedation (histamine blockade), anticholinergic effects (muscarinic blockade), and hypotension (α-blockade). Key side effects include:

- **Extrapyramidal symptoms:** See Table 2.14–3.
- **Hyperprolactinemia:** Amenorrhea, gynecomastia, galactorrhea.
- **Anticholinergic effects:** Dry mouth, urinary retention, constipation, etc.
- **Neuroleptic malignant syndrome:** Fever, muscle rigidity, autonomic instability, clouded consciousness, increased CPK, leukocytosis. To treat, stop neuroleptic and give dantrolene/bromocriptine and IV fluids (EM.41).
- **Other:** Seizures (neuroleptics lower seizure threshold), ECG changes.

Atypical Antipsychotics

Currently first-line treatment for schizophrenia. Act through 5-HT$_2$ and DA antagonism with varying receptor profiles. Benefits are fewer EPS and anticholinergic effects as well as efficacy for positive and negative symptoms and treatment-refractory patients. May cause **weight gain, type 2 diabetes mellitus, and QT prolongation.**

- **Clozapine:** Reserved for treatment-resistant patients or those with severe tardive dyskinesia (TD) or EPS. Good for negative symptoms. May cause **agranulocytosis** (0.5–1.0% incidence; weekly CBCs required), fever, excessive salivation, and eosinophilia.
- **Risperidone:** May cause insomnia, agitation, orthostasis, and reflex tachycardia. Higher doses may cause EPS, hyperprolactinemia, palpitations, and sexual effects.
- **Olanzapine:** Effective for negative symptoms and agitation. **Somnolence and weight gain are common.** Rare hyperglycemia, orthostasis, DKA, and transaminase elevations.

> **Evolution of EPS:**
>
> **4 hours:** Acute dystonia
> **4 days:** Akinesia
> **4 weeks:** Akathisia
> **4 months:** Tardive dyskinesia

TABLE 2.14–3. Extrapyramidal Symptoms and Treatment

EPS	Description	Treatment
Acute dystonia	Involuntary muscle contraction or spasm (e.g., torticollis, oculogyric crisis).	Give an anticholinergic (benztropine) or diphenhydramine. To prevent, give prophylactic benztropine with antipsychotic.
Akathisia	Subjective/objective restlessness.	Decrease neuroleptic and try β-blockers (propranolol). Benzodiazepines or anticholinergics may help.
Dyskinesia	Pseudoparkinsonism (e.g., shuffling gait, cogwheel rigidity).	Give an anticholinergic (benztropine) or DA agonist (amantadine). Decrease dose of neuroleptic or discontinue (if tolerated).
Tardive dyskinesia	Stereotypic oral-facial movements. Likely from DA receptor sensitization. Often irreversible (50%).	Discontinue or reduce dose of neuroleptic, attempt treatment with more appropriate drugs, and consider changing neuroleptic (e.g., to clozapine or risperidone). **Giving anticholinergics or decreasing neuroleptic may initially worsen TD.**

Atypical antipsychotics have fewer extrapyramidal and anticholinergic side effects.

- **Quetiapine:** Side effects include somnolence, orthostasis, and dizziness. Weight gain and transaminase elevations are rare. May increase risk of **cataracts (eye exams recommended).**
- **Ziprasidone:** Rarely causes somnolence, dizziness, nausea, prolactin elevation, and **QT prolongation. No weight gain.**

SUBSTANCE-RELATED DISORDERS

SUBSTANCE ABUSE/DEPENDENCE

Substance abuse is diagnosed if a person continues to use despite ≥ 1 of the following substance-related problems over one year: failure to fulfill major obligations, use in physically hazardous situations, and legal problems. **Substance dependence** is diagnosed if a person continues to use despite ≥ 3 of the following problems in one year: tolerance, withdrawal, using larger amounts than intended, desire/attempts to cut down, significant energy spent obtaining substance, and withdrawal from activities. More than 15% of the U.S. adult population has a serious substance use problem. Comorbid psychiatric disorders are common.

Differential

Rule out other Axis I disorders and delirium. See Table 2.14–4 for signs and symptoms of substance abuse for selected drugs.

Evaluation/Treatment

Drug use is often denied or underreported, so seek out collateral information from family and friends. Check urine and blood tox screens, LFTs, and Breathalyzer or serum EtOH level. Offer HIV testing (especially to IV drug users). Management of intoxication for selected drugs is described in Table 2.14–4.

UCV *Psych.18,19,22,24,25*

ALCOHOLISM

The male-to-female ratio is 4:1. Prevalence is highest in males aged 21–34, but incidence in females is increasing. Alcohol is the most commonly abused substance (apart from tobacco and caffeine). Family history increases an individual's risk.

History/PE

See Table 2.14–4 for symptoms of intoxication and Selected Topics in Emergency Medicine for symptoms and signs of alcohol withdrawal.

Evaluation

Screen with the **CAGE** questionnaire. Monitor vital signs for evidence of withdrawal. Look for palmar erythema or telangiectasias. Lab tests may reveal elevated SGOT, GGT, LDH, HDL, and MCV.

CAGE questions:

1. Have you ever felt the need to **C**ut down on your drinking?
2. Have you ever felt **A**nnoyed by criticism of your drinking?
3. Have you ever felt **G**uilty about drinking?
4. Have you ever had to take a morning **E**ye opener?

More than one "yes" answer makes alcoholism likely.

TABLE 2.14–4. Signs and Symptoms of Substance Abuse

Drug	Intoxication	Withdrawal
Alcohol	Disinhibition, emotional lability, slurred speech, ataxia, aggression, hypoglycemia, blackouts (retrograde amnesia), coma.	Tremor, tachycardia, HTN, malaise, nausea, seizures, DTs, agitation, hallucinations.
Opioids	CNS depression, nausea, vomiting, constipation, **pupillary constriction,** seizures, respiratory depression (life threatening in overdose). Naloxone/naltrexone will block opioid receptors and reverse effects (beware of antagonist clearing before opioid, particularly with long-acting opioids such as methadone).	Anxiety, insomnia, anorexia, diaphoresis, dilated pupils, fever, rhinorrhea, piloerection, nausea, stomach cramps, diarrhea, yawning.
Amphetamines	Psychomotor agitation, impaired judgment, HTN, **pupillary dilation,** tachycardia, fever, euphoria, prolonged wakefulness/attention, arrhythmias, delusions, hallucinations. Can give haloperidol for severe agitation and symptom-targeted medications (e.g., antiemetics, NSAIDs)	Post-use "crash" with anxiety, lethargy, headache, stomach cramps, hunger, fatigue, depression/dysphoria, sleep disturbance.
Cocaine	Psychomotor agitation, euphoria, impaired judgment, tachycardia, **pupillary dilation,** HTN, paranoia, angina, hallucinations, sudden death. Treat with haloperidol for severe agitation and symptom-targeted medications.	Post-use "crash" with hypersomnolence, depression, malaise, severe craving, suicidality.
Phencyclidine hydrochloride (PCP)	Belligerence, psychosis, violence, impulsiveness, psychomotor agitation, fever, tachycardia, **vertical/horizontal nystagmus,** ataxia, delirium. Give benzodiazepines for severe symptoms; otherwise reassure.	Recurrence of intoxication symptoms due to reabsorption in the GI tract; sudden onset of severe, random violence.
LSD	Marked anxiety or depression, delusions, visual hallucinations, flashbacks, pupil dilation. Give benzodiazepines or traditional antipsychotics for severe symptoms.	
Marijuana	Euphoria, slowed sense of time, impaired judgment, social withdrawal, increased appetite, dry mouth, conjunctival injection, hallucinations, anxiety, paranoia, amotivational syndrome.	
Barbiturates	Low safety margin, respiratory depression.	Anxiety, seizures, delirium, life-threatening cardiovascular collapse.
Benzodiazepines	Interactions with alcohol, amnesia, ataxia, somnolence, mild respiratory depression.	Rebound anxiety, seizures, tremor, insomnia, HTN, tachycardia.
Caffeine	Restlessness, insomnia, diuresis, muscle twitching, arrhythmias.	Headache, lethargy, depression, weight gain.
Nicotine	Restlessness, insomnia, anxiety, arrhythmias.	Irritability, headache, anxiety, weight gain, craving, tachycardia.

Treatment

- Rule out medical complications; correct electrolyte abnormalities.
- Start benzodiazepine taper (e.g., chlordiazepoxide) for withdrawal symptoms.
- Give **multivitamins and folic acid; give thiamine** before glucose (which depletes thiamine) to prevent Wernicke's encephalopathy.
- Give $MgSO_4$ or anticonvulsants to patients with seizure history. Avoid neuroleptics, which decrease seizure threshold.
- Alcohol dependence can be treated with group therapy (Alcoholics Anonymous), disulfiram, or naltrexone.

Complications

DTs are a medical emergency with a mortality rate of 15–20%.

GI bleeding (e.g., gastritis, varices, Mallory-Weiss tears), **pancreatitis, liver disease,** DTs *(Psych.20)*, alcohol-induced psychosis, peripheral neuropathy, cerebellar degeneration, Wernicke's encephalopathy (ophthalmoplegia, ataxia, confusion) and Korsakoff's psychosis (amnesia, disorientation) *(Psych.3)*.

UCV *Psych.17*

MISCELLANEOUS DISORDERS

GENDER IDENTITY DISORDERS

Defined by **strong, persistent cross-gender identification** and **discomfort with one's assigned sex** in the absence of intersexual disorders (e.g., pseudohermaphroditism). Differentiate from **transvestic fetishism** (i.e., **cross-dressing,** usually for **heterosexual arousal**). Transsexuals seek medical or surgical treatment to change sex. These disorders are more common in men.

UCV *Psych.38*

SOMATOFORM DISORDERS

Physical signs/symptoms are not fully explained by a medical cause. Patients have **no conscious control over symptoms** and should not be told they are imagining them (see Table 2.14–5).

FACTITIOUS DISORDERS AND MALINGERING

Consider malingering in any case with litigation or potential for secondary gain.

Patients are conscious that symptoms are faked, but their motivations differ. In **factitious disorders** (e.g., Munchausen syndrome), patients produce physical or psychological symptoms **to assume the "sick role" (primary gain).** Munchausen by proxy is the production of symptoms in another person (usually in a child by a parent). These disorders are more common in men and **health care workers. Malingerers** intentionally simulate illness for **concrete benefits** such as money, food, or shelter **(secondary gain).**

UCV *Psych.36,37*

TABLE 2.14–5. Somatoform Disorders

Somatization disorder *Psych.53*	Multiple, chronic symptoms from different organ systems. Frequent clinical contacts and/or surgeries. Significant functional impairment. Male-to-female ratio is 1:20. Manage with regular appointments.
Conversion disorder *Psych.51*	Symptoms or deficits of voluntary motor or sensory function (e.g., blindness, seizure) suggest a condition incompatible with medical processes. Close temporal relationship to stress or intense emotion. More common in young females and in lower socioeconomic and less educated groups.
Hypochondriasis *Psych.52*	Preoccupation with or fear of having a serious disease despite medical reassurance. Causes significant distress/impairment. Often history of prior physical disease. Men and women are equally affected. Onset in adulthood.
Body dysmorphic disorder *Psych.50*	Preoccupation with imagined physical defect or abnormality causes significant distress/impairment. Often presents to dermatologists or plastic surgeons. Slight female predominance. May be associated with depression, and SSRIs may help.
Pain disorder	Intensity or profile of pain symptoms is inconsistent with physiologic processes. More common in females. May be associated with depression.

SEXUAL AND PHYSICAL ABUSE

Up to 200,000 sexual abuse cases are reported in the United States each year. Abusers are usually **male,** are commonly **known to the victim,** and are often **family members.** Incidence is highest in children aged 9–12. Risk factors include single-parent households, marital discord, substance abuse, and crowded living conditions. Children may exhibit precocious sexual behavior, **genital or anal trauma, STDs,** UTIs, and psychiatric problems. If abuse is suspected, doctors must protect the patient and **report the case to the appropriate authority.**

Sexual abusers are usually male, often known to the victim and often family members.

Domestic physical abuse, most commonly by males against females, is also prevalent. Many battered women are eventually killed by husbands or boyfriends. **Pregnant women are at increased risk.** In elder abuse cases, victims typically live with their abusers, who are often their children. Elder abuse must be reported. See the Pediatrics chapter for further discussion of child abuse.

UCV *Psych.13*

SUICIDALITY

Suicide is the third leading cause of death (after homicide and accidents) among 15- to 24-year-olds in the United States. Risk factors include psychiatric disorders, recent severe stressors, family suicide history, recent recovery from a first schizophrenic episode or severe depression, and factors outlined in the mnemonic **SAD PERSONS.** Risk is higher in police officers and doctors than in the general population and is higher in whites than in nonwhites. Women are more likely to attempt suicide, but men are more likely to use violent methods and to succeed.

Women are more likely to attempt suicide, while men are more likely to commit suicide.

Suicide risk factors—

SAD PERSONS
Sex (male)
Age (older)
Depression
Previous attempt
Ethanol/substance abuse
Rational thought
Sickness (chronic illness)
Organized plan
No spouse
Social support lacking

Evaluation/Treatment

Perform a mental status exam. Ask about family history, previous attempts, ambivalence toward death, and hopelessness. **Ask directly about suicidal ideation, intent, and plan** and look for available means. A patient who expresses a desire to kill himself, or who you believe may do so, requires **emergent inpatient hospitalization** even against his will (involuntary hospitalization). Consider ECT in actively suicidal patients refractory to medication and psychotherapy. Suicide risk may be greater in the first few weeks after beginning antidepressant medication because a patient's energy may return before depressed mood lifts.

The following clinical questions and accompanying answers are reproduced, with permission, from Mancini-Mezzacappa GM, *PreTest: Psychiatry*, 9th ed., New York: McGraw-Hill, 2001.

Questions

1. A 25-year-old man's teaching career has been abruptly terminated by a psychiatric illness. During a psychiatric evaluation he is asked the meaning of the proverb "People in glass houses should not throw stones." The patient replies, "They will break the windows." This response is an example of

   a. Idiosyncratic thinking
   b. Concrete thinking
   c. Formal operation
   d. Loose associations
   e. Autistic thinking

Items 2 and 3

Match the symptoms with the most appropriate diagnosis.

   a. Conversion disorder
   b. Specific phobia
   c. Agoraphobia
   d. Narcissistic personality disorder
   e. Body dysmorphic disorder
   f. Schizophrenia
   g. Borderline personality disorder
   h. Dissociative amnesia

2. The career of a young executive who needs to travel often for his business is much impaired because, due to his overwhelming fear of flying, he refuses all the jobs that require traveling by plane.

3. A young woman who has ambivalent feelings about separating from her family wakes up paralyzed on the morning she is scheduled to go back to college.

4. A 27-year-old woman has been sad for the past two weeks. She is fatigued and has a hard time concentrating at work. Just a few weeks earlier she was energetic and enthusiastic, and was able to work 10–12 hours a day with little sleep and go dancing at night. Her husband wants a divorce because he is tired of "these constant ups and downs." The most accurate diagnosis is
   a. Borderline personality disorder
   b. Seasonal mood disorder
   c. Dissociative identity disorder
   d. Cyclothymic disorder
   e. Recurrent major depression

Answers

1. **The answer is b.** Patients who present with concrete thinking have lost the ability to form abstract concepts, such as metaphors, and focus instead on actual things and facts. Concrete thinking is the norm in children and is seen in cognitive disorders (mental retardation, dementia) and schizophrenia.

2–3. **The answers are 2-b, 3-a.** Fear of flying is one of the many presentations of specific phobias. Phobic individuals have an excessive or unreasonable fear of an object, an animal, or a situation. When exposed to the feared stimulus, they experience severe anxiety that can reach the level of panic attack. Characteristically, phobic patients go to great lengths to avoid whatever they fear and this phobic avoidance can greatly interfere with functioning.

   Conversion disorder is characterized by the sudden appearance of often dramatic neurological symptoms that are not associated with the usual diagnostic signs and test results. Conversion disorder occurs in the context of a psychosocial stressor or an insoluble interpersonal or intrapsychic conflict. The psychological distress is not consciously acknowledged but it is expressed through a metaphorical body dysfunction. In the vignette example, the young woman who was torn between leaving home and becoming independent found a temporary solution in her paralysis, which prevented her from leaving her home without having to consciously acknowledge her conflict.

4. **The answer is d.** Cyclothymic disorder is characterized by recurrent periods of mild depression alternating with periods of hypomania. This pattern has to have been present for at least two years (one year for children and adolescents) before the diagnosis can be made. During these two years, the symptom-free intervals should not be longer than two months. Cyclothymic disorder usually starts during adolescence or early adulthood and tends to have a chronic course. The marked shifts in mood of cyclothymic disorder can be confused with the affective instability of borderline personality disorder or may suggest a substance abuse problem.

Pulmonary

Lung—physical findings

Abnormality	Breath Sounds	Resonance	Fremitus	Tracheal Deviation
Bronchial obstruction	Absent over area	↓	↓	Toward side of lesion
Pleural effusion	↓ over effusion	Dullness	↓	—
Pneumonia (lobar)	May have bronchial breath sounds over lesion	Dullness	↑	—
Pneumothorax	↓	Hyperresonant	Absent	Away from side of lesion

Lung volumes

1. Residual volume (RV)—air in lung at maximal expiration
2. Expiratory reserve volume (ERV)—air that can still be breathed out after normal expiration
3. Tidal volume (TV)—air that moves into lung with each quiet inspiration, typically 500 mL
4. Inspiratory reserve volume (IRV)—air in excess of tidal volume that moves into lung on maximum inspiration
5. Vital capacity (VC)—TV + IRV + ERV
6. Functional reserve capacity (FRC)—RV + ERV (volume in lungs after a normal respiration)
7. Inspiratory capacity (IC)—IRV + TV
8. Total lung capacity—TLC = IRV + TV + ERV + RV

Vital capacity is everything but the residual volume.

A capacity is a sum of ≥ 2 volumes.

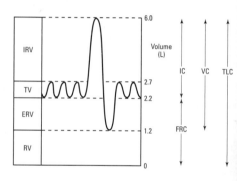

Obstructive vs. restrictive lung disease

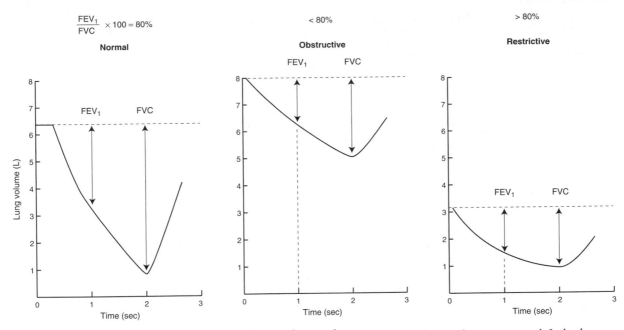

$$\frac{FEV_1}{FVC} \times 100 = 80\%$$

Normal

< 80%

Obstructive

> 80%

Restrictive

Note: Obstructive lung volumes > normal (↑ TLC, ↑ FRC, ↑ RV); restrictive lung volumes < normal. In both obstructive and restrictive, FEV_1 and FVC are reduced, but in obstructive, FEV_1 is more dramatically reduced, resulting in a ↓ FEV_1/FVC ratio.

V/Q mismatch

Zone 1		$P_A > P_a > P_v$
Zone 2		$P_a > P_A > P_v$
Zone 3		$P_a > P_v > P_A$

Ideally, ventilation is matched to perfusion (i.e., V/Q = 1) in order for adequate oxygenation to occur efficiently.

Lung zones:
1. Apex of the lung—V/Q = 3 (wasted ventilation)
2. Base of the lung—V/Q = 0.6 (wasted perfusion)

Both ventilation and perfusion are greater at the base of the lung than at the apex of the lung.

With exercise (↑ cardiac output), there is vasodilation of apical capillaries, resulting in a V/Q ratio that approaches 1.

Certain organisms that thrive in high O_2 (e.g., TB) flourish in the apex.

V/Q → 0 = airway obstruction.

V/Q → ∞ = blood flow obstruction.

Asthma drugs

Nonspecific beta agonists	**Isoproterenol**—relaxes bronchial smooth muscle (β_2). Adverse effect is tachycardia (β_1).
β_2 agonists	**Albuterol**—relaxes bronchial smooth muscle (β_2). Use during acute exacerbation.
	Salmeterol—long-acting agent for prophylaxis. Adverse effects are tremor and arrhythmia.
Methylxanthines	**Theophylline**—likely causes bronchodilation by inhibiting phosphodiesterase, thereby $\downarrow$ cAMP hydrolysis. The usage is limited because of narrow therapeutic index (cardiotoxicity, neurotoxicity).
Muscarinic antagonists	**Ipratropium**—competitive block of muscarinic receptors, preventing bronchoconstriction.
Cromolyn	Prevents release of mediators from mast cells. Effective only for the prophylaxis of asthma. Not effective during an acute asthmatic attack. Toxicity is rare.
Corticosteroids	**Beclomethasone, prednisone**—inhibits the synthesis of virtually all cytokines. Inactivates NF-κB, the transcription factor that induces the production of TNFα, among other inflammatory agents. 1st-line therapy for chronic asthma.
Antileukotrienes	**Zileuton**—A 5-lipoxygenase pathway inhibitor. Blocks conversion of arachidonic acid to leukotrienes.
	Zafirlukast—blocks leukotriene receptors.

Exposure to antigen
(dust, pollen, etc.)

Avoidance

Antigen and IgE
on mast cells

Cromolyn
Steroids

Mediators
(leukotrienes, histamine, etc.)

Steroids

Beta-agonist
Theophylline
Muscarinic
antagonists

Late response:
inflammation

Early response:
bronchoconstriction

Bronchial
hyperreactivity

Symptoms

Treatment strategies in asthma

Bronchodilation

ATP

AC ← (+) **Beta-agonists**

(+) ← cAMP

Bronchial tone

PDE ← (−) **Theophylline**

→ AMP

Acetylcholine → (+) → ← (+) ← Adenosine

Muscarinic antagonists (−)   (−) **Theophylline**

Bronchoconstriction

(Adapted, with permission, from Katzung BG, Trevor AJ. *Examination & Board Review: Pharmacology*, 5th ed. Stamford, CT: Appleton & Lange, 1998:159, 161.)

Acute respiratory failure with refractory **hypoxemia, decreased lung compliance,** and **noncardiogenic pulmonary edema.** Its underlying pathogenesis is thought to be endothelial injury. ARDS commonly occurs in the setting of sepsis, aspiration, infection, multiple blood transfusions, inhaled/ingested toxins, trauma, multiorgan failure, or shock. Overall mortality is > 50%.

ARDS occurs in the setting of aspiration, infection, shock, or sepsis.

History/PE

Presents with acute onset (12–48 hours) of tachypnea, dyspnea, tachycardia, fever, cyanosis, labored breathing, diffuse, high-pitched rales, and hypoxemia. There is usually a progression of symptoms:

- **Phase 1:** Acute injury—normal physical exam, respiratory alkalosis.
- **Phase 2:** 6–48 hours after injury—hyperventilation, hypocapnia, widening alveolar-arterial (A-a) oxygen gradient.
- **Phase 3:** Acute respiratory failure, tachypnea, dyspnea, decreased lung compliance, scattered rales, diffuse chest infiltrates on CXR (see Figure 2.15–1).
- **Phase 4:** Severe hypoxemia unresponsive to therapy; increased intrapulmonary shunting; metabolic and respiratory acidosis.

Differential

Cardiogenic pulmonary edema, pneumonia, bronchiolitis obliterans with organizing pneumonia, pulmonary hemorrhage.

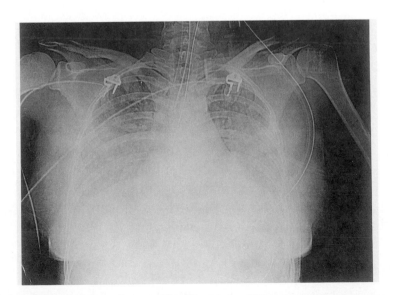

FIGURE 2.15–1. Acute respiratory distress syndrome. Note the diffuse, extensive bilateral interstitial and alveolar infiltrates on PA CXR. (Reproduced, with permission, from Isselbacher KJ. *Harrison's Principles of Internal Medicine,* 13th ed. Stamford, CT: McGraw-Hill, 1994:1241, Fig. 230–1.)

HIGH-YIELD FACTS

Pulmonary

Evaluation

The criteria for ARDS diagnosis (the American-European Consensus Conference definition) are as follows:

- Acute onset of respiratory distress.
- **PaO_2/FIO_2 ratio $\leq$ 200 mmHg.**
- Bilateral pulmonary infiltrates on CXR.
- **No evidence of cardiac origin** (normal capillary wedge pressure = 18 mmHg).

Treatment

There is no standard successful treatment. **Treat the underlying disease and maintain adequate perfusion and O_2 delivery to organs.** Use mechanical ventilation with low PEEP (because of decreased lung compliance) and increased inspiratory times. Maintain oxygenation with a goal of $FIO_2 < 0.6$, PaO_2 of > 60 mmHg, and $SaO_2 > 90\%$. Support cardiac output with inotropes and cautious fluid administration. Steroids have been shown to increase mortality in patients with sepsis and ARDS.

UCV *IM2.42*

ASTHMA

Asthma triggers include allergens, URIs, cold air, exercise, and stress.

Reversible airway obstruction secondary to bronchial **hyperreactivity,** airway **inflammation, mucous plugging,** and **smooth muscle hypertrophy** of the airways. Triggers include allergens (dust, animal hair, odors), URIs, cold air, exertion, and stress. Note that chronic airway inflammation is a consistent feature of all asthma.

History

Beware — all that wheezes is not asthma.

Presents with **cough,** dyspnea, **episodic wheezing,** and/or chest tightness along with a history of frequent ER visits, intubations, and PO steroid use. Symptoms often worsen at night or early in the morning. Male sex and older age are additional historical risk factors.

PE

Exam reveals tachypnea, tachycardia, decreased breath sounds, **wheezing, prolonged expiratory duration** (decreased I/E ratio), decreased O_2 saturation (late sign), hyperresonance, **accessory muscle use,** and possibly pulsus paradoxus.

Differential

Asthma should be suspected in children with multiple episodes of croup and URIs associated with dyspnea.

- **Children:** Aspiration, bronchiolitis, bronchopulmonary dysplasia, CF, GERD, vascular rings, pneumonia.
- **Adults:** CHF, COPD, GERD, pulmonary embolism (PE), foreign body, tumor, sleep apnea, anaphylaxis.

Evaluation

- **ABG: Mild hypoxia** and **respiratory alkalosis.** Normalizing P_{CO_2} in acute exacerbation warrants close observation, as it may indicate fatigue of ventilatory muscles and impending respiratory failure.
- **Spirometry/pulmonary function tests (PFTs): Peak flow** is **diminished** during acute exacerbation. Decreased 1-second forced expiratory volume (FEV_1).
- **CBC: Eosinophilia.**
- **CXR: Hyperinflation.**
- **Methacholine challenge:** Tests for bronchial hyperresponsiveness. Allows definitive diagnosis (when the patient is not acutely ill).

Treatment

In general, avoid allergens or any potential exacerbating factor. The medications used for asthma treatment can be remembered using the mnemonic **ASTHMA.**

- **Acute management:** Treat with O_2, **bronchodilating agents** (β-agonists; first-line therapy), ipratropium (never used alone), and **steroids** (systemic steroids if severe). Positive airway pressure and Heliox may be used to avoid intubation in severe cases.
- **Chronic management:** Measurements of lung function using FEV_1, peak flow, and (in severe exacerbations) ABGs are essential to guide management. Administer regularly inhaled **bronchodilators** and/or steroids, systemic **steroids,** cromolyn, or **theophylline. Montelukast** and other leukotriene antagonists are oral agents that may serve as adjuncts to inhalant therapy (see Table 2.15–1).

Medications used to treat asthma exacerbations—

ASTHMA
Albuterol
Steroids
Theophylline
Humidified O_2
Magnesium
Anti-leukotrienes

TABLE 2.15–1. Medications for Chronic Treatment of Asthma

Type	Symptoms (day/night)	FEV$_1$	Medications
Severe persistent	Continual Frequent	≤ 60%	High-dose inhaled corticosteroids + long-acting inhaled β$_2$-agonists. Possible PO steroids. prn short-acting bronchodilator.
Moderate persistent	Daily > 1 night/week	60 – 80%	Low- to medium-dose inhaled corticosteroids + long-acting inhaled β$_2$-agonists. prn short-acting bronchodilator.
Mild persistent	> 2/week but < 1/day > 2 nights/month	≥ 80%	Low-dose inhaled corticosteroids. prn short-acting bronchodilator.
Mild intermittent	≤ 2 days/week ≤ 2 nights/month	≥ 80%	No daily medications. prn short-acting bronchodilator.

UCV *IM2.44*

A disease of the bronchi and bronchioles involving cycles of infection and inflammation that result in permanent remodeling and **dilatation of bronchi** with suppuration.

History/PE

Usually follows pneumonia. Presents with yellow or green **sputum, cough,** dyspnea, and possible hemoptysis and halitosis. Associated with a history of pulmonary infections (e.g., *Pseudomonas, Haemophilus,* TB), hypersensitivity (allergic bronchopulmonary aspergillosis), CF, immunodeficiency, aspiration, autoimmune disease (e.g., rheumatoid arthritis, SLE), or inflammatory bowel disease. Physical exam reveals rales, wheezes, rhonchi purulent mucus, and occasional hemoptysis.

Differential

COPD, atelectasis, asthma, bronchitis, pneumonia.

Evaluation

CXR may show increased bronchovascular markings from peribronchial fibrosis and intrabronchial secretions; crowding from an atelectatic lung; **tram lines** (parallel lines outlining dilated bronchi due to peribronchial inflammation and fibrosis); and areas of **honeycombing. High-resolution CT** shows **dilatation of the airway,** varicose constriction, lack of airway taper, and ballooned cysts at the end of the bronchus, primarily affecting the lower lobes. IgG, IgA, and IgM studies may show specific subclass deficiency. Spirometry shows a reduced FEV_1/FVC ratio.

Treatment

Give antibiotics (erythromycin, fluoroquinolone, inhaled aminoglucosides, and others) if bacterial and possibly inhaled corticosteroids. Maintain bronchopulmonary hygiene (cough control, postural drainage, chest physiotherapy, thinning of secretions). Lobectomy or lung transplantation considered for severe disease.

CHRONIC OBSTRUCTIVE PULMONARY DISEASE

Causes of obstructive
pulmonary disease:
COPD (emphysema, bronchitis)
Asthma
Bronchiectasis
Cystic fibrosis
Tracheal or bronchial
*   obstruction*

A chronic, progressive disease characterized by decreased lung function with airflow obstruction. COPD is generally due to chronic bronchitis or emphysema. **Chronic bronchitis** is a productive cough lasting at least three months per year for two consecutive years. **Emphysema** is a pathologic diagnosis of terminal airway destruction due to smoking (centrilobular) or inherited α_1-**antitrypsin deficiency** (panlobular). Most patients have components of both centrilobular and panlobular, and **nearly all are smokers.** COPD is the fourth most common cause of death in the United States.

History/PE

Symptoms are often minimal or nonspecific until the disease is advanced (with loss of > 50% of lung function):

- **Emphysema ("pink puffer"): Dyspnea, pursed lips,** minimal cough, decreased breath sounds, late hypercarbia/hypoxia. Pure emphysematous patients tend to have less reactive airways between exacerbations.
- **Chronic bronchitis ("blue bloater"): Productive cough,** cyanotic but with mild dyspnea; frequently overweight with peripheral edema, rhonchi, and early hypercarbia/hypoxia. Patients may not demonstrate the hyperinflation and sparse lung markings on CXR.

Also look for barrel chest, use of accessory chest muscles, JVD, end-expiratory **wheezing,** or muffled breath sounds.

Differential

Acute bronchitis, asthma, bronchiectasis, CHF, CF, bronchogenic carcinoma.

Evaluation

- **CXR:** Classically shows decreased markings with flat diaphragms, **hyperinflated lungs,** and a thin-appearing heart and mediastinum. Parenchymal **bullae** or subpleural **blebs** may be noted and are pathognomonic of emphysema (see Figure 2.15–2).
- **PFTs:** Diagnostic (see Table 2.15–2).
- **ABG:** During an acute exacerbation, will show **hypoxemia** with **acute respiratory acidosis** (increased P_{CO_2}; however, patients have baseline increased P_{CO_2}).

Rising P_{CO_2} may indicate fatigue and impending respiratory failure.

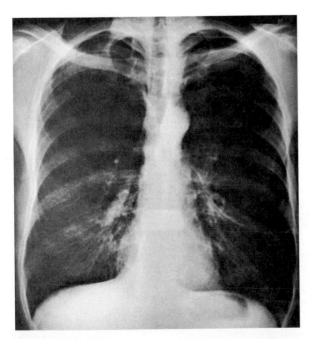

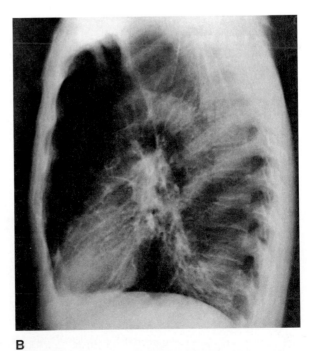

A　　　　　　　　　　　　　　　**B**

FIGURE 2.15–2. Chronic obstructive pulmonary disease. Note the hyperinflated and hyperlucent lungs, flat diaphragms, increased AP diameter, narrow mediastinum, and large upper lobe bullae on (A) AP and (B) lateral CXRs. (Reproduced, with permission, from Stobo JD et al. *Principles and Practice of Medicine,* 23rd ed. Stamford, CT: Appleton & Lange, 1997:135, Fig. 2.3–2.)

TABLE 2.15–2. PFTs in Obstructive and Restrictive Lung Disease		
Measurement[a]	**Obstructive**	**Restrictive**
Spirometry		
FEV_1	↓ or N (asthma between exacerbations)	N or ↓
FEV_{25-75}	↓	N or ↓
FEV_1/FVC	↓	N or ↑
Lung volumes		
FVC	N or ↓	↓
VC	N or ↓	↓
TLC	N or ↑ (emphysema, asthma)	↓
RV	↑ (in air trapping)	N, ↓, or ↑

[a]FVC = forced vital capacity; VC = vital capacity; TLC = total lung capacity; RV = residual volume.
(Adapted, with permission, from Tierney LM. *Current Medical Diagnosis & Treatment.* Stamford, CT: Appleton & Lange, 1997:239.)

- **Blood cultures:** If patient is febrile.
- **Gram stain and sputum culture:** Obtain if the patient is febrile or has a productive cough.

> *"CO$_2$ retainers" occasionally do worse with supplemental O$_2$ because they lose their hypoxemic drive to breathe and acutely increase their PCO$_2$.*

Treatment

- **Acute exacerbations:** O$_2$, inhaled β-agonists (albuterol) and **anticholinergics** (ipratropium), IV steroids, antibiotics.
- **Chronic: Smoking cessation,** supplemental O$_2$, inhaled β-agonists (albuterol), anticholinergics (ipratropium) and steroids. Pneumococcal and **flu vaccines.** Severe cases may benefit from noninvasive ventilation.

Complications

Chronic respiratory failure, cor pulmonale, pneumonia, bronchogenic carcinoma.

UCV *IM2.45,46*

CYSTIC FIBROSIS

An **autosomal-recessive (chromosome 7)** disorder caused by mutations in the CFTR gene (chloride channel) and characterized by widespread **exocrine gland dysfunction.** CF is the most common severe genetic disease in the United States and is most frequently found in **Caucasians.** It was previously considered a childhood disease, but life expectancy has increased such that many CF patients are treated well into adulthood.

History

- **Respiratory: Recurrent pulmonary infections** (especially with *Pseudomonas* and *S. aureus*), cyanosis, digital clubbing, cough, dyspnea, **bronchiectasis,** hemoptysis, chronic sinusitis.
- **GI:** Fifteen percent of infants present with **meconium ileus.** Patients usually have greasy stools and flatulence. **Malabsorption syndromes,** failure to thrive (FTT), pancreatitis, rectal prolapse, esophageal varices, and biliary cirrhosis may be seen.
- **Other: Abnormal glucose tolerance,** type 2 diabetes, "salty taste," unexplained hyponatremia. Most males are infertile. Fifty percent of patients present with FTT or respiratory compromise.

PE

Presents with cough, rhonchi, rales, hyperresonance to percussion, and nasal polyposis. Growth retardation and digital clubbing are also seen.

Differential

Immunodeficiency, asthma, celiac sprue, GERD, poor caloric intake.

Evaluation

Sweat chloride test > 60 mEq/L for those < 20 years of age, > 80 mEq/L in adults; genetic testing.

Treatment

Pulmonary manifestations are managed with **chest physical therapy, bronchodilators, anti-inflammatory agents, antibiotics,** and **DNase.** Administer **pancreatic enzymes** and **fat-soluble vitamins A, D, E, and K** for malabsorption. Nutritional counseling and support are essential to health maintenance in cystics. Patients with severe disease (but who can tolerate surgery) may be candidates for lung or pancreas transplants.

DIFFUSE INTERSTITIAL PULMONARY FIBROSIS

The most common restrictive pulmonary disease; characterized by thickening of the interstitium of the alveolar wall leading to cystic spaces formed by dilated terminal and respiratory bronchioles. Most common in the elderly.

History/PE

Presents with **shallow, rapid breathing;** dyspnea with exercise; and nonproductive **cough.** Exam reveals cyanosis worsened by exercise. Patients may have fine rales and finger clubbing.

Drugs associated with interstitial lung disease: busulfan, nitrofurantoin, amiodarone, bleomycin, radiation, long-term high O_2 concentration (ventilator).

Differential

Other causes of restrictive lung disease **(PAINT).** Also consider hypersensitivity pneumonitis, TB, pulmonary histiocytosis X, and fungal infection.

Evaluation

A **honeycomb** pattern is seen on **CXR** with severe disease. Otherwise, CXR shows a reticular pattern that is usually more pronounced at the bases. TLC and FVC are low, and FEV_1/FVC is increased.

Treatment

Treatment is supportive. Possibly steroids, cytotoxic agents, and immunomodulatory substances.

HYPERSENSITIVITY PNEUMONITIS

A type III hypersensitivity reaction affecting the lung parenchyma secondary to inhaled organic material. The types and causes of hypersensitivity pneumonitis are summarized in Table 2.15–3. Alveolar walls thicken with lymphocytic plasma cells and histiocytes, forming small granulomas. Fibrosis is seen in the chronic form.

History

- **Acute:** Dyspnea, fever, shivering, cough starting 4–6 hours after exposure.
- **Chronic:** Progressive dyspnea.

PE

Exam reveals fine bilateral rales.

TABLE 2.15–3. Antigens of Hypersensitivity Pneumonitis

Disorder	Antigen
Farmer's lung	Spores of actinomycetes from moldy hay
Bird fancier's lung	Antigens from feathers, excreta, serum
Mushroom worker's lung	Spores of actinomycetes from compost
Malt worker's lung	Spores of *Aspergillus clavatus*
Grain handler's lung	Grain weevil dust
Bagassosis	Spores of actinomycetes from sugarcane
Air conditioner lung	Spores of actinomycetes from air conditioners

Differential

Diffuse interstitial pulmonary fibrosis, scleroderma, sarcoidosis.

Evaluation

CXR shows miliary nodular infiltrate to normal findings in the acute phase and fibrosis in the upper lobes in the chronic phase.

Treatment

Avoid ongoing exposure. Possible treatments include steroids, cytotoxic agents, and immunomodulatory substances.

HYPOXEMIA

Defined as a decreased blood O_2 content due to **alveolar hypoventilation.** This can in turn be due to a right-to-left shunt, hyperventilation, increased blood velocity, **decreased inspired O_2 tension,** an airway obstruction or **ventilation-perfusion mismatch,** or a **diffusion impairment.**

Causes of hypoxemia:

Right-to-left shunt

Hypoventilation

Low inspired O_2 tension

Ventilation-perfusion mismatch

Diffusion defect

↑ blood velocity

History/PE

Physical findings depend on the etiology but are always significant for **decreased HbO_2 saturation.** Other signs and symptoms may include cyanosis, tachypnea, shortness of breath, pleuritic chest pain, and altered mental status.

Differential

Almost all of the diseases listed in this chapter may cause hypoxemia. Think of the differential based on the different pathophysiological mechanisms of hypoxemia described above. Acutely, think of ARDS, PE, atelectasis, and asthma. Chronically, think of COPD and diffuse interstitial pulmonary fibrosis.

Evaluation

Pulse oximetry will demonstrate decreased Hb O_2 saturation. Obtain a **CXR** to rule out ARDS, atelectasis, or an infiltrative process (i.e., pneumonia) and to look for signs of PE (see "Pulmonary Embolism," p. 442). Obtain an **ABG** to evaluate PaO_2 and to calculate an **A-a gradient** $[(P_{atm} - 47) \times FIO_2] - [(PaCO_2/0.8) - PaO_2]$. An elevated A-a gradient suggests a V/Q mismatch or a diffusion impairment.

Treatment

Treatment should be in accordance with the underlying etiology. Always give a hypoxemic patient O_2 before initiating any evaluation. If a patient is on a ventilator, O_2 saturation can be increased by **increasing FIO_2, increasing PEEP,** or increasing the I/E ratio.

Always give a hypoxic patient oxygen.

Note that hypercapnic patients are treated by increasing minute ventilation. This is done by either increasing tidal volume or increasing the respiratory rate.

Abnormal accumulation of fluid in the pleural space. Pleural effusions are classified as **transudative** or **exudative.**

History/PE

Often **asymptomatic,** but patients may present with **dyspnea** and **pleuritic chest pain.** Physical exam is marked by decreased breath sounds, dullness to percussion, and **decreased** tactile fremitus.

Differential

Transudative and exudative pleural effusions may be differentiated as follows:

	Pleural/Serum Protein	**Pleural/Serum LDH**
Transudate	< 0.5	< 0.6
Exudate	> 0.5	> 0.6

- **Transudative effusion: Intact capillaries** lead to protein-poor pleural fluid that is an ultrafiltrate of plasma. Common causes of pleural fluid transudates include **CHF, nephrotic syndrome, cirrhosis,** and **protein-losing enteropathy.**
- **Exudative effusion:** Inflammation leads to **leaky capillaries,** resulting in protein-rich pleural fluid. Common causes of exudative pleural effusions include **malignancy, TB, bacterial infection** (parapneumonic effusion and empyema), viral infection, pulmonary emboli with infarct, collagen vascular disease, pancreatitis, hemothorax, chylothorax, and traumatic tap. Note that CHF can also produce an exudative effusion.

Evaluation

- **CXR: Blunting of the costophrenic angles.** A decubitus CXR will determine whether the fluid is free flowing or loculated.
- **Pleural fluid analysis: LDH** and **protein** analysis, as above. Obtain a Gram stain and a CBC with differential and culture for evidence of infection or trauma (increased RBCs). Increased **amylase** suggests malignancy or pancreatitis. Cytology may reveal malignant cells.
- Needle biopsy of pleura diagnoses TB effusion.
- Definitive diagnosis is made by thoracocentesis or open biopsy.

Treatment

- **Transudative:** Treat the underlying condition. Perform therapeutic thoracocentesis if the patient is dyspneic.
- **Malignant:** Consider pleurodesis (injection of an irritant into the pleural cavity to scar the two pleural layers together) in symptomatic patients who are unresponsive to chemotherapy and radiation therapy. Alternatives include therapeutic thoracocentesis, pleuroperitoneal shunting, and surgical pleurectomy.

- **Parapneumonic:** Pleural effusion in the presence of pneumonia. If there is evidence of empyema (frank pus, pH < 7.2, glucose < 40 mg/dL, positive Gram stain), initiate chest tube drainage. Here the aim of fluid analysis is to identify **complicated** parapneumonic effusion.
- **Hemothorax:** Chest tube.

An occupational lung injury affecting the pulmonary interstitium. Typically, interstitial lung disease develops after long-term, high-concentration exposure to particles that are inhaled and induce inflammation and fibrosis. The risk of disease increases with the level and duration of exposure. Now becoming rare in developed countries owing to the enforcement of safety regulations.

History/PE

See Table 2.15–4 for the history, diagnosis, and complications of pneumoconioses.

TABLE 2.15–4. Pneumoconioses

	History	Diagnosis	Complications
Asbestosis	Work involving manufacture of tile or brake linings, insulation, construction, demolition, or building maintenance. Presents 15–20 years after initial exposure.	CXR: linear opacities at lung bases and pleural plaques. Biopsy: asbestos bodies.	Increased risk of mesothelioma and lung cancer, worse in smokers.
Coal mine disease	Work in underground coal mines.	CXR: small nodular opacities (< 1 cm) in upper lung zones. Spirometry: consistent with restrictive disease.	Progressive massive fibrosis.
Silicosis	Work in mines or quarries or with glass, pottery, silica.	CXR: small (< 1 cm) nodular opacities in upper lung zones. **Eggshell calcifications.** Spirometry: consistent with restrictive disease.	Increased risk of TB; need annual TB skin test. Progressive massive fibrosis.
Berylliosis	Work in high-technology fields such as aerospace, nuclear, and electronics plants; ceramics industries; foundries; plating facilities; dental material sites; and die manufacturing.	CXR: diffuse infiltrates, hilar adenopathy.	Requires chronic steroid treatments.

Evaluation

CXR may show linear or nodular opacification. A **high-resolution CT** scan is used in patients with a normal CXR who are suspected of having pneumoconiosis.

Treatment

There is no cure for pneumoconioses. Treatment generally involves supportive therapy and O_2 supplementation. Patients should quit smoking, as it can have an additive detrimental effect. Physicians who diagnose these conditions should alert the appropriate agency.

UCV *IM2.43,49*

PNEUMOTHORAX

A collection of air in the pleural space that can lead to pulmonary collapse.

- **Primary spontaneous** pneumothorax is due to rupture of subpleural apical blebs (usually in **tall, thin young males**).
- **Secondary** causes of pneumothorax include COPD, TB, trauma, *Pneumocystis carinii* pneumonia (PCP), and iatrogenesis (thoracocentesis, subclavian line placement, positive-pressure mechanical ventilation, or bronchoscopy).
- **Tension** pneumothorax occurs when a pulmonary or chest wall defect acts as a **one-way valve,** drawing air into the pleural space during inspiration but trapping air during expiration. Etiologies include penetrating trauma, infection, CHF, and positive-pressure mechanical ventilation. Tension pneumothorax is a **life-threatening condition** that proceeds to shock and death unless it is immediately recognized and treated.

Tension pneumothorax is a medical emergency.

History/PE

Unilateral pleuritic chest pain and **dyspnea.** Physical exam reveals tachypnea, **diminished/absent breath sounds, hyperresonance,** and **decreased tactile fremitus.** Suspect tension pneumothorax if you see respiratory distress, falling O_2 saturation, hypotension, distended neck veins, and **tracheal deviation.**

Differential

MI, pulmonary emboli, pneumonia, pericardial tamponade, pleural effusion.

Evaluation

CXR often shows a visceral pleural line and/or **lung retraction** from the chest wall (best seen in end-expiratory films; see Figure 2.15–3).

Treatment

Small pneumothoraces may reabsorb spontaneously. Supplemental O_2 therapy may be helpful. Large, symptomatic pneumothoraces require chest tube place-

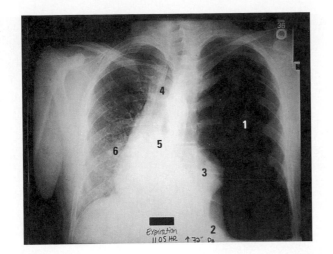

FIGURE 2.15–3. Tension pneumothorax. Note the hyperlucent lung field (1), hyperexpanded lower diaphragm (2), collapsed lung (3), tracheal deviation (4), mediastinal shift (5), and compression of the opposite lung (6) on AP CXR.

ment and/or pleurodesis. **Tension pneumothorax is an emergency** requiring immediate needle decompression in the second intercostal space at the midclavicular line. Do not wait for a CXR! After initial decompression, insert a chest tube.

UCV *IM2.47*

PULMONARY EDEMA

Abnormal accumulation of fluid in extravascular space. See Table 2.15–5 for common causes and precipitating events.

History

Dyspnea, orthopnea, paroxysmal nocturnal dyspnea, Cheyne-Stokes breathing, cough, cyanosis.

TABLE 2.15–5. Causes of Pulmonary Edema

Mechanism	Precipitating events
Increased capillary hydrostatic pressure	MI, mitral stenosis, fluid overload, heart failure
Increased capillary permeability	Sepsis, radiation, oxygen toxicity, ARDS, toxins
Reduced lymph drainage	Increased central venous pressure
Decreased interstitial pressure	Rapid removal of pleural effusion
Decreased colloid pressure	Hypoalbuminemia
Other etiologies	High altitude, neurogenic, overinflation, narcotics

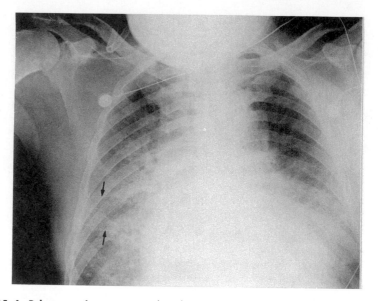

FIGURE 2.15–4. Pulmonary edema. Interstitial and air-space pulmonary edema. (Reproduced, with permission, from Novelline RA. *Squire's Fundamentals of Radiology,* 5th ed. Cambridge, MA: Harvard University Press, 1997:187, Fig. 10–22.)

PE

Rales on inspiration, musical rhonchi, possible murmurs if cardiogenic.

Differential

ARDS, cardiogenic pulmonary edema, neurogenic pulmonary edema, aspiration, pneumonia.

Evaluation

CXR reveals an enlarged heart, prominent pulmonary vessels, **Kerley B lines,** "bat's-wing" appearance of hilar shadows, and perivascular and peribronchial cuffing (see Figure 2.15–4).

Treatment

Treat the underlying cause. Diuretics. Arrhythmia management, inotropes and afterload reduction may be necessary in selected cases.

PULMONARY EMBOLISM (PE)

Occlusion of the pulmonary vasculature, typically by a blood clot. Ninety-five percent of emboli originate from DVTs in the deep leg veins. Pulmonary thromboembolism often leads to pulmonary infarction, right heart failure (RHF), and hypoxia. Risk factors for DVT and subsequent pulmonary thromboembolism include **Virchow's triad:**

- **Stasis:** Immobility, CHF, obesity, surgery, increased CVP.
- **Endothelial injury:** Trauma, surgery, recent fracture, previous DVT.

- **Hypercoagulable states:** Pregnancy/postpartum, OCP use, coagulation disorders such as protein C/protein S deficiency, factor V Leiden, malignancy, severe burns.

History

Sudden-onset dyspnea, **pleuritic chest pain, low-grade fever,** cough, and, rarely, hemoptysis or hypotension and syncope.

PE

- **Pulmonary embolism:** Hypoxia with hypocarbia with resulting respiratory alkalosis. Tachypnea, tachycardia, fever. Loud P2. Prominent jugular a waves with RHF.
- **Venous thrombosis:** Homans' sign (calf pain on forced dorsiflexion), cords on the calf. Neither is sensitive.

Differential

Pneumonia, MI, CHF, pericarditis, intracardiac shunt, other intrapulmonary shunt.

Evaluation

Dyspnea, tachycardia, and a normal CXR in a hospitalized and/or bedridden patient should raise suspicion of PE.

Consider pulmonary embolism in any dyspneic hospitalized patient.

- **ABG: Respiratory alkalosis** (due to hyperventilation), with $P_{O_2} < 80$ mm (90% sensitive). The A-a gradient may be elevated with arterial hypoxemia.
- **CXR:** Usually normal, but may show a pleural effusion, **Hampton's hump** (wedge-shaped infarct), or **Westermark's sign** (oligemia in the embolized lung zone). Most common abnormal finding is simply atelectasis.
- **ECG:** Not diagnostic. Most commonly reveals **sinus tachycardia.** The classic triad of **"S1Q3T3"**—acute right heart strain with an S in lead I, a Q wave in lead III, and an inverted T-wave in lead III—is uncommon.
- **V/Q scan:** May reveal segmental areas of mismatch. Results are reported with a designated probability of pulmonary embolism (low, indeterminate, high) and are interpreted on the basis of clinical suspicion.
- **Helical (spiral) CT with IV contrast:** Sensitive for pulmonary embolism in the proximal pulmonary arteries but less so in the distal segmental arteries.
- **Pulmonary angiogram:** Gold standard but is more invasive (see Figure 2.15–5).
- See Figure 2.15–6 for the diagnostic algorithm.

Treatment

- **Heparin:** Bolus and then weight-based continuous infusion.
- **Warfarin:** For long-term anticoagulation, usually 3–6 months of therapy unless the underlying predisposing factor persists (then indefinitely). Follow INR; maintain between 2 and 3.

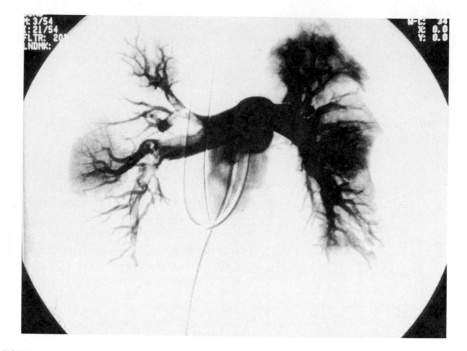

FIGURE 2.15–5. Pulmonary embolus. A large filling defect in the pulmonary artery is evident on pulmonary angiogram. (Reproduced from Le T. *First Aid for the USMLE Step 2*, 3rd ed. New York: McGraw-Hill, 2001:404, Fig 2.15–1.)

DVT prophylaxis is an often overlooked issue in the hospital and a major cause of morbidity and mortality.

- **IVC filter:** Indicated if anticoagulation is contraindicated or if the patient has recurrent emboli while anticoagulated.
- **Thrombolysis:** Indicated only in severe cases.
- **DVT prophylaxis:** Treat bedridden medical patients and surgical patients, use **low-dose subcutaneous heparin,** low-molecular-weight heparin (LMWH), intermittent pneumatic compression of the lower extremities (less effective), and **early ambulation (most effective).** LMWH,

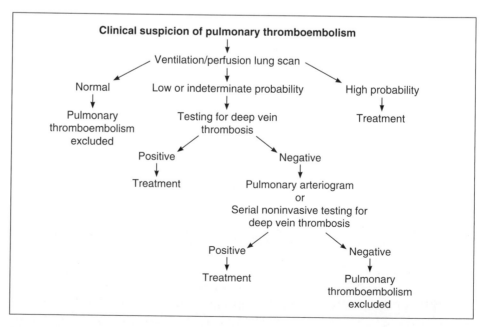

FIGURE 2.15–6. Diagnostic approach to pulmonary embolism. (Reproduced, with permission, from Tierney LM. *Current Medical Diagnosis & Treatment,* 39th ed. New York: McGraw-Hill, 2000:326, Fig. 9–2.)

which is administered subcutaneously and does not require monitoring of bleeding times, has a reduced risk of complications such as GI bleeding. LMWH is now accepted as an alternative means of anticoagulation on an outpatient basis.

SARCOIDOSIS

A systemic disease of unknown etiology characterized by **noncaseating granulomas.** In the United States, sarcoid is most common in **black females** and usually presents in the third or fourth decade of life.

History/PE

Presents with **fever, cough, malaise,** weight loss, dyspnea, and **arthritis,** commonly of the knees and ankles. The lungs, liver, eyes, skin (erythema nodosum), nervous system, heart, and kidney may be affected. The symptoms can be **GRUELING.**

> **Features of sarcoid—**
>
> **GRUELING**
> **G**ranulomas
> **R**heumatoid arthritis
> **U**veitis
> **E**rythema nodosum
> **L**ymphadenopathy
> **I**nterstitial fibrosis
> **N**egative TB test
> **G**ammaglobulinemia

Differential

TB, fungal infections, foreign body reaction, lymphoma, berylliosis.

Evaluation

A **diagnosis of exclusion** (steroid treatment for sarcoid will exacerbate TB or other infections):

- **CXR:** Bilateral hilar lymphadenopathy and/or pulmonary infiltrates.
- **Biopsy:** Transbronchial or video-assisted thoracoscopic biopsy reveals **noncaseating granulomas.**
- **PFTs:** Decreased volumes and diffusion capacity (a restrictive pattern).
- **Other findings:** Elevated serum ACE levels (neither sensitive nor specific), **hypercalcemia,** hypercalciuria, elevated alkaline phosphatase (with liver involvement), and lymphopenia.
- **Kveim skin test:** Often positive (performed by injecting protein from human sarcoid tissue) but rarely done.

Treatment

Systemic **corticosteroids.**

UCV *IM2.48*

SLEEP APNEA

May be **obstructive** or **central.** Patients with obstructive sleep apnea (OSA) have recurrent episodes of partial or complete closure of the upper airway during sleep, during which respiratory efforts continue. Patients with central (nonobstructive) apnea have episodic cessation of both airflow and respiratory efforts due to loss of central drive. Mixed apnea, with both obstructive and central elements, may also occur. The cause is unknown but may include abnormalities in the feedback control of breathing during sleep or decreased sensitivity of upper airway muscles or muscles of inspiration to stimulation. **Anatomic abnormalities** of the upper airway are also a possible cause. Risk factors include **male** gender (four times greater incidence in males), **obesity,** use of **sedatives for sleep,** nasal obstruction, hypothyroidism, macroglossia, micrognathia, and acromegaly.

History/PE

Daytime sleepiness and fatigue, impaired concentration, loud **snoring,** gasping or choking during sleep, and recurrent arousals from sleep. Patients may be otherwise normal, with normal PFTs.

Evaluation

Sleep studies (polysomnography) document number of arousals, obstructions, and episodes of decreased O_2 saturation. In addition, sleep studies can identify associated issues, such as movement disorders, seizures, and abnormal sleep architecture. Most significantly, sleep studies can separate central and obstructive events and aid in titration of therapy.

Treatment

Sleep-related disorders, after alcohol, are a leading cause of vehicular accidents in the United States.

- Early treatment is essential. Depending on the severity and positional nature of the disease, options include weight loss, continuous positive airway pressure (CPAP, usually via the nasal route), mandibular advancement devices, body repositioning, surgery (not first line), and weight loss. Patients with OSA must avoid alcohol and sedating/hypnotic medications.
- In children, the vast majority of cases are due to tonsillar/adenoidal hypertrophy and can be corrected early by surgical means.
- Other associated/complicating factors include GERD, myxedema of hypothyroidism (low frequency), and HTN (which is frequently associated).

SOLITARY PULMONARY NODULE

Forty percent of solitary pulmonary nodules are malignant.

A lung nodule < 3 cm in size that is discovered on CXR or CT. Solitary pulmonary nodules have a 40% likelihood of being malignant.

History/PE

Often asymptomatic. There may be chronic cough, dyspnea, and shortness of breath.

Differential

Granuloma (e.g., old or active TB infection, fungal infection, foreign body reaction), carcinoma, hamartoma, metastasis (usually multiple), bronchial adenoma (95% carcinoid tumors), pneumonia.

Evaluation

- **Compare serial CXRs:** Determine the nature, location, progression, and extent of the nodule. Biopsy or resection if diagnosis is in doubt.
- **Chest CT:** Obtain to determine the nature, location, extent, and infiltrating nature of the nodule.
- **Characteristics favoring carcinoma:** Age > 45–50 years; lesions new or larger in comparison to old films; absence of calcification or irregular calcification; size > 2 cm; irregular margins.
- **Characteristics favoring a benign lesion:** Age < 35 years; no change from old films; central/uniform/laminated calcification; smooth margins; size < 2 cm; regular margins.

Older age and larger size of nodule favor malignancy.

Treatment

A nodule in a patient > 35 years old should be resected unless there is radiologic proof that the lesion has not changed in size or appearance in at least two years. If the patient is young, if the lesion is unchanged, or if the patient objects, the lesion can be followed with a **second study in 3–6 months.** Resect lesions that change in size or character. Surgical excision is preferred over biopsy.

PRIMARY LUNG CANCER

The leading cause of cancer death. Risk factors include tobacco smoke (except for bronchoalveolar carcinoma) and radon and asbestos exposure.

Lung cancer is the leading cause of cancer death.

- **Small cell lung cancer (SCLC):** Highly related to **cigarette exposure. Central location. Neuroendocrine origin;** associated with paraneoplastic syndromes (see Table 2.15–6). Commonly presents with metastases (brain, livers, bone).
- **Non–small cell lung cancer (NSCLC): Less propensity to metastasize** (bone, adrenals).
  - **Adenocarcinoma:** Most common lung cancer, **peripheral** location.
  - **Bronchoalveolar type of adenocarcinoma:** Associated with multiple nodules, interstitial infiltration, and prolific sputum production.
  - **Squamous cell carcinoma:** Central location; associated with hypercalcemia.
  - **Large cell/neuroendocrine carcinomas:** Least common.

History

Presents with cough, hemoptysis, chest pain, and weight loss.

PE

Physical exam is usually unremarkable but may reveal abnormalities on respiratory exam (crackles, atelectasis). Other findings include **Horner's syndrome** (miosis, ptosis, anhidrosis) in patients with Pancoast's tumor and many **paraneoplastic syndromes** (see Table 2.15–6).

TABLE 2.15–6. Paraneoplastic Syndromes of Lung Cancer

Classification	Syndrome	Histologic Type
Endocrine/metabolic	Cushing's syndrome	Small cell
	SIADH	Small cell
	Hypercalcemia	Squamous cell
	Gynecomastia	Large cell
Connective tissue	Hypertrophic pulmonary osteoarthropathy	Non–small cell
Neuromuscular	Peripheral neuropathy	Small cell
	Subacute cerebellar degeneration	Small cell
	Myasthenia (Eaton-Lambert syndrome)	Small cell
	Dermatomyositis	All
Cardiovascular	Thrombophlebitis	Adenocarcinoma
	Nonbacterial verrucous endocarditis	Adenocarcinoma
Hematologic	Anemia	All
	DIC	All
	Eosinophilia	All
	Thrombocytosis	All
Cutaneous	Acanthosis nigricans	All
	Erythema gyratum repens	All

Differential

TB/other granulomatous diseases, fungal disease (aspergillus, histoplasmosis), lung abscess, metastasis, benign tumor (bronchial adenoma), hamartoma.

Evaluation

Lung cancer is usually first noted as a nodule on CXR and is best seen with **lung CT.** Fine needle aspiration under CT guidance or bronchoscopy with either biopsy or brushing can usually establish the diagnosis. Mediastinoscopy may be necessary for biopsy of hilar nodes. Thoracoscopic biopsy may be performed, with conversion to open thoracotomy if the lesion is found to be malignant.

Treatment

Lesions are grouped into NSCLC and SCLC for the purposes of treatment.

- **SCLC** is **not considered resectable** and often responds initially to radiation and chemotherapy but usually recurs, carrying a much lower median survival rate than NSCLC.
- **NSCLC** should be treated with **surgical resection** in early stages (IA, IB, IIA, IIB). Stage IIIA may be resectable, but Stage IIIB is not. The decision is based on lesion size, the presence of metastases, and the patient's age, general health, and lung function. Accompany surgery with radiation or chemotherapy (depends on stage). Unresectable disease may be treated palliatively with radiation and chemotherapy if the patient is symptomatic.

Complications

Always remember the **SPHERE** of lung cancer complications. Other complications include airway obstruction, lung abscess, and chronic interstitial fibrosis. Treat superior vena cava (SVC) syndrome with radiation. Symptoms of pain, dyspnea, and hemoptysis may respond to radiotherapy.

Lung cancer—

SPHERE of complications
Superior vena cava syndrome
Pancoast's tumor
Horner's syndrome
Endocrine (paraneoplastic)
Recurrent laryngeal symptoms (hoarseness)
Effusions (pleural or pericardial)

HIGH-YIELD FACTS

Pulmonary

Questions reproduced, with permission, from Reteguiz J, *PreTest: Physical Diagnosis*, 4th ed., New York: McGraw Hill, 2001.

Questions

1. A 39-year-old woman presents with the sudden onset of pleuritic chest pain and shortness of breath. She has been in good health until three days ago, when she noticed some swelling of her left lower extremity. She is not a smoker and denies any recent trauma. On physical examination, she is afebrile but has a respiratory rate of 32/min. Her heart rate is 120/min and her blood pressure is normal. An accentuated (loud) S2 is heard on heart auscultation. The left lower extremity is swollen, tender to palpation, and erythematous. Dorsiflexion of the left foot **(Homans' sign)** causes severe calf discomfort. Lung examination and chest radiograph are normal. Arterial blood analysis on room air shows a PC_{O_2} of 30 mmHg and a P_{O_2} of 58 mmHg. Which of the following is the most appropriate next diagnostic step?
   a. Transesophageal echocardiogram
   b. Transthoracic echocardiogram
   c. Cardiac catheterization
   d. Ventilation/perfusion scan
   e. D-dimer assay

2. A 14-year-old boy presents with a history of chronic sinusitis and frequent pneumonias. On physical examination, the patient has normal vital signs and is afebrile. He has mild frontal maxillary sinus tenderness with palpation. Transillumination of the sinuses is normal. Heart sounds are best heard on the right side of the chest. The boy is coughing copious amounts of yellowish sputum. Which of the following is the most likely diagnosis?
   a. Cystic fibrosis
   b. Kartagener syndrome
   c. Pulmonary dysplasia
   d. Tuberculosis
   e. Pulmonary hypertension

3. A 70-year-old man with a history of chronic obstructive pulmonary disease (COPD) presents complaining of worsening shortness of breath for the last several days. He is coughing large amounts of yellow-colored sputum and is receiving no relief from his β_2-agonist and ipratropium aerosolized pumps. On physical examination, the patient's respiratory rate is 40/min and his heart rate is 110/min. His blood pressure is 150/85 mmHg. The patient is afebrile. He is using his accessory muscles of respiration (sternocleidomastoids and intercostals) to assist in breathing. Lung examination reveals inspiratory and expiratory diffuse wheezing. Which of the following is the most likely diagnosis?
   a. Acute exacerbation of COPD
   b. α_1-antitrypsin deficiency
   c. Chronic bronchitis
   d. Exacerbation of asthma
   e. Pneumonia

4. A man is stabbed and arrives at the emergency room within 30 minutes. You notice that the trachea is deviated away from the side of the chest with the puncture. The most likely lung finding on physical examination of the traumatized side is which of the following?
   a. Increased fremitus
   b. Increased breath sounds
   c. Dullness to percussion
   d. Hyperresonant percussion
   e. Wheezing
   f. Stridor

Answers

1. **The answer is d.** The most frequent presenting clinical sign of **pulmonary embolus (PE)** is shortness of breath. Patients may also present with pleuritic chest pain, hemoptysis, and tachycardia. An excellent clue to the diagnosis of PE is deep venous thrombosis (DVT), but absence of signs of DVT does not exclude the diagnosis of PE. Embolus from a thrombus in the lower extremities (DVT) is the most common cause of PE. Common settings for PE include prolonged immobilization, use of oral contraceptives, obesity, recent surgery, burns, severe trauma, congestive heart failure, malignancy, pregnancy, sickle cell anemia, polycythemias, inherited deficiencies of the anticoagulating proteins (protein C, protein S, antithrombin III), and the Leiden factor V mutation. Chest radiograph in PE may be normal but may demonstrate a peripheral wedge-shaped density above the diaphragm **(Hampton's hump)**, focal oligemia **(Westermark sign)**, or abrupt occlusion of a vessel **(cutoff sign)**. A loud **S2** is often heard in disorders that cause pulmonary hypertension, such as pulmonary embolism. The next best step in making the diagnosis would be to order a ventilation/perfusion (V/Q) scan. If the V/Q scan results are of low or indeterminate probability, the patient may need further studies, such as pulmonary arteriogram or venous ultrasonography of the lower extremity. **D-dimer assays** will result in future changes to existing diagnostic strategies for pulmonary embolism, but the marker is still in the investigative stages (the absence of this product is evidence against thromboembolism). **Helical (spiral) CT** scans are comparable to V/Q scans and may be the first step in diagnosing pulmonary embolus.

2. **The answer is b.** **Kartagener syndrome** is the inheritable disorder of dextrocardia, chronic sinusitis (with the formation of nasal polyps), and bronchiectasis. Patients may also present with **situs inversus.** The disorder is due to a defect that causes the cilia within the respiratory tract epithelium to become immotile. Cilia of the sperm are also affected.

3. **The answer is a.** **COPD** is defined as a condition where there is chronic obstruction to airflow due to chronic bronchitis or emphysema. An exacerbation of COPD occurs when the patient develops the acute onset of marked dyspnea and tachypnea requiring the use of accessory muscles that is unresponsive to medications. **α_1-antitrypsin deficiency** should be suspected in nonsmokers who present with COPD of the lung bases in their fifties without any predisposing history, such as occupational exposure to support the diagnosis. α_1-antitrypsin deficiency is rare in African Americans and Asian–Pacific Islanders.

4. **The answer is d.** The patient has a **tension pneumothorax,** which is evidenced by the trachea deviating away from the side of the traumatized lung. This occurs secondary to trauma or during mechanical ventilation. Breath sounds will be faint or distant, percussion will be hyperresonant, and fremitus will be decreased. The increased air on the affected side is in the pleural space, not in the lung. As an attempt is made to inflate the lung, air moves into the pleural space from the puncture site, resulting in a collapsed lung with a large pleural space. The contralateral lung is also at risk for collapse. Any time the trachea is deviated from the involved side, it is considered a medical emergency and the tension pneumothorax must be relieved or the patient will die from hypoxemia or inadequate cardiac output.

Renal/Genitourinary

Acid-base physiology

	pH	P_{CO_2}	$[HCO_3^-]$	Cause	Compensatory response
Metabolic acidosis	↓	↓	**↓**	Diabetic ketoacidosis, diarrhea, lactic acidosis, salicylate OD, acetazolamide	Hyperventilation
Respiratory acidosis	↓	**↑**	↑	COPD, airway obstruction	Renal $[HCO_3^-]$ reabsorption
Respiratory alkalosis	↑	**↓**	↓	High altitude, hyperventilation	Renal $[HCO_3^-]$ secretion
Metabolic alkalosis	↑	↑	**↑**	Vomiting	Hypoventilation

$$\text{Henderson-Hasselbalch equation: pH} = pKa + \log \frac{[HCO_3^-]}{0.03\, P_{CO_2}}$$

Key: **↑ ↓** = primary disturbance; ↓ ↑ = compensatory response.

Diuretics: site of action

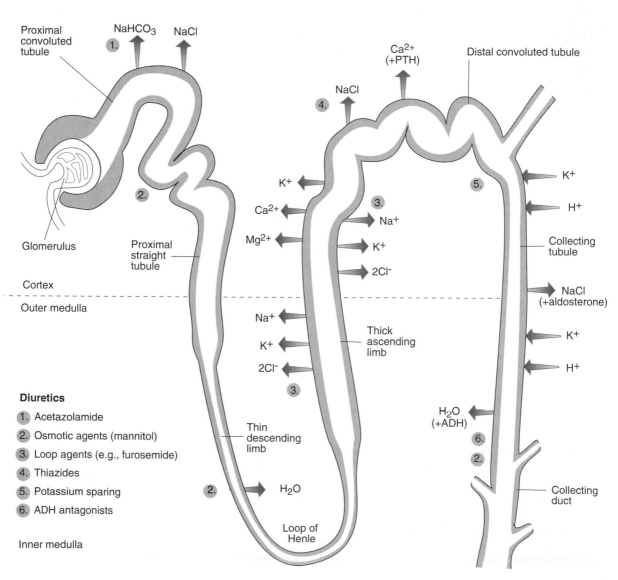

Diuretics

1. Acetazolamide
2. Osmotic agents (mannitol)
3. Loop agents (e.g., furosemide)
4. Thiazides
5. Potassium sparing
6. ADH antagonists

(Adapted, with permission, from Katzung BG. *Basic and Clinical Pharmacology,* 7th ed. Stamford, CT: Appleton & Lange, 1997:243.)

Acidosis/alkalosis

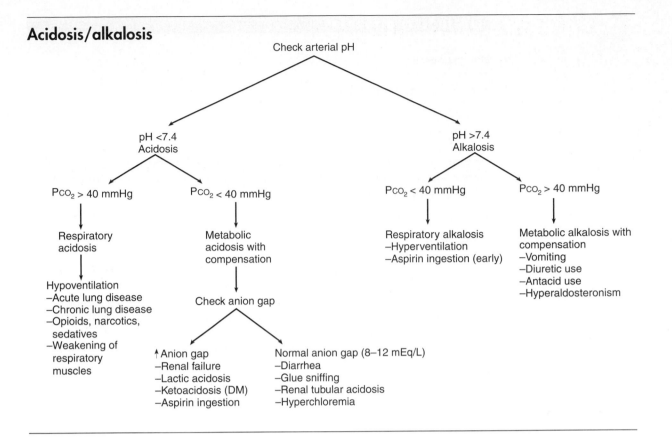

Check arterial pH

pH <7.4
Acidosis

pH >7.4
Alkalosis

P_{CO_2} > 40 mmHg

P_{CO_2} < 40 mmHg

P_{CO_2} < 40 mmHg

P_{CO_2} > 40 mmHg

Respiratory
acidosis

Metabolic
acidosis with
compensation

Respiratory alkalosis
–Hyperventilation
–Aspirin ingestion (early)

Metabolic alkalosis with
compensation
–Vomiting
–Diuretic use
–Antacid use
–Hyperaldosteronism

Hypoventilation
–Acute lung disease
–Chronic lung disease
–Opioids, narcotics,
 sedatives
–Weakening of
 respiratory
 muscles

Check anion gap

↑Anion gap
–Renal failure
–Lactic acidosis
–Ketoacidosis (DM)
–Aspirin ingestion

Normal anion gap (8–12 mEq/L)
–Diarrhea
–Glue sniffing
–Renal tubular acidosis
–Hyperchloremia

HYPERNATREMIA

Serum sodium > 145 mEq/L.

History/PE

May report **thirst** and oliguria or polyuria (depending on etiology) as well as mental status changes, weakness, focal neurologic deficits, and seizures. Physical exam may show **"doughy" skin.**

Evaluation

Assess volume status by clinical exam and measure urine volume and osmolality. Hypervolemic hypernatremia suggests **increased aldosterone** or excess sodium (e.g., IV saline). A minimal volume (approximately 500 mL/day) of maximally concentrated urine (> 400 mOsm/kg) suggests adequate renal response without adequate free water replacement. Fluid loss may be due to decreased intake, diuretics, glycosuria, or third spacing. Large volumes of dilute urine suggest **diabetes insipidus (DI,** central or nephrogenic).

Treatment

Treat underlying causes and replace free water deficit with hypotonic saline, D5W, or oral water depending on volume status. Correction of hypernatremia should occur **gradually over 48–72 hours** to prevent neurologic damage secondary to cerebral swelling.

HYPONATREMIA

Serum sodium < 135 mEq/L.

History/PE

May be asymptomatic or may present with **confusion, lethargy,** muscle cramps, and nausea. Hyponatremia may progress to seizures, status epilepticus, or coma.

Evaluation

Hyponatremia can be classified by serum osmolality, volume status (by clinical exam), and urinary sodium. Osmolality is classified as:

- **High (> 295 mEq/L):** Hyperglycemia, hypertonic (e.g., mannitol) infusion.
- **Normal (280–295 mEq/L):** Hyperlipidemia, hyperproteinemia (pseudohyponatremia).
- **Low (< 280 mEq/L):** Hypotonic etiologies (see Table 16.2–1).

Hypernatremia may result in patients who do not drink enough free water to replace insensible losses.

TABLE 16.2–1. Evaluation and Treatment of Hypotonic Hyponatremia

Volume Status	Etiologies	Treatment
Hypervolemic	Renal failure, nephrotic syndrome, cirrhosis, CHF.	Salt and water restriction.
Euvolemic	SIADH, hypothyroidism, renal failure, drugs, psychogenic polydipsia, adrenal insufficiency.	Salt and water restriction.
Hypovolemic	Diuretics, vomiting, diarrhea, third spacing, dehydration.	Replete volume with normal saline.

Treatment

Specific treatments are defined in Table 16.2–1. Chronic hyponatremia should be corrected slowly in order to prevent central pontine myelinolysis (quadriplegia and pseudobulbar palsy).

> Hypervolemic hyponatremia is caused by "nephr**OSIS**, cirrh**OSIS**, cardi**OSIS**."

HYPERKALEMIA

Serum potassium > 5 mEq/L.

History/PE

May be asymptomatic or may present with nausea, vomiting, **intestinal colic, areflexia, weakness,** flaccid paralysis, and paresthesias. Causes include:

- **Spurious:** Hemolysis (e.g., during blood draw), fist clenching during blood draw, extreme leukocytosis or thrombocytosis, rhabdomyolysis.
- **Decreased excretion:** Renal insufficiency, drugs (e.g., spironolactone, triamterene, ACE inhibitors (ACEIs), trimethoprim, NSAIDs), mineralocorticoid deficiency/type 4 renal tubular acidosis (RTA).
- **Cellular shifts:** Tissue injury, insulin deficiency, drugs (e.g., succinylcholine, digitalis, arginine, β-blockers).
- **Iatrogenic.**

QRS prolongation   Peaked T
PR prolongation
ECG:
Low P

FIGURE 16.2–1. Hyperkalemia. Electrocardiographic manifestations include peaked T waves, PR prolongation, and a widened QRS complex. (Reproduced, with permission, from Cogan MG, *Fluid and Electrolytes,* 1st ed., Stamford, CT: Appleton & Lange, 1991: p. 170, Fig. 9–4.)

Evaluation

First verify hyperkalemia with a **repeat blood draw** unless suspicion is already high. ECG findings may include **tall peaked T waves,** PR prolongation, wide QRS, loss of P waves that can progress to **sine waves** (see Figure 16.2–1), ventricular fibrillation, and cardiac arrest.

Treatment

Values > 6.5 mEq/L or ECG changes (especially PR prolongation or wide QRS) require emergent treatment. The mnemonic **C BIG K** summarizes the treatment of hyperkalemia.

- **Calcium gluconate** for cardiac cell membrane stabilization.
- **Bicarbonate or insulin and glucose** to temporarily shift potassium into cells.

> **Treatment of hyperkalemia—**
>
> **C BIG K**
> **C**alcium
> **B**icarbonate
> **I**nsulin
> **G**lucose
> **K**ayexalate

- **Kayexalate** and loop diuretics (e.g., furosemide) to remove potassium from the body.
- Dialysis for patients with renal failure or severe, refractory cases.

UCV *IM2.34*

HYPOKALEMIA

Serum potassium < 3.5 mEq/L. Etiologies include:

- **Transcellular shifts:** Insulin, β_2-agonists, alkalosis, periodic paralysis.
- **GI losses:** Diarrhea, chronic laxative abuse, vomiting, NG suction.
- **Renal K+ losses:** Diuretics (e.g., loop or thiazide), primary mineralocorticoid excess or secondary hyperaldosteronism (decreased circulating volume, Bartter's syndrome), drugs (e.g., gentamicin, amphotericin), DKA, hypomagnesemia, type 1 RTA.

History/PE

May present with fatigue, **muscle weakness or cramps, ileus,** hyporeflexia, paresthesias, and flaccid paralysis, if severe.

Evaluation

Twenty-four-hour or spot urine potassium may distinguish renal from GI losses. ECG may show **T-wave flattening, U waves** (additional wave after the T wave), and ST depression followed by atrioventricular (AV) block and subsequent cardiac arrest. Consider RTA in the setting of metabolic acidosis.

Treatment

Treat the underlying disorder. Administer oral and/or IV **potassium repletion.** Replace magnesium, as this deficiency makes potassium repletion more difficult. Monitor ECG and plasma potassium levels frequently during replacement.

HYPERCALCEMIA

Serum calcium > 10.2 mg/dL. The most common causes are **hyperparathyroidism and malignancy** (e.g., squamous cell cancers myeloma). Common causes are summarized in the mnemonic **CHIMPANZEES.**

History/PE

May present with "**bones** (fractures), **stones** (kidney stones), abdominal **groans** (anorexia, vomiting, constipation), and **psychiatric overtones** (weakness, fatigue, altered mental status)."

Evaluation

Order an ECG (may show **short QT interval**), total/ionized calcium, albumin, phosphate, PTH, PTHrP (parathyroid hormone–related peptide), vitamin D, TSH, and serum immunoelectrophoresis.

Causes of hypercalcemia—

CHIMPANZEES
Calcium supplementation
Hyperparathyroidism
Iatrogenic (e.g., thiazides)/**I**mmobility
Milk alkali syndrome
Paget's disease
Addison's disease/**A**cromegaly
Neoplasm
Zollinger-Ellison syndrome (e.g., multiple endocrine neoplasia [MEN] I)
Excess vitamin A
Excess vitamin D
Sarcoidosis and other granulomatous disease

Treatment

Treat with **IV hydration** (watch for CHF) followed by **furosemide.** Calcitonin, bisphosphonates (e.g., pamidronate), glucocorticoids, and dialysis are used for severe or refractory cases. **Avoid thiazide diuretics,** which increase tubular reabsorption of calcium.

"Loops (furosemide) lose calcium."

HYPOCALCEMIA

Serum calcium < 8.5 mg/dL. Etiologies include hypoparathyroidism (post-surgery, idiopathic), malnutrition, hypomagnesemia, acute pancreatitis, medullary thyroid cancer (excess calcitonin), vitamin D deficiency, pseudo-hypoparathyroidism, and renal insufficiency.

Serum calcium may be falsely low in hypoalbuminemia.

History/PE

Abdominal muscle cramps, dyspnea, **tetany, perioral and acral paresthesias,** and convulsions may be present. Facial spasm while tapping the facial nerve (**Chvostek's sign**) and carpal spasm after arterial occlusion by a BP cuff (**Trousseau's sign**) are classic findings on physical exam. ECG may show a **prolonged QT interval.**

The classic case is a patient who develops cramps and tetany following thyroidectomy.

Evaluation

Order an ionized Ca^{2+}, Mg^+, PTH, albumin, and possibly, calcitonin. If post-thyroidectomy, review operative note to determine number of parathyroid glands removed.

Treatment

Treat the underlying disorder. Administer oral **calcium supplements;** give IV calcium if symptoms are severe.

HYPOMAGNESEMIA

Serum magnesium < 1.5 mEq/L. Etiologies include:

- **Decreased intake:** Malnutrition, **alcoholism,** malabsorption, short bowel syndrome, TPN.
- **Increased loss:** Diuretics, diarrhea, vomiting.
- **Miscellaneous: DKA,** pancreatitis.

History/PE

Symptoms are generally related to concurrent hypocalcemia and hypokalemia and include anorexia, nausea, vomiting, muscle cramps, and weakness. At very low levels, symptoms include paresthesias, irritability, confusion, lethargy, seizures, and arrhythmias.

Evaluation

Labs may show concurrent hypocalcemia and hypokalemia. ECG may show prolonged PR and QT intervals.

Treatment

IV and oral supplements are available. Hypokalemia and hypocalcemia will not correct without magnesium correction.

ACUTE RENAL FAILURE (ARF)

An abrupt decrease in renal function leading to the retention of Cr and BUN. Decreased urine output (i.e., oliguria, defined as < 500 cc/day) is not required for ARF. ARF is categorized as **prerenal, intrinsic,** or **postrenal.** Prerenal failure is caused by decreased renal plasma flow. Intrinsic renal failure results from injury within the nephron unit. Postrenal failure is caused by urinary outflow obstruction. Generally, both kidneys must be obstructed in order to cause a significant increase in BUN and Cr. Table 16.2–2 outlines etiologies of ARF.

History/PE

In acute tubular necrosis (ATN), there may be a recent history of contrast or aminoglycoside use; papillary necrosis can be associated with DM, analgesic abuse, and sickle cell anemia. Patients may present with malaise, fatigue, oliguria, anorexia, and nausea secondary to **uremia.** Exam might reveal a **pericardial friction rub, asterixis, HTN,** decreased urine output, and increased RR either from compensation of metabolic acidosis or from pulmonary edema due to volume overload. Hypovolemia and orthostasis suggest a prerenal etiology. Fever and rash support an acute interstitial nephritis (methicillin is classically associated). Patients with postrenal etiologies may have a distended bladder.

Evaluation

Renal ischemia, toxins, hemoglobinuria, or myoglobinuria may cause ATN.

FE_{Na} < 1% indicates that kidneys are conserving Na^+ and suggests a prerenal etiology.

Examine the urine for RBCs, WBCs, casts (see Table 16.2–3), **urine eosinophils,** and check serum electrolytes. A urinary catheter and renal U/S can help rule out obstruction; a renal U/S can also identify kidneys that are reduced in size, as with chronic renal failure. In patients with oliguria, the fractional excretion of sodium (FE_{Na}) can help identify prerenal failure:

$$FE_{Na} = (U_{Na}/P_{Na})/(U_{Cr}/P_{Cr})$$

A FE_{Na} < 1%, a U_{Na} < 20, or a BUN/Cr ratio > 20 suggests a prerenal etiology.

TABLE 16.2–2. Causes of Acute Renal Failure

Prerenal	Renal (Intrinsic)	Postrenal
Hypovolemia (dehydration, hemorrhage)	ATN	Prostate disease
Cardiogenic shock	Acute/allergic interstitial nephritis	Nephrolithiasis
Sepsis	Glomerulonephritis	Pelvic tumors
Drugs (e.g., NSAIDs)	Thromboembolism	Recent pelvic surgery
Renal artery stenosis		

TABLE 16.2–3. Findings on Microscopic Urine Examination in Acute Renal Failure

Urine Sediment	Etiology
Hyaline casts	Normal finding, but increased amount suggests prerenal condition.
Red cell casts, red cells	Glomerulonephritis.
White cells, white cell casts	Pyelonephritis.
White cells, eosinophils	Allergic interstitial nephritis.
Granular casts, renal tubular cells, "muddy brown casts"	ATN (intrinsic).

Treatment

- Balance fluids and electrolytes.
- Adjust/discontinue offending medications in acute/allergic interstitial nephritis.
- Dialyze if indicated (**AEIOU** mnemonic).
- Give corticosteroids or cytotoxic agents for some causes of glomerulonephritis.

Complications

Chronic renal failure may result, requiring dialysis to prevent the buildup of **K⁺, H⁺, and toxic metabolites.** Patients who are dialysis-dependent are at increased risk for a number of diseases, including CAD.

UCV *IM2.32, 33*

> **Indications for dialysis—**
>
> **AEIOU**
> **A**cidosis
> **E**lectrolyte abnormalities (hyperkalemia)
> **I**ngestions
> **O**verload (fluid)
> **U**remic symptoms (pericarditis, encephalopathy, bleeding, nausea, pruritus, myoclonus)

DIURETICS

Table 16.2–4 summarizes the actions and side effects of commonly used diuretics.

GLOMERULAR DISEASE

NEPHRITIC SYNDROME

Also called glomerulonephritis, nephritic syndrome is a disorder of glomerular inflammation. Proteinuria may be present but is usually mild. Causes are summarized in Table 16.2–5.

Think nephritic syndrome if the patient has hematuria, HTN, and oliguria.

History/PE

Patients may present with the classic findings of oliguria, macroscopic hematuria (smoky-brown urine), HTN, and possibly with **edema in low-pressure regions** such as the periorbital and scrotal areas.

Evaluation

UA will show hematuria and possibly, mild proteinuria. Patients have a reduced GFR with elevated BUN and Cr. Complement, ANA, ANCA, and

TABLE 16.2–4. Mechanism of Action and Side Effects of Diuretics

Type	Drugs	Site of Action	Mechanism of Action	Side Effects
Carbonic anhydrase inhibitors	Acetazolamide	Proximal convoluted tubule.	Inhibits carbonic anhydrase, increases H^+ reabsorption.	Hyperchloremic metabolic acidosis, sulfa allergy.
Osmotic agents	Mannitol, urea	Entire tubule.	Increases tubular fluid osmolarity.	Pulmonary edema, due to CHF and anuria.
Loop agents	Furosemide, ethacrynic acid, bumetanide, torsemide	Ascending loop of Henle.	Inhibits $Na^+/K^+/2\ Cl^-$ transporter.	Water loss, metabolic alkalosis, $\downarrow K^+$, $\downarrow Ca^{2+}$, **ototoxicity**, sulfa allergy (e.g., except ethacrynic acid).
Thiazide agents	Hydrochlorothiazide, chlorothiazide	Distal convoluted tubule.	Inhibits Na^+/Cl^- cotransporter.	Water loss, metabolic alkalosis, $\downarrow Na^+$, $\downarrow K^+$, $\uparrow$ glucose, $\uparrow Ca^{2+}$, $\uparrow$ uric acid, sulfa allergy, pancreatitis.
K^+-sparing agents	Spironolactone, triamterene, amiloride	Cortical collecting tubule.	Aldosterone receptor antagonist (spironolactone), block sodium channel (triamterene, amiloride).	Metabolic acidosis, $\uparrow K^+$, anti-androgenic effects including gynecomastia (spironolactone).

anti-GBM (anti-glomerular basement membrane) antibody levels should be measured to determine the underlying etiology. Renal biopsy may be useful for histologic evaluation.

Treatment

Treat HTN, fluid overload, and uremia with salt and water restriction, diuretics, and, if necessary, dialysis. **Corticosteroids** are useful in reducing glomerular inflammation in some cases.

Proteinuria, hypoalbuminemia, edema, hyperlipidemia, and hyperlipiduria are due to the initial increased permeability of the glomerulus to protein.

NEPHROTIC SYNDROME

Defined as **proteinuria (≥ 3.5 grams/day), generalized edema, hypoalbuminemia, hyperlipidemia.** Also predisposes patients to a **hypercoagulable state.** Approximately one-third of all cases are the result of systemic diseases such as diabetes mellitus (DM), systemic lupus erythematosus (SLE), or amyloidosis. Causes are summarized in Table 16.2–6.

TABLE 16.2–5. Causes of Nephritic Syndrome

	Description	History and PE	Labs and Histology	Treatment and Prognosis
Postinfectious glomerulo-nephritis	Often associated with a recent **streptococcal infection** (group A β-hemolytic).	Oliguria, edema, HTN, smoky-brown urine.	Low serum C3, increased anti-streptolysin O (ASO) titer, **lumpy-bumpy immuno-fluorescence (IF).**	Supportive. Almost all children and most adults have complete recovery.
IgA nephropathy (Berger's disease)	**Most common type;** associated with upper respiratory or GI infections; commonly in young men.	Gross hematuria.	May see increased serum IgA level. Biopsy and IF will show mesangial IgA deposits.	Glucocorticoids for select patients; 20% progress to end-stage renal disease (ESRD).
Wegener's granulomatosis	Granulomatous inflammation of the respiratory tract and kidney with necrotizing vasculitis; a paucimmune form of rapidly progressive glomerulonephritis (RPGN).	Fever, weight loss, hematuria, respiratory and sinus symptoms; cavitary pulmonary lesions bleed and cause **hemoptysis.**	Presence of **c-ANCA** (cell-mediated immune response).	High-dose corticosteroids and cytotoxic agents. Patients tend to have frequent relapses.
Alport's syndrome	Hereditary glomerulonephritis; presents in boys 5–20 years old.	Asymptomatic hematuria associated with **nerve deafness** and eye disorders.	GBM splitting on electron microscopy.	Progresses to renal failure. Anti-GBM nephritis may recur after transplant.
Goodpasture's syndrome	Glomerulonephritis with pulmonary hemorrhage; peak incidence in men in their mid-20s; an immune form of RPGN.	**Hemoptysis,** dyspnea, possible respiratory failure.	**Linear anti-GBM deposits** on IF, iron-deficiency anemia, hemosiderin-filled macrophages in sputum, pulmonary infiltrates on CXR.	Plasma exchange therapy, pulsed steroids. May progress to ESRD.

History/PE

Patients present with **generalized edema** and may report **foamy urine.** In severe cases, dyspnea and ascites may develop. Patients have an increased susceptibility to infection as well as venous thrombosis and pulmonary embolism.

TABLE 16.2–6. Causes of Nephrotic Syndrome

	Description	History and PE	Labs and Histology	Treatment and Prognosis
Minimal change disease (IM2.36)	Common in children; idiopathic etiology.	Tendency toward infections and thrombotic events.	Light microscopy appears **normal.** Electron microscopy shows **fusion of epithelial foot processes** with lipid-laden renal cartices.	Steroids; excellent prognosis.
Focal segmental glomerulo-sclerosis (FSGS)	Idiopathic, IVDU, HIV infection.	Typical patient is young black male with uncontrolled HTN.	Microscopic hematuria; biopsy shows sclerosis in capillary tufts.	Prednisone, cytotoxic therapy.
Membranous nephropathy (IM2.35)	**Most common Caucasian adult nephropathy;** an immune complex disease.	Associated with HBV, syphilis, **malaria,** and gold.	**"Spike and dome"** appearance due to granular deposits of IgG and C3 at basement membrane.	Prednisone and cytotoxic therapy for severe disease.
Diabetic nephropathy	Two characteristic forms: diffuse hyalinization and nodular glomerulosclerosis **(Kimmelstiel-Wilson lesions).**	Generally have long-standing, poorly controlled DM.	Thickened GBM; **increased mesangial matrix.**	Tight control of blood sugar; protein restriction; ACEIs.
Lupus nephritis	Classified as WHO types I–V. Both nephrotic and nephritic. Severity of renal disease often determines overall prognosis.	Proteinuria or RBCs on UA may be found during evaluation of SLE patients.	Mesangial proliferation; subendothelial immune complex deposition.	Prednisone and cytotoxic therapy may reduce disease progression.
Renal amyloidosis	Primary (plasma cell dyscrasia) and secondary (infectious or inflammatory) are the most common.	Patients may have multiple myeloma or a chronic inflammatory disease (e.g., RA, TB).	Abdominal fat biopsy; seen with **Congo red stain; apple green** birefringence under polarized light.	Prednisone and melphalan. BMT may be used for multiple myeloma.
Membrano-proliferative nephropathy (MPGN)	Can also be a nephritic syndrome.	Slow progression to renal failure.	**"Tram-track"** double-layered basement membrane. Type I has subendothelial deposits; type II involves a C3 nephritic factor and decreased C3.	Corticosteroids and cytotoxic agents may help.

Evaluation

UA will show **proteinuria** (≥ 3.5 g/day) and lipiduria. Blood chemistry will show **decreased albumin** (< 3 g/dL) and hyperlipidemia. Renal biopsy is used to diagnose the underlying etiology in some cases.

Treatment

Protein and salt restriction, diuretic therapy, and antihyperlipidemics. **ACEIs** decrease proteinuria and diminish the progression of renal disease. Vaccinate with 23-polyvalent pneumococcus vaccine (PPV23), as patients are at increased risk of *Streptococcus pneumoniae* infection.

NEPHROLITHIASIS

Most commonly occurs in older males. Risk factors include a positive family history, **low fluid intake,** gout, postcolectomy/ileostomy, specific enzyme disorders, RTA, and hyperparathyroidism. Stones are most commonly calcium oxalate but may also be calcium phosphate, struvite, uric acid, or cystine (see Table 16.2–7).

History/PE

Acute onset of severe, colicky flank pain that may **radiate to the testes or vulva** and may be associated with nausea and vomiting. Patients are unable to get comfortable and shift position frequently (as opposed to those with peritonitis who are still).

TABLE 16.2–7. Types of Nephrolithiasis

Type	Frequency	Etiology and Characteristics	Treatment
Calcium oxalate/ calcium phosphate	83%	Most common causes are **idiopathic hypercalciuria,** elevated urine uric acid secondary to diet, and primary hyperparathyroidism. Alkaline urine. Radiopaque.	Hydration, thiazide diuretic.
Struvite ($Mg\text{-}NH_4\text{-}PO_4$)	9%	"Triple phosphate stones." Associated with urease-producing organisms (e.g., *Proteus*). Form staghorn calculi. Alkaline urine. Radiopaque.	Hydration, treat UTI if present.
Uric acid	7%	Associated with gout and high purine turnover states. Acidic urine (pH < 5.5). **Radiolucent.**	Hydration, alkalinize urine with citrate, which is converted to HCO_3^- in the liver.
Cystine	1%	Due to a defect in renal transport of certain amino acids (COLA—cystine, ornithine, lysine, and arginine). **Hexagonal crystals.** Radiopaque.	Hydration, alkalinize urine, penicillamine.

Evaluation

UA may show gross or **microscopic hematuria** and **an altered urine pH.** Obtain a **KUB** and possibly a **renal U/S.** An **IVP** can be used to confirm the diagnosis if there is a lack of contrast filling below the stone. **Noncontrast abdominal CT scans** may diagnose stones and other causes of flank pain.

Treatment

Hydration and analgesia are the initial treatment; additional treatment is based on the size of the stone. Kidney stones < 5 mm in diameter can pass through the urethra; stones < 3 cm in diameter can be treated with **extracorporeal shock wave lithotripsy (ESWL)** or percutaneous nephrolithotomy. Preventive measures include hydration; other prophylaxis is composition-dependent.

UCV *ER.30*

POLYCYSTIC KIDNEY DISEASE (PCKD)

Most commonly autosomal dominant (AD) and usually asymptomatic until patients are > 30 years old. One-half of autosomal-dominant PCKD patients will have ESRD requiring dialysis by age 60. Autosomal-recessive (AR) PCKD is less common but more severe. It presents in infants and young children with renal failure, liver fibrosis, and portal HTN and may lead to death in the first few years of life.

History/PE

Pain and hematuria are the most common presenting symptoms. Sharp, localized pain may result from cyst rupture, infection, or passage of renal calculi. Additional findings include **HTN, hepatic cysts, cerebral berry aneurysms,** and mitral valve prolapse. Patients may also have large, palpable kidneys on abdominal exam.

Evaluation

Diagnosis can be based on U/S or CT scan. Multiple bilateral cysts will be present throughout the renal parenchyma, and renal enlargement will be visualized.

Treatment

Prevent complications and decrease the rate of progression to ESRD. Early management of UTIs is critical to prevent renal cyst infection. BP control is necessary to reduce HTN-induced renal damage. Dialysis and renal transplantation are used to manage patients with ESRD.

RENAL TUBULAR ACIDOSIS

A net decrease in either tubular H^+ secretion or HCO_3^- reabsorption that produces a **non-anion gap metabolic acidosis.** There are three main types of RTA. **Type IV (distal) is the most common form** (see Table 16.2–8).

UCV *IM2.37*

TABLE 16.2–8. Types of RTA

	Type I (distal)	Type II (proximal)	Type IV (distal)
Defect	H+ secretion.	HCO_3^- reabsorption.	Aldosterone deficiency or resistance → defects in Na+ reabsorption, H+ and K+ excretion.
Serum K+	High or low.	Low.	High.
Urinary pH	> 5.3.	> 5.3 initially; < 5.3 once serum is acidic.	< 5.3.
Etiologies (most common)	Hereditary, amphotericin, collagen vascular disease, cirrhosis, nephrocalcinosis.	Hereditary, carbonic anhydrase inhibitors, Fanconi's syndrome.	Hyporeninemic hypoaldosteronism with DM, HTN, chronic interstitial nephritis.
Treatment	Potassium citrate.	Potassium citrate.	Furosemide, kayexelate.
Complications	Nephrolithiasis.	Rickets, osteomalacia.	Hyperkalemia.

URETERAL REFLUX

Retrograde projection of urine from the bladder to the ureters and kidneys. Often caused by insufficient tunneling of ureters into submucosal bladder tissue, resulting in ineffective restriction of retrograde urine flow during bladder contraction. Patients present with **recurrent UTIs.** Perform a **voiding cystourethrogram (VCUG)** to detect abnormalities at ureteral insertion sites and to classify the grade of reflux. Treat infections aggressively. Mild reflux (no ureteral or renal pelvic dilatation) often resolves spontaneously. Moderate to severe reflux (ureteral dilatation with associated calyceal blunting in severe cases) requires surgical intervention (ureteral reimplantation).

DIABETES INSIPIDUS

Central or nephrogenic in origin. In **central DI,** the posterior pituitary fails to secrete ADH. Causes include **tumor,** ischemia (Sheehan's syndrome), or traumatic cerebral injury, infection, and autoimmune disorders. In **nephrogenic DI,** the kidneys fail to respond to circulating ADH. Causes include renal diseases and drugs (e.g., **lithium,** demeclocycline).

History/PE

Patients have **polydipsia, polyuria,** and **persistent thirst** with a dilute urine. Patients may present with hypernatremia and dehydration, but if given unlimited access to water, they are typically normonatremic.

Evaluation

Patients with DI continue to excrete a high volume of dilute urine during a **water deprivation test.** In central DI, a DDAVP (desmopressin acetate) challenge will **reduce urine output and increase urine osmolarity.** In nephrogenic DI, a DDAVP challenge will not significantly reduce urine output. MRI may show a pituitary or hypothalamic mass in central DI.

Treatment

- **Central DI:** DDAVP, a synthetic analog of ADH, is administered intranasally.
- **Nephrogenic DI:** Salt restriction and increased water intake are the primary treatment. Thiazide diuretics are used to promote mild volume depletion and stimulate proximal reabsorption of salt and water. Address the underlying cause.

SIADH

A common cause of euvolemic hyponatremia that results from **nonosmotically stimulated ADH release.** SIADH is associated with **CNS disease** (e.g., head injury, tumor), **pulmonary disease** (e.g., sarcoid, pneumonia), ectopic tumor production/paraneoplastic syndrome (e.g., small cell carcinoma), drugs (e.g., antipsychotics, antidepressants), or surgery.

Evaluation

Diagnose on the basis of urine osmolality > 50–100 mOsm/kg with concurrent serum hyposmolarity in the absence of a physiologic reason for increased ADH (e.g., CHF, cirrhosis, hypovolemia). **Urinary sodium ≥ 20 mEq/L** is used to demonstrate that the patient is not hypovolemic.

Treatment

Restrict fluid and address the underlying cause. If the patient is symptomatic as a result of hyponatremia, give hypertonic saline followed by furosemide. Chronic correction depends on treatment of the underlying disorder; **demeclocycline** can help normalize serum sodium by antagonizing the action of ADH in the collecting duct.

UCV *IM1.28*

BENIGN PROSTATIC HYPERPLASIA (BPH)

Enlargement of the prostate that is a normal part of the aging process and is seen in **> 80% of individuals by age 80.** Most commonly presents in patients **> 50 years of age.**

History/PE

In BPH, the enlarged prostate may cause irritative and obstructive symptoms:

- **Obstructive:** Hesitancy, weak stream, intermittent stream, incomplete emptying, urinary retention, bladder fullness.
- **Irritative:** Nocturia, daytime frequency, urge incontinence, opening hematuria.

On digital rectal exam (DRE), the prostate is uniformly enlarged with a rubbery texture. If the prostate is hard or has irregular lesions, suspect cancer. BPH most commonly occurs in the central zone of the prostate and may not be detected on exam.

Differential

Bladder calculi, bladder tumor, neurogenic bladder, prostatitis, prostate cancer, urethral stricture, urethritis.

Evaluation

Potentially dangerous causes of urinary symptoms must be ruled out before diagnosing BPH.

- **DRE** to screen for masses; if findings are suspicious, evaluate for prostate cancer.
- **UA and urine culture** to rule out infection and hematuria.
- **Cr levels** to rule out obstructive uropathy and renal insufficiency.
- PSA testing and cystoscopy are not recommended for BPH monitoring.

Treatment

- **Reassurance** for mild symptoms.
- **Medical therapy** with α-blockers (terazosin) and 5α-reductase inhibitors (finasteride) to reduce mild to moderate symptoms.
- Transurethral resection of the prostate [TURP] or open prostatectomy.
- **Surgery** for patients with moderate to severe symptoms.

UCV *Surg.35*

PROSTATE CANCER

The **most common cancer in men** and the **second leading cause of cancer death** in men (after lung cancer). Risk factors include advanced age and a positive family history.

Prostate cancer is the most common cancer and the second leading cause of cancer death in men.

History/PE

Usually **asymptomatic,** but may present with **urinary retention,** a decrease in the force of the urine stream, lymphedema due to obstructing metastases, constitutional symptoms, and **back pain.** DRE might reveal a **palpable nodule** or an area of induration. Early carcinoma is usually not detectable on exam. A tender prostate suggests prostatitis.

Differential

BPH, prostatitis, urethral stricture, neurogenic bladder.

Evaluation

Diagnosis is suggested by clinical findings and/or a markedly **elevated PSA** (mild elevations in PSA may be seen with BPH or prostatitis). Diagnosis is made with **U/S-guided transrectal biopsy.** Tumors are graded by the **Gleason histologic system,** which sums the scores (from 1 to 5) of the two most dysplastic samples; 10 is the highest grade. Look for metastases with CXR and **bone scan.**

Treatment

- Treatment is controversial, as many cases of prostate cancer are slow to progress. Treatment choice is based on the aggressiveness of the tumor and the patient's risk of dying from the disease.
- **Watchful waiting** may be the best approach for elderly patients with low-grade tumors.
- **Radical prostatectomy** and **radiation therapy** (e.g., brachytherapy or external beam) are associated with an increased risk of incontinence and/or impotence.
- **PSA,** while controversial as a screening test, is used to follow patients post-treatment to evaluate for disease recurrence.
- Treat metastatic disease with **androgen ablation** (e.g., GnRH agonists, orchiectomy, flutamide) and chemotherapy.

Prevention

Annual DRE after the age of 50 is the current screening method for prostate cancer.

- All males > 50 years of age should have an **annual DRE.** Screening should begin earlier in African American males and in men with a first-degree relative with prostate cancer.
- Screening with PSA is common, but its utility is controversial.

UCV *Surg.37*

BLADDER CANCER

The second most common urologic cancer and **the most frequent malignant tumor of the urinary tract.** Bladder cancer is usually a **transitional cell carcinoma.** It's most prevalent in men during the sixth and seventh decades. Risk factors include smoking, chronic bladder infections (e.g., schistosomiasis), calculous disease, and exposure to aniline dye (a benzene derivative) or hair dye.

History/PE

Gross hematuria is the most common presenting symptom. Other urinary symptoms, such as frequency, urgency, and dysuria, can also occur, but most patients are asymptomatic in the early stages of disease.

Differential

Strictures, stones, infection, inflammation, infarction, tumor, trauma, TB ($S^2I^3T^3$).

Differential for hematuria—

$S^2I^3T^3$
Strictures
Stones
Infection
Inflammation
Infarction
Tumor
Trauma
TB

Evaluation

- **UA** is the most basic evaluation and often shows hematuria (macro- or microscopic); cytology may show dysplastic cells.
- **IVP** can examine the upper urinary tracts as well as defects in bladder filling.
- **Cystoscopy with biopsy is diagnostic.**
- U/S, MRI, and pelvic CT scan may be used.

Treatment

Treatment depends on the extent of spread beyond the bladder mucosa.

- **Carcinoma in-situ (CIS):** Intravesicular chemotherapy.
- **Superficial cancers:** Complete transurethral resection or intravesicular chemotherapy with mitomycin-C or BCG (the vaccine for TB).
- **Large, high-grade recurrent lesions:** Intravesicular chemotherapy.
- **Invasive cancers without metastases:** Aggressive surgery, radiotherapy, or both.
- **Patients with distant metastases:** Chemotherapy alone.

UCV *Surg.36*

RENAL CELL CARCINOMA (RCC)

An adenocarcinoma from tubular epithelial cells that causes 80–90% of all malignant tumors of the kidney. Risk factors include **male gender, smoking, and von Hippel–Lindau disease.** Can spread along the renal vein to the IVC and metastasize to lung and bone.

History/PE

Presents with a triad of **hematuria, flank pain, and a palpable flank mass.** Many patients have **fever** or other constitutional symptoms. **Polycythemia** due to increased erythropoietin production is seen in 5–10% of patients.

The classic triad of RCC = hematuria, flank pain, and a palpable flank mass.

Treatment

Surgical resection may be curative in localized disease. Response rates from chemotherapy are only 15–30%.

UCV *Surg.38*

TESTICULAR CANCER

A heterogeneous group of neoplasms, 95% of testicular tumors derive from **germ cells,** and **virtually all are malignant.** Most common malignancy in 25–34-year-old men. **Cryptorchidism** is associated with increased risk of neoplasia in both testes. **Klinefelter's syndrome** is also a risk factor.

History/PE

Patients most often present with **painless enlargement of the testis.** Most testicular cancers occur between the ages of 15 and 30, but seminomas have a peak incidence between ages 40 and 50.

Evaluation

β-hCG = choriocarcinoma.

AFP = endodermal sinus tumor.

Tumor markers are useful in diagnosis. β-hCG is always elevated in choriocarcinoma and is elevated in 10% of seminomas; α-fetoprotein (AFP) is often elevated in nonseminomatous germ cell tumors, particularly endodermal sinus (yolk sac) tumors.

Treatment

Seminomas are **exquisitely radiosensitive** and also respond to chemotherapy. Platinum-based chemotherapy is used for nonseminomatous germ cell tumors.

UCV *Surg.39*

CRYPTORCHIDISM

Failure of the testes to fully descend into the scrotum. Prematurity is a risk factor for the disorder, and bilateral cryptorchidism is associated with oligospermia and infertility. On exam, testes **cannot be manipulated into the scrotal sac** with gentle pressure (unlike retracted testes) and may be palpated anywhere along the inguinal canal or in the abdomen. Treat with **orchiopexy** after age one (in all but 1% males, testes will descend by this age) but before age five (to preserve fertility). If discovered later in life, treat with orchiectomy to avoid risk of testicular cancer.

ERECTILE DYSFUNCTION (ED)

Found in 10–25% of middle-aged and elderly men, ED has a significant impact on the well-being of affected individuals. Risk factors include **DM, atherosclerosis, medications** (e.g., β-blockers, SSRIs), HTN, heart disease, surgery or radiation for prostate cancer, and spinal cord injury. The pathophysiology is classified as failure to initiate (e.g., psychological, endocrinologic, neurologic), failure to fill (e.g., arteriogenic), or failure to store (e.g., venoocclusive dysfunction).

History/PE

Because patients rarely volunteer this complaint, physicians should make a specific inquiry. Ask about risk factors, **medication use,** recent life changes, and psychological stressors. The distinction between psychological and organic ED is based on the presence of **nocturnal or early-morning erections** and on **situation dependence** (i.e., occurring with only one partner). If patients can have a normal erection, the problem is not organic. Evaluate for **neurologic dysfunction** (e.g., anal tone, lower extremity sensation) and for **hypogonadism** (e.g., small testes, loss of secondary sexual characteristics).

Evaluation

Testosterone and gonadotropin levels may be abnormal. Check prolactin, as elevated **prolactin** can cause decreased androgen activity.

Treatment

Patients with psychological ED may benefit from psychotherapy or sex therapy involving discussion and exercises with the appropriate partner. Oral **sildenafil (Viagra)** is a phosphodiesterase–5 (PDE5) inhibitor that causes prolonged action of cyclic GMP-mediated smooth muscle relaxation and increased blood flow in the corpora cavernosa. Sildenafil is effective for a broad range of etiologies, including psychogenic, diabetic, vasculogenic, or the result of prostatectomy or spinal cord injury. **Testosterone** is useful therapy for patients with hypogonadism of testicular or pituitary origin; it is discouraged for patients with normal testosterone levels. Vacuum pumps, intracavernosal injections, and surgical implantation of semirigid or inflatable penile prostheses are alternatives for patients who fail sildenafil therapy.

The following clinical questions and accompanying answers are reproduced, with permission, from Berk SL, *PreTest: Medicine*, 9th ed., New York: McGraw-Hill, 2001.

Questions

1. A 70-year-old male with a history of UTI and CHF was admitted to the hospital for sepsis and pulmonary edema. He was treated with clindamycin and tobramycin and also received intravenous furosemide. After several days, the signs of sepsis improved, but his BUN rose to 60 mg/dL and the creatinine to 5.0 mg/dL. His blood pressure was stable at 120/70, pulse 70, and there were no postural changes. Weight was unchanged throughout the hospital course. The most likely cause of the patient's deteriorating renal function is
   a. Prerenal azotemia
   b. Acute tubular necrosis
   c. Interstitial nephritis
   d. Hypercalcemic nephropathy

2. The best evidence to support the diagnosis of ATN in this patient would be
   a. Urine Na^+ of 25 mEq/L
   b. Renal tubular epithelial cells and muddy brown casts in urine sediment
   c. A negative renal ultrasound
   d. An IVP showing abnormalities of the medulla

3. Under what circumstances would this patient require acute hemodialysis?
   a. BUN and creatinine do not return to normal after three days
   b. The patient produces < 200 cc of urine a day following the development of ATN
   c. The patient develops hyperkalemia with peaked T waves and widening of the QRS complex
   d. Urine sodium is > 40 mEq/L

4. A 70-year-old is found to be hypotensive in his home. He appears volume-depleted. Initial blood gases show a pH of 7.2, P_{CO_2} 35 (mmHg). Other electrolytes are

Na^+ 136 mEq/L	Cl^- 114
K^+ 4.0	HCO_3 14

   The primary acid–base disorder in this patient is
   a. Respiratory acidosis
   b. Metabolic acidosis
   c. Respiratory alkalosis
   d. Metabolic alkalosis with compensation

5. A 30-year-old male with HIV presents with complaints of flank pain and hematuria that have occurred suddenly. The patient, while being examined, is writhing in pain. A urinalysis shows many red blood cells without casts and few white blood cells. The most likely diagnosis is
   a. Urolithiasis
   b. Streptococcal glomerulonephritis
   c. Bladder tumor
   d. Pyelonephritis

Answers

1. **The answer is b.** Since there is no clinical evidence of prerenal azotemia, it is most likely that this patient's ARF is secondary to aminoglycoside toxicity and ATN.

2. **The answer is b.** The urine sediment in ATN is usually abnormal, with renal tubular epithelial cells, debris, and muddy brown casts. The high urine sodium, particularly if the patient has been getting a diuretic, is less specific. A U/S would rule out obstruction as a cause of renal failure, but would not be helpful in distinguishing prerenal from intrinsic renal failure. An IVP is contraindicated in the setting of acute renal failure.

3. **The answer is c.** Hyperkalemia with cardiotoxicity is an indication for acute hemodialysis. The BUN and creatinine would not be expected to return to normal within days, and the patient may remain oliguric for several days or longer. The urine sodium is not a measure of recovery in ATN.

4. **The answer is b.** The pH of 7.2 shows this to be a severe acidosis. The P_{CO_2} is < 40 mmHg; hence there is no CO_2 retention to suggest respiratory acidosis. The patient has a metabolic acidosis.

5. **The answer is a.** The patient presents with clinical features of a renal stone, which is supported by the findings of red blood cells in the urine sediment. Red blood cell casts would be expected in glomerular disease, white blood cells in pyelonephritis. The patient's symptoms are not consistent with bladder cancer.

Selected Topics in Emergency Medicine

Table 2.17–1 summarizes some major drug side effects.

TABLE 2.17–1. Drug Side Effects

Drug	Side Effects
ACE Inhibitors (ACEIs)	Cough, rash, proteinuria, angioedema, taste changes, teratogenic effects.
Amantadine	Ataxia, **livido reticularis.**
Aminoglycosides	Ototoxicity, nephrotoxicity (ATN).
Amiodarone	Pulmonary fibrosis, peripheral deposition causing bluish discoloration, arrhythmias, hypo-/hyper-thyroidism, corneal deposition.
Amphotericin	Fever/chills, nephrotoxicity, bone marrow suppression, anemia.
Antipsychotics	Sedation, acute dystonic reaction, akathisia, parkinsonism, tardive dyskinesia, **neuroleptic malignant syndrome** *(EM.41).*
-Azoles (e.g, fluconazole)	Inhibition of P450 enzymes.
AZT	Thrombocytopenia, megaloblastic anemia.
β-blockers	Asthma exacerbation, masking of hypoglycemia, impotence.
Benzodiazepines	Sedation, dependence, respiratory depression.
Bile acid resins	GI upset, malabsorption of vitamins and medications.
Calcium channel blockers	Peripheral edema, constipation, cardiac depression.
Carbamazepine	Induction of P450 enzymes, **agranulocytosis,** aplastic anemia.
Chloramphenicol	**Gray baby syndrome,** aplastic anemia.
Cisplatin	Nephrotoxicity, acoustic nerve damage.
Clonidine	Dry mouth, **severe rebound headache,** rebound HTN.
Clozapine	Agranulocytosis.
Corticosteroids	Mania (acute), immunosuppression, bone mineral loss, thin skin, easy bruising, myopathy (chronic), cataracts.
Cyclophosphamide	Myelosuppression, **hemorrhagic cystitis.**
Digoxin	GI disturbance, **yellow visual changes, arrhythmias** (e.g., junctional supraventricular tachycardia [SVT]).
Doxorubicin	**Cardiotoxicity (cardiomyopathy).**
Ethyl alcohol	Renal dysfunction.
Fluoroquinolones	Cartilage damage in children, Achilles tendon rupture in adults.
Furosemide	Ototoxicity, hypokalemia, nephritis.
Gemfibrozil	Myositis, reversible increase in LFTs.
Gold	Renal dysfunction, leukopenia, rash.
Halothane	Hepatotoxicity, **malignant hyperthermia.**
HMG-CoA reductase inhibitors	Myositis, reversible increase in LFTs.

TABLE 2.17–1 *(continued).* **Drug Side Effects**

Drug	Side Effects
Hydralazine	Drug-induced systemic lupus erythematosus (SLE).
Hydrochlorothiazide (HCTZ)	Hypokalemia, hyperuricemia, hyperglycemia.
Hydroxychloroquine	Retinopathy.
INH	Peripheral neuropathy **(prevent with vitamin B$_6$),** hepatotoxicity, inhibition of P450 enzymes, seizures with overdose.
MAOIs	**Hypertensive tyramine reaction, serotonin syndrome** (with meperidine).
Methanol	Blindness *(EM.48).*
Methotrexate	Hepatic fibrosis, pneumonitis, anemia.
Methyldopa	Positive Coombs' test, drug-induced SLE.
Metronidazole	Disulfiram reaction, vestibular dysfunction, **metallic taste.**
Niacin	**Cutaneous flushing.**
Nitroglycerin	Hypotension, tachycardia, headache, tolerance.
Pencillin/β-lactams	Hypersensitivity reactions.
Penicillamine	Drug-induced SLE.
Phenytoin	Nystagmus, diplopia, ataxia, **gingival hyperplasia,** hirsutism.
Prazosin	First-dose hypotension.
Procainamide	Drug-induced SLE.
Propylthiouracil (PTU)	Agranulocytosis.
Quinidine	Cinchonism (headache, tinnitus), thrombocytopenia, arrhythmias (e.g., **torsades de pointes**).
Reserpine	Depression.
Rifampin	Induction of P450 enzymes, **orange-red body secretions.**
Salicylates	Fever, hyperventilation with **respiratory alkalosis and metabolic acidosis,** dehydration, diaphoresis, hemorrhagic gastritis *(EM.49).*
Selective serotonin reuptake inhibitors (SSRIs)	Anxiety, **sexual dysfunction.**
Succinylcholine	**Malignant hyperthermia.**
Tetracyclines	Tooth discoloration, photosensitivity, Fanconi's syndrome.
Tricyclic antidepressants (TCAs)	Sedation coma, anticholinergic effects, seizures and arrhythmias *(EM.42).*
Valproic acid	Neural tube defects.
Vancomycin	Nephrotoxicity, ototoxicity, **"red man syndrome"** (histamine release; not an allergy).
Vinblastine	Severe myelosuppression.
Vincristine	Peripheral neuropathy.

HIGH-YIELD FACTS

Emergency Medicine

Table 2.17–2 summarizes drug withdrawal symptoms and treatment.

TABLE 2.17–2. Management of Drug Withdrawal

Drug	Withdrawal Symptoms	Treatment
Alcohol	Tremor (6–12 hours), tachycardia, HTN, agitation, seizures (within 48 hours), hallucinations, **delirium tremens (DTs;** severe autonomic instability, including tachycardia, HTN, delirium, and death) within 2–7 days. Mortality is 15–20%.	Benzodiazepines; haloperidol for hallucinations; thiamine, folate, and multivitamin replacement (these will not affect withdrawal, but most alcoholics are malnourished).
Barbiturates	Anxiety, seizures, delirium, tremor, cardiac and respiratory depression.	Mainstay of treatment is **benzodiazepines.**
Benzodiazepines	Rebound anxiety, seizures, tremor, insomnia.	Mainstay of treatment is benzodiazepines. Watch out for DTs.
Cocaine/ amphetamines (EM.40)	Depression, hyperphagia, hypersomnolence.	Supportive treatment. Avoid pure β-blockers (results in excess unhibited cardiac activation).
Opioids (EM.39)	Anxiety, insomnia, **flu-like symptoms,** sweating, piloerection, fever, rhinorrhea, nausea, stomach cramps, diarrhea, mydriasis.	Clonidine and/or buprenorphine for moderate withdrawal. Methadone for severe symptoms. Naltrexone for patients who are drug free for 7–10 days.

Table 2.17–3 describes some common drug interactions.

TABLE 2.17–3. Drug Interactions

Interaction/Reaction	Drugs
Induction of P450 enzymes	Barbiturates, phenytoin, carbamazepine, rifampin.
Inhibition of P450 enzymes	Cimetidine, ketoconazole, INH.
Metabolism by P450 enzymes	Benzodiazepines, amide anesthetics, metoprolol, propranolol, nifedipine, phenytoin, quinidine, theophylline, warfarin, barbiturates.
Increasing risk of digoxin toxicity	Quinidine, cimetidine, amiodarone, calcium channel blockers.
Competition for albumin binding sites	Warfarin, ASA, phenytoin.
Blood dyscrasias	Ibuprofen, quinidine, methyldopa, chemotherapeutic agents.
Hemolysis in G6PD-deficient patients	Sulfonamides, INH, ASA, ibuprofen, nitrofurantoin, primaquine.
Gynecomastia	Cimetidine, ketoconazole, spironolactone.
Stevens-Johnson syndrome	Ethosuximide, sulfonamides (EM.7).
Photosensitivity	Tetracycline, amiodarone, sulfonamides.
Drug-induced SLE	Procainamide, hydralazine, INH, penicillamine.

HIGH-YIELD FACTS

Emergency Medicine

Table 2.17–4 summarizes the antidotes for various substance overdoses.

TABLE 2.17–4. Specific Antidotes

Toxin	Antidote/Treatment
Acetaminophen	N-acetylcysteine.
Anticholinesterases, organophosphates	Atropine, pralidoxime.
Antimuscarinic, anticholinergic agents	Physostigmine.
Black widow bite	Calcium gluconate.
Iron salts	Deferoxamine.
Methanol, ethylene glycol (antifreeze)	EtOH, fomepizole, dialysis.
Lead	Succimer, CaEDTA, dimercaprol.
Arsenic, mercury, gold	Succimer, dimercaprol.
Copper, arsenic, lead, gold	Penicillamine.
Cyanide	Nitrite, sodium thiosulfate.
Salicylates	Urine alkalinization, dialysis, activated charcoal.
Heparin	Protamine sulfate.
Methemoglobin	Methylene blue.
Opioids	Naloxone.
Benzodiazepines	Flumazenil.
Barbiturates (phenobarbital)	Urine alkalinization, dialysis, activated charcoal.
TCAs	Sodium bicarbonate for QRS prolongation, diazepam or lorazepam for seizures, cardiac monitor for arrhythmias.
Warfarin	Vitamin K, FFP (EM.24).
Carbon monoxide	100% O_2, hyperbaric O_2.
Digitalis	Stop digitalis, normalize K^+, lidocaine (for torsades), anti-digitalis Fab.
β-blockers	Glucagon.
Tissue plasminogen activator (tPA), streptokinase	Aminocaproic acid.
Phencyclidine hydrochloride (PCP)	NG suction.
Theophylline	Activated charcoal.
Acid/alkali ingestion	Upper endoscopy to evaluate for stricture.

Table 2.17–5 summarizes the signs and symptoms of key vitamin deficiencies.

TABLE 2.17–5. Vitamin Functions and Deficiencies

Vitamin	Signs/Symptoms of Deficiency
Vitamin A	Night blindness, dry skin.
Vitamin B$_1$ (thiamine)	Beriberi (polyneuritis, dilated cardiomyopathy, high-output CHF, edema), Wernicke-Korsakoff.
Vitamin B$_2$ (riboflavin)	Angular stomatitis, cheilosis, corneal vascularization.
Vitamin B$_3$ (niacin)	Pellagra (diarrhea, dermatitis, dementia).
Vitamin B$_5$ (pantothenate)	Dermatitis, enteritis, alopecia, adrenal insufficiency.
Vitamin B$_6$ (pyridoxine)	Convulsions, hyperirritability; required during administration of INH.
Vitamin B$_{12}$ (cobalamin)	Macrocytic, megaloblastic anemia; neurologic symptoms (e.g., optic neuropathy, subacute combined degeneration, paresthesia); glossitis.
Vitamin C	Scurvy (e.g., swollen gums, bruising, anemia, poor wound healing).
Vitamin D	Rickets in children (bending bones), osteomalacia in adults (soft bones), hypocalcemic tetany.
Vitamin E	Increased fragility of RBCs.
Vitamin K	Neonatal hemorrhage; increased PT and aPTT, normal BT.
Biotin	Dermatitis, enteritis. Can be caused by ingestion of **raw eggs.**
Folic acid	**Most common vitamin deficiency in the United States.** Sprue; macrocytic, megaloblastic anemia without neurologic symptoms.
Magnesium	Weakness, muscle cramps, exacerbation of hypocalcemic tetany, CNS hyperirritability leading to tremors, choreoathetoid movement, positive Babinski sign.
Selenium	Keshan's syndrome (cardiomyopathy).

Aspects of a pain history—

OPQRST
Onset
Precipitating factors
Quality
Radiation
Symptoms
Temporal
quality/**T**reatment
modalities

If the patient remembers the exact time of pain onset, consider perforation.

All abdominal pain is not GI pain.

All female patients with an acute abdomen require a pelvic exam and a pregnancy test to rule out PID, ectopic pregnancy, and ovarian torsion.

Acute-onset abdominal pain is associated with many potential etiologies and may require immediate surgical intervention.

History/PE

A complete history should include all aspects of the **OPQRST** mnemonic.

- **Character of pain:** Pain quality and intensity, onset, and radiation must be considered. Sharp pain implies parietal (peritoneal) pain; dull, diffuse pain is commonly visceral (organ) pain.
  - **Perforation:** Sudden onset of diffuse, severe pain.
  - **Obstruction:** Acute onset of severe, radiating, colicky pain.
  - **Inflammation:** Gradual onset (over 10–12 hours) of constant, ill-defined pain.
- **Location of pain:** Figure 2.17–1 differentiates the causes of acute abdomen by quadrant.
- **Associated symptoms:** Anorexia, nausea, vomiting, changes in bowel habits, hematochezia, and melena may suggest GI etiologies. Hematuria or costovertebral angle (CVA) tenderness suggest a GU etiology. Association with meals points to mesenteric ischemia. A family history of abdominal pain may suggest familial Mediterranean fever or acute intermittent porphyria. A prior history of pain may suggest vasculitides, SLE, DKA, or sickle cell disease. A full gynecologic history must always be taken in females; ask about the patient's last menstrual period, the possibility of pregnancy, and the presence of STD symptoms.

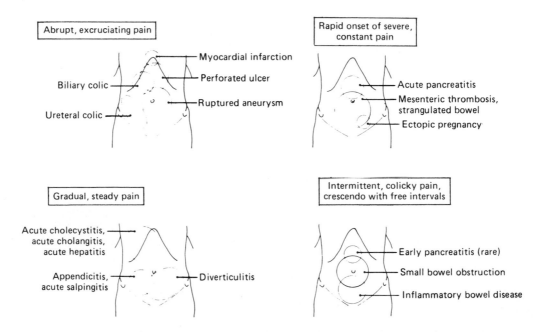

FIGURE 2.17–1. Acute abdomen. The location and character of pain are helpful in the differential diagnosis of the acute abdomen. (Reproduced, with permission, from Way L. *Current Surgical Diagnosis & Treatment,* 10th ed. Stamford, CT: Appleton & Lange, 1994:444, Fig. 21–3.)

Evaluation

First assess the stability of the patient. If peritoneal signs, impending shock, or shock is present, emergent surgical treatment with an exploratory laparotomy is necessary. If the patient is stable, a complete physical exam, including a rectal exam and, in women, a pelvic exam, is mandatory. Order electrolytes, LFTs, amylase, lipase, **urine β-hCG,** UA, and a CBC with differential. Radiologic studies can include a KUB or contrast studies. **Avoid contrast studies if a complete large bowel obstruction is suspected.** In women, U/S can be used to evaluate for ectopic pregnancy and ovarian torsion.

Treatment

Patients who are hemodynamically unstable must have an **emergent exploratory laparotomy.** If the patient is stable, expectant management may include NPO status, NG tube, IV fluids, placement of a Foley (to monitor urine output and fluid status), and vital sign monitoring with serial abdominal exams and serial labs. Type and cross all patients.

APPENDICITIS

Must **always** be considered in the differential of acute abdomen. Approximately 7% of people in the United States will develop appendicitis, with the peak age of presentation in the teens and mid-20s. Etiologies include luminal obstruction by hypertrophied lymphoid tissue (55–65%), fecalith (35%), foreign body, tumor (e.g., carcinoid tumor), or parasite. Obstruction results in overdistention and eventually, with increased pressure, ischemia and necrosis.

Appendicitis must always be considered in a patient with acute abdomen.

History/PE

Patients present with a history of dull, vague pain originating at the umbilicus and lasting 1–12 hours. Pain is then followed by nausea, vomiting, and anorexia ("hamburger sign"). Mild fever may be present. As the irritation becomes visceral, a sharper pain will localize to the RLQ at McBurney's point. The psoas, obturator, and Rovsing's signs are insensitive tests that may be positive. If a patient has a perforated appendix, he may state that the pain decreases, but peritoneal signs (e.g., rebound, guarding, hypotension, high WBC count, high fever) will ultimately develop. Children and the elderly can have atypical presentations, as can patients who are pregnant or who have retrocecal appendices.

"Hamburger sign" — If a patient wants to eat, consider a diagnosis other than appendicitis.

McBurney's point is located two-thirds of the distance from the anterior superior iliac spine to the umbilicus.

Differential

The differential diagnosis includes the etiologies summarized in Figure 2.17–1.

Evaluation

Obtain a full H&P, as the diagnosis is commonly clinical. Patients might have mild fever, mild leukocytosis (11,000–15,000 cells/μL) with a left shift, and a UA with a few RBCs or WBCs. Radiographically, a KUB may show a fecalith or a loss of psoas shadow; U/S may be useful in female patients to rule out gynecologic abnormalities. Abdominal CT can help rule out abscesses.

Rovsing's sign = deep palpation of the LLQ causes referred pain in the RLQ.

Psoas sign = passive extension of the hip causes RLQ pain.

Obturator sign = passive internal rotation of the hip causes RLQ pain.

Don't forget about atypical presentations of appendicitis in children, pregnant women, and the elderly.

Treatment

Immediately perform an open or laparoscopic appendectomy on patients in whom appendicitis is strongly suspected. A 15–20% false positive rate for appendectomy is generally accepted. If appendicitis is not found on operative exam, do a complete exploration of the abdomen through the same incision. Prior to surgery, patients should be held NPO, receive IV fluids, and receive antibiotics for anaerobic coverage for 24 hours. If perforation occurs, antibiotic use should continue until the patient is afebrile and the WBC count normalizes; the wound should be closed by delayed primary closure on POD 5. If an abscess is present, broad-spectrum antibiotics should be given and the abscess percutaneously drained (by U/S or CT); 6–8 weeks later, an elective appendectomy should be performed.

Complications

The risk of perforation and mortality increases with the amount of time the appendicitis is present; the risk approaches 75% at 48 hours.

UCV *Surg.20*

ACUTE MANAGEMENT OF A TRAUMA PATIENT

Acute management of a trauma patient can be remembered with the mnemonic **ABCDE.**

Workup of a trauma patient—

ABCDE
Airway
Breathing
Circulation
Disability
Exposure

Evaluation/Treatment

Airway patency and adequacy of ventilation take precedence over other treatment.

- Start with supplemental O_2 by nasal cannula or face mask for conscious patients. Use a chin-lift or jaw-thrust maneuver to reposition the tongue in an unconscious patient. An oropharyngeal or nasopharyngeal airway may help bag-mask ventilation.
- Perform early intubation in patients with apnea, decreased mental status, impending airway compromise (e.g., significant maxillofacial trauma, inhalation injury in fires), severe closed head injuries, or failed bag-mask ventilation.
- Perform a surgical airway (i.e., cricothyroidectomy) in patients who cannot be intubated or in whom there is significant maxillofacial trauma.
- Maintain cervical-spine stabilization in trauma patients, but **never allow this concern to delay airway management.**

Immediately evaluate trauma patients for tension pneumothorax, cardiac tamponade, open pneumothorax, massive hemothorax, and airway obstruction.

Adequacy of breathing should next be addressed. Thorough cardiac and pulmonary exams will help identify the five thoracic causes of immediate death that **must not be missed: tension pneumothorax, cardiac tamponade, open pneumothorax, massive hemothorax, and airway obstruction.**

Circulation may then be evaluated. If possible, two 16-gauge IVs should be placed in the antecubital fossae. Fluid resuscitation should include a fluid bolus (1–2 L in adults). Vitals should then be rechecked and repletion should continue as indicated by fluid status. Remember that isotonic (LR or NS) fluids and blood should be repleted in a **3:1 ratio (fluid to blood).**

After the ABCs, the patient's disability (e.g., CNS dysfunction) should be quantified with the Glasgow Coma Scale. Exposure assesses temperature status and other missed findings.

The primary survey is followed by the secondary survey, which includes additional x-rays and a full examination. Do not forget to order a trauma series (i.e., AP chest, AP pelvis, and AP/lateral C-spine, including the T1 vertebra) and to place a Foley catheter during the primary survey (after urethral injury has been ruled out; see "Pelvic Fractures," p. 490).

AORTIC DISRUPTION

A **rapid deceleration injury** seen most commonly after high-speed motor vehicle accidents (MVAs), falls from great heights, and ejection from vehicles. Since complete aortic rupture is rapidly fatal (85% die at the scene), trauma patients with an aortic injury usually have a contained hematoma within the adventitia. Laceration usually occurs at the ligamentum arteriosum.

Evaluation

Obtain an **immediate CXR,** which may reveal a **widened mediastinum** (> 8 cm), **loss of aortic knob, pleural cap,** deviation of the trachea to the right, and depression of the left main stem bronchus. **Always suspect aortic disruption if there are sternal or first and second rib fractures. Aortography is the gold standard for evaluation.** CT evaluation remains controversial, although spiral CT is finding more widespread use. Transesophageal echocardiography (TEE) should also be performed prior to going to the OR.

Aortic disruption is often associated with first and second rib and sternal fractures.

Treatment

If a patient survives the initial insult, he should proceed to the OR emergently for defect repair.

AORTIC DISSECTION

Occurs when an intimal tear allows blood to enter the aortic media, splitting the medial lamellae and causing a **second "false" lumen** to form. Stanford **type A** dissections involve the ascending aorta; **type B** are distal to the left subclavian artery. Risk factors include **HTN,** trauma, coarctation of the aorta, syphilis, pregnancy, Ehlers-Danlos syndrome, and **Marfan's syndrome.**

History/PE

Presents with acute onset of severe **"tearing" or "ripping" chest** or back pain. Occlusion of aortic branch vessels may lead to asymmetric or decreased peripheral pulses, syncope, stroke, MI, or paraplegia. Aortic regurgitation with diastolic murmur may occur in a type A dissection. Shock may develop as the condition worsens.

Patients classically present with a sudden onset of tearing chest pain radiating to the back.

Differential

MI, pulmonary embolus, angina, thoracic aortic aneurysm, esophageal rupture.

Evaluation

CXR findings are similar to those in aortic disruption. Diagnose via **CT with IV contrast,** TEE, MRI/MRA, or **angiography** (the gold standard). An intimal flap or pseudolumen may be seen. Workup should also include an ECG (look for LVH and ischemic changes).

Treatment

- Stabilize high or low blood pressure. Treat high blood pressure with **IV nitrates and β-blockers.** Nitrates (e.g., sublingual nitroglycerin) may cause hypotension, so exercise caution. Goal is systolic BP < 120 mmHg and HR < 70 bpm to reduce shear stress.
- Type A dissections require **emergent surgery.** Consider medical management for type B dissections in stable patients.

Complications

MI, CHF, future dissection or aneurysm formation, cardiac tamponade, postoperative hemorrhage, death.

BASICS OF CARDIAC LIFE SUPPORT

Table 2.17–6 summarizes the basic management of cardiac arrhythmias in an acute setting.

BURNS

The **second leading cause of death in children.**

History/PE

Patients may present with obvious skin wounds, but do not underestimate the degree of nonvisible deep destruction, especially with electrical burns. Perform a thorough airway and lung exam.

Evaluation

Always assess the ABCs. If airway compromise is impending, intubate. Be aware of the possibility of shock, inhalation injury, and carbon monoxide (CO) poisoning. Evaluate the percentage of body surface area (%BSA) involved. Burns can be categorized by depth of destruction:

- **First degree:** The epidermis is involved. Area is painful, blisters are not present, and capillary refill is intact.
- **Second degree:** The epidermis and superficial dermis are involved. Area is painful and blisters are present.
- **Third degree:** The epidermis and dermis are involved. Area is painless, white, and charred.

TABLE 2.17–6. Management of Cardiac Arrhythmias

Arrhythmia	Treatment
Asystole	Epinephrine, Atropine.
Ventricular fibrillation (EM.6)	Desynchronized shock with 200, 300, and 360 J → epinephrine or vasopressin → shock → lidocaine or amiodarone → shock → procainamide or magnesium.
Ventricular tachycardia	If unstable and pulseless, desynchronized shock; if stable, give lidocaine or amiodarone.
Pulseless electrical activity	Identify and treat the underlying cause. Consider epinephrine and/or atropine.
Atrial fibrillation/ atrial flutter	If unstable, shock starting at 100 J. If stable, control rate (calcium channel blockers, digoxin, or β-blockers), convert rhythm (if < 48 hours, convert electrically or chemically; if > 48 hours, anticoagulate or do a TEE prior to conversion), and anticoagulate.
SVT	Control rate with maneuvers such as Valsalva, carotid sinus massage, or cold stimulus. If resistant, consider adenosine.
Bradycardia	If symptomatic, consider atropine. If Mobitz II or third-degree heart block is present, install a pacemaker. Acutely, give unstable or resistant patients atropine or dopamine (DA), dobutamine, or transvenous pacing.

Treatment

Treatment is supportive. Although silver sulfadiazine and mafenide can be used, there is no proven benefit associated with the use of PO/IV antibiotics or steroids. Repletion of fluids by the **Parkland formula** is critical, but adjust repletion based on additional insensible losses. Maintain at least 1 cc/kg/hr of urine output.

Complications

Shock and superinfection, with the latter most likely due to *Pseudomonas.*

UCV EM.21

CARBON MONOXIDE (CO) POISONING

A **hypoxemic poisoning syndrome** seen in patients exposed to automobile exhaust, smoke inhalation, barbecues in poorly ventilated locations, or old appliances.

History/PE

Hypoxemia, **cherry-red skin,** confusion, and **headaches.** Coma or seizures occur in severe cases. Chronic low-level exposure may cause **flu-like symptoms** with generalized myalgias, nausea, and headaches. **Suspect smoke inhalation in the presence of singed nose hairs, facial burns, hoarseness, wheezing, or carbonaceous sputum.**

Evaluation

Pulse oximetry will be falsely elevated in CO poisoning.

Check an ABG; the normal serum carboxyhemoglobin level is < 5% in non-smokers and < 10% in smokers. Perform laryngoscopy or bronchoscopy if smoke inhalation is suspected. Check an ECG in the elderly and in patients with a history of cardiac disease.

Treatment

Treat with 100% O_2 (use **hyperbaric O_2** for pregnant patients, those with neurologic symptoms, or those with severely elevated carboxyhemoglobin) to facilitate displacement of CO from Hb. Patients with **smoke inhalation** may require early intubation, since upper airway edema can rapidly progress to complete obstruction.

Intubate early if you suspect CO poisoning.

UCV EM.47

PELVIC FRACTURES

Most common after a trauma such as an MVA. Pelvic fractures require immediate attention by the orthopedist owing to their potentially life-threatening nature.

Evaluation/Treatment

After the initial ABC trauma survey, the secondary survey may reveal an unstable pelvis upon compression. AP pelvic x-rays may confirm the fracture; when the patient is stable, a CT pelvis will better define the extent of damage. If hypotension and shock are present, an exsanguinating hemorrhage is likely. In the field, MAST (military anti-shock trousers; rarely used today) can be used to maintain adequate BP and organ perfusion. In the hospital, treatment options include embolization of bleeding vessels, emergent external pelvic fixation, or, in a hemodynamically stable patient, internal fixation. With a pelvic fracture, remember the following:

Never place a Foley in a patient who has suspected urethral damage.

- Pelvic injuries can be associated with urethral injury. Make note of **blood at the urethral meatus, a high-riding, "ballotable" prostate, or the lack of a prostate.** These findings suggest urethral injury, and a **retrograde urethrogram** must be ordered to rule out injury before a Foley catheter is placed.
- Never explore a pelvic or retroperitoneal hematoma. Follow with serial Hb and HCT.

Evaluation and treatment depend on the location and extent of the injury.

- **Neck:** Intubate early. Evaluation can include aortography for zone 1 injuries and aortography, tracheobronchoscopy, and esophagoscopy for zone 3 injuries. Surgically explore injuries to zone 2, if the platysma is penetrated (though at some institutions, angiography and triple endoscopy are also being used for injuries to this zone; see Figure 2.17–2).
- **Chest:** Unstable patients with penetrating thoracic injuries require immediate **intubation** and bilateral **chest tubes.** Thoracotomy may be necessary if a patient remains unstable despite resuscitative efforts. Leave any impaled objects in place until the patient is taken to the OR, as such objects may tamponade further blood loss. Beware of pneumothorax, hemothorax, cardiac tamponade, aortic disruption, diaphragmatic tear, and esophageal injury. If a previously stable chest trauma patient suddenly dies, suspect **air embolism.** *(EM.19)*
- **Abdomen:** The absence of pain does not completely rule out an abdominal injury.
  - Gunshot wound → immediate exploratory laparotomy.
  - Stab wound or blunt injury in a patient who is hemodynamically unstable or who has peritoneal signs or evisceration → immediate exploratory laparotomy.
  - Stab wound or blunt injury in a hemodynamically stable patient → CT scan or focused abdominal sonography for trauma (FAST scan) is preferred to diagnostic peritoneal lavage (DPL).
  - The **spleen is the most common abdominal organ injured in blunt trauma.** Suspect splenic injury if there are left lower rib fractures *(EM.18)*.
- **Musculoskeletal:** If there is no neurovascular injury, debride and repair. If injury is suspected, do an arteriogram first.
  - **Early wound irrigation** and **tissue debridement,** not antibiotic therapy, constitute the most important steps in the treatment of contaminated wounds. However, do administer antibiotics and tetanus prophylaxis.

Leave any impaled objects in place until the person is taken to the OR.

Suspect air embolism when a previously stable chest trauma patient suddenly dies.

HIGH-YIELD FACTS

Emergency Medicine

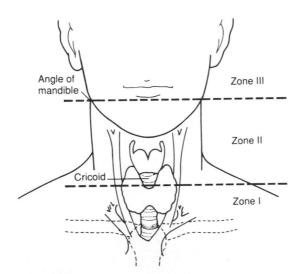

FIGURE 2.17–2. Zones of the neck. (Reproduced, with permission, from Way L. *Current Surgical Diagnosis & Treatment,* 10th ed. Stamford, CT: Appleton & Lange, 1994:223, Fig. 13–9.)

5 W's of post operative fever—

Wind → atelectasis, pnemonia
Water → UTI
Walking → DVT
Wounds → wound infection, abscess
Wonder drugs → drug reaction

POSTOPERATIVE FEVER

Remember the mnemonic **"wind, water, walking, wounds, and wonder drugs."** Decrease the risk of postoperative fever with incentive spirometry, pre- and post-operative antibiotics (when indicated), short-term Foley catheter use, early ambulation, and DVT prophylaxis (e.g., anticoagulation, compression stockings). Fevers before POD 3 are unlikely to be infectious unless *Clostridium* or β-hemolytic streptococcus are involved.

SHOCK

Defined as **inadequate perfusion to maintain vital organ function,** shock takes many forms that are differentiated by their cardiovascular states and treatment options (see Table 2.17–7).

TABLE 2.17–7. Types of Shock

Type of Shock[c]	Major Causes	Cardiac Output	PCWP[a]	PVR[b]	Treatment
Hypovolemic	Trauma, blood loss, inadequate fluid repletion, third spacing, burns.	↓	↓	↑	Replete with isotonic solution (e.g., LR or NS) and blood in a 3:1 (fluid-to-blood) ratio.
Cardiogenic	Tension pneumothorax, CHF, cardiac tamponade, arrhythmia, structural heart disease (severe MR, VSD), MI (> 40% of LV function).	↓	↑	↑	Identify the cause and treat if possible. Give pressors such as **dobutamine** and, if necessary, DA or norepinephrine (NE).
Septic (EM.26)	Bacteremia, especially gram-negative organisms.	↑	↓	↓	Administer fluid and antibiotics. Consider a Swan-Ganz catheter. Give DA or NE.
Anaphylactic (EM.28)	Bee stings, medication, food allergies.	↑	↓	↓	Give diphenhydramine. If severe, administer 1:1000 epinephrine.

[a]PCWP = pulmonary capillary wedge pressure.
[b]PVR = peripheral vascular resistance.
[c]Type of shock = neurogenic shock, which is characterized by **hypotension with bradycardia,** is different from Cushing's triad (increased intracranial pressure), which involves **HTN with bradycardia.**

Rapid Review

Classic ECG finding in atrial flutter.	"Sawtooth" P waves
Definition of unstable angina.	Angina is new, is worsening, or occurs at rest
Antihypertensive for a diabetic patient with proteinuria.	ACE inhibitor (ACE I)
Patient develops Mobitz type 1 heart block following an MI with ECG changes in leads II, III, and aVF. Treatment?	Atropine (inferior MI)
Beck's triad for cardiac tamponade.	Hypotension, distant heart sounds, and JVD
Drugs that slow AV node transmission.	β-blockers, digoxin, Ca^{2+} channel blockers
Hypercholesterolemia treatment that causes flushing and pruritus.	Niacin
Treatment for atrial fibrillation (AF).	Anticoagulation, rate control, cardioversion
Treatment for ventricular fibrillation (VF).	Immediate cardioversion
Autoimmune complication occurring 2–4 weeks post-MI.	Dressler's syndrome: fever, pericarditis, increased ESR
IVDU with JVD and holosystolic murmur at left sternal border. Treatment?	Treat existing heart failure and replace tricuspid valve
Diagnostic test for hypertrophic cardiomyopathy.	Echocardiogram (showing thickened LV wall and outflow obstruction)
Fall in systolic BP of > 10 mmHg with inspiration.	Pulsus paradoxus (seen in cardiac tamponade)
Classic ECG findings in pericarditis.	Low-voltage, diffuse ST-segment elevation
Definition of HTN.	BP > 140/90 mmHg on three separate occasions two weeks apart
Eight surgically correctable causes of HTN.	Renal artery stenosis, coarctation of the aorta, pheochromocytoma, Conn's syndrome, Cushing's syndrome, unilateral renal parenchymal disease, hyperthyroidism, hyperparathyroidism
Evaluation of a pulsatile abdominal mass and bruit.	Abdominal U/S
Indications for surgical repair of abdominal aortic aneurysm.	> 5 cm, rapidly enlarging, symptomatic, or ruptured
Treatment for acute coronary syndrome.	O_2, sublingual nitroglycerin, ASA, IV β-blockers (metoprolol), heparin, and clopidogrel
What is the metabolic syndrome?	Abdominal obesity, high triglycerides, low HDL, HTN, insulin resistance, prothrombotic or proinflammatory states
Appropriate diagnostic test? ■ A 50-year-old male with angina can exercise to 85% of maximum predicted HR. ■ A 65-year-old woman with left bundle branch block and severe osteoarthritis has unstable angina.	Exercise stress treadmill with ECG Pharmacologic stress test (e.g., dobutamine echo)

Target LDL in a patient with diabetes.	< 100
Signs of active ischemia during stress testing.	Angina, ST-segment changes on ECG, or decreased BP
ECG findings suggesting an MI.	ST-segment elevation (depression means ischemia), flattened T waves, and Q waves
Young patient has angina at rest with ST-segment elevation. Cardiac enzymes are normal.	Prinzmetal's angina
Common symptoms associated with silent MIs.	CHF, shock, and altered mental status
Diagnostic test for pulmonary embolism (PE).	V/Q scan (plus pulmonary angiogram if indeterminate)
Agent that reverses the effects of heparin.	Protamine
Coagulation parameter affected by warfarin.	PT
Young patient with a family history of sudden death collapses and dies while exercising.	Hypertrophic cardiomyopathy
Endocarditis prophylaxis regimens.	Oral surgery: amoxicillin; GI or GU procedures: ampicillin and gentamicin before and amoxicillin after
Most common cause of HTN in young women.	OCPs
Most common cause of HTN in young men.	Excessive EtOH

DERMATOLOGY

"Stuck-on" appearance.	Seborrheic keratosis
Red plaques with silvery-white scales and sharp margins. Biopsy shows thickened epidermis and neutrophils in the stratum corneum (Munro microabcesses).	Psoriasis
Most common type of skin cancer; lesion is a pearly-colored papule with a translucent surface and telangectasias.	Basal cell carcinoma
Honey-crusted lesions.	Impetigo
Febrile patient with a history of diabetes presents with a red, swollen, painful lower extremity. Diagnosis? Treatment?	Cellulitis. Treat as outpatient with cephalexin, which has activity against group A streptococci and staphylocci
Positive Nikolsky's sign.	Pemphigus vulgaris
A 55-year-old obese patient presents with dirty, velvety patches on the back of the neck. Diagnosis? Workup?	Acanthosis nigricans. Check fasting blood sugar to rule out diabetes
Dermatomal distribution.	Varicella zoster virus
Flat-topped papules.	Lichen planus
Iris-like target lesions.	Erythema multiforme
Lesion characteristically occurring in a linear pattern in areas where skin comes into contact with clothing or jewelry.	Contact dermatitis

HIGH-YIELD FACTS

Rapid Review

Presents with herald-patch, Christmas-tree pattern.	Pityriasis rosea
"Target" lesions with a red center, pale zone, and dark outer ring appearing on the palms and soles with a prodrome of malaise and myalgias.	Erythema multiforme
A 16-year-old presents with an annular patch of alopecia with broken-off stubby hairs. Diagnosis? Treatment?	Alopecia areata (autoimmune process). Treat with topical steroids
Pinkish, scaling flat lesions on the chest and back. KOH prep has "spaghetti-and-meatballs" appearance. Diagnosis? Treatment?	Pityriasis versicolor. Use topical antifungal agent
Risk factors for squamous cell carcinoma.	Exposure to sun or radiation, actinic keratosis, immunosuppression, arsenic, industrial carcinogens
Child presents with shiny, annular papules on the dorsum of the hand. Biopsy shows chronic inflammation with "palisading histiocytes."	Granuloma annulare. Treat with reassurance and topical/intralesional steroids
Four characteristics of a nevus suggestive of melanoma.	Asymmetry, border irregularity, color variation, large diameter
Beefy-red patches and satellite pustules appearing in intertriginous areas. How to diagnose?	Candidal intertrigo; KOH prep of satellite lesion scraping reveals pseudohyphae
Stress-related hair loss. Treatment?	Telogen effluvium. Reassurance
Child with flesh-colored, umbilicated lesions on the face. When occurring in adults, where do the lesions appear?	Molluscum contagiosum appears in perigenital and perianal area in adults
Sharply demarcated, pruritic red macules with maceration, commonly found on the toe web spaces.	Erythrasma. Diagnose with coral-red fluorescence with Wood's lamp
Premalignant lesion from sun exposure that can lead to SCC.	Actinic keratosis
"Dew drop on a rose petal."	Lesions of primary varicella
Smooth, dome-shaped nodule lacking central punctum, primarily found on the scalp. Biopsy shows lack of granular layer.	Pilar cyst
Causative agent for pityriasis versicolor.	*Malassezia furfur*

ENDOCRINOLOGY

Most common cause of hypothyroidism.	Hashimoto's thyroiditis
Exophthalmos, pretibial myxedema, and decreased TSH.	Graves' disease

First-line treatment for growth hormone–secreting pituitary adenoma.	Transsphenoidal surgical resection
Source of lesion in Cushing's syndrome with high ACTH levels.	Either ectopic or pituitary
Most common cause of Cushing's syndrome.	Iatrogenic steroid administration. Second most common cause is Cushing's disease
Patient presents with signs of hypocalcemia, high phosphorus, and low PTH.	Hypoparathyroidism
"Stones, bones, groans, psychiatric overtones."	Signs and symptoms of hypercalcemia
Patient complains of headache, weakness, and polyuria; exam reveals HTN and tetany. Labs reveals hypernatremia, hypokalemia, and metabolic alkalosis.	Primary hyperaldosteronism due to Conn's syndrome or bilateral adrenal hyperplasia
Patient presents with tachycardia, wild swings in BP, headache, diaphoresis, altered mental status, and a sense of panic.	Pheochromocytoma
Should α- or β-antagonists be used first in treating pheochromocytoma?	α-antagonists (phentolamine and phenoxybenzamine)
Patient with a history of lithium use presents with copious amounts of dilute urine.	Nephrogenic diabetes inspidus (DI)
Diagnostic test that helps differentiate central from nephrogenic DI.	Administration of DDAVP and measurement of urine osmolality
Postoperative patient with significant pain presents with hyponatremia and normal volume status.	SIADH due to stress
The only indication for administering hypertonic saline to a patient with SIADH.	Active seizures
Antidiabetic agent associated with lactic acidosis.	Metformin
Morning hyperglycemia that is a rebound response to nighttime hypoglycemia, not a need for more insulin. Treatment?	Somogyi effect. Reduce PM insulin dose
Patient presents with weakness, nausea, vomiting, weight loss, and new skin pigmentation. Labs show hyponatremia and hyperkalemia. Treatment?	Addison's disease. Treat with replacement glucocorticoids and mineralocorticoids
Goal hemoglobin A_{1c} for a patient with diabetes mellitus (DM).	< 7.0
Treatment of DKA.	Fluids, insulin, and aggressive replacement of electrolytes (e.g., K^+)
In obese patients with this disorder, weight loss may completely eliminate the need for medication.	Type 2 DM
Why are β-blockers contraindicated in diabetics?	They can mask symptoms of hypoglycemia
Most common cause of pathologic fractures in elderly, thin women.	Osteoporosis

Bias introduced into a study when a clinician is aware of what type of treatment his patient received.	Observational bias
Bias introduced when screening detects a disease earlier and thus lengthens the time from diagnosis to death.	Lead-time bias
If you want to know if race affects infant mortality rate but most of the variation in infant mortality is predicted by socioeconomic status, then socioeconomic status is a _____.	Confounding variable
True positives divided by number of patients with the disease.	Sensitivity. Sensitive tests have few false negatives and are used to rule out a disease
PPD reactivity is used as a screening test for TB because most people with TB (except those who are anergic) will have a positive PPD. Highly sensitive or specific?	Highly sensitive
Chronic diseases like systemic lupus erythematosus SLE—higher prevalence or incidence?	Higher prevalence
Epidemics such as influenza—higher prevalence or incidence?	Higher incidence
Cross-sectional survey—incidence or prevalence?	Prevalence
Cohort study—incidence or prevalence?	Incidence
Case-control study—incidence or prevalence?	Neither
Describe a test that consistently gives identical results, but the results are wrong.	High reliability, low validity
Difference between a cohort and a case-control study.	Cohort studies are prospective and can be used to calculate relative risk (RR) and incidence. Case-control studies are retrospective and can be used to calculate an odds ratio (OR)
Attributable risk?	Incidence rate (IR) of disease in exposed—IR of disease in unexposed
Relative risk?	IR of a disease in a population exposed to a particular factor/IR of those not exposed to the factor
Odds ratio?	Likelihood of exposure to a risk factor in individuals with and without the disease
Number needed to treat?	1/incidence
In which patients do you initiate colorectal cancer screening early?	Patients with inflammatory bowel disease (IBD), familial adenomatous polyposis (FAP)/hereditary nonpolyposis colorectal cancer (HNPCC), first-degree relatives with adenomatous polyps (< 60 years old) or colorectal cancer

HIGH-YIELD FACTS

Rapid Review

Most common cancer in men and most common cause of death from cancer in men.	Prostate cancer is the most common, but lung cancer causes more deaths
Percentage of cases within one standard deviation (SD) of the mean? Two SDs? Three SDs?	68%, 95.5%, 99.7%
Birth rate?	Number of live births per 1,000 population
Fertility rate?	Number of live births per 1,000 women 15–44 years old
Mortality rate?	Number of deaths per 1,000 population
Neonatal mortality?	Number of deaths from birth to 28 days per 1,000 *live* births
Postnatal mortality?	Number of deaths from 28 days to one year per 1,000 *live* births
Infant mortality?	Neonatal + postnatal mortality
Fetal mortality?	Number of deaths from 20 weeks' gestation to birth per 1,000 total births
Perinatal mortality?	Number of deaths from 20 weeks' gestation to one month of life per 1,000 total births
Maternal mortality?	Number of deaths during pregnancy to 90 days postpartum per 100,000 *live* births

ETHICS

True or false: Once patients sign a statement giving consent, they must continue treatment.	False. Patients may change their minds at any time
Exceptions to the requirement of informed consent.	Emergency situations, patients without decision-making capacity, and patients who sign waivers to the right of informed consent
A 15-year-old pregnant girl requires hospitalization for preeclampsia. Should parents be informed?	No. Parental consent is not necessary for medical treatment of pregnant minors
Doctor refers a patient for an MRI at a facility he owns.	Conflict of interest
Involuntary psychiatric hospitalization can be undertaken for which three reasons?	Patient is a danger to self, a danger to others, or gravely disabled (unable to provide for basic needs)
True or false: Withdrawing life-sustaining care is a more serious measure than withholding care.	False. Withdrawing and withholding life-sustaining care are the same from an ethical standpoint
When can a physician refuse to continue treating a patient on the grounds of futility?	When there is no rationale for treatment, maximal intervention is failing, a given intervention has already failed, and treatment will not achieve the goals of care
An 8-year-old child is in a serious accident. She requires emergent transfusion, but her parents are not present.	Treat immediately. Consent is implied in emergency situations

Conditions in which confidentiality must be overridden.	Real threat of harm to third parties, suicidality, certain contagious diseases, and elder and child abuse
Involuntary commitment or isolation for medical treatment may be undertaken for what reason?	Treatment noncompliance represents a serious danger to public health (e.g., active TB)
A 10-year-old child presents in status epilepticus, but her parents refuse treatment on religious grounds.	Treat because the disease represents an immediate threat to the child's life. Then seek a court order
A son asks that his mother not be told about her recently discovered cancer.	A patient's family cannot require that a doctor withhold information from the patient

GASTROINTESTINAL

Patient presents with sudden onset of severe, diffuse abdominal pain. Exam reveals peritoneal signs and abdominal (AXR) reveals free air under the diaphragm. Management?	Emergent laparotomy to repair perforated viscus, likely stomach
Most likely cause of acute lower GI bleed in patients > 40 years old.	Diverticulosis
Can cause GI bleeding?	No
Diagnostic modality used when U/S is equivocal for cholecystitis.	HIDA scan
Sentinel loop on AXR.	Acute pancreatitis
Risk factors for cholelithiasis.	Fat, female, fertile, forty, flatulent
Inspiratory arrest during palpation of the RUQ.	Murphy's sign, seen in acute cholecystitis
Identify key organisms causing diarrhea: ■ Most common organism ■ Recent antibiotic use ■ Camping ■ Traveler's diarrhea ■ Church picnics/mayonnaise ■ Uncooked hamburgers ■ Fried rice ■ Poultry/eggs ■ Raw seafood ■ AIDS ■ Pseudoappendicitis	*Campylobacter* *Clostridium difficile* *Giardia* ETEC *Staphylococcus aureus* *Escherichia coli* O157:H7 *Bacillus cereus* *Salmonella* *Vibrio*, HAV *Isospora, Cryptosporidium, Mycobacterium avium complex* (MAC) *Yersinia*
A 25-year-old Jewish male presents with pain and watery diarrhea after meals. Exam shows fistulas between the bowel and skin and nodular lesions on his tibias.	Crohn's disease
Inflammatory disease of the colon with increased risk of colon cancer.	Ulcerative colitis

Extraintestinal manifestations of IBD.	Uveitis, ankylosing spondylitis (AS), pyodema gangrenosum, erythema nodosum, primary sclerosing cholangitis
Medical treatment for IBD.	5-aminosalicylic acid +/– sulfasalazine and steroids during acute exacerbations
Difference between Mallory-Weiss and Boerhaave tears.	Mallory-Weiss: Superficial tear in the esophageal mucosa Boerhaave: Full-thickness esophageal rupture
Charcot's triad.	RUQ pain, jaundice, and fever/chills in the setting of ascending cholangitis
Reynold's pentad.	Charcot's triad plus shock and mental status changes, with suppurative ascending cholangitis
Medical treatment for hepatic encephalopathy.	Decreased protein intake, lactulose, neomycin
First step in the management of a patient with acute GI bleed.	Establish the ABCs
A four-year-old child presents with oliguria, petechiae, and jaundice following an illness with bloody diarrhea. Most likely diagnosis and cause?	Hemolytic uremic syndrome due to *E. coli* O157:H7
Post-HBV exposure treatment.	HBV immunoglobulin
Classic causes of drug-induced hepatitis.	TB medications (INH, rifampin, pyrazinamide), acetaminophen, and tetracycline
A 40-year-old obese female with elevated alkaline phosphatase, elevated bilirubin, pruritus, dark urine, and clay-colored stools.	Biliary tract obstruction
Hernia with highest risk of incarceration— indirect, direct, or femoral?	Femoral hernia
A 50-year-old man with a history of alcohol abuse presents with boring epigastric pain that radiates to the back and is relieved by sitting forward. Management?	Confirm the diagnosis of acute pancreatitis with elevated amylase and lipase. Make patient NPO and give IV fluids, O_2, analgesia, and "tincture of time"

HEMATOLOGY/ONCOLOGY

Four causes of microcytic anemia.	**TICS**—**T**halassemia, **I**ron deficiency, anemia of **C**hronic disease, and **S**ideroblastic anemia
Elderly male with hypochromic, microcytic anemia is asymptomatic. Diagnostic tests?	FOBT and sigmoidoscopy; suspect colorectal cancer
Precipitants of hemolytic crisis in patients with G6PD deficiency.	Sulfonamides, antimalarial drugs, fava beans
Most common inherited hemolytic anemia.	Hereditary spherocytosis
Diagnostic test for hereditary spherocytosis.	Osmotic fragility test
Pure RBC aplasia.	Diamond-Blackfan anemia

Anemia associated with absent radii and thumbs, diffuse hyperpigmentation, café-au-lait spots, microcephaly, and pancytopenia.	Fanconi's anemia
Medications and viruses that cause aplastic anemia.	Chloramphenicol, sulfonamides, radiation, HIV, chemotherapeutic agents, hepatitis, parvovirus B19, EBV
How to distinguish polycythemia vera from secondary polycythemia.	Both have increased HCT and RBC mass, but polycythemia vera should have normal O_2 saturation and low erythropoietin level.
Thrombotic thrombocytopenic purpura (TTP) pentad?	Anemia/splenomegaly, thrombocytopenia, fever, acute renal failure (ARF), and neurologic changes
Hemolytic-uremic syndrome (HUS) triad?	Anemia, thrombocytopenia, and ARF
Treatment for TTP.	Emergent large-volume plasmapheresis, corticosteroids, antiplatelet drugs
Treatment for ITP in children.	Usually resolves spontaneously; may require IVIG and/or corticosteroids
Which of the following are elevated in DIC: fibrin split products, D-dimer, fibrinogen, platelets, and HCT.	Fibrin split products and D-dimer are elevated; platelets, fibrinogen, HCT are decreased
An 8-year-old boy presents with hemarthrosis and increased PTT with normal PT and BT. Diagnosis? Treatment?	Hemophilia A or B; consider desmopressin (for hemophilia A) or factor VIII or IX supplements
A 14-year-old girl presents with prolonged bleeding after dental surgery and with menses, normal PT, normal or increased PTT, and increased BT. Diagnosis? Treatment?	von Willebrand's disease; treat with desmopressin, FFP, or cryoprecipitate
A 60-year-old African-American male presents with bone pain. Workup for multiple myeloma might reveal?	Monoclonal gammopathy, Bence Jones proteinuria, "punched-out" lesions on x-ray of skull and long bones
Reed-Sternberg cells	Hodgkin's lymphoma
A 10-year-old boy presents with fever, weight loss, and night sweats. Exam shows anterior mediastinal mass. Suspected diagnosis?	Non-Hodgkin's lymphoma
Microcytic anemia with decreased serum iron, decreased total iron-binding capacity (TIBC), and normal or increased ferritin.	Anemia of chronic disease.
Microcytic anemia with decreased serum iron, decreased ferritin, and increased TIBC.	Iron-deficiency anemia
An 80-year-old man presents with fatigue, lymphadenopathy, splenomegaly, and isolated lymphocytosis. Suspected diagnosis?	Chronic lymphocytic leukemia (CLL)
Late, life-threatening complication of chronic myelogenous leukemia (CML).	Blast crisis (fever, bone pain, splenomegaly, pancytopenia)
Auer rods on blood smear.	Acute myelogenous leukemia (AML)

AML subtype associated with DIC.	M3
Electrolyte changes in tumor lysis syndrome.	Decreased Ca^{2+}, increased K^+, increased phosphate, increased uric acid
Treatment for AML M3.	Retinoic acid
A 50-year-old male presents with early satiety, splenomegaly, and bleeding. Cytogenetics show t(9,22). Diagnosis?	CML
Heinz bodies?	Intracellular inclusions seen in thalassemia, G6PD deficiency, and postsplenectomy
Autosomal-recessive disorder with a defect in the GPIIbIIIa platelet receptor and decreased platelet aggregation.	Glanzmann's thrombasthenia
Virus associated with aplastic anemia in patients with sickle cell anemia.	Parvovirus B19
A 25-year-old African-American male with sickle cell anemia has sudden onset of bone pain. Management of pain crisis?	O_2, analgesia, hydration, and if severe, transfusion
Significant cause of morbidity in thalassemia patients. Treatment?	Iron overload; use deferoxamine

INFECTIOUS DISEASE

Three most common causes of fever of unknown origin (FUO).	Infection, cancer, and autoimmune disease
Four signs and symptoms of streptococcal pharyngitis.	Fever, pharyngeal erythema, tonsillar exudate, lack of cough
Nonsuppurative complication of streptococcal infection that is not altered by treatment of primary infection.	Postinfectious glomerulonephritis
Asplenic patients are particularly susceptible to these organisms.	Encapsulated organisms—pneumococcus, meningococcus, *Haemophilus influenzae*, *Klebsiella*
Number of bacterial culture on clean-catch specimen to diagnose a UTI.	10^5 bacteria/mL
Which healthy population is susceptible to UTIs?	Pregnant women. Treat this group aggressively because of potential complications
Patient from California or Arizona presents with fever, malaise, cough, and night sweats. Diagnosis? Treatment?	Coccidioidomycosis. Fluconazole
Nonpainful chancre.	Primary syphilis
"Blueberry-muffin" rash is characteristic of what congenital infection?	Rubella
Meningitis in neonates. Causes? Treatment?	Group B strep, *E. coli*, *Listeria*. Treat with gentamicin and ampicillin
Meningitis in infants. Causes? Treatment?	Pneumococcus, meningococcus, *H. influenzae*. Treat with cefotaxime and vancomycin

What should always be done prior to LP?	Check for increased intracranial pressure (ICP). Look for papilledema
CSF findings: • Low glucose, PMN predominance. • Normal glucose, lymphocytic predominance. • Numerous RBCs in serial CSF samples. • Increased gammaglobulins.	Bacterial meningitis Aseptic (viral) meningitis Subarachnoid hemorrhage (SAH) Multiple sclerosis
Initially presents with a pruritic papule with regional lymphadenopathy and evolves into black eschar after 7–10 days. Treatment?	Anthrax. Treat with ampicillin
Findings in tertiary syphilis.	Tabes dorsalis, general paresis, gummas, Argyll-Robertson pupil, aoritis, aortic root aneurysms
Region where Lyme disease is endemic.	North American northeast
Characteristics of secondary Lyme disease.	Arthralgias, migratory polyarthropathies, Bell's palsy, myocarditis
Cold agglutinins.	*Mycoplasma*
A 24-year-old male presents with soft white plaques on his tongue and the back of his throat. Diagnosis? Workup?	Candidal thrush. Workup should include HIV test
Begin *Pneumocystis carinii* (PCP) prophylaxis in HIV-positive patient at what CD4 count? MAC prophylaxis?	≤ 200 for PCP (with TMP); ≤ 100 for MAC (with clarithromycin/azithromycin)
Risk factors for pyelonephritis.	Pregnancy, vesicoureteral reflux, anatomic anomalies, indwelling catheters, and kidney stones
Neutropenic nadir post-chemotherapy.	7–10 days
Treatment for HSV meningitis.	Acyclovir
Antigen test to confirm the diagnosis of Rocky Mountain spotted fever rickettsial disease.	Weil-Felix test
Erythema migrans.	Lesion of primary Lyme disease
Classic physical findings for endocarditis.	Fever, heart murmur, Osler's nodes, splinter hemorrhages, Janeway lesions, Roth's spots
Most common infection from a blood transfusion.	HCV
Name the organism: • Branching rods in oral infection. • Painful chancroid. • Dog or cat bite. • Meningitis in adults. • Meningitis in elderly. • Alcoholic with pneumonia. • Currant jelly sputum. • Infection in burn victims. • Osteomyelitis from foot wound puncture. • Osteomyelitis in sickle cell patient.	*Actinomyces israelii* *Haemophilus ducreyi* *Pasteurella multocida* *Neisseria meningitidis* *Streptococcus pneumoniae* *Klebsiella* *Klebsiella* *Pseudomonas* *Pseudomonas* *Salmonella*

Patient presents with pain on passive movement, pallor, poikilothermia, paresthesias, paralysis, and pulselessness. Treatment?	All-compartment fasciotomy for suspected compartment syndrome
Back pain that is exacerbated by standing and walking and relieved with sitting and hyperflexion of the hips.	Spinal stenosis
Joints in the hand affected in rheumatoid arthritis (RA).	Metacarpophalangeal (MCP) and PIP joints; DIP joints are spared
Joint pain and stiffness that worsen over the course of the day and are relieved by rest.	Osteoarthritis
Genetic disorder associated with multiple fractures and commonly mistaken for child abuse.	Osteogenesis imperfecta
Hip and back pain along with stiffness that improves with activity over the course of the day and worsens at rest. Diagnostic test?	Suspect ankylosing spondylitis. Check HLA-B27
Arthritis, conjunctivitis, and urethritis in young men. Associated organisms?	Reiter's arthritis. *Campylobacter, Shigella, Salmonella, Chlamydia,* or *Ureaplasma*
A 55-year-old man has sudden, excruciating first metatarsophalangeal (MTP) joint pain after a night of drinking red wine. Diagnosis, workup, and chronic treatment?	Gout. Needle-shaped, negatively birefringent crystals are seen on joint fluid aspirate. Chronic treatment with allopurinol and probenecid
Rhomboid-shaped, positively birefringent crystals on joint fluid aspirate.	Pseudogout
Elderly man complains of bony pain; he mentions frontal bossing and adds that his favorite hat no longer fits.	Paget's disease
Elderly female presents with pain and stiffness of the shoulders and hips; she cannot lift her arms above her head. Labs show anemia and elevated ESR.	Polymyalgia rheumatica
Active 13-year-old boy has anterior knee pain. Diagnosis?	Osgood-Schlatter
Bone is fractured in fall on outstretched hand.	Distal radius (Colles' fracture)
Complication of scaphoid fracture.	Avascular necrosis (AVN)
Signs suggesting radial nerve damage with humeral fracture.	Wrist drop, loss of thumb abduction
Young child presents with proximal muscle weakness, waddling gait, and pronounced calf muscles.	Duchenne muscular dystrophy (DMD)
First-born female who was born in breech position is found to have asymmetric skin folds on her newborn exam. Diagnosis? Treatment?	Developmental dysplasia of the hip. If severe, consider Pavlik harness to maintain abduction

HIGH-YIELD FACTS

Rapid Review

An 11-year-old obese, African American boy presents with sudden onset of limp. Diagnosis? Workup?	Slipped capital femoral epiphyses. AP and frog-leg lateral view
Most common primary malignant tumor of bone.	Multiple myeloma
Xerostomia with paratoid enlargement and anti-LLa antibodies.	Sjögren's syndrome
Joint pain associated with a heliotropic rash around the eyelids.	Dermatomyositis
Small vessel vasculitides.	Wegener's granulomatosis and Henoch-Schönlein purpura (HSP)
Medium vessel vasculitides.	Churg-Strauss and polyarteritis nodosa
Large vessel vasculitides.	Temporal arteritis and Takayasu's arteritis
Palpable purpura, abdominal pain, and asymmetric periarticular swelling.	HSP
A 45-year-old woman presents with calcinosis, Raynaud's phenomenon, esophageal dysmotility, sclerodactyly, and telangiectasis.	CREST syndrome of scleroderma
Most specific SLE antibodies.	Anti-Sm and anti-dsDNA
Anticentromere antibodies.	Scleroderma
Antihistone antibodies.	Drug-induced SLE
Anti-La (SSB) antibodies.	Sjögren's syndrome
c-ANCA.	Wegener's granulomatosis
p-ANCA.	Polyarteritis nodosa
Sarcoma associated with "onion skinning."	Ewing's sarcoma
Sarcoma associated with "sunburst" pattern.	Osteosarcoma
Radiographic "bamboo spine."	AS

NEUROLOGY

Unilateral, severe periorbital headache with tearing and conjunctival erythema.	Cluster headache
Prophylactic treatment for migraine.	β-blockers, Ca^{2+} channel blockers, TCAs
Most common pituitary tumor. Treatment?	Prolactinoma. Dopamine agonists (DA) (e.g., bromocriptine)
A 55-year-old patient presents with acute "broken speech." What type of aphasia? What lobe and vascular distribution? First step in workup?	Broca's aphasia. Frontal lobe, left middle cerebral artery (MCA) distribution. Head CT to rule out a hemorrhage

Most common cause of SAH.	Trauma; second most common is berry aneurysm
Crescent-shaped hyperdensity on CT that does not cross the midline.	Subdural hematoma
History significant for initial altered mental status with an intervening lucid interval. Diagnosis? Most likely etiology? Treatment?	Epidural hematoma. Middle meningeal artery. Neurosurgical evacuation.
CSF findings with SAH.	Elevated ICP, RBCs, xanthochromia
Albuminocytologic dissociation	Guillain-Barré (increased protein in CSF with only modest increase in cell count)
A 61-year-old patient in the ICU is awake and alert but cannot move anything but the eyes and eyelids.	Locked-in syndrome
Cold water is flushed into a patient's ear, and the fast phase of the nystagmus is toward the opposite side. Normal or pathological?	Normal
Most common primary sources of metastases to the brain.	Lung, breast, skin (melanoma), kidney, GI tract
Dysequilibrium associated with tinnitus and hearing loss and often treated with acetazolamide.	Ménière's disease
Most frequent presentation of intracranial neoplasm.	Headache
Most common cause of seizures in children (age 2–10 years).	Infection, febrile seizures, trauma, idiopathic
Most common cause of seizures in young adults (18–35 years).	Trauma, alcohol withdrawal, brain tumor
Mainstay of treatment for myasthenia gravis.	Immunosuppressants (e.g., prednisone)
First-line medication for status epilepticus.	IV benzodiazepine
Most common intracranial malignancy.	Metastatic
What % lesion is an indication for carotid endarterectomy?	70% if stenosis is symptomatic
Most common causes of dementia.	Alzheimer's and multi-infarct
Atrophy of the mammillary bodies.	Wernicke's encephalopathy
Combined upper and lower motor neuron disorder.	Amyotrophic lateral sclerosis (ALS)
Rigidity and stiffness with resting tremor and masked facies.	Parkinson's disease
Mainstay of Parkinson's therapy.	Levodopa/carbidopa
Treatment for Guillain-Barré syndrome.	IVIG or plasmapheresis
Rigidity and stiffness that progress to choreiform movements, accompanied by moodiness and altered behavior.	Huntington's disease

A six-year-old girl presents with a port-wine stain in the V2 distribution, mental retardation, seizures, and leptomeningeal angioma.	Sturge-Weber syndrome. Treat symptomatically. Possible focal cerebral resection of affected lobe
Café-au-lait spots on skin.	Neurofibromatosis 1
Hyperphagia, hypersexuality, hyperorality, and hyperdocility.	Klüver-Bucy syndrome (amygdala)
Administer to symptomatic patient to diagnose myasthenia gravis.	Edrophonium

OBSTETRICS

Treatment for breast-feeding mastitis.	Continue breast-feeding and give PO antibiotics
Most common cause of nonobstetric postpartum death.	Thromboembolic disease
Characteristics of postmaturity syndrome.	Oligohydramnios and passage of meconium in utero; "scrawny" neonate with dry, peeling skin
Cardinal movements of labor.	Engagement, Descent, Flexion, Internal rotation, Extension, Restitution (External rotation), Expulsion
A pregnant woman has an HCT of 10 g/dL. Is this the normal anemia of pregnancy?	No. An HCT < 11 g/dL should raise suspicions for iron deficiency
Tests used to assess neural tube defects.	α-fetoprotein (AFP) or amniocentesis
Test used in the tenth week of gestation to screen for chromosomal abnormalities.	Chorionic villus sampling
Appropriate antihypertensive in a patient with severe preeclampsia.	Hydralazine and/or β-blocker (e.g., labetolol)
Abnormal HR pattern in contraction stress test.	Late decelerations, indicating fetal hypoxia
Discrepancy exists between fundal height and gestational age; biparietal diameter is normal but abdominal circumference is decreased.	Asymmetric IUGR
Seizure prophylaxis in severe preeclampsia.	IV magnesium sulfate
HELLP syndrome.	Hemolysis, elevated LFTs, and low platelets; a variant of preeclampsia with a poor prognosis
Cure for preeclampsia/eclampsia.	Delivery
Cause of erythroblastosis fetalis.	Maternal antibodies against infant's Rh-positive RBCs result in fetal RBC hemolysis
Cause of hydrops fetalis.	Decreased protein production by the fetal liver, resulting in decreased oncotic pressure, edema, and high-output cardiac failure
Preeclampsia in the first trimester is pathognomonic for what condition?	Hydatidiform mole

HIGH-YIELD FACTS

Rapid Review

Primary causes of third-trimester bleeding	Placental abruption and placenta previa
Classic U/S and gross appearance of complete hydatidiform mole.	Snowstorm on U/S. "Cluster-of-grapes" appearance on gross examination
Chromosomal pattern of a complete mole.	46,XX
Molar pregnancy containing fetal tissue.	Partial mole
Symptoms of placental abruption.	Continuous, painful vaginal bleeding
Symptoms of placenta previa.	Self-limited, painless vaginal bleeding
When should a vaginal exam be performed with suspected placenta previa?	Never
Antibiotics with teratogenic effects.	Tetracycline, fluoroquinolones, aminoglycosides, sulfonamides
Shortest AP diameter of the pelvis.	Obstetric conjugate: between the sacral promontory and midpoint of the symphysis pubis
Medication given to accelerate fetal lung maturity.	Betamethasone or dexamethasone × 48 hours
Most common cause of postpartum hemorrhage.	Uterine atony
Treatment for postpartum hemorrhage.	Uterine massage; if that fails, give oxytocin
Typical antibiotics for group B streptococcus (GBS) prophylaxis.	IV penicillin or ampicillin
Patient fails to lactate after an emergency C-section with marked blood loss.	Sheehan's syndrome (postpartum pituitary necrosis)

GYNECOLOGY

First test to perform when a woman presents with amenorrhea.	β-hCG; the most common cause of amenorrhea is pregnancy
Term for heavy bleeding during and between menstrual periods.	Menometrorrhagia
Cause of amenorrhea with normal prolactin, no response to estrogen-progesterone challenge, and a history of D&C.	Asherman's syndrome
Therapy for polycystic ovarian syndrome.	Weight loss and OCPs
Medication used to induce ovulation.	Clomiphene citrate
Diagnostic step required in a postmenopausal woman who presents with vaginal bleeding.	Endometrial biopsy
Indications for medical treatment of ectopic pregnancy.	Stable, unruptured ectopic pregnancy of < 3.5 cm at < 6 weeks' gestation
Medical options for endometriosis.	OCPs, danazol, GnRH agonists
Uterine bleeding at 18 weeks' gestation; no products expelled; cervical os closed.	Threatened abortion

HIGH-YIELD FACTS

Rapid Review

Uterine bleeding at 18 weeks' gestation; no products expelled; membranes ruptured; cervical os open.	Inevitable abortion
Laparoscopic findings in endometriosis.	"Chocolate cysts," powder burns
Most common location for an ectopic pregnancy.	Ampulla of the oviduct
How to diagnose and follow a leiomyoma.	U/S
Natural history of a leiomyoma.	Regresses after menopause
Patient has increased vaginal discharge and petechial patches in the upper vagina and cervix.	*Trichomonas* vaginitis
Treatment for bacterial vaginosis.	Oral or topical metronidazole
Most common cause of bloody nipple discharge.	Intraductal papilloma
Contraceptive methods that protect against PID.	OCP and barrier contraception
Unopposed estrogen is contraindicated in which cancers?	Endometrial or estrogen receptor-positive breast cancer
Patient with recent PID with RUQ pain.	Consider Fitz-Hugh–Curtis syndrome
Breast malignancy presenting as itching, burning, and erosion of the nipple.	Paget's disease
Annual screening for women with strong family history of ovarian cancer.	CA-125 and transvaginal U/S
A 50-year-old woman leaks urine when laughing or coughing. Nonsurgical options?	Kegel exercises, estrogen, pessaries for stress incontinence
A 30-year-old woman has unpredictable urine loss. Exam is normal. Medical options?	Anticholinergics (oxybutynin) or β-adrenergics (metaproterenol) for urge incontinence.
Lab values suggestive of menopause.	Elevated serum FSH
Most common cause of female infertility.	Endometriosis
Two consecutive findings of atypical squamous cells of undetermined significance (ASCUS) on Pap smear. Followup evaluation?	Colposcopy and endocervical curettage
Breast cancer type that increases future risk of invasive carcinoma in both breasts.	Lobular carcinoma in situ

PEDIATRICS

Nontender abdominal mass associated with elevated VMA and HVA.	Neuroblastoma
Most common type of tracheoesophageal fistula (TEF). Diagnosis?	Esophageal atresia with distal TEF (85%). Unable to pass NG tube
Not contraindications to vaccination.	Mild illness and/or low-grade fever, current antibiotic therapy, and prematurity

Tests to rule out shaken baby syndrome.	Ophthalmologic exam, CT, and MRI
A neonate has meconium ileus.	Cystic fibrosis or Hirschsprung's disease
Bilious emesis within hours after the first feeding.	Duodenal atresia
A two-month-old presents with nonbilious, projectile emesis. First step in management?	Correct metabolic abnormalities. Then correct pyloric stenosis with pyloromyotomy
Most common primary immunodeficiency.	Selective IgA deficiency
Infant has a high fever and onset of rash as fever breaks. What is he at risk for?	Febrile seizures (roseola infantum)
What is the immunodeficiency? ■ Boy has chronic respiratory infections. Nitroblue tetrazolium test is positive. ■ Child has eczema, thrombocytopenia, and high levels of IgA. ■ A four-month-old boy has life-threatening *Pseudomonas* infection.	Chronic granulomatous disease Wiskott-Aldrich syndrome Bruton's X-linked agammaglobulinemia
Acute-phase treatment for Kawasaki disease.	High-dose aspirin for inflammation and fever, IVIG to prevent coronary artery aneurysms
A one-year-old is able to cruise, use two-finger pincer grasp, babble, and imitate actions. Diagnosis?	Suspected language delay
Treatment for mild and severe unconjugated hyperbilirubinemia.	Phototherapy (mild) or exchange transfusion (severe)
Sudden onset of mental status changes, emesis, and liver dysfunction after taking aspirin.	Reye's syndrome
Child has loss of red light reflex. Diagnosis?	Suspect retinoblastoma
Vaccinations at a six-month well-child visit.	HBV, DTaP, Hib, IPV, PCV
Tanner stage III in a six-year-old female.	Precocious puberty
Infection of small airways with epidemics in winter and spring.	RSV bronchiolitis
Cause of neonatal RDS.	Surfactant deficiency
Condition associated with red "currant-jelly" stools.	Intussusception
Congenital heart disease that causes secondary HTN.	Coarctation of the aorta
First-line treatment for otitis media.	Amoxicillin × 10 days
Most common pathogen causing croup.	PIV type 1
Homeless child is small for his age and has peeling skin and a swollen belly.	Kwashiorkor (protein malnutrition)
Defect in an X-linked syndrome with mental retardation, gout, self-mutilation, and choreoathetosis.	Lesch-Nyhan syndrome (purine salvage problem with HGPRTase deficiency)
Newborn female has continuous "machinery murmur."	Patent ductus arteriosus (PDA)

First-line pharmacotherapy for depression.	Selective serotonin reuptake inhibitors (SSRIs)
Antidepressants associated with hypertensive crisis.	MAOIs
Preferred antidepressant for patients with comorbid medical conditions.	Citalopram (few drug interactions)
Benzodiazepines to use in patients with liver dysfunction.	Lorazepam, oxazepam, and temazepam (non-P450 metabolism)
A 17-year-old female has left arm paralysis after her boyfriend dies in a car crash. No medical cause is found.	Conversion disorder
Name the defense mechanism: ▪ A mother who is angry at her husband yells at her child. ▪ A pedophile enters a monastery. ▪ A woman calmly describes a grisly murder. ▪ A hospitalized 10-year-old begins to wet his bed.	Displacement Reaction formation Isolation Regression
A 35-year-old male has recurrent episodes of palpitations, diaphoresis, and fear of going crazy.	Panic disorder
Most serious side effect of clozapine.	Agranulocytosis
A 21-year-old male has three months of social withdrawal, worsening grades, flattened affect, and concrete thinking.	Schizophreniform disorder (diagnosis of schizophrenia requires $\geq$ 6 months of symptoms)
Key side effects of atypical antipsychotics.	Weight gain, type 2 DM, QT prolongation
Young weight lifter receives IV haloperidol and complains that his eyes are deviated sideways. Diagnosis? Treatment?	Acute dystonia (oculogyric crisis). Treat with benztropine or diphenhydramine
Medication to avoid in patients with a history of alcohol withdrawal seizures.	Neuroleptics
A 13-year-old male has a history of theft, vandalism, and violence toward family pets.	Conduct disorder
A five-month-old girl has decreasing head growth, truncal dyscoordination, and decreased social interaction.	Rett's disorder
Common therapy for phobias, obsessive-compulsive disorder (OCD), and panic disorder.	Cognitive behavioral therapy (CBT)
Patient hasn't slept for days, lost $20,000 gambling, is agitated, and has pressured speech. Diagnosis? Treatment?	Acute mania. Start a mood stabilizer (e.g., lithium)
After a minor fender bender, a man wears a neck brace and requests permanent disability.	Malingering
Nurse presents with severe hypoglycemia; blood analysis reveals no elevation in C peptide.	Factitious disorder (Munchausen syndrome)

Patient continues to use cocaine after being in jail, losing his job, and not paying child support.	Substance abuse
Violent patient has vertical and horizontal nystagmus.	Phencyclidine hydrochloride (PCP) intoxication
Woman who was abused as a child frequently feels outside of or detached from her body.	Depersonalization disorder
Man has repeated, intense urges to rub his body against unsuspecting passengers on a bus.	Frotteurism (a paraphilia)
Schizophrenic patient takes haloperidol for one year and develops uncontrollable tongue movements. Diagnosis? Treatment?	Tardive dyskinesia. Decrease or discontinue haloperidol and consider other antipsychotic (e.g., risperidone, clozapine)
Man unexpectedly flies across country, takes a new name, and has no memory of his prior life.	Dissociative fugue

PULMONARY

Risk factors for DVT.	Stasis, endothelial injury and hypercoagulability
Hampton's hump on x-ray.	PE
Criteria for exudative effusion.	Pleural/serum protein > 0.5; pleural/serum LDH > 0.6
Causes of exudative effusion.	Think of leaky capillaries. Malignancy, TB, bacterial or viral infection, PE with infarct, and pancreatitis
Causes of transudative effusion.	Think of intact capillaries. CHF, liver or kidney disease, and protein-losing enteropathy
Pulmonary lesion of sarcoidosis.	Noncaseating granulomas
Normalizing P_{CO_2} in a patient having an asthma exacerbation may indicate?	Fatigue and impending respiratory failure
Dyspnea, lateral hilar lymphodenopathy on CXR, increased ACE, and hypercalcemia.	Sarcoidosis
Treatment for child presenting with acute asthma attack.	IV steroids
Curschmann's spirals (whorled mucous plugs).	Bronchial asthma
PFT showing decreased FEV_1/FVC.	Obstructive pulmonary disease (e.g., asthma)
PFT showing increased FEV_1/FVC.	Restrictive pulmonary disease
Infant with failure to thrive, frequent pulmonary infections, and greasy stools. Diagnostic test?	Sweat chloride test > 60 mEq/L = CF (in children)
Common pathogens in CF patients.	*Pseudomonas* and *S. aureus*
Honeycomb pattern on CXR. Diagnosis? Treatment?	Diffuse interstitial pulmonary fibrosis. Supportive care. Steroids may help

Treatment for superior vena cava syndrome.	Radiation
Treatment for mild, persistent asthma.	Inhaled β-agonists and inhaled corticosteroids
Acid-base disorder in pulmonary embolism.	Hypoxia and hypocarbia
Non–small cell lung cancer (NSCLC) associated with hypercalcemia.	SCC
Lung cancer associated with SIADH.	Small cell lung cancer (SCLC)
Lung cancer highly related to cigarette exposure.	SCLC
Tall, white male presents with acute shortness of breath. Diagnosis? Treatment?	Spontaneous pneumothorax. Spontaneous regression. Supplemental O_2 may be helpful
Treatment of tension pneumothorax.	Immediate needle thoracostomy
Characteristics favoring carcinoma in an isolated pulmonary nodule.	Age > 45–50 years; lesions new or larger in comparison to old films; absence of calcification or irregular calcification; size > 2 cm; irregular margins
Hypoxemia and pulmonary edema with normal pulmonary capillary wedge pressure.	Acute respiratory distress syndrome (ARDS)
Increased risk of what infection with silicosis?	*Mycobacterium tuberculosis*
Causes of hypoxemia.	Right-to-left shunt, hypoventilation, low inspired O_2 tension, diffusion defect, ventilation-perfusion mismatch
Classic CXR findings for pulmonary edema.	Cardiomegaly, prominent pulmonary vessels, Kerley B lines, "bat's-wing" appearance of hilar shadows, and perivascular and peribronchial cuffing

RENAL/GENITOURINARY

Renal tubular acidosis (RTA) associated with abnormal H^+ secretion and nephrolithiasis.	Type I (distal) RTA
RTA associated with abnormal HCO_3^- and rickets.	Type II (proximal) RTA
RTA associated with aldosterone defect.	Type IV (distal) RTA
"Doughy skin."	Hypernatremia
Differential of hypervolemic hyponatremia.	Cirrhosis, CHF, nephritic syndrome
Chvostek's and Trousseau's signs.	Hypocalcemia
Most common causes of hypercalcemia.	Malignancy and hyperparathyroidism
T-wave flattening and U waves.	Hypokalemia
Peaked T waves and widened QRS.	Hyperkalemia
First-line treatment for moderate hypercalcemia.	IV hydration and loop diuretics (furosemide)

Type of ARF in patient with $FE_{Na} < 1\%$.	Prerenal
A 49-year-old male presents with acute-onset flank pain and hematuria.	Nephrolithiasis
Most common type of nephrolithiasis.	Calcium oxalate
A 20-year-old man presents with a palpable flank mass and hematuria. U/S shows bilateral enlarged kidneys with cysts. Associated brain anomaly?	Cerebral berry aneurysms (AD PcKD)
Hematuria, HTN, and oliguria.	Nephritic syndrome
Proteinuria, hypoalbuminemia, hyperlipidemia, hyperlipiduria, edema.	Nephrotic syndrome
Most common form of nephritic syndrome.	Membranous glomerulonephritis
Most common form of glomerulonephritis.	IgA nephropathy (Berger's disease)
Glomerulonephritis with deafness.	Alport's syndrome
Glomerulonephritis with hemoptysis.	Wegener's granulomatosis and Goodpasture's syndrome
Presence of red cell casts in urine sediment.	Glomerulonephritis/nephritic syndrome
Eosinophils in urine sediment.	Allergic interstitial nephritis
Waxy casts in urine sediment and Maltese crosses (seen with lipiduria).	Nephrotic syndrome
Drowsiness, asterixis, nausea, and a pericardial friction rub.	Uremic syndrome seen in patients with renal failure
A 55-year-old man is diagnosed with prostate cancer. Treatment options?	Wait, surgical resection, radiation and/or androgen suppression
Low urine specific gravity in the presence of high serum osmolality.	DI
Treatment of SIADH?	Fluid restriction, demeclocycline
Hematuria, flank pain, and palpable flank mass.	Renal cell carcinoma (RCC)
Testicular cancer associated with β-hCG, AFP.	Choriocarcinoma
Most common type of testicular cancer.	Seminoma—a type of germ cell tumor
Most common histology of bladder cancer.	Transitional cell carcinoma
Complication of overly rapid correction of hyponatremia.	Central pontine myelinolysis
Salicylate ingestion results in what type of acid-base disorder?	Anion gap acidosis and primary respiratory alkalosis due to central respiratory stimulation
Acid-base disturbance commonly seen in pregnant women.	Respiratory alkalosis
Three systemic diseases causing nephrotic syndrome.	DM, SLE, and amyloidosis
Elevated erythropoietin level, elevated HCT, and normal O_2 saturation suggest?	RCC or other erythropoietin-producing tumor; evaluate with CT scan

A 55-year-old man presents with irritative and obstructive urinary symptoms. Treatment options?	Likely BPH. Options include no treatment, terazosin, finasteride, or surgical intervention (TURP)

SELECTED TOPICS IN EMERGENCY MEDICINE

Class of drugs that may cause syndrome of muscle rigidity, hyperthermia, autonomic instability, and extrapyramidal symptoms.	Antipsychotics (neuroleptic malignant syndrome)
Side effects of corticosteroids.	Acute mania, immunosuppression, thin skin, osteoporosis, easy bruising, myopathies
Treatment for DTs.	Benzodiazepines
Treatment for acetaminophen overdose.	N-acetylcysteine
Treatment for opioid overdose.	Naloxone
Treatment for benzodiazepine overdose.	Flumazenil
Treatment for iron overdose.	Deferoxamine
Treatment for neuroleptic malignant syndrome.	Dantrolene or bromocriptine
Treatment for malignant HTN.	Nitroprusside
Treatment of AF.	Rate control, rhythm conversion, and anticoagulation
Treatment of supraventricular tachycardia (SVT).	Rate control with carotid massage or other vagal stimulation
Causes of drug-induced SLE.	INH, penicillamine, hydralazine, procainamide
Macrocytic, megaloblastic anemia with neurologic symptoms.	B_{12} deficiency
Macrocytic, megaloblastic anemia without neurologic symptoms.	Folate deficiency
Burn patient presents with cherry-red flushed skin and coma. SaO_2 is normal, but carboxyhemoglobin is elevated. Treatment?	Treat CO poisoning with 100% O_2 or with hyperbaric O_2 if severe poisoning or pregnant
Blood in the urethral meatus or high-riding prostate.	Bladder rupture or urethral injury
Test to rule out urethral injury.	Retrograde cystourethrogram
Radiographic evidence of aortic disruption or dissection.	Widened mediastinum (> 8 cm), loss of aortic knob, pleural cap, tracheal deviation to the right, depression of left main stem bronchus
Radiographic indications for surgery in patients with acute abdomen.	Free air under the diaphragm, extravasation of contrast, severe bowel distention, space-occupying lesion (CT), mesenteric occlusion (angiography)

Most common organism in burn-related infections.	*Pseudomonas*
Method of calculating fluid repletion in burn patients.	Parkland formula
Acceptable urine output in a trauma patient.	50 cc/hour
Acceptable urine output in a stable patient.	30 cc/hour
Cannon "a" waves.	Third-degree heart block
Signs of neurogenic shock.	Hypotension and bradycardia
Signs of increased ICP (Cushing's triad).	HTN, bradycardia, and abnormal respirations
Decreased CO, decreased pulmonary capillary wedge pressure (PCWP), increased peripheral vascular resistance (PVR).	Hypovolemic shock
Decreased CO, increased PCWP, increased PVR.	Cardiogenic shock
Increased CO, decreased PCWP, decreased PVR.	Septic or anaphylactic shock
Treatment of septic shock.	Fluids and antibiotics
Treatment of cardiogenic shock.	Identify cause; pressors (e.g., dobutamine)
Treatment of hypovolemic shock.	Identify cause; fluid and blood repletion
Treatment of anaphylactic shock.	Diphenhydramine or epinephrine 1:1000
Supportive treatment for ARDS.	Continuous positive airway pressure (CPAP)
Signs of air embolism.	A patient with chest trauma who was previously stable suddenly dies
Trauma series.	AP chest, AP/lateral C-spine, AP pelvis

HIGH-YIELD FACTS

Rapid Review

Clinical Images

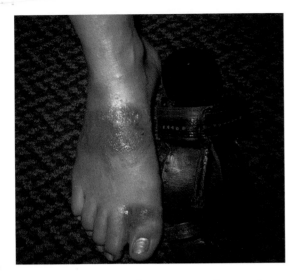

Contact dermatitis. Erythematous papules, vesicles, and serous weeping localized to areas of contact with the offending agent are characteristic. (Reproduced, with permission, from Hurwitz RM, *Pathology of the Skin: Atlas of Clinical–Pathological Correlation,* 1st ed. Stamford, CT: Appleton & Lange, 1991: p. 3, Fig. 1–5.)

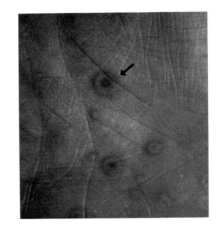

Erythema multiforme. The classic target lesion has a dull red center, pale zone, and darker outer ring (arrow). This acute self-limited reaction may occur with infection, antibiotic use, exposure to radiation or chemicals, or malignancy. (Reproduced, with permission, from Bondi EE, *Dermatology: Diagnosis and Therapy,* 1st ed., Stamford, CT: Appleton & Lange, 1991: p. 392, Fig. 19.)

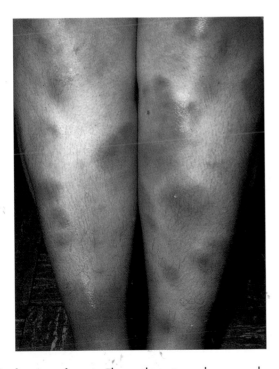

Erythema nodosum. The erythematous plaques and nodules are commonly located on pretibial areas. Lesions are painful and indurated and heal spontaneously without ulceration. (Reproduced, with permission, from Hurwitz RM, *Pathology of the Skin: Atlas of Clinical–Pathological Correlation,* 1st ed., Stamford, CT: Appleton & Lange, 1991: p. 132, Fig. 10-1A.)

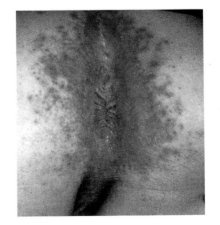

Candidial intertrigo. Erythematous areas surrounded by satellite pustules are restricted to warm, moist intertriginous areas. (Reproduced, with permission, from Bondi EE, *Dermatology: Diagnosis and Therapy,* 1st ed., Stamford, CT: Appleton & Lange, 1991: p. 390, Fig. 11.)

1

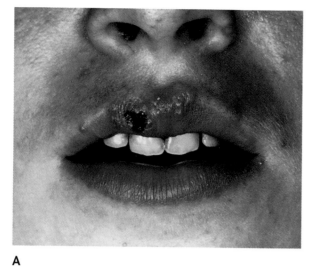

A

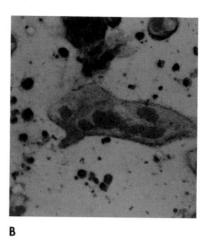

B

Herpes simplex. (A) Primary infection. Grouped vesicles on an erythematous base on the patient's lips and oral mucosa may progress to pustules before resolving. (B) Tzanck smear. The multinucleated giant cells from vesicular fluid provide a presumptive diagnosis of HSV infection. However, the Tzanck smear cannot distinguished between HSV and VZV infection. (Reproduced, with permission, from Hurwitz RM, *Pathology of the Skin: Atlas of Clinical–Pathological Correlation*, 1st ed., Stamford, CT: Appleton & Lange, 1991: p. 145, Fig. 11–9 and Bondi EE, *Dermatology: Diagnosis and Therapy*, 1st ed., Stamford, CT: Appleton & Lange, 1991: p. 396, Fig. 47.)

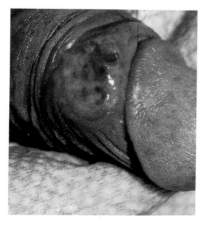

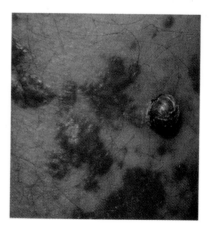

Primary syphilis. The chancre, which appears at the site of infection, is an ulcerated papule with a smooth, clean base; raised, indurated borders; and scant discharge. (Reproduced, with permission, from Bondi EE, *Dermatology: Diagnosis and Therapy*, 1st ed., Stamford, CT: Appleton & Lange, 1991: p. 394, Fig. 33.)

Kaposi's sarcoma. Manifests as red to purple nodules and surrounding pink to red macules. The latter appear most often in immunosuppressed patients. (Reproduced, with permission, from Bondi EE, *Dermatology: Diagnosis and Therapy*, 1st ed., Stamford, CT: Appleton & Lange, 1991: p. 393, Fig. 25.)

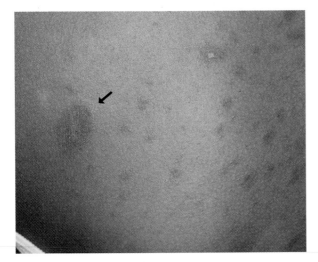

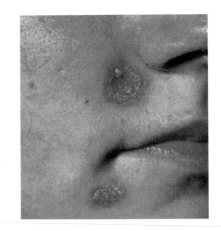

Pityriasis rosea. The round to oval erythematous plaques are often covered with a fine white scale ("cigarette paper") and are often found on the trunk ("Christmas tree distribution") and proximal extremities. The plaques are often preceded by a larger herald patch (arrow). (Reproduced, courtesy of the Yale Department of Dermatology.)

Impetigo. Dried pustules with superficial golden-brown crust are most commonly found around the nose and mouth. (Reproduced, with permission, from Bondi EE, *Dermatology: Diagnosis and Therapy*, 1st ed., Stamford, CT: Appleton & Lange, 1991: p. 390, Fig. 12.)

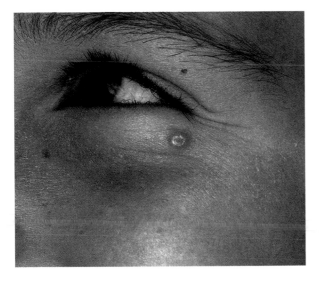

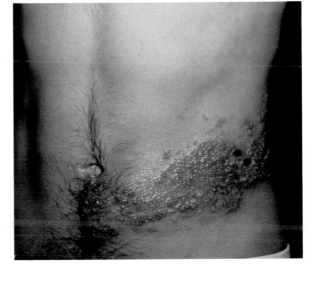

Molluscum contagiosum. The dome-shaped, fleshy, umbilicated papule on the child's eyelid is characteristic. (Reproduced, with permission, from Hurwitz RM, *Pathology of the Skin: Atlas of Clinical–Pathological Correlation*, 1st ed., Stamford, CT: Appleton & Lange, 1991: p. 149, Fig. 11–19.)

Herpes zoster. The unilateral dermatomal distribution of the grouped vesicles on an erythematous base is characteristic. (Reproduced, courtesy of the Yale Department of Dermatology.)

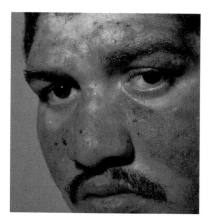

Malar rash of systemic lupus erythematosus. The malar rash is a red to purple continuous plaque extending across the bridge of the nose and to both cheeks. (Reproduced, with permission, from Bondi EE, *Dermatology: Diagnosis and Therapy,* 1st ed., Stamford, CT: Appleton & Lange, 1991: p. 395, Fig. 38.)

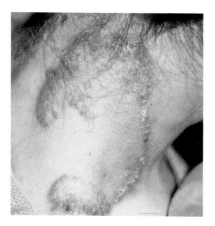

Tinea corporis. Ring-shaped, erythematous, scaling macules with central clearing are characteristic. (Reproduced, with permission, from Bondi EE, *Dermatology: Diagnosis and Therapy,* 1st ed., Stamford, CT: Appleton & Lange, 1991: p. 389, Fig. 4.)

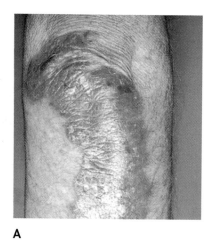

A

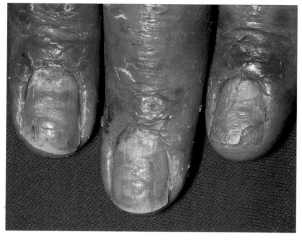

B

Psoriasis. (A) Skin changes. The classic sharply demarcated dark red plaques with silvery scales are commonly located on extensor surfaces (e.g., elbows, knees). (B) Nail changes. Note the pitting, onycholysis, and oil spots. (Reproduced, with permission, from Bondi EE, *Dermatology: Diagnosis and Therapy,* 1st ed., Stamford, CT: Appleton & Lange, 1991: p. 389, Fig. 1 and Hurwitz RM, *Pathology of the Skin: Atlas of Clinical–Pathological Correlation,* 1st ed., Stamford, CT: Appleton & Lange, 1991: p. 15, Fig. 1–55.)

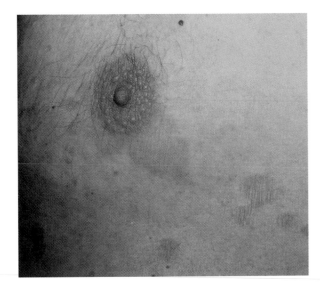

Tinea versicolor. These pinkish scaling macules commonly appear on the chest and back. Lesions may also be lightly pigmented or hypopigmented depending on the patient's skin color and sun exposure. (Reproduced, courtesy of the Yale Department of Dermatology.)

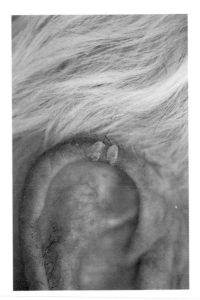

Actinic keratosis. The discrete patch has an erythematous base and rough white scaling. Actinic keratosis is a premalignant lesion that may progress to squamous cell carcinoma. It is most commonly found in sun-exposed areas. (Reproduced, with permission, from Hurwitz RM, *Pathology of the Skin: Atlas of Clinical–Pathological Correlation,* 1st ed., Stamford, CT: Appleton & Lange, 1991: p. 354, Fig. 31–3.)

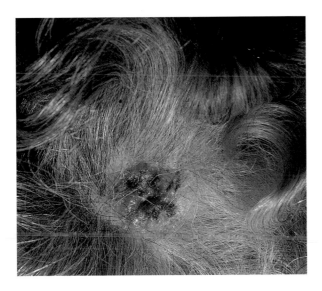

Squamous cell carcinoma. Note the crusting and ulceration of this erythematous plaque. Most lesions are exophytic nodules with erosion or ulceration. (Reproduced, with permission, from Hurwitz RM, *Pathology of the Skin: Atlas of Clinical–Pathological Correlation,* 1st ed., Stamford, CT: Appleton & Lange, 1991: p. 360, Fig. 31–20.)

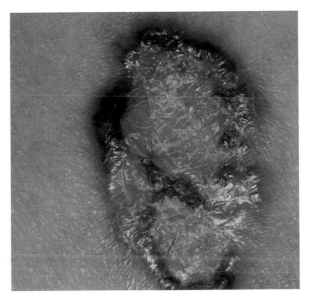

Basal cell carcinoma. Note the pearly, translucent surface (often covered with fine telangectasias), rolled border, and central ulceration. (Reproduced, courtesy of the Yale Department of Dermatology.)

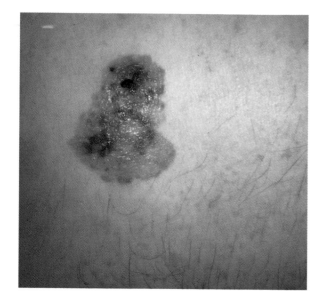

Melanoma. Note the **a**symmetry, **b**order irregularity, **c**olor variation, and large **d**iameter of this plaque. (Reproduced, with permission, from Hurwitz RM, *Pathology of the Skin: Atlas of Clinical–Pathological Correlation*, 1st ed., Stamford, CT: Appleton & Lange, 1991: p. 432, Fig. 36–8.)

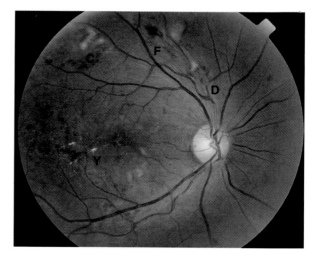

Nonproliferative diabetic retinopathy. Flame hemorrhages (F), dot-blot hemorrhages (D), cotton-wool spots (C), and yellow exudate (Y) result from small vessel damage and occlusion. (Reproduced, courtesy of the Washington University Department of Ophthalmology.)

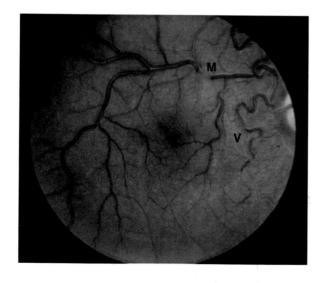

Hypertensive retinopathy. Note the tortuous retinal veins (V) and venous microaneurysms (M). Other findings include hemorrhages, retinal infarcts, detachment of the retina, and disk edema. (Reproduced, courtesy of the Washington University Department of Ophthalmology.)

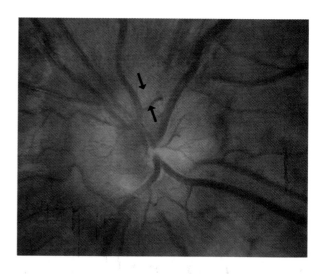

Papilledema. Look for blurred disk margins due to edema of the optic disk (arrows). (Reproduced, courtesy of the Washington University Department of Ophthalmology.)

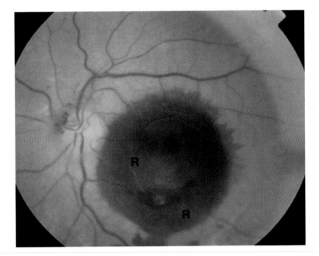

Subretinal hemorrhage. Note the preretinal blood and overlying retinal vessels (R). Subretinal hemorrhages may be seen in any condition with abnormal vessel proliferation (e.g., diabetes, hypertension) or in trauma. (Reproduced, courtesy of the Washington University Department of Ophthalmology.)

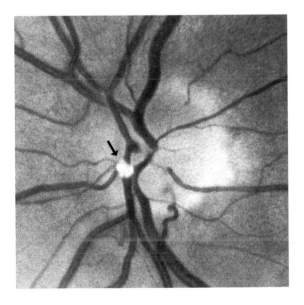

Cholesterol emboli. Cholesterol emboli (Hollenhorst plaque; arrow) usually arise in atherosclerotic carotid arteries and often lodge at the bifurcation of retinal arteries. (Reproduced, with permission, from Vaughan D, *General Ophthalmology,* 14th ed., Stamford, CT: Appleton & Lange, 1995: p. 299, Fig. 15–6.)

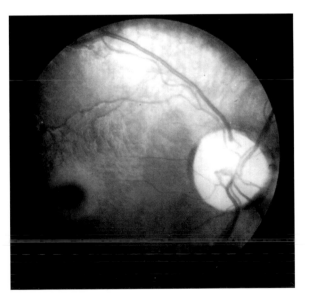

Tay–Sachs. Cherry-red spot. The red spot in the macula may be seen in Tay–Sachs disease, Niemann–Pick disease, central retinal artery occlusion, and methanol toxicity. (Reproduced, with permission, from Vaughan D, *General Ophthalmology,* 14th ed., Stamford, CT: Appleton & Lange, 1995: p. 293, Fig. 14–29.)

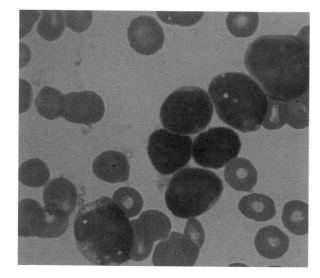

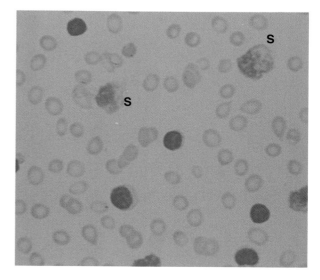

Acute lymphoblastic leukemia. Peripheral blood smear reveals numerous large, uniform lymphoblasts with fine granular cytoplasm and faint nucleoli. (Reproduced, courtesy of Dr. Peter McPhedran, Yale Department of Hematology.)

Chronic lymphocytic leukemia. The numerous, small, mature lymphocytes and smudge cells (S; fragile malignant lymphocytes are disrupted during blood smear preparation) are characteristic. (Reproduced, courtesy of Dr. Peter McPhedran, Yale Department of Hematology.)

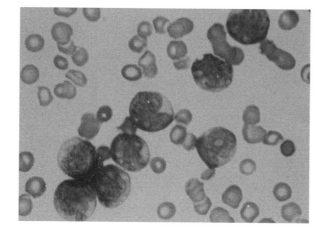

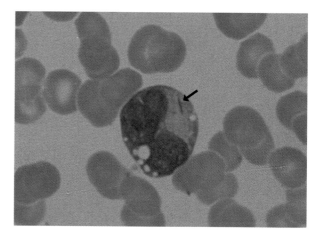

Acute myelocytic leukemia. Large, uniform myeloblasts with notched nuclei and prominent nucleoli are characteristic. (Reproduced, courtesy of Dr. Peter McPhedran, Yale Department of Hematology.)

Auer rod in acute myelocytic leukemia. The red rod-shaped structure (arrow) in the cytoplasm of the myeloblast is pathognomonic. (Reproduced, courtesy of Dr. Peter McPhedran, Yale Department of Hematology.)

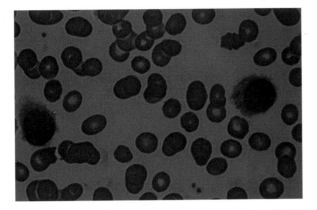

Hairy cell leukemia. Note the hairlike cytoplasmic projections from neoplastic lymphocytes. (Reproduced, courtesy of Dr. Peter McPhedran, Yale Department of Hematology.)

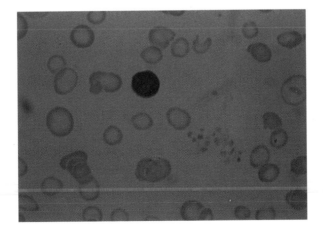

Iron deficiency anemia. Note the microcytic, hypochromic red blood cells ("doughnut cells") with enlarged areas of central pallor. (Reproduced, courtesy of Dr. Peter McPhedran, Yale Department of Hematology.)

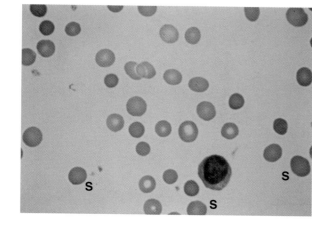

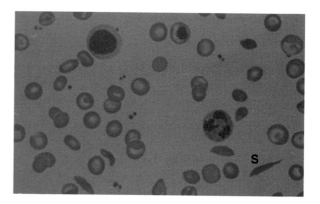

Spherocytes. These RBCs (S) lack areas of central pallor. Spherocytes are seen in autoimmune hemolysis and hereditary spherocytosis. (Reproduced, courtesy of Dr. Peter McPhedran, Yale Department of Hematology.)

Sickle cells. Sickle-shaped RBCs (S) may appear during infection, dehydration, or hypoxia. Anisocytosis, poikilocytosis, target cells, and nucleated RBCs are also seen in sickle cell disease. (Reproduced, courtesy of Dr. Peter McPhedran, Yale Department of Hematology.)

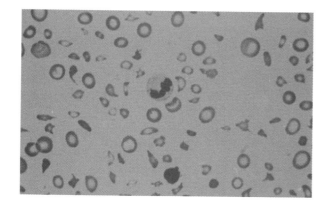

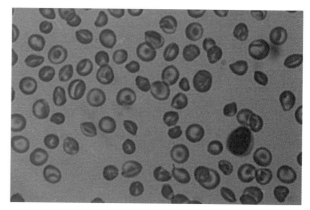

Schistocytes. These fragmented red blood cells may be seen in microangiopathic hemolytic anemia and mechanical hemolysis. (Reproduced, courtesy of Dr. Peter McPhedran, Yale Department of Hematology.)

Target cells. The dense zone of hemoglobin in the RBC center is characteristic. Target cells are seen in hemoglobin C or S disease and thalassemia, or they may be an artifact. (Reproduced, courtesy of Dr. Peter McPhedran, Yale Department of Hematology.)

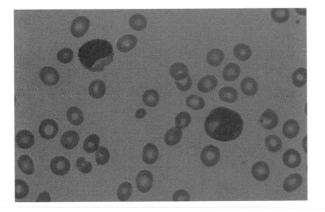

Mononucleosis. These lymphocytes, with enlarged nuclei and prominent nucleoli, are seen in EBV and CMV infections. (Reproduced, courtesy of Dr. Peter McPhedran, Yale Department of Hematology.)

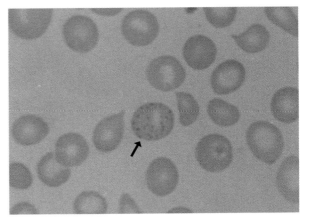

Basophilic stippling. The basophilic granules (arrow) within the red blood cells are a nonspecific finding that may suggest megaloblastic anemia, lead poisoning, or a benign condition. (Reproduced, courtesy of Dr. Peter McPhedran, Yale Department of Hematology.)

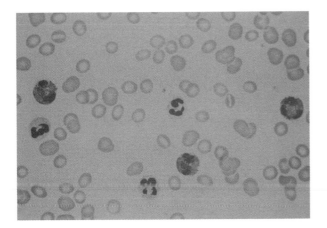

Eosinophilia. Eosinophils have red-staining cytoplasmic granules. Eosinophilia may be seen in allergic reactions, parasitic infections, collagen vascular diseases, malignancies such as Hodgkin's disease, and adrenal insufficiency. (Reproduced, courtesy of Dr. Peter McPhedran, Yale Department of Hematology.)

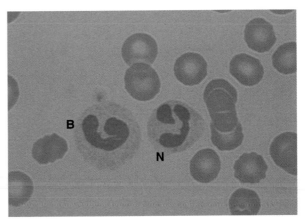

Neutrophil (N) and band (B). The more immature band form has a U-shaped rather than a segmented nucleus. (Reproduced, courtesy of Dr. Peter McPhedran, Yale Department of Hematology.)

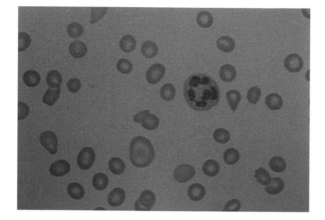

Hypersegmentation. The nucleus of this hypersegmented neutrophil has six lobes (six or more nuclear lobes are required). This is a characteristic finding of megaloblastic anemia. (Reproduced, courtesy of Dr. Peter McPhedran, Yale Department of Hematology.)

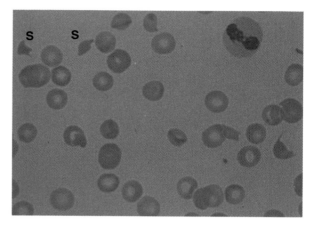

Thrombotic thrombocytopenic purpura (TTP). Note the schistocytes (S) and paucity of platelets. TTP is characterized by microangiopathic hemolytic anemia, thrombocytopenia, fever, neurologic abnormalities, and renal failure. (Reproduced, courtesy of Dr. Peter McPhedran, Yale Department of Hematology.)

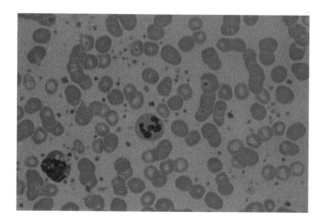

Thrombocytosis. Numerous clumps of platelets are seen in myeloproliferative disorders, severe iron deficiency anemia, acute bleeding, inflammation, malignancy, and postsplenectomy states. (Reproduced, courtesy of Dr. Peter McPhedran, Yale Department of Hematology.)

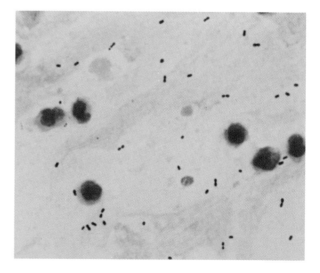

Streptococcus pneumoniae. This is a sputum sample from a patient with pneumonia. Note the characteristic lancet-shaped gram-positive diplococci. (Reproduced, courtesy of Vinnie Piscitelli, Yale Microbiology Lab.)

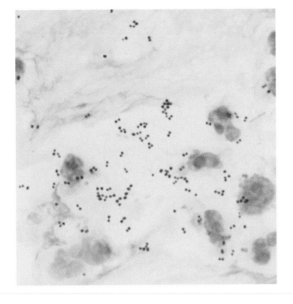

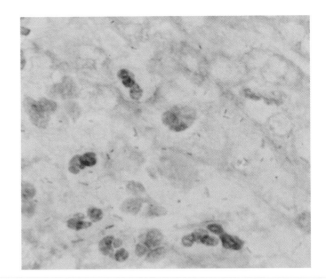

Staphylococcus aureus. These clusters of gram-positive cocci were isolated from the sputum of a patient with pneumonia. (Reproduced, courtesy of Vinnie Piscitelli, Yale Microbiology Lab.)

Pseudomonas aeruginosa. This sputum sample from a patient with pneumonia revealed gram-negative rods. The large number of neutrophils and relative paucity of epithelial cells indicate that this sample is not contaminated with oropharyngeal flora. (Reproduced, courtesy of Vinnie Piscitelli, Yale Microbiology Lab.)

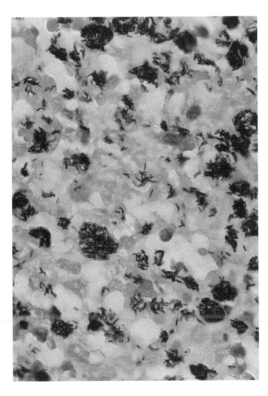

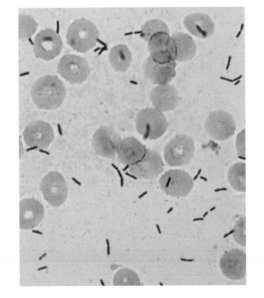

Listeria. These numerous rod-shaped bacilli were isolated from the blood of a patient with *Listeria* meningitis. (Reproduced, courtesy of Vinnie Piscitelli, Yale Microbiology Lab.)

Tuberculosis (AFB smear). Note the red color of the tubercle bacilli an acid-fast staining of a sputum sample ("red snappers"). (Reproduced, with permission, from Milikowski C, *Color Atlas of Basic Histopathology*, 1st ed., Stamford, CT: Appleton & Lange, 1997: p. 193, Fig. 9–10.)

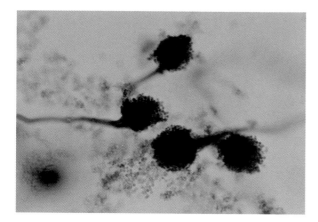

Aspergillosis. Note the characteristic appearance of *Aspergillus* spores in radiating columns. (Reproduced, courtesy of Vinnie Piscitelli, Yale Microbiology Lab.)

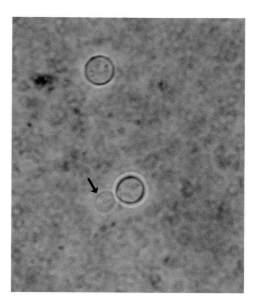

Cryptococcus. Note the budding yeast (arrow) and wide capsule of cryptococcus isolated from CSF. (Reproduced, courtesy of Vinnie Piscitelli, Yale Microbiology Lab.)

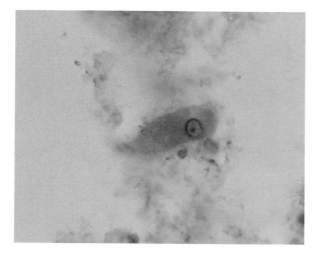

Entamoeba. *Entamoeba* cysts have large nuclei. This is a sample from diarrheal stool. (Reproduced, courtesy of Vinnie Piscitelli, Yale Microbiology Lab.)

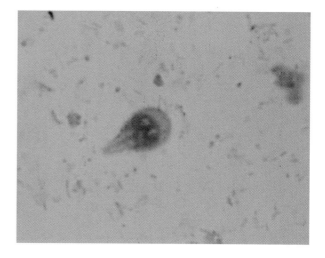

Giardia trophozoite in stool. The trophozoite exhibits a classic pear shape with two nuclei imparting an owl's-eye appearance. (Reproduced, courtesy of Vinnie Piscitelli, Yale Microbiology Lab.)

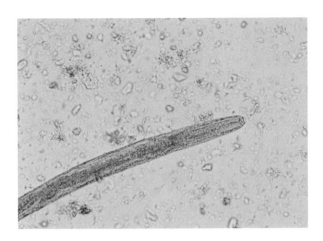

Strongyloides. These filarial larva were found in the stool of a patient watery diarrhea. (Reproduced, courtesy of Vinnie Piscitelli, Yale Microbiology Lab.)

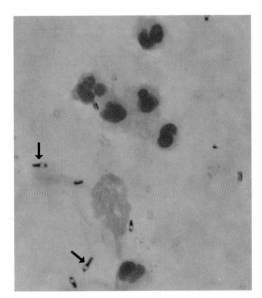

***Clostridium* wound infection.** The lucency at the end of each gram-positive bacillus is the terminal spore (arrow). This sample was isolated from an infected wound site. (Reproduced, courtesy of Vinnie Piscitelli, Yale Microbiology Lab.)

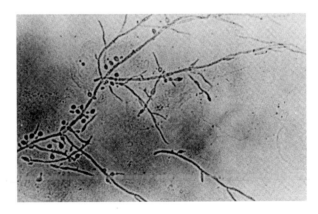

Candidal vaginitis. Branched and budding *Candida albicans* are evident on KOH preparation of vaginal discharge. (Reproduced, with permission, from DeCherney A, *Current Obstetrics and Gynecology Diagnosis and Treatment*, 8th ed., Stamford, CT: Appleton & Lange, 1994: p. 692, Fig. 34–4.)

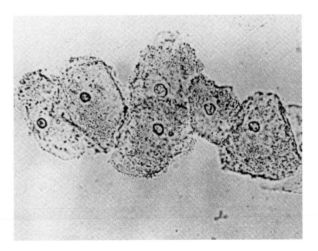

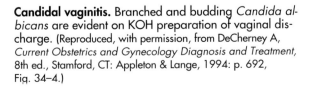

Gardnerella vaginalis. Saline wet mount of vaginal fluid reveals granulations on vaginal epithelial cells ("clue cells") due to adherence of *G. vaginalis* organisms to the cell surface. (Reproduced, with permission, from DeCherney A, *Current Obstetrics and Gynecology Diagnosis and Treatment*, 8th ed., Stamford, CT: Appleton and Lange, 1994: p. 692, Fig. 34–2.)

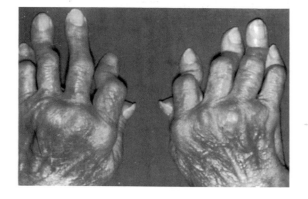

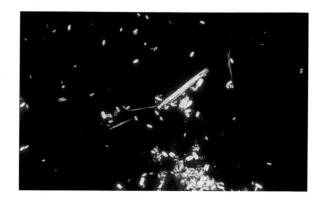

Rheumatoid arthritis. The swan-neck deformities of the digits and severe involvement of the proximal interphalangeal joints are characteristic. (Reproduced, with permission, from Chandrasoma P, *Concise Pathology*, 3rd ed., Stamford, CT: Appleton & Lange, 1998: p. 978, Fig. 68–2.)

Gout. Negatively birefringent crystals. (Reproduced, with permission, from Milikowshi C, *Color Atlas of Basic Histopathology*, 1st ed., Stamford, CT: Appleton & Lange, 1997: p. 546.)

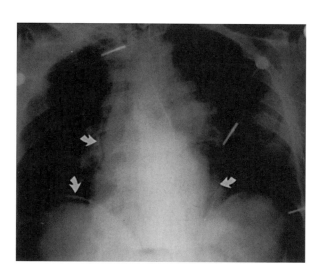

Pneumomediastinum. The lucency outlining the left heart border on chest x-ray suggests air in the mediastinum. (Reproduced, with permission, from Goldfrank LR, *Toxic Emergencies*, 6th ed., Stamford, CT: Appleton & Lange, 1998: p. 285, Fig. 8–2A.)

Pneumoperitoneum. The lucency outlining small bowel on abdominal x-ray indicated the abnormal presence of air. (Reproduced, with permission, from Goldfrank LR, *Toxic Emergencies*, 6th ed., Stamford, CT: Appleton & Lange, 1998: p. 285, Fig. 8–2B.)

Database of Clinical Science Review Resources

This section is a database of current clinical science review books, sample examination books, and commercial review courses marketed to medical students studying for the USMLE Step 2. For each book, we list the **Title** of the book, the **First Author** (or editor), the **Current Publisher**, the **Copyright Year**, the **Edition**, the **Number of Pages**, the **ISBN Code**, the **Approximate List Price**, the **Format** of the book, and the **Number of Test Questions.** Most entries also include Summary Comments that describe their style and utility for studying. Finally, each book receives a **Rating.** The books are sorted into a comprehensive section as well as into sections corresponding to the seven clinical disciplines (internal medicine, neurology, OB/GYN, pediatrics, preventive medicine, psychiatry, and surgery).Within each section, books are arranged first by Rating, then by Author, and finally by Title.

For this fourth edition of *First Aid for the USMLE Step 2*, the database of review books has been completely revised, with in-depth summary comments on more than 100 books and software. A letter rating scale with ten different grades reflects the detailed student evaluations. Each book receives a rating as follows:

A+	Excellent for boards review.
A	
A–	Very good for boards review; choose among the group.
B+	
B	Good, but use only after exhausting better sources.
B–	
C+	
C	Fair, but many better books in the discipline, or low-yield subject material.
C–	
N	Not rated.

The **Rating** is meant to reflect the overall usefulness of the book in preparing for the USMLE Step 2 examination. This is based on a number of factors, including:

- The cost of the book
- The readability of the text
- The appropriateness and accuracy of the book
- The quality and number of sample questions
- The quality of written answers to sample questions
- The quality and appropriateness of the illustrations (e.g., graphs, diagrams, photographs)
- The length of the text (longer is not necessarily better)
- The quality and number of other books available in the same discipline
- The importance of the discipline on the USMLE Step 2 examination

Please note that **the rating does not reflect the quality of the book for purposes other than reviewing for the USMLE Step 2 examination.** Many books with low ratings are well written and informative but are not ideal for boards preparation. We have also avoided listing or commenting on the wide variety of general textbooks available in the clinical sciences.

Evaluations are based on the cumulative results of formal and informal surveys of hundreds of medical students from medical schools across the country. The summary comments and overall ratings represent a consensus opinion, but there may have been a large range of opinions or limited student feedback on any particular book.

Please note that the data listed are subject to change because:

- Publishers' prices change frequently.
- Individual bookstores often charge an additional markup.
- New editions come out frequently, and the quality of updating varies.
- The same book may be reissued through another publisher.

We actively encourage medical students and faculty to submit their opinions and ratings of these clinical science review books so that we may update our database (see "How to Contribute," p. xv). In addition, we ask that publishers and authors submit review copies of clinical science review books, including new editions and books not included in our database, for evaluation. We also solicit reviews of new books or suggestions for alternate modes of study that may be useful in preparing for the examination, such as flash cards, computer-based tutorials, commercial review courses, and World Wide Web sites.

Disclaimer/Conflict of Interest Statement

No material in this book, including the ratings, reflects the opinion or influence of the publisher. All errors and omissions will gladly be corrected if brought to the attention of the authors through the publisher. Please note that the *Underground Clinical Vignette* series are publications by the authors of this book.

A ## NMS Review for USMLE Step 2

$36.95   Test/900 q

Gruber

Lippincott Williams & Wilkins, 1999, 2nd edition, 470 pages, ISBN 0683302833

Comprehensive review book in question-and-answer format. **Pros:** Level of difficulty, content, and style of questions best approximate those seen on the Step 2 exam. Clear, concise, excellent coverage of high-yield topics. Complete explanations. **Cons:** Lacks illustrations or images. **Summary:** Best single source of Step 2-style questions with appropriate format and content. Highly recommended.

A⁻ ## Boards & Wards

$27.95   Review

Ayala

Blackwell Science, 2000, 1st edition, 363 pages, ISBN 0632044934

Concise book in outline format, packed with key information across the various fields of medicine. **Pros:** Very high yield. Nice use of tables and charts. Good for quick study and last-minute review. **Cons:** Small print; few explanations. Not tremendously detailed, but covers many topics. Few images. **Summary:** Good, comprehensive review, although it lacks some details.

A⁻ ## Crush the Boards: The Ultimate USMLE Step 2 Review

$28.00   Review

Brochert

Hanley & Belfus, 2000, 1st edition, 224 pages, ISBN 1560533668

Comprehensive review of many high-yield topics, organized by specialty. **Pros:** Good emphasis on key points. Conversational style is easy to read. Good use of charts and diagrams. **Cons:** Not comprehensive. No practice questions or vignettes. **Summary:** An excellent review of key points and frequently tested topics. Should probably be supplemented with other review material and practice tests.

A⁻ ## USMLE Step 2 Mock Exam

$29.00   Test/750 q

Brochert

Hanley & Belfus, 2001, 1st edition, 328 pages, ISBN 1560534621

Consists of 750 vignette-style questions in 15 timed test blocks. **Pros:** Questions are case based and offer a good approximation of real boards questions. Questions cover high-yield topics, and explanations are terse but adequate. Many questions also include images and associated laboratory findings. **Cons:** Explanations may not be adequate for those who require an in-depth review of certain topics. **Summary:** Excellent vignette-type questions in mock exam format.

REVIEW RESOURCES

Comprehensive

A⁻ **NMS Review for USMLE Step 2**   **$49.95**   Software/900 q

Gruber

Lippincott Williams & Wilkins, 2000, V3.0, ISBN 0781729440
Comprehensive question bank with complete explanations. Question style
is similar to that of *NMS Review for USMLE Step 2* text. **Pros:** Provides
added benefit of mimicking the CBT format of the actual boards. Offers
mock exams or exams focused on certain areas. **Cons:** Some find the interface awkward or confusing. **Summary:** Quality questions in boards-type
setting, but somewhat difficult to navigate.

A⁻ **Cracking the Boards**   **$29.95**   Review

Mariani

Random House, 2000, 2nd edition, 304 pages, ISBN 0375761640
Clinical vignette review organized by specialty with more than 400
vignette-style questions. **Pros:** Well organized, with uniform format
throughout the book and lots of charts. Appropriate emphasis on treatment. Questions reflect the style of the Step 2 exam. **Cons:** Few images.
Summary: Useful review that follows the emphasis of Step 2 on clinical
vignettes.

B⁺ **Step 2 Exam, General Clinical Sciences**   **$32.00**   Test/800 q

Alario

Mosby–Year Book, 1999, 1st edition, 417 pages, ISBN 081513715X
Boards-type questions in both integrated and topic-based test sections.
Pros: Questions have appropriate content and level of difficulty. Explanations of both correct and incorrect answers are provided. **Cons:** Makes little use of images (radiographic, patient photos, pathology, or ECG). **Summary:** Decent practice questions approximating the boards.

B⁺ **Underground Clinical Vignettes: Nine-Volume Set**   **$199.95**   Review

Bhushan

Blackwell Science, 2001, 2nd edition, ISBN 0632045779
Nine-volume set containing clinical case scenarios of the various specialties, including OB/GYN, neurology, internal medicine, surgery, emergency
medicine, psychiatry, and pediatrics, along with an extensive color atlas
supplement. **Pros:** Well organized by focus points: pathogenesis, epidemiology, management, complications, and associated diseases. Well illustrated, and the new edition includes "mini-cases" and updated treatment
and management guidelines. **Cons:** Expensive for the nine-volume set.
Not comprehensive; use as a supplement to review. **Summary:** Organized
and easy to read. Excellent as a supplement to studying, but not sufficient
by itself. More economical to purchase the nine-volume set than individual volumes.

B+   **USMLE Step 2 Secrets**   **$33.00**   Review

Brochert

Hanley & Belfus, 2000, 1st edition, 257 pages, ISBN 1560534516

Typical Secrets series format, with questions and answers organized by specialty. **Pros:** Concise review of many high-yield topics. Good use of clinical images, including patient photos, blood smears, and radiographs. **Cons:** No clinical vignettes; simply lists of questions that might be posed on the wards. Does not follow Step 2 format and may leave out important information. Expensive. Content is redundant with other books by Brochert. **Summary:** Overall, good content for self-quizzing and study, but does not substitute for a formal review or practice tests. Portable book that stresses relevant topics in a quick, easy format.

B+   **A&L's Review for the USMLE Step 2**   **$39.95**   Test/1060 q

Chan

McGraw-Hill, 2002, 4th edition, 372 pages, ISBN 007137728X

Review questions organized by specialty along with two comprehensive practice exams. **Pros:** Overall question content good, with broad coverage of high-yield topics. Well illustrated. New edition contains more vignette-type questions. **Cons:** Vignettes are brief. Some questions do not reflect Step 2 style and format. **Summary:** Good overall review questions on high-yield topics make it well suited for focused specialty review. Good buy for the number of questions.

B+   **Rx: Prescription for the Boards USMLE Step 2**   **$33.95**   Review

Feibusch

Lippincott Williams & Wilkins, 2002, 3rd edition, 515 pages, ISBN 0781734002

Comprehensive text review based on the widely used USMLE content outline. **Pros:** Comprehensive coverage of high-yield core and specialty topics. New edition offers tips for the computer-based exam and provides more illustrations. Well-designed format. **Cons:** Too detailed in several cases. Lacks tables and diagrams to facilitate studying. Facts outlining the next step in management are often not discussed. Lengthy. **Summary:** Good single source for Step 2 review. Requires time commitment.

B+   **Advanced Life Support for the USMLE Step 2**   **$18.95**   Review

Flynn

Lippincott Williams & Wilkins, 1999, 2nd edition, 142 pages, ISBN 0781719763

Brief outline format with high-yield topics described in tables or illustrations. **Pros:** Quick, easy read. Emphasis on high-yield facts. Amusing cartoons highlight key concepts and excellent mnemonics. Great last-minute review. **Cons:** Not adequate for in-depth review. **Summary:** Worthwhile review for the night before the exam.

B+ **A&L's Practice Tests: USMLE Step 2**   **$36.95** Test/900 q
Goldberg

McGraw-Hill, 2003, 2nd edition, 253 pages, ISBN 0071377409
Comprehensive test questions. **Pros:** Great source of high-yield questions
covering all topics. Most questions reflect the vignette format of Step 2.
Many questions include radiographs and photographs of pathology. Adequate explanations. **Cons:** Some questions are not vignette style and do
not reflect boards format. **Summary:** Good compilation of test questions
that focus on high-yield material, but some questions still do not reflect
boards style.

B+ **A&L's Flash Facts for the USMLE Steps 2 and 3**   **$26.50** Test/200 q
Kaiser

McGraw-Hill, 1997, 1st edition, 220 pages, ISBN 0838526063
More than 200 clinically based questions presented on flash cards. Answers and discussions are on the reverse side of each card. **Pros:** Quick
case-based review. Covers high-yield topics in core specialties. Focuses on
key aspects of management and diagnosis. Useful for on-the-go review.
Cons: Style may not suit all students. Expensive for a limited number of
topics. Awkward reference system. No index. **Summary:** High-quality material, but expensive and limited in scope. Use with other comprehensive
resources.

B+ **PreTest Clinical Vignettes for the USMLE Step 2**   **$24.95** Test/400 q
McGraw-Hill

McGraw-Hill, 2001, 2nd edition, 309 pages, ISBN 0071364536
Vignette-style question book with answers organized by subject. A collection of the "best of" from the PreTest question books. **Pros:** Broad coverage of Step 2 topics. Good variety. Detailed explanations. **Cons:** Some
questions are too picky or lack the appropriate emphasis for boards review.
Some questions are too simplistic and straightforward. **Summary:** Good
source of practice questions; strongest of the PreTest series.

B **Medical Boards Step 2 Made Ridiculously Simple**   **$24.95** Review
Carl

MedMaster, 2002, 2nd edition, 363 pages, ISBN 0940780550
General review of topics for the Step 2 exam. Outline format with tables
and brief discussions. **Pros:** Quick review. Useful in areas that might otherwise be overlooked, e.g., ophthalmology, dermatology, and ENT. Helpful
for last-minute review. New edition has an updated management section.
Cons: Often lacks substantive details. Some errors. **Summary:** Highlights
most high-yield topics. Should not be used as a sole source for review.

B **USMLE Step 2: The Stanford Solutions to the NBME Computer-Based Sample Test Questions**

$18.95   Test/150 q

Kush

Planet Med Publishing, 1999, 1st edition, 152 pages, ISBN 1893730255

Detailed answers to questions provided on the NBME sample test. **Pros:** Inexpensive review with good discussion of topics and page references to standard textbooks of medicine. Answers are thoroughly explained. **Cons:** Questions are not reprinted in the book, giving no references for the answers provided. **Summary:** By nature, not a systematic or well-organized review, but a welcome solution for those who take the NBME practice test.

B **Medical Student USMLE Parts II and III Pearls of Wisdom**

$32.00   Review

Plantz

Boston Medical Publishing, 1998, 1st edition, 331 pages, ISBN 1890369101

Comprehensive review with many questions. **Pros:** A good job approximating the questions on Step 2 of the boards, with similar clinical emphasis and distribution across various specialties. **Cons:** Lacks illustrations, including images to aid in diagnosis. **Summary:** Easy-to-read, compact review designed for self-testing.

B⁻ **A&LERT USMLE Step 2**

$74.95   Software/1200+ q

Appleton & Lange

McGraw-Hill, 1998, 1st edition, ISBN 0838584470

Computerized test bank based on *A&L's Review for the USMLE Step 2*. Users can take timed exams that are scored automatically. **Pros:** Quick way to review selected topics with use of search function and bookmarks. Allows users to simulate a timed exam. Questions and answers may be printed out for further review. **Cons:** Very costly. Some questions are too specific. Interface does not reflect the new CBT. **Summary:** Good-quality questions, but the interface differs from the actual CBT.

B⁻ **A&LERT USMLE Step 2 Deluxe**

$95.00   Software/3400 q

Appleton & Lange

McGraw-Hill, 1998, 1st edition, ISBN 0838503748

Question bank includes questions from *A&L's Review for the USMLE Step 2* and from A&L's MEPC series. Otherwise identical to *A&LERT USMLE Step 2*. **Pros:** Large collection of questions will keep you busy. **Cons:** Includes lower-yield "second-tier" questions that do not accurately reflect USMLE style. **Summary:** Worth considering if you need a large collection of computerized questions.

Comprehensive

B− Mosby's Ace the Boards: General Clinical Sciences Step 2

$41.95 Review/1000+ q

Bollet

Mosby–Year Book, 1996, 1st edition, 530 pages, ISBN 0815107234

Detailed review of Step 2. Features questions in book and on disk. **Pros:** Comprehensive review of most major Step 2 topics. Explanations to questions are generally complete. **Cons:** Dense, overly detailed text makes for difficult reading. Few clinical vignette questions in non-boards style. Poorly illustrated. **Summary:** Comprehensive review is too dense and detailed for boards review or wards preparation.

B− REA's Interactive Flashcards USMLE Step 2

$8.95 Flash card

Fogiel

REA, 1998, 1st edition, 500 pages, ISBN 0878911685

Flash-card review in book format. **Pros:** Cheap. Has fill-in-the-blank format. **Cons:** Cannot remove pages to use as flash cards. Fairly random questions; some picky and low-yield questions. **Summary:** Not very helpful for review given non-boards-style questions and low-yield topics.

B− A&L's Outline Review for the USMLE Step 2

$39.95 Review

Goldberg

McGraw-Hill, 1999, 3rd edition, 680 pages, ISBN 0838503543

General outline of major clinical topics. "Cram facts" are scattered throughout. **Pros:** Information is presented by symptoms, diagnosis, pathology, and treatment. Many classic photos. Covers most relevant topics. **Cons:** Coverage varies widely from topic to topic. Difficult to extract key points. Time-consuming. **Summary:** Large, well-illustrated book that is sometimes light on meaningful content.

B− MEPC USMLE Step 2 Review

$32.95 Test/1000+ q

Jacobs

McGraw-Hill, 1996, 410 pages, ISBN 0838562701

Question-and-answer format with explanations. **Pros:** Relatively quick review. Numerous photographs of classic findings. Appropriate coverage of high-yield topics. Answers highlight important buzzwords. **Cons:** Discussions of answers are sometimes brief. Relatively simple vignettes do not reflect current boards format. **Summary:** Fair source of additional questions that may be read quickly. Well illustrated.

B− **Classic Presentations and Rapid Review**
for USMLE Step 2 $25.00   Review

O'Connell

J&S, 1999, 1st edition, 215 pages, ISBN 1888308052

Light overview organized by specialty, with emphasis on "classic" presentations of commonly seen conditions. In bulleted-point format. **Pros:** Good for last-minute studying. **Cons:** Neither comprehensive nor consistent in the material provided on each topic. Information is not overly detailed. No clinical images, ECGs, or clinical case examples. **Summary:** Quick and superficial review.

B− **Insider's Guide to the USMLE Step 2** $39.95   Review/450 q

Stang

Saunders, 1999, 1st edition, 426 pages, ISBN 0721682790

Contains case-based questions with explanations and includes suggested review topics. **Pros:** "Pop quizzes" after each section encourage retention. Practice test has detailed explanations to answers. **Cons:** Sparse information; may serve as a study guide rather than a review book. Some topics are not relevant for boards. Questions do not reflect the vignette format on Step 2. **Summary:** Well-organized but not overly detailed comprehensive review. Some content is irrelevant to Step 2.

C+ **Step 2 of the Boards: Clinical Problem Solving** $299.00 Audio review
and Advanced Internal Medicine

Gold Standard Board Preparation Systems

Gold Standard, 1997–1999, 54 tapes

Audio review organized into the following topics: differential diagnosis, drugs of choice, urgent care, surgery, pediatrics, OB/GYN, advanced cardiac life support, cardiology and EKGs, and diabetes and hypertension. Also includes an in-depth review of internal medicine with tapes on pulmonary medicine, hematology, genitourinary disorders, heart failure, cardiac arrhythmias, gastrointestinal disease, and endocrinology. **Pros:** Offers a novel study method. Question-and-answer format keeps the listener engaged. **Cons:** Lacks adequate emphasis on diagnosis and management. Focuses on low-yield topics; sometimes overly simplistic. Expensive. No CD format available. **Summary:** Useful as a supplemental review source but relatively expensive, with some focus on low-yield material.

C+ **Clinical Science Question Bank for the USMLE Step 2**   **$28.00**   Test/500 q

Zaslau

FMSG, 1997, 1st edition, 135 pages, ISBN 1886468168

Review-question book with five 100-question exams. Includes lengthy
clinical vignettes as well as figures and images. **Pros:** Questions focus on
high-yield topics. **Cons:** Questions are of variable quality. Some questions
lack explanations. Illustrations are not representative of Step 2. Relatively
expensive. **Summary:** Covers appropriate topics, but many questions are
poorly written.

C+ **Step 2 Virtual Reality**   **$20.00**   Test/320 q

Zaslau

FMSG, 1998, 1st edition, 170 pages, ISBN 1886468249

Two practice exams with discussions of correct and incorrect responses.
Pros: Lengthy question stems approximate those of Step 2. Questions also
reflect emphasis on management and treatment decisions. Generally
good-quality content. **Cons:** Not much material covered. Explanations of
incorrect answers are very superficial. **Summary:** Limited number of good-
quality questions.

C **USMLE Success**   **$38.00**   Review/540 q

Zaslau

FMSG, 1996, 3rd edition, 280 pages, ISBN 1886468095

General overview for Steps 1, 2, and 3 in outline format. Contains simulated exams for both Step 1 and Step 2. **Pros:** Many clinical vignette
questions with appropriate emphasis on diagnosis and management. Quick
read. **Cons:** Scanty facts; outdated book recommendations. Poorly written
explanations. Few illustrations. Expensive for the amount and quality of
material. **Summary:** Inadequate source for any Step review. Questions
may be helpful, but explanations are poorly written.

C– **Clinical Science Review Success**   **$22.00**   Review

Zaslau

FMSG, 1997, 1st edition, 132 pages, ISBN 188646815X

General overview of core clinical rotations. Notes are printed straight
from the author's PowerPoint presentation. There is added information on
the Match and residency. **Pros:** Overview of high-yield topics may be
quickly reviewed. "Most common" list may be useful for quick cramming.
Cons: Mostly superficial coverage. PowerPoint printout is difficult to read.
Summary: Inadequate, superficial, poorly formatted content review with
an expensive price tag.

REVIEW RESOURCES

Comprehensive

A⁻ Kaplanmedical.com $129–$329
Kaplan

Compilation of online programs for Step 2 review. **Pros:** Questions can be arranged by topic or randomly to simulate the real exam. Tests are timed to simulate boards conditions. Extensive number of questions in vignette format. Content level of questions reflects the boards test. Explanations are thorough. Allows students to identify strong and weak points. **Cons:** Very expensive. Online lectures can be difficult to watch for extensive periods of time. **Summary:** Excellent source of questions with thorough explanations, but the price may be prohibitive for many.

A⁻ Medrevu.com $34.95–$179
Lippincott Williams & Wilkins

Comprehensive question bank with complete explanations. Similar in style to the *NMS Review for USMLE Step 2* software described above. **Pros:** Mimics the CBT format of the actual boards. Can purchase subscriptions of different durations. Offers mock or focused exams on areas of weakness. **Cons:** Interface can be awkward, confusing, and at times difficult to navigate. **Summary:** Quality questions are given in a boards-type setting but are somewhat difficult to navigate. Good exam simulation with appropriate-style questions.

REVIEW RESOURCES

Online Review

REVIEW RESOURCES

Internal Medicine

A– **Underground Clinical Vignettes: Internal Medicine, Vol. I.**   **$19.95**   Review

Bhushan

Blackwell Science, 2002, 2nd edition, 100 pages, ISBN 0632045639

Clinical vignette review of common topics in internal medicine. **Pros:** Well organized by focus points: pathogenesis, epidemiology, management, complications, and associated diseases. Well illustrated, and the new edition includes high-yield updates on nearly every case, new and updated "mini-cases," and links to the UCV Clinical/Basic Color Atlas. **Cons:** Not comprehensive; use as a supplement. **Summary:** Organized and easy-to-read supplement to studying.

A– **Underground Clinical Vignettes: Internal Medicine, Vol. II**   **$21.95**   Review

Bhushan

Blackwell Science, 2002, 2nd edition, 100 pages, ISBN 0632045655

Clinical vignette review of common topics in internal medicine. **Pros:** Well organized by focus points: pathogenesis, epidemiology, management, complications, and associated diseases. Well illustrated, and the new edition includes high-yield updates on nearly every case, new and updated "mini-cases," and links to the UCV Clinical/Basic Color Atlas. **Cons:** Not comprehensive; use as a supplement. **Summary:** Organized and easy-to-read supplement to studying.

A– **Platinum Vignettes: Internal Medicine**   **$24.95**   Review

Brochert

Hanley & Belfus, 2002, 1st edition, 102 pages, ISBN 1560535318

Clinical vignette review of common topics in internal medicine. **Pros:** Well-written cases similar to boards-type vignettes. Well illustrated. Discussion is organized by pathophysiology, diagnosis and treatment, and more high-yield facts. **Cons:** Not comprehensive; use as a supplement. **Summary:** Organized and easy-to-read supplement to studying.

A– **Platinum Vignettes: Internal Medicine Subspecialties** **$24.95**   Review

Brochert

Hanley & Belfus, 2002, 1st edition, 105 pages, ISBN 1560535377

Clinical vignette review of common topics in internal medicine. **Pros:** Well-written cases similar to boards-type vignettes. Well illustrated. Discussion is organized by pathophysiology, diagnosis and treatment, and more high-yield facts. **Cons:** Not comprehensive; use as a supplement. **Summary:** Organized and easy-to-read supplement to studying.

A⁻ **Blueprints in Medicine** $29.95 Review/89 q

Young

Blackwell Science, 2000, 2nd edition, 354 pages, ISBN 0632044845

Text review of internal medicine organized by common diseases and common symptoms. Question-and-answer section with explanations. **Pros:** Well-organized, concise review. Engaging, easy reading. Symptom approach is helpful for boards review. Good charts and diagrams. **Cons:** Few illustrations. Not a quick read. Has some superfluous details; some areas are too broad and simplistic. **Summary:** Good primary boards review for internal medicine, although poorly illustrated.

B⁺ **Medicine Recall** $9.95 Review

Bergin

Lippincott Williams & Wilkins, 1997, 1st edition, 928 pages, ISBN 0683180983

Standard Recall series question-and-answer format, organized by medical specialty. **Pros:** Addresses a broad range of high-yield clinical topics. Good format for self-quizzing. Appropriate level of detail. **Cons:** No vignettes and no images; requires time commitment. **Summary:** Style may be more conducive to wards than to boards preparation. Use as a supplement to other resources. New edition not yet reviewed.

B⁺ **PreTest Medicine** $24.95 Test/500 q

Berk

McGraw-Hill, 2001, 9th edition, 238 pages, ISBN 0071359605

Question-and-answer format organized by medical subspecialty. **Pros:** Organization by subspecialty helps pinpoint weak areas. Decent number of vignette-style questions, with detailed explanations. **Cons:** Many questions are more detailed than needed for the boards, and some questions are too simplistic. Few illustrations. **Summary:** Solid source of challenging review questions.

B⁺ **Underground Clinical Vignettes: Emergency Medicine** $21.95 Review

Bhushan

Blackwell Science, 2002, 2nd edition, 100 pages, ISBN 0632045612

Clinical vignette review of emergency medicine topics. **Pros:** Well organized by focus points: pathogenesis, epidemiology, management, complications, and associated diseases. Well illustrated, and the new edition includes high-yield updates on nearly every case, new and updated "mini-cases," and links to the UCV Clinical/Basic Color Atlas. **Cons:** Not comprehensive; use as a supplement. **Summary:** Organized and easy-to-read supplement to studying.

B+ A&L's Review of Internal Medicine
Goldlist

$34.95   Test/1100+ q

McGraw-Hill, 2003, 3rd edition, 276 pages, ISBN 007138524X

General review with questions and answers divided by subspecialty. **Pros:** Well-written vignette questions reflect boards format. Representative of the content of the boards. Complete explanations. Well illustrated. New edition has updated questions to reflect current standard of practice. **Cons:** Questions are shorter, and some nonvignette questions are more straightforward than those on the exam. **Summary:** Good source of questions that accurately reflect the multistep nature of boards questions.

B+ High-Yield Internal Medicine
Nirula

$18.95   Review

Lippincott Williams & Wilkins, 1997, 1st edition, 197 pages, ISBN 0683180444

Core review of internal medicine in outline format. **Pros:** Focus is on high-yield diseases and symptoms. Quick and easy read. **Cons:** Some mistakes in formulas. Needs more illustrations. No index. **Summary:** Good, fast review presented in a format that allows for quick and repetitive readings. Use as a supplement, not as a primary study source.

B+ Medical Secrets
Zollo

$39.95   Review

Lippincott Williams & Wilkins, 2001, 3rd edition, 564 pages, ISBN 1560534761

Question-discussion style typical of the Secrets series. **Pros:** Covers a great deal of clinically relevant information. Concise answers with pearls, tips, and memory aids. **Cons:** Too lengthy and detailed for USMLE review. No images or vignettes. **Summary:** May be most appropriate for wards use. Not a focused review.

B Blueprints Q & A Step 2 Medicine
Clement

$12.95   Test/100 q

Blackwell Science, 2002, 1st edition, 97 pages, ISBN 0632046023

One hundred vignette-style questions. **Pros:** Nice companion to the Blueprints series. Focuses on high-yield topics. Explanations are easy to follow. **Cons:** Not comprehensive; use as a supplement for review. Sparse images. Some questions are esoteric and not boards-like. Expensive; number of questions few for the cost of the book. **Summary:** Organized and easy-to-read supplement. Adds clinical correlates to the Blueprints series.

B **Outpatient Medicine Recall**   **$29.95**   Review

Franko

Lippincott Williams & Wilkins, 1998, 1st edition, 350 pages, ISBN
0683180185

Question-and-answer format typical of Recall series books, focused on outpatient management. **Pros:** Well-written material; good for self-testing.
Cons: Not as concise or focused as other boards resources. No vignettes or
images. **Summary:** Style is not ideal for boards review, but may be a useful
adjunct.

B **Blueprints Clinical Cases in Medicine**   **$18.95**   Test/200 q

Gandhi

Blackwell Science, 2002, 1st edition, 143 pages, ISBN 0632046031
Compendium of vignette-type cases arranged by symptom followed by related questions and answers. **Pros:** Excellent companion to the Blueprints
series. Focuses on high-yield cases. Easy to read with nice illustrations and
review of management. **Cons:** Not comprehensive; use as a supplement
for review. **Summary:** Organized and easy-to-read supplement. Adds clinical correlates to the Blueprints series. Best if used with the Blueprints text.

B **Internal Medicine Pearls**   **$45.00**   Review

Heffner

Lippincott Williams & Wilkins, 2000, 2nd edition, 249 pages, ISBN
1560534044

Detailed clinical vignettes with laboratory and radiographic findings followed by a discussion and emphasis of clinically important pearls. **Pros:**
High-quality, realistic vignettes. Questions focus on decision making and
management. **Cons:** Selected topics; not comprehensive. Discussions may
be too detailed for purposes of review. Miscellaneous details. **Summary:**
Good, clinically focused supplement for review.

B **Blueprints Clinical Cases in Family Medicine**   **$18.95**   Test/200 q

Lesko

Blackwell Science, 2002, 1st edition, 135 pages, ISBN 0632046546
Compendium of vignette-type cases arranged by symptom followed by related questions and answers. **Pros:** Excellent companion to the Blueprints
series. Focuses on high-yield cases. Easy to read with nice illustrations and
review of management. **Cons:** Not comprehensive; use as a supplement
for review. **Summary:** Organized and easy-to-read supplement. Adds clinical correlates to the Blueprints series. Best if used with the Blueprints text.

B Physical Diagnosis Secrets $38.00 Review

Mangione

Lippincott Williams & Wilkins, 1999, 1st edition, 350 pages, ISBN 1560531649

Secrets series question-and-answer format. **Pros:** Concise review of many high-yield topics. Good use of clinical images. **Cons:** No clinical vignettes; simply lists of questions that might be posed on the wards. Does not have a structured format and may leave out important information. Expensive for the amount of material. **Summary:** Overall, good content for self-quizzing and study, but does not substitute for a formal review or practice tests.

B PreTest Physical Diagnosis $21.95 Review/500 q

Reteguiz

McGraw-Hill, 2001, 4th edition, 328 pages, ISBN 0071360980

Vignette-style question book with answers organized by subject. Questions serve as a primer for review before moving on to the other PreTest series books. **Pros:** Broad coverage of vignette-style questions with detailed explanations. **Cons:** Some questions are too picky and are more focused on how to diagnose disease. **Summary:** Good tool to begin review of Step 2. Overall, low yield.

B First Aid for the Emergency Medical Clerkship $29.95 Review

Stead

McGraw-Hill, 2002, 1st edition, 470 pages, ISBN 0071364269

High-yield review of symptoms and diseases. **Pros:** Comprehensive review; well organized by symptoms with good illustrations, scenarios, diagrams, algorithms, and mnemonics. **Cons:** May not cater to the reader who prefers information arranged in text form. **Summary:** Excellent review of emergency medicine, and nice presentation of high-yield topics for Step 2 preparation but not intended for boards review.

B First Aid for the Medical Clerkship $29.95 Review

Stead

McGraw-Hill, 2002, 1st edition, 405 pages, ISBN 0071364218

High-yield review of symptoms and diseases. **Pros:** Comprehensive review; well organized by symptoms with good illustrations, scenarios, diagrams, algorithms, and mnemonics. **Cons:** May not cater to the reader who prefers information arranged in text form. **Summary:** Excellent review of medicine, but lengthy for boards review.

C+ **Saint-Frances Guide to Inpatient Medicine** $23.95 Review

Frances

Lippincott Williams & Wilkins, 1997, 1st edition, 533 pages, ISBN 0683075470

General review of high-yield medicine topics in outline format. **Pros:** Readable, concise, and well organized with mnemonics and "hot keys" emphasized. Portable. **Cons:** Brief coverage of some important topics. Lacks images. Requires time commitment. **Summary:** Comprehensive but designed for use on the wards; less useful for studying for Step 2.

C+ **Saint-Frances Guide to Outpatient Medicine** $23.95 Review

Frances

Lippincott Williams & Wilkins, 2000, 1st edition, 713 pages, ISBN 0781726123

General review of high-yield outpatient medicine topics in outline format. **Pros:** Readable, concise, and well organized with mnemonics and "hot keys" emphasized. Portable. **Cons:** Brief coverage of some important topics. Lacks images. Requires time commitment. More relevant for clerkship study. **Summary:** Solid medicine review, but fewer high-yield topics than *Saint-Frances Guide to Inpatient Medicine*.

B+

Underground Clinical Vignettes: Neurology
$24.95 Review

Bhushan

Blackwell Science, 2001, 2nd edition, 100 pages, ISBN 0632045671
Clinical vignette review of high-yield topics in neurology. **Pros:** Well organized by focus points: pathogenesis, epidemiology, management, complications, and associated diseases. Well illustrated, and the new edition has additional "mini-cases," links to a color atlas supplement, and updated treatments. **Cons:** Not comprehensive; use as a supplement to review. **Summary:** Organized and easy-to-read supplement to studying. Lengthy for dedicated review of neurology.

B+

PreTest Neurology
$21.95 Test/500 q

Elkind

McGraw-Hill, 2001, 4th edition, 292 pages, ISBN 0071373500
Question-and-answer review of neurology. **Pros:** Thorough coverage of neurology topics with good number of clinical vignettes. Good emphasis on common topics. **Cons:** Some questions may be more detailed than the level needed for the boards. Poorly illustrated. **Summary:** Good source of test questions for rapid review of neurology.

B+

Blueprints in Neurology
$29.95 Review

Joshi

Blackwell Science, 2002, 1st edition, 232 pages, ISBN 0632045396
Review of neurology by disease and symptom with a brief exam. **Pros:** Reviews high-yield topics and is easy to follow. Good use of tables, images, and diagrams. **Cons:** Lengthy. **Summary:** Excellent review of high-yield material for the wards and Step 2.

B

Blueprints Clinical Cases in Neurology
$19.95 Review

Joshi

Blackwell Science, 2002, 1st edition, 135 pages, ISBN 0632046139
Compendium of vignette-type cases organized by symptom followed by related question and answers. **Pros:** Excellent companion to the Blueprints subspecialty series. Focuses on high-yield cases. Easy to read, with nice illustrations and review of management. **Cons:** Not comprehensive; use as a supplement. Few illustrations. **Summary:** Organized and easy to read. Adds clinical correlates to the Blueprints series.

B | Neurology Recall

$28.00   Review

Miller

Lippincott Williams & Wilkins, 1997, 1st edition, 340 pages, ISBN 0683182161

Brief question-and-answer format. **Pros:** Many important facts are reviewed; useful for self-quizzing. **Cons:** Not a comprehensive review. Lengthy and lacks illustrations. Concepts are not integrated. **Summary:** Good for review of some high-yield concepts, but not a standalone resource for this topic.

B | Neurology Secrets

$39.95   Review

Rolak

Lippincott Williams & Wilkins, 2001, 3rd edition, 438 pages, ISBN 1560534656

Secrets series question-and-answer format. **Pros:** Concise review of many high-yield topics. Good use of clinical images. Quick question-and-answer approach. **Cons:** No clinical vignettes; instead lists of questions that might be posed on the wards. Does not have a structured format and leaves out important information. Relatively expensive, lengthy. Not a reference book. **Summary:** Overall, good content for self-quizzing and study, but does not substitute for a formal review or practice tests. More appropriate for clerkship than for boards review.

B | Neurology Pearls

$45.00   Review

Waclawik

Lippincott Williams & Wilkins, 2000, 1st edition, 250 pages, ISBN 1560532610

Detailed clinical vignettes, including laboratory and test results and radiographic findings, followed by a discussion of diagnosis and emphasis on important pearls. **Pros:** High-quality vignettes on many important neurologic conditions. **Cons:** Requires an investment in time. A number of entries are devoted to closure disease entities. **Summary:** Challenging clinical scenarios to supplement a more structured topic review.

B- | The Resident's Neurology Book

$26.95   Review

Devinsky

F. A. Davis, 1997, 1st edition, 276 pages, ISBN 0803601867

Thorough summary of neurology by topic. **Pros:** Good review. Well written and easy to read. **Cons:** Not organized for boards review. Few illustrations and diagrams. Some areas are not covered extensively. **Summary:** Good overview, but not designed for boards review.

Oklahoma Notes Neurology and Clinical Neuroscience

$19.95   Review/100 q

Brumback

Springer-Verlag, 1996, 2nd edition, 186 pages, ISBN 0387946357
General topics in clinical neurology reviewed in brief outline format.
Pros: Some illustrations. Inexpensive. Easy read. **Cons:** Not updated in several years, so not as reflective of the evolving Step 2 format. Outline has poor coverage of risk factors and management. Clinical vignette questions are too easy. **Summary:** Limited review of neuroscience topics with no emphasis on differential diagnosis, risk factors, or management.

 Case Studies in Neuroscience

$28.95   Review

Jozefowicz

F. A. Davis, 1999, 1st edition, 230 pages, ISBN 0803603045
Case studies followed by essay questions and answers. **Pros:** Vignettes present material in an interesting and challenging manner. Adequate explanations, and good use of images, diagrams, and definitions of key terms. Good way to self-assess knowledge. **Cons:** Does not cover every topic, and questions posed are too challenging for boards review. **Summary:** Challenging clinical scenarios, often beyond the scope of the boards.

A⁻ **Underground Clinical Vignettes: OB/GYN**   **$24.95** Review

Bhushan

Blackwell Science, 2001, 2nd edition, 100 pages, ISBN 0632045698

Clinical vignette review of frequently tested diseases in obstetrics and gynecology. **Pros:** Well organized by focus points: pathogenesis, epidemiology, management, complications, and associated diseases. Well illustrated. Easy read and stresses high-yield facts. New edition includes "mini-cases" to broaden subject material. **Cons:** Not comprehensive; use as a supplement. **Summary:** Well-organized and easy-to-read practice vignettes.

A⁻ **Platinum Vignettes: Obstetrics and Gynecology**   **$24.95** Review

Brochert

Hanley & Belfus, 2002, 1st edition, 102 pages, ISBN 1560535326

Clinical vignette review of common topics in obstetrics and gynecology. **Pros:** Well-written cases similar to boards-type vignettes. Well illustrated. Discussion is organized by pathophysiology, diagnosis and treatment, and more high-yield facts. **Cons:** Not comprehensive; use as a supplement. **Summary:** Organized and easy-to-read supplement to studying.

A⁻ **Blueprints in Obstetrics and Gynecology**   **$34.95** Review/149 q

Callahan

Blackwell Science, 2000, 2nd edition, 207 pages, ISBN 0632044845

Text review with tables and illustrations. Includes a short exam with explanations. **Pros:** Strong emphasis on high-yield topics with concise text, clear diagrams, and many classic illustrations. Easy read. **Cons:** Some overly detailed material is included, and some are not detailed enough. Lengthy text. **Summary:** Overall, good choice for boards and wards preparation, although some material is not for last-minute Step 2 review.

B **Obstetrics and Gynecology Secrets**   **$39.95** Review

Badu

Lippincott Williams & Wilkins, 2003, 3rd edition, 378 pages, ISBN 1560534753

Secrets series question-and-answer format, organized by topics within OB/GYN. **Pros:** Good coverage of many high-yield, clinically relevant topics. **Cons:** Detailed; not useful for rapid review. No vignettes; few illustrations and images. **Summary:** Good clinical context, but does not serve as a formal topic review.

B NMS Obstetrics and Gynecology   **$32.00**   Review/500 q

Beck

Lippincott Williams & Wilkins, 1997, 4th edition, 510 pages, ISBN
0683180150

Detailed outline of OB/GYN with few tables and diagrams. **Pros:** Comprehensive review for both wards and boards. Final exam is relatively good with complete explanations. **Cons:** Dense and lengthy OB/GYN review. Many questions do not reflect boards format. Lacks illustrations. **Summary:** Complete review with questions and discussion. Too ambitious for exam prep alone; more helpful if used throughout clerkship.

B Blueprints Clinical Cases in Obstetrics   **$18.95**   Test/200 q
and Gynecology

Caughey

Blackwell Science, 2002, 1st edition, 138 pages ISBN 0632046112

Compendium of vignette-type cases arranged by symptom followed by related questions and answers. **Pros:** Excellent companion to the Blueprints series. Focuses on high-yield cases. Easy to read with nice illustrations and review of management. **Cons:** Not comprehensive; use as a supplement. **Summary:** Organized and easy-to-read supplement. Adds clinical correlates to the Blueprints series.

B PreTest Obstetrics and Gynecology   **$24.95**   Test/500 q

Evans & Ginsburg

McGraw-Hill, 2001, 9th edition, 263 pages, ISBN 0071359613

Question-and-answer review with detailed explanations for OB/GYN. **Pros:** Organization by subtopic may be useful for studying weak areas. Good content emphasis. Generally well illustrated. **Cons:** Some questions are too difficult or detailed. Vignette-based questions are short and simplistic compared to Step 2 content, which has recently had an emphasis on this topic. **Summary:** Decent source of questions to supplement topic study, especially to address specific areas of weakness.

B Blueprints Q & A Step 2 Obstetrics & Gynecology   **$12.95**   Test/100 q

Mouer

Blackwell Science, 2002, 1st edition, 82 pages ISBN 0632045949

One hundred vignette-style questions. **Pros:** Nice companion to the Blueprints series. Focuses on high-yield topics. Explanations are easy to follow. **Cons:** Not comprehensive; use as a supplement for review. Sparse images. Some questions are esoteric and not boards-like. Expensive: number of questions few for the cost of the book. **Summary:** Organized and easy-to-read supplement. Adds clinical correlates to the Blueprints series.

BRS Obstetrics and Gynecology

$32.95   Review/500 q

Sakala

Lippincott Williams & Wilkins, 2000, 2nd edition, 443 pages, ISBN 0683307436

General review text with questions at the ends of the chapters and a comprehensive exam at the end of the book. **Pros:** Appropriate content for boards and wards study. New edition offers more detail on pregnancy complications and a new STD chapter. **Cons:** Some sections are overly detailed with few diagrams. Questions offer few clinical vignettes. **Summary:** Appropriate content review, but more helpful for wards than for boards.

First Aid For the OB/GYN Clerkship

$29.95   Review

Stead

McGraw-Hill, 2002, 1st edition, 280 pages, ISBN 0071364234

High-yield review of symptoms and diseases. **Pros:** Comprehensive review with nice diagrams, images, charts, algorithms, and mnemonics. **Cons:** Lengthy review. **Summary:** Excellent review of OB/GYN, but lengthy for boards review.

Case Files: Obstetrics and Gynecology

$34.95   Review

Toy

McGraw-Hill, 2003, 1st edition, 488 pages, ISBN 0071402845

Review of OB/GYN in case format with questions and answers following each vignette. **Pros:** Cases reflect high-yield topics and are arranged in an easy-to-follow format. **Cons:** Some topics are either not covered or given only brief treatment. Few diagrams and images. Lengthy and time-consuming for one topic. Explanations terse. **Summary:** Comprehensive review with emphasis on vignette-style case presentation, but some areas not very detailed.

Obstetrics and Gynecology Recall

$28.00   Review/350 q

Bourgeois

Lippincott Williams & Wilkins, 1997, 1st edition, 528 pages, ISBN 0683182145

Recall series question-and-answer style. **Pros:** Two-column format makes it useful for self-quizzing. Reviews many high-yield concepts and facts. **Cons:** Questions emphasize individual facts but do not integrate concepts. No vignettes or images. Spotty coverage of some topics. **Summary:** Useful for review of selected concepts, but not a comprehensive source for USMLE preparation. More appropriate for clerkship than for boards.

B⁻ **Obstetrics and Gynecology: Review for the New National Boards**   **$25.00**   Test/530 q

Kramer

J&S, 1996, 1st edition, 190 pages, ISBN 0963287397

General review of OB/GYN in question-and-answer format. **Pros:** Good U/S images and fetal heart tracings. Appropriate depth of coverage. **Cons:** As many as 40 questions per vignette stem with corresponding multiple-page explanations. Focuses on some low-yield topics. **Summary:** Below-average source of questions. Does not reflect Step 2 format or style.

B⁻ **A&L's Review of Obstetrics and Gynecology**   **$39.95**   Test/1600+ q

Vontver

McGraw-Hill, 2000, 6th edition, 400 pages, ISBN 0838503233

Detailed review of OB/GYN in question-and-answer format. **Pros:** Some high-yield sections such as clinical endocrinology. Lots of questions. **Cons:** Overall emphasis is not appropriate for Step 2 preparation. May be more appropriate for specialty preparation. **Summary:** Far more detailed than required for Step 2. New edition not yet reviewed. Scheduled for release in 2003.

C⁺ **Clinical Obstetrics and Gynecology: A Problem-Based Approach**   **$32.95**   Review

Burnett

Blackwell Science, 2001, 1st edition, 450 pages, ISBN 0632043539

Comprehensive review of OB/GYN by subject matter. **Pros:** Extensive reference with detailed explanations of pathophysiology, diagnosis, and treatment. Clinical correlates added to make the text more reader friendly. **Cons:** Lengthy for boards review. Not a fast read. Few illustrations. **Summary:** Comprehensive review of OB/GYN, but too detailed and lengthy for boards review. Better used as a reference.

C **MEPC Obstetrics and Gynecology**   **$19.95**   Test/765 q

Ross

McGraw-Hill, 1997, 411 pages, ISBN 0838563287

Question-and-answer format with explanation. **Pros:** Another source of questions that may be quickly reviewed. Content of questions is appropriate for Step 2. Most explanations are thorough and well written. **Cons:** Few vignette-based questions. Few illustrations. **Summary:** Average source of additional questions that may be read quickly. Appropriate content emphasis, but questions do not reflect boards-style format.

REVIEW RESOURCES

OB/GYN

Underground Clinical Vignettes: Pediatrics

$24.95 Review

Bhushan

Blackwell Science, 2001, 2nd edition, 100 pages, ISBN 063204571X

Clinical vignette review of frequently tested topics in pediatrics. **Pros:** Well organized by focus points: pathogenesis, epidemiology, management, complications, and associated diseases. Well illustrated, and the new edition includes "mini-cases" to broaden subject material and present more high-yield information. **Cons:** Not comprehensive; use as a supplement text review. **Summary:** Well organized and easy to read, but meant as a supplement for review.

Platinum Vignettes: Pediatrics

$24.95 Review

Brochert

Hanley & Belfus, 2002, 1st edition, 104 pages, ISBN 1560535334

Clinical vignette review of common topics in pediatrics. **Pros:** Well-written cases similar to boards-type vignettes. Well illustrated. Discussion is organized by pathophysiology, diagnosis and treatment, and more high-yield facts. **Cons:** Not comprehensive; use as a supplement. **Summary:** Organized and easy-to-read supplement to studying.

A&L's Review of Pediatrics

$34.95 Test/1000+ q

Lorin

McGraw-Hill, 1997, 5th edition, 222 pages, ISBN 0838503039

Question-and-answer review of pediatrics with detailed explanations. **Pros:** Questions are focused on boards-relevant content. Last chapter includes excellent vignette-based questions. Thorough, well-written explanations. Nice primer on test-taking strategies. **Cons:** Non-vignette-based questions are shorter and more straightforward than those on Step 2. Some questions may be too detailed for Step 2 preparation. Poorly illustrated. **Summary:** Excellent, concise review with appropriate content and good discussions, but the majority of questions do not reflect Step 2 style.

PreTest Pediatrics

$21.95 Test/500 q

Yetman

McGraw-Hill, 2001, 9th edition, 295 pages, ISBN 0071359559

Question-and-answer review with detailed discussion. **Pros:** Organization by organ system is useful for pinpointing weaknesses. Strong, thorough explanations. Fair number of vignette-style questions. Well illustrated. **Cons:** Some questions are too detailed or emphasize low-yield topics. **Summary:** Good source of questions and review for pediatrics. Appropriate content with good illustrations, although not entirely in Step 2 format.

B+ Blueprints in Pediatrics

$29.95   Review/1269 q

Marino

Blackwell Science, 2000, 2nd edition, 246 pages, ISBN 0632044861

Text review of pediatrics with tables and diagrams. Question-and-answer section with explanations included. **Pros:** Appropriate focus on high-yield topics. **Cons:** Relatively dense text with few illustrations. Overly detailed. **Summary:** Good for the motivated student.

B+ Pediatrics: Review for USMLE Step 2

$25.00   Test/545 q

Paulson

J&S, 2000, 1st edition, 273 pages, ISBN 1888308087

Test booklet with many clinical vignettes covering a broad range of topics within pediatrics. **Pros:** Organized by topic; informative answer explanations. Not too dense for last-minute review. **Cons:** Few images; includes non-boards-type questions ("except" and K-type answers). **Summary:** Good content review; does not replicate boards style.

B Blueprints Clinical Cases in Pediatrics

$8.95   Test/200 q

Caughey

Blackwell Science, 2002, 1st edition, 138 pages, ISBN 0632046112

Compendium of vignette-type cases arranged by symptom followed by related questions and answers. **Pros:** Excellent companion to the Blueprints series. Focuses on high-yield cases. Easy to read with nice illustrations and review of management. **Cons:** Not comprehensive; use as a supplement for review. **Summary:** Organized and easy-to-read supplement. Adds clinical correlates to the Blueprints series.

B Blueprints Q & A Step 2 Pediatrics

$12.95   Test/100 q

Clement

Blackwell Science, 2002, 1st edition, 76 pages, ISBN 0632045981

One hundred vignette-style questions. **Pros:** Nice companion to the Blueprints series. Focuses on high-yield topics. Explanations are easy to follow. **Cons:** Not comprehensive; use as a supplement for review. Sparse images. Some questions are esoteric and not boards-like. Expensive: number of questions few for the cost of the book. **Summary:** Organized and easy-to-read supplement. Adds clinical correlates to the Blueprints series.

B Pediatrics Recall

$28.00   Review

McGahren

Lippincott Williams & Wilkins, 1997, 1st edition, 459 pages, ISBN 068305855X

Concise question-and-answer format typical of the Recall series. **Pros:** Two-column format makes self-quizzing easy. Emphasizes diagnosis and management. **Cons:** Requires time commitment. Not all topics are covered thoroughly. No vignettes. **Summary:** Useful material, but does not provide a systematic review or substitute for practice tests.

B− NMS Pediatrics
Dworkin

$33.00   Review/166+ q

Lippincott Williams & Wilkins, 2000, 4th edition, ISBN 0683306375
General review of pediatrics in outline format. Questions at the end of each chapter. **Pros:** Thorough, detailed review of pediatrics. Boldfacing highlights key points. Case studies and comprehensive exam (also provided on CD-ROM) at the end of the book are helpful. Good discussion. **Cons:** Dense, lengthy text. Lacks good illustrations of any kind. **Summary:** Thorough review, but more appropriate for clerkships than for Step 2 review.

B− MEPC Pediatrics
Hansbarger

$19.95   Test/700 q

McGraw-Hill, 1995, 9th edition, 248 pages, ISBN 083856223X
Question-and-answer format with brief discussion. **Pros:** Appropriate content emphasis. Quick read. **Cons:** Not updated in several years. Few vignette questions. Scanty explanations. Poor illustrations. **Summary:** Below-average source of questions with poor discussion of answers.

B− Pediatric Secrets
Polin

$39.00   Review

Lippincott Williams & Wilkins, 2001, 3rd edition, 731 pages, ISBN 1560534567
Question-and-answer format typical of the Secrets series, organized by pediatric subspecialty. **Pros:** Thorough discussion of a wide variety of clinical topics. **Cons:** Detailed content geared for the wards; requires a large time investment. No images or illustrations. **Summary:** Too detailed for USMLE review. Better suited for clerkship.

C+ Oklahoma Notes Pediatrics
Puls

$19.95   Review/126 q

Springer-Verlag, 1996, 2nd edition, 390 pages, ISBN 0387946349
General outline format of pediatrics. **Pros:** Well organized by system. Good tables. **Cons:** Not updated in several years. Poorly illustrated. Incomplete explanations. Focuses on some low-yield topics. Questions lack clinical vignettes or explanations. **Summary:** Well-organized review of pediatrics with incomplete text. Above average for series.

C USMLE Step 2 Board Certification Review: Pediatrics and Medical Ethics
Kanjilal

$69.95   Review

Rivercross, 2001, 1st edition, 427 pages, ISBN 1581410565
Boards review text focusing on pediatrics and medical ethics. **Pros:** Comprehensive review of topic matter. Highly detailed, with helpful hints on how to score well on the exam. **Cons:** Lengthy and too detailed at times. Not an easy read. Very costly. **Summary:** Although comprehensive, too cumbersome and expensive for boards review.

REVIEW RESOURCES

Preventative Medicine

B+ PreTest Preventive Medicine and Public Health
Ratelle

$21.95 Test/500 q

McGraw-Hill, 2001, 9th edition, 238 pages, ISBN 0071359621

Question-and-answer review of epidemiology, biostatistics, and preventive medicine. **Pros:** Majority of test questions appropriately simulate boards content and difficulty. Good explanations. **Cons:** Some questions are too calculation heavy. Biostatistics chapter is too detailed. Few vignettes. **Summary:** Good question-and-answer review for a low-yield topic.

B− MEPC Preventive Medicine and Public Health
Hart

$21.95 Review/700 q

McGraw-Hill, 1996, 265 pages, ISBN 0838563198

Question-and-answer review with discussions. **Pros:** Appropriate level of biostatistics review. **Cons:** Few clinical vignettes. Many questions are too picky. Brief explanations with poor detail. **Summary:** Adequate content review, but questions do not follow boards format. Explanations are poor.

C+ STARS Epidemiology, Biostatistics, and Preventive Medicine Review
Katz

$21.95 Review/350 q

Saunders, 1997, 249 pages, ISBN 0721640842

Detailed text review of epidemiology and biostatistics. **Pros:** Good tables and diagrams. **Cons:** Small print makes it difficult to read. Text is too detailed for quick review. Questions do not reflect boards style and format. Discussions of questions are too detailed. Requires time commitment. **Summary:** Too detailed for Step 2 review.

C+ NMS Clinical Epidemiology and Biostatistics
Knapp

$28.00 Review/300 q

Lippincott Williams & Wilkins, 1992, 435 pages, ISBN 0683062069

Detailed outline review of epidemiology and biostatistics. **Pros:** Exhaustive coverage. **Cons:** Too much detail for a small subject area. Not updated in several years for the new style of the boards. Very slow read. Questions focus on low-yield topics. **Summary:** Inappropriate for Step 2 review. Better suited for an epidemiology student.

C NMS Preventive Medicine and Public Health
Cassens

$28.00 Review/450 q

Lippincott Williams & Wilkins, 1992, 2nd edition, 497 pages, ISBN 068306262X

Detailed review of preventive medicine and public health. **Pros:** Highly comprehensive review. Questions have thorough explanations. **Cons:** Too long and detailed for boards review. Too much low-yield material. **Summary:** Not ideal for Step 2 review. Better suited for a public health student.

A **Blueprints in Psychiatry** $26.95 Review/74 q

Murphy

Blackwell Science, 2000, 2nd edition, 128 pages, ISBN 0632044888

Brief text review of psychiatry with DSM-IV criteria. Brief question-and-answer section at the end of the book. **Pros:** Clear, concise review of psychiatry with helpful tables. Good coverage of high-yield topics, including pharmacology section. Quick read. **Cons:** Relatively expensive and some areas are not detailed enough. **Summary:** Rapid review with appropriate coverage of high-yield topics.

A⁻ **Underground Clinical Vignettes: Psychiatry** $24.95 Review

Bhushan

Blackwell Science, 2001, 2nd edition, 100 pages, ISBN 0632045736

Clinical vignette review of frequently tested topics in psychiatry. **Pros:** Well organized by focus points: pathogenesis, epidemiology, management, and associated diseases. Well illustrated, and the new edition includes "mini-cases" to broaden subject material and present more high-yield information **Cons:** Not comprehensive; use as a supplement. **Summary:** Organized and easy-to-read practice vignettes.

A⁻ **Platinum Vignettes: Psychiatry** $24.95 Review

Brochert

Hanley & Belfus, 2002, 1st edition, 102 pages, ISBN 1560535342

Clinical vignette review of common topics in pediatrics. **Pros:** Well-written cases similar to boards-type vignettes. Well illustrated. Discussion is organized by pathophysiology, diagnosis and treatment, and more high-yield facts. **Cons:** Not comprehensive; use as a supplement. **Summary:** Organized and easy-to-read supplement to studying.

A⁻ **High-Yield Psychiatry** $21.95 Review

Fadem

Lippincott Williams & Wilkins, 2001, 2nd edition, 125 pages, ISBN 0781730848

Brief outline-format review of psychiatry. **Pros:** Quick read with clinical vignettes scattered throughout. Concise tables. Good supplement to *Blueprints in Psychiatry*. **Cons:** Not enough detail for in-depth review. **Summary:** Excellent, quick review of psychiatry, but may lack depth. Book is similar to *High-Yield Behavioral Sciences* by same author.

B+ PreTest Psychiatry

$21.95 Test/500 q

Mezzacappa

McGraw-Hill, 2001, 9th edition, 255 pages, ISBN 0071361553

Question-and-answer review of topics in psychiatry. **Pros:** Questions are well written and organized. Most questions have appropriate content level. Good explanations. **Cons:** Too few vignette-type questions. Some questions are too detailed. **Summary:** Good source of questions and review for psychiatry, although the format may not reflect the actual test.

B+ A&L's Review of Psychiatry

$34.95 Test/900+ q

Oransky

McGraw-Hill, 2003, 7th edition, 336 pages, ISBN 0071402535

General review of psychiatry with questions and answers. **Pros:** Includes 114 vignette-style questions appropriate for boards review. Appropriate content emphasis; thorough explanations. New edition features updated treatment and management sections. **Cons:** Questions are shorter and more straightforward than those of the boards. **Summary:** Decent boards review for psychiatry, but does not reflect boards format.

B+ NMS Psychiatry

$32.95 Review/500 q

Scully

Lippincott Williams &Wilkins, 2001, 4th edition, 339 pages, ISBN 0683307916

General review of topics in outline format with questions at the end of each chapter and a comprehensive final exam. **Pros:** Well-written text with concise disease discussions. Expanded pharmacology section. Questions test appropriate content and have complete explanations, and the new edition offers more vignette-style questions. Good companion text for clerkship. **Cons:** Not enough vignette-style questions. Lengthy for purposes of boards review. **Summary:** Detailed review that requires time commitment. Good single choice for clerkship study and boards review.

B Blueprints Clinical Cases in Psychiatry

$18.95 Test/200 q

Caughey

Blackwell Science, 2002, 1st edition, 138 pages, ISBN 0632046112

Compendium of vignette-type cases arranged by symptom followed by related questions and answers. **Pros:** Excellent companion to the Blueprints series. Focuses on high-yield cases. Easy to read with nice illustrations and review of management. **Cons:** Not comprehensive; use as a supplement for review. **Summary:** Organized and easy-to-read supplement. Adds clinical correlates to the Blueprints series.

B Blueprints Q & A Step 2 Psychiatry

$12.95 Test/100 q

Clement

Blackwell Science, 2002, 1st edition, 82 pages, ISBN 0632045949

One hundred vignette-style questions. **Pros:** Nice companion to the Blueprints series. Focuses on high-yield topics. Explanations are easy to follow. **Cons:** Not comprehensive; use as a supplement for review. Sparse images. Some questions are esoteric and not boards-like. Expensive: number of questions few for the cost of the book. **Summary:** Organized and easy-to-read supplement. Adds clinical correlates to the Blueprints series.

B Psychiatry Recall

$28.00 Review

Fadem

Lippincott Williams & Wilkins, 1997, 1st edition, 250 pages, ISBN 0683180045

Quick question-and-answer format of the Recall series. **Pros:** Two-column format is conducive to self-quizzing. Covers many high-yield facts and concepts necessary for the USMLE. **Cons:** Lacks vignettes, so does not substitute for practice tests. **Summary:** Requires time commitment. Some topics are glossed over. Use as a supplement to other resources.

B Behavioral Science/Psychiatry: Review for the New National Boards

$25.00 Test/521 q

Frank

J&S, 1998, 1st edition, 248 pages, ISBN 1888308001

General review of psychiatry in question-and-answer format. **Pros:** Includes some vignette-based questions with complete explanations. **Cons:** Does not emphasize high-yield topics. Does not follow boards format or style. Some questions are too short and easy. **Summary:** Mixed-quality questions with generally complete explanations.

B Psychiatry Made Ridiculously Simple

$12.95 Review

Good

MedMaster, 1999, 3rd edition, 93 pages, ISBN 0940780224

Part of the "Made Ridiculously Simple" series. **Pros:** Comprehensive. Fast read with nice tables and entertaining illustrations to highlight key points. **Cons:** Some areas are not detailed enough; other areas are too verbose. Not boards oriented. **Summary:** Good, fast review, but more helpful for clerkship than for boards.

BRS Psychiatry
Shaner

$26.95   Review/400 q

Lippincott Williams & Wilkins, 2000, 2nd edition, 448 pages, ISBN 0863307665

Comprehensive review of psychiatry in outline format. Vignette-style questions follow each chapter. **Pros:** Thorough, systematic review of clinical psychiatry. Clear, concise definitions provided. Good pharmacology section. **Cons:** Great deal of information for single-topic review. **Summary:** Good material, but requires a large time investment; not for last-minute review of all topics.

B **First Aid for the Psychiatry Clerkship**
Stead

$29.95   Review

McGraw-Hill, 2002, 1st edition, 181 pages, ISBN 007136420X

High-yield review of symptoms and diseases. **Pros:** Comprehensive review that includes DSM-IV criteria with nice mnemonics and scenarios. **Cons:** May not appeal to readers who prefer information in text format. **Summary:** Good review of high-yield topics in psychiatry, but better suited for the wards than to the Step 2 exam.

B− **Psychiatric Secrets**
Jacobson

$39.00   Review

Lippincott Williams & Wilkins, 2000, 2nd edition, 500 pages, ISBN 1560534184

Question-discussion format of the Secrets series, organized by topic. **Pros:** Clear explanations of important concepts in psychiatry. Good wards reading. **Cons:** Too detailed and lengthy for review purposes. Lacks vignettes. **Summary:** Requires significant time to read; not for rapid, focused review.

 B− **Saint-Frances Guide to Psychiatry**
McCarthy

$23.95   Review

Lippincott Williams & Wilkins, 2001, 3rd edition, 279 pages, ISBN 0683306618

Comprehensive text review of psychiatry. **Pros:** Thorough. Outline format is easy to read and follow. Portable. Clinical correlates stress key points. **Cons:** Lengthy. Some areas have superfluous information. Not geared toward boards. **Summary:** Nice review of psychiatry with helpful correlates that emphasize key points, but may be more helpful for clerkship than for boards.

MEPC Psychiatry

C+

$19.95   Test/700 q

Chan

McGraw-Hill, 1995, 10th edition, 259 pages, ISBN 0838557805

Question-and-answer format organized by topics in psychiatry. **Pros:** Last chapter has many good clinical vignette questions. **Cons:** Not updated in several years. Most questions are not vignette based. Some questions are picky and focus on low-yield topics. Many explanations are brief. **Summary:** Below-average source of review questions.

Psychiatry at a Glance

C+

$19.95   Review

Katona

Blackwell Science, 2000, 2nd edition, 96 pages, ISBN 0632055545

Discussion of some common psychiatric and neuropsychiatric conditions, with multiple-choice questions. **Pros:** Easy to read. Most important psychiatric conditions are covered. **Cons:** Text is written as an introduction of the topics, so simplistic or generalized at times. Lacks emphasis on high-yield facts or concepts. No vignettes. No explanations. **Summary:** More useful for overview or introduction than for focused USMLE review.

Oklahoma Notes Psychiatry

C+

$19.95   Review/103 q

Shaffer

Springer-Verlag, 1996, 2nd edition (revised), 247 pages, ISBN 0387946330

Outline-format review of clinical psychiatry. **Pros:** Inexpensive, quick read. **Cons:** Haphazard text lacks tables and details. Matching-style questions do not reflect Step 2 format or content. **Summary:** Below-average review of psychiatry.

NMS Behavioral Sciences in Psychiatry

C

$30.00   Review/300 q

Wiener

Lippincott Williams & Wilkins, 1995, 3rd edition, 375 pages, ISBN 0683062034

Outline review of behavioral science in psychiatry. **Pros:** Clear outline format. Case studies highlight differential diagnosis and management. **Cons:** Focuses on many low-yield topics with little emphasis on clinical syndromes. **Summary:** Poor choice for Step 2 review. Lacks adequate clinical emphasis for wards.

A⁻ **Blueprints in Surgery**

Karp

$29.95 Review/62 q

Blackwell Science, 2000, 2nd edition, 160 pages, ISBN 063204487X

Short text review of general surgery with tables and diagrams. Brief question-and-answer section is included. **Pros:** Well organized. Easy to read with strong focus on high-yield topics. Clear diagrams. **Cons:** Some sections are overly detailed (e.g., anatomy). Some information is simplistic. Few illustrations. **Summary:** Concise review of surgery with appropriate emphasis on high-yield topics.

B⁺ **Underground Clinical Vignettes: Surgery**

Bhushan

$21.95 Review

Blackwell Science, 2001, 2nd edition, 100 pages, ISBN 0632045752

Clinical vignette review of frequently tested surgical topics. **Pros:** Well organized by focus points: pathogenesis, epidemiology, management, complications, and associated diseases. Well illustrated, and the new edition includes "mini-cases" to broaden subject material and present more high-yield information. **Cons:** Not comprehensive; use as a supplement to review. **Summary:** Well-organized and easy-to-read practice vignettes.

B⁺ **Platinum Vignettes: Surgery and Trauma**

Brochert

$24.95 Review

Hanley & Belfus, 2002, 1st edition, 102 pages, ISBN 1560535350

Clinical vignette review of common topics in surgery and trauma medicine. **Pros:** Well-written cases similar to boards-type vignettes. Well illustrated. Discussion is organized by pathophysiology, diagnosis and treatment, and more high-yield facts. **Cons:** Not comprehensive; use as a supplement. **Summary:** Organized and easy-to-read supplement to studying.

B⁺ **Platinum Vignettes: Surgical Subspecialties**

Brochert

$24.95 Review

Hanley & Belfus, 2002, 1st edition, 105 pages, ISBN 1560535385

Clinical vignette review of common topics in internal medicine. **Pros:** Well-written cases similar to boards-type vignettes. Well illustrated. Discussion is organized by pathophysiology, diagnosis and treatment, and more high-yield facts. **Cons:** Not comprehensive; use as a supplement. **Summary:** Organized and easy-to-read supplement to studying.

REVIEW RESOURCES

Surgery

B+ BRS General Surgery

$29.95   Review/375 q

Crabtree

Lippincott Williams & Wilkins, 2000, 1st edition, 564 pages, ISBN 0683306367

Comprehensive review in outline format, organized by topic or organ. **Pros:** Appropriate clinical emphasis for boards and wards. Vignette-style review questions at the end of each chapter. **Cons:** Lengthy for single-topic review. Some information is not specific enough to be useful. Few images or illustrations. **Summary:** Overall, a strong review resource. Requires time commitment, so may not be suited to rapid review.

B+ High-Yield Surgery

$21.95   Review

Nirula

Lippincott Williams & Wilkins, 2000, 1st edition, 160 pages, ISBN 068330691X

Outline review of most common general surgery topics. **Pros:** Concise; useful for quick topic review. Well organized. **Cons:** Information can be superficial. Some topics are omitted. No practice questions. **Summary:** Lean text for rapid review.

B+ A&L's Review of Surgery

$34.95   Test/1000+ q

Wapnick

McGraw-Hill, 2002, 4th edition, 320 pages, ISBN 0071378146

General review of surgery with questions and answers. **Pros:** Good clinical emphasis. Many vignette-style questions. Explanations are thorough. **Cons:** Some questions are shorter, and style does not reflect that of the Step 2 exam. Questions are highly variable in difficulty. Few illustrations. **Summary:** Good content for exam, but some questions are picky.

B Surgical Recall

$32.95   Review

Blackbourne

Lippincott Williams & Wilkins, 2002, 3rd edition, 745 pages, ISBN 0781729734

Question-and-answer format as with other Recall series books. **Pros:** Questions emphasize important, high-yield clinical concepts. Columns allow self-testing. Fast review. Good preparation for "pimping" on rounds. **Cons:** Not boards-type questions. Poorly organized. Spotty coverage of some topics. **Summary:** Useful adjunct to a more organized topic review. More appropriate for clerkship than for boards review.

Blueprints Q & A Step 2 Surgery
Clement

$12.95 Test/100 q

Blackwell Science, 2002, 1st edition, 56 pages, ISBN 0632045965
One hundred vignette-style questions. **Pros:** Nice companion to the Blueprints series. Focuses on high-yield topics. Explanations are easy to follow. **Cons:** Not comprehensive; use as a supplement for review. Sparse images. Some questions are esoteric and not boards-like. Expensive: number of questions few for the cost of the book. **Summary:** Organized and easy-to-read supplement. Adds clinical correlates to the Blueprints series.

B **Surgery: Review for the New National Boards**
Geelhoed

$25.00 Test/562 q

J&S, 1995, 1st edition, 246 pages, ISBN 0963287354
Question-and-answer review of surgery. **Pros:** Good focus on high-yield topics. Very good explanations. Classic illustrations. **Cons:** Lacks the lengthy clinical vignette style typical of Step 2. **Summary:** Appropriate review of Step 2-relevant content, but questions do not reflect current USMLE format.

B **PreTest Surgery**
Geller

$21.95 Test/500 q

McGraw-Hill, 2001, 9th edition, 328 pages, ISBN 0070525331
Question-and-answer-format review of topics in general surgery. **Pros:** Predominantly case based. Well organized by subspecialty. **Cons:** Many questions are too detailed or esoteric and do not reflect boards style. Some explanations are overly detailed. **Summary:** Thorough review, but questions may be beyond the level needed for Step 2 preparation.

B **NMS Surgery**
Jarrell

$31.95 Review/350 q

Lippincott Williams & Wilkins, 2000, 4th edition, 720 pages, ISBN 0683306154
Outline review of general surgery and surgical subspecialties. **Pros:** Well organized and thorough. Vignette-style questions after each chapter, with good explanations. **Cons:** Dense, detailed text. Few tables or illustrations. **Summary:** Comprehensive surgery review, but very time-consuming. More appropriate for clerkship than for boards review.

B Surgery 1

$32.00   Review/120 q

Lavelle-Jones

Saunders, 1997, 1st edition, 207 pages, ISBN 0443051720

Text review of general surgery with illustrations and questions. **Pros:** Concise, well-organized text. Excellent illustrations and radiographs. Illustrative case vignettes. **Cons:** Need *Surgery 2* to complete review of surgery. Questions are not boards style. Not updated in several years. **Summary:** Excellent review with classic illustrations, but incomplete without *Surgery 2* title.

B Blueprints Clinical Cases in Surgery

$18.95   Test/200 q

Li

Blackwell Science, 2002, 1st edition, 134 pages, ISBN 0632046074

Compendium of vignette-type cases arranged by symptom followed by related questions and answers. **Pros:** Excellent companion to the Blueprints series. Focuses on high-yield cases. Easy to read with nice illustrations and review of management. **Cons:** Not comprehensive; use as a supplement for review. Few illustrations. **Summary:** Organized and easy-to-read supplement. Adds clinical correlates to the Blueprints series.

B− BRS Surgical Specialties

$25.95   Review/150 q

Crabtree

Lippincott Williams & Wilkins, 2000, 1st edition, 288 pages, ISBN 0781727715

Focused review of topics in the surgical subspecialties in outline format. **Pros:** Good emphasis for boards and wards. Good use of illustrations. Vignette-style review questions. **Cons:** Some information may be redundant from review of other topics. Some information may be beyond the scope of the Step 2 exam. **Summary:** For the advanced surgery student.

B− Abernathy's Surgical Secrets

$39.00   Review

Harken

Lippincott Williams & Wilkins, 2000, 4th edition, 300 pages, ISBN 1560533633

Question-and-answer Secrets series format. **Pros:** Discussions are up to date and thorough. **Cons:** Too detailed for purposes of the USMLE, yet not comprehensive. **Summary:** Not a well-organized review. Better suited to clerkship than to boards preparation.

B− Pocket Surgery

$24.95   Review

Wrightson

Blackwell Science, 2002, 1st edition, 291 pages, ISBN 0632046155

Review of high-yield surgical material in outline format. **Pros:** Fast, easy read. Portable. Highlights high-yield information in "fact boxes." **Cons:** Some material is not detailed enough. No illustrations. **Summary:** Good for rapid review during clerkship. Does not contain enough detailed information to be used as a single study source for the boards.

Surgery at a Glance   **$26.95**   Review

Grace

Blackwell Science, 2002, 2nd edition, 176 pages, ISBN 0632059885

Review of clinical presentations and surgical diseases in outline format.
Pros: Images and tables easy to follow. Nice review of differential diagnoses and management. **Cons:** Pathophysiology of disease is not covered in detail. Information frequently sparse or vague. No vignettes or illustrations. Outline format may not be suitable for everyone. **Summary:** Good review in rapid manner.

 Oklahoma Notes General Surgery   **$19.95**   Review/168 q

Jacocks

Springer-Verlag, 1996, 2nd edition, 189 pages, ISBN 0387946373

Outline format for surgery. **Pros:** Inexpensive, quick read. **Cons:** Text lacks high-yield details and illustrations. Questions lack vignettes and explanations. **Summary:** Below-average resource for this subject.

MEPC Surgery   **$21.95**   Test/700 q

Metzler

McGraw-Hill, 1995, 11th edition, 317 pages, ISBN 0838561950

Question-and-answer self-examination for surgery. **Pros:** Questions have appropriate focus. Good explanations. Well illustrated. **Cons:** Questions do not reflect current boards format. **Summary:** Adequate source of questions for review, but does not follow boards format.

A− First Aid for the International Medical Graduate $29.95   Review
Chandler

McGraw-Hill, 2002, 1st edition, 295 pages, ISBN 0071385320
High-yield review for the IMG on how to pass the USMLE boards and
adapt to medical culture in the United States. **Pros:** Comprehensive,
well-organized review. **Cons:** May need to obtain additional information
from other sources. **Summary:** Excellent review of material for the IMG.
Best used as a primer for boards review.

A− The IMG's Guide to Mastering the USMLE $29.95   Test/500 q
& Residency
Chandler

McGraw-Hill, 2000, 1st edition, 310 pages, ISBN 0071347240
Comprehensive guide for IMGs that navigates the complicated process of
training in the United States. Includes information on visas, USMLE and
TOEFL exams, the CSA exam, and applying to residencies, with emphasis
on overcoming the many obstacles that IMGs face along the way. Also
provides practical advice on establishing a home in the United States, residency survival skills, and finding a job.

N Dermatology for Boards and Wards $25.00   Review
Ayala

Blackwell Science, 2001, 96 pages, ISBN 0632045728
Not yet reviewed or rated.

N Immunology for Boards and Wards $15.00   Review
Ayala

Blackwell Science, 2001, 80 pages, ISBN 0632045744
Not yet reviewed or rated.

REVIEW RESOURCES

Miscellaneous

REVIEW RESOURCES

Miscellaneous

Commercial Review Courses

Commercial preparation courses can be helpful for some students, but these courses are expensive and require significant time commitment. They are usually effective in organizing study material for students who feel overwhelmed by the volume of material. Note that multiweek courses may be quite intense and may thus leave limited time for independent study. Also note that some commercial courses are designed for first-time test takers while others focus on students who are repeating the examination. In addition, some courses focus on IMGs who want to take all three Steps in a limited amount of time. Student experience and satisfaction with review courses are highly variable. We suggest that you discuss options with recent graduates of the review courses you are considering. Course content and structure can change rapidly. Some student opinions can be found in discussion groups on the World Wide Web. Below is contact information for some Step 2 commercial review courses.

Kaplan Medical　　　　　　　　　　　　$129–$999　　Center/Online
700 South Flower Street
Los Angeles, CA 90017
800-KAP-TEST (800-527-8378)
800-533-8850
www.kaplanmedical.com/usmle

Kaplan Medical offers a compilation of center-based and online programs for USMLE Step 2 review. Courses include diagnostic testing with computer feedback and comprehensive lecture notes. Questions can be arranged by topic. Tests are timed to simulate boards conditions. An extensive number of questions are in vignette format. The content level of questions reflects boards tests. Explanations are thorough and allow student to identify strong and weak points. In summary, one of the best question-and-answer tools to prepare for Step 2, but very costly.

Northwestern Medical Review　　　　　　$860　　　　　Center
P.O. Box 22174
East Lansing, MI 48909-2174
866-MedPass (866-633-7277)
contact@northwesternmedicalreview.com
www.northwesternmedicalreview.com

Northwestern Medical Review offers an eight-day, eight-hour-per-day USMLE review program designed for current medical students, graduating MDs, and IMGs. In addition to a comprehensive clinical review, the course targets high-yield subjects, concepts, and notions that are likely to be tested on the exam. Review subjects of the course are internal medicine, obstetrics and gynecology, pediatrics, preventive medicine, public health, epidemiology, psychiatry, neurology, surgery, and practice tests.

Postgraduate Medical Review Education (PMRE)　$980　　　　　Books/Audiotapes
407 Lincoln Road, Suite 12E
Miami Beach, FL 33139
800-433-3539
sales@pmre.com
www.pmre.com

PMRE has been preparing medical students for its licensing exams for 26 years. The program offers live classes, video classes, audio tapes, books, and tutorial classes. The home study materials have key topics and mnemonics that make learning easy. The material is written by professors from schools such as Harvard, Yale, New York University, and Columbia University. Some of these professors have written questions and answers for boards exams.

REVIEW RESOURCES

Commercial Courses

Youel's Prep, Inc.
P.O. Box 4605
West Palm Beach, FL 33402
800-645-3985
Fax: 561-366-8628
YouelsPrep@bellsouth.net
www.youelsprep.com

Youel's Prep, Inc., has specialized in medical board preparation for more than 25 years. Preparation includes webcasts, videotapes, audiotapes, books, live lectures, and tutorials for small groups and for individuals. Courses focus on test-relevant topics, including high-yield facts and how to remember those facts and use them during test time. Courses includes 40 hours of videotaped or audiotaped lectures and two books. Lectures are held at select medical schools at the invitation of the school and students. The program includes telephone tutoring by Dr. Youel.

REVIEW RESOURCES

Commercial Courses

Abbreviations and Symbols

Abbreviation	Meaning
ABC	airway, breathing, circulation
ABG	arterial blood gas
ABI	ankle-brachial index
ACA	anterior cerebral artery
ACE	angiotensin-converting enzyme
ACEI	ACE inhibitor
ACh	acetylcholine
ACL	anterior cruciate ligament
Acom	anterior communicating artery
ACTH	adrenocorticotropic hormone
AD	Alzheimer's disease
ADA	Americans with Disabilities Act
ADH	antidiuretic hormone
ADHD	attention-deficit hyperactivity disorder
AF	atrial fibrillation
AFI	amniotic fluid index
AFP	α-fetoprotein
AIDS	acquired immunodeficiency syndrome
ALL	acute lymphocytic leukemia
ALS	amyotrophic lateral sclerosis
ALT	alanine transaminase
AML	acute myelogenous leukemia
ANA	antinuclear antibody
ANCA	antineutrophil cytoplasmic antibody
AP	anteroposterior
AR	attributable risk
ARC	Appalachian Regional Commission
ARDS	acute respiratory distress syndrome
ARF	acute renal failure
AS	ankylosing spondylitis
ASA	acetylsalicylic acid [aspirin]
ASCUS	atypical squamous cells of undetermined significance
ASD	atrial septal defect
ASO	antistreptolysin O
AST	aspartate transaminase
AT	angiotensin
ATN	acute tubular necrosis
ATPase	adenosine triphosphatase
AV	arteriovenous, atrioventricular
AVM	arteriovenous malformation
AVN	avascular necrosis
AXR	abdominal x-ray
AZT	azidothymidine [zidovudine]
BCG	bacille Calmette-Guérin
bid	twice a day
BMA	bone marrow aspiration
BMT	bone marrow transplant
BP	blood pressure
BPH	benign prostatic hyperplasia
BPP	biophysical profile
BPPV	benign paroxysmal positional vertigo
BRBPR	bright red blood per rectum
BSA	body surface area

Abbreviation	Meaning
BSE	breast self-examination
BUN	blood urea nitrogen
CABG	coronary artery bypass graft
CAD	coronary artery disease
CAH	congenital adrenal hyperplasia
CBC	complete blood count
CBGD	cortical-basal ganglionic degeneration
CBT	cognitive-behavioral therapy, computer-based test
CF	cystic fibrosis
CGD	chronic granulomatous disease
CHF	congestive heart failure
CIN	Candidate Identification Number, cervical intraepithelial neoplasia
CIS	carcinoma in situ
CJD	Creutzfeldt-Jakob disease
CK	creatine phosphokinase
CK-MB	creatine phosphokinase, MB fraction
CLL	chronic lymphocytic leukemia
CML	chronic myelogenous leukemia
CMT	cervical motion tenderness
CMV	cytomegalovirus
CN	cranial nerve
CNS	central nervous system
COGME	Council on Graduate Medical Education
COM	communication
COPD	chronic obstructive pulmonary disease
COX	cyclooxygenase
CP	cerebral palsy
CPAP	continuous positive airway pressure
CPR	cardiopulmonary resuscitation
Cr	creatinine
CSA	Clinical Skills Assessment
CSD	combined system disease
CSF	cerebrospinal fluid
CST	contraction stress test
CT	computed tomography
CVA	cerebrovascular accident, costovertebral angle
CVP	central venous pressure
CVS	chorionic villus sampling
CXR	chest x-ray
D&C	dilatation and curettage
DA	dopamine
DBP	diastolic blood pressure
DCIS	ductal carcinoma in situ
DDAVP	1-deamino-8-D-arginine vasopressin
DDH	developmental dysplasia of the hip
DES	diethylstilbestrol
DEXA	dual-energy x-ray absorptiometry
DG	data gathering
DHEA	dehydroepiandrosterone
DHEAS	dehydroepiandrosterone sulfate
DI	diabetes insipidus

Abbreviation	Meaning	Abbreviation	Meaning
DIC	disseminated intravascular coagulation	GDM	gestational diabetes mellitus
DIP	distal interphalangeal [joint]	GERD	gastroesophageal reflux disease
DJD	degenerative joint disease	GFR	glomerular filtration rate
DKA	diabetic ketoacidosis	GGT	gamma glutamyl transferase
DM	diabetes mellitus	GI	gastrointestinal
DMD	Duchenne muscular dystrophy	GMP	guanosine monophosphate
DNI	do not intubate	GNR	gram-negative rod
DNR	do not resuscitate	GnRH	gonadotropin-releasing hormone
DOE	dyspnea on exertion	GTD	gestational trophoblastic disease
DPL	diagnostic peritoneal lavage	GTT	glucose tolerance test
DPOA	durable power of attorney	GU	genitourinary
DRE	digital rectal examination	GVHD	graft-versus-host disease
DS	double strength	H&P	history and physical
DTaP	diphtheria, tetanus, pertussis [vaccine]	HAV	hepatitis A virus
DTs	delirium tremens	Hb	hemoglobin
DTR	deep tendon reflex	HBV	hepatitis B virus
DUB	dysfunctional uterine bleeding	hCG	human chorionic gonadotropin
DVT	deep venous thrombosis	HCT	hematocrit
DWI	diffusion-weighted imaging	HCV	hepatitis C virus
EBV	Epstein-Barr virus	HDL	high-density lipoprotein
EC	endocervical curettage	HDV	hepatitis D virus
ECFMG	Educational Commission for Foreign Medical Graduates	HGPRT	hypoxanthine-guanine phosphoribosyltransferase
ECG	electrocardiogram	HHNK	hyperosmolar hyperglycemic nonketotic [coma]
ECMO	extracorporeal membrane oxygenation	HHS	[U.S. Department of] Health and Human Services
ECT	electroconvulsive therapy		
ED	erectile dysfunction	HHV	human herpesvirus
EDD	estimated date of delivery	Hib	*Haemophilus influenzae* type B
EEG	electroencephalogram	HIDA	hepato-iminodiacetic acid [scan]
EF	ejection fraction	HIV	human immunodeficiency virus
EGD	esophagogastroduodenoscopy	HLA	human leukocyte antigen
ELISA	enzyme-linked immunosorbent assay	HMG-CoA	hydroxymethylglutaryl-coenzyme A
EMB	endometrial biopsy	HNPCC	hereditary nonpolyposis colorectal cancer
EMG	electromyogram		
EPS	extrapyramidal symptoms	HPA	hypothalamic-pituitary axis
ERAS	Electronic Residency Application Service	hpf	high-power field
		HPL	human placental lactogen
ERCP	endoscopic retrograde cholangiopancreatography	HPSA	Health Professional Shortage Area
		HPV	human papillomavirus
ESR	erythrocyte sedimentation rate	HR	heart rate
ESRD	end-stage renal disease	HRT	hormone replacement therapy
EtOH	ethanol	HSIL	high-grade squamous intraepithelial lesion
FAP	familial adenomatous polyposis		
Fe$_{Na}$	fractional excretion of sodium	HSV	herpes simplex virus
FEV	forced expiratory volume	5-HT	5-hydroxytryptamine
FFP	fresh frozen plasma	HTLV	human T-cell leukemia virus
FHR	fetal heart rate	HTN	hypertension
FMG	foreign medical graduate	HUS	hemolytic-uremic syndrome
FNA	fine-needle aspiration	HVA	homovanillic acid
FOBT	fecal occult blood test	IBD	inflammatory bowel disease
FSH	follicle-stimulating hormone	IBS	irritable bowel syndrome
FSMB	Federation of State Medical Boards	ICE	Integrated Clinical Encounter
FTA-ABS	fluorescent treponemal antibody-absorbed	ICP	intracranial pressure
		ICU	intensive care unit
FTT	failure to thrive	IDDM	insulin-dependent diabetes mellitus
5-FU	5-fluorouracil	IE	infective endocarditis
FUO	fever of unknown origin	IFN	interferon
FVC	forced vital capacity	IGF	insuline-like growth factor
G6PD	glucose-6-phosphate dehydrogenase	IHSS	idiopathic hypertrophic subaortic stenosis
GA	gestational age		
GAD	generalized anxiety disorder	IMA	inferior mesenteric artery
GBM	glioblastoma multiforme, glomerular basement membrane	IMG	international medical graduate
		INH	isoniazid
GBS	group B streptococcus, Guillain-Barré syndrome	INR	International Normalized Ratio

Abbreviation	Meaning	Abbreviation	Meaning
INS	Immigration and Naturalization Service	MMPI	Minnesota Multiphasic Personality Inventory
IPV	inactivated polio vaccine	MMR	measles, mumps, rubella [vaccine]
IR	incidence rate	MoM	multiple of the median
ISA	intrinsic sympathomimetic activity	MR	mental retardation
ITP	idiopathic thrombocytopenic purpura	MRA	magnetic resonance angiography
IUD	intrauterine device	MRI	magnetic resonance imaging
IUGR	intrauterine growth retardation	MS	multiple sclerosis
IV	intravenous	MSA	multiple-system atrophy
IVC	inferior vena cava	MSAFP	maternal serum α-fetoprotein
IVDU	IV drug use, IV drug user	MTP	metatarsophalangeal [joint]
IVIG	intravenous immunoglobulin	MVA	motor vehicle accident
IVP	intravenous pyelogram	NBME	National Board of Medical Examiners
IWA	Interactive Web Application	NCV	nerve conduction velocity
JG	juxtaglomerular	NE	norepinephrine
JVD	jugular venous distention	NF	neurofibromatosis
KOH	potassium hydroxide	NG	nasogastric
KUB	kidney, ureter, bladder	NIDDM	non-insulin-dependent diabetes mellitus
LA	left atrial	NNT	number needed to treat
LAD	left anterior descending [artery]	NPH	normal pressure hydrocephalus
LAP	leukocyte alkaline phosphatase	NPO	nil per os [nothing by mouth]
LBBB	left bundle branch block	NS	normal saline
LBO	large bowel obstruction	NSAID	nonsteroidal anti-inflammatory drug
LBP	low back pain	NSCLC	non–small cell lung cancer
LCIS	lobular carcinoma in situ	NST	nonstress test
LCL	lateral collateral ligament	NYHA	New York Heart Association
LCME	Liaison Committee for Medical Education	O_2	oxygen
LCP	Legg-Calvé-Perthes disorder	OA	osteoarthritis
LDH	lactate dehydrogenase	OCD	obsessive-compulsive disorder
LDL	low-density lipoprotein	OCP	oral contraceptive pill
LEEP	loop electrosurgical excision procedure	OPV	oral polio vaccine
LES	lower esophageal sphincter	OR	odds ratio, operating room
LFT	liver function test	ORIF	open reduction and internal fixation
LH	luteinizing hormone	PCA	posterior cerebral artery
LHF	left heart failure	PCKD	polycystic kidney disease
LLQ	left lower quadrant	PCL	posterior cruciate ligament
LMN	lower motor neuron	PCOS	polycystic ovarian syndrome
LMP	last menstrual period	Pcom	posterior communicating artery
LMWH	low-molecular-weight heparin	PCP	phencyclidine hydrochloride, *Pneumocystis carinii* pneumonia
LOC	loss of consciousness		
LP	lumbar puncture	PCR	polymerase chain reaction
LR	lactated Ringer's	PCV	pneumococcal conjugate vaccine
LSIL	low-grade squamous intraepithelial lesion	PD	posterior descending [artery]
		PDA	patent ductus arteriosus
LUQ	left upper quadrant	PE	pulmonary embolism
LV	left ventricle, left ventricular	PEA	pulseless electrical activity
LVEDP	left ventricular end-diastolic pressure	PEEP	positive end-expiratory pressure
LVH	left ventricular hypertrophy	PFT	pulmonary function test
MAOI	monoamine oxidase inhibitor	PG	prostaglandin
MAST	military anti-shock trousers	PID	pelvic inflammatory disease
MAT	multifocal atrial tachycardia	PIP	proximal interphalangeal [joint]
MCA	middle cerebral artery	PIV	parainfluenza virus
MCL	medial collateral ligament	PMI	point of maximal impulse
MCP	metacarpophalangeal [joint]	PMN	polymorphonuclear [leukocyte]
MCTD	mixed connective tissue disease	PMR	polymyalgia rheumatica
MCV	mean corpuscular volume	PN	patient note
MDD	major depressive disorder	PND	paroxysmal nocturnal dyspnea
MDE	major depressive episode	PO	per os [by mouth]
MEN	multiple endocrine neoplasia	POC	products of conception
$MgSO_4$	magnesium sulfate	POD	postoperative day
MGUS	monoclonal gammopathy of undetermined significance	PPD	purified protein derivative [of tuberculin]
		PPI	proton pump inhibitor
MHA-TP	microhemagglutination assay-*Treponema pallidum*	prn	as needed
		PROM	premature rupture of membranes
MI	myocardial infarction	PSA	prostate-specific antigen

Abbreviation	Meaning	Abbreviation	Meaning
PSP	progressive supranuclear palsy	SV	stroke volume
PT	prothrombin time	SVT	supraventricular tachycardia
PTCA	percutaneous transluminal coronary angioplasty	T_3	triiodothyronine
		T_4	thyroxine
PTH	parathyroid hormone	TA	temporal arteritis
PTSD	post-traumatic stress disorder	TAH-BSO	total abdominal hysterectomy and bilateral salpingo-oophorectomy
PTT	partial thromboplastin time		
PTU	propylthiouracil	TB	tuberculosis
PUBS	percutaneous umbilical blood sampling	TBG	thyroxine-binding globulin
PUD	peptic ulcer disease	TCA	tricyclic antidepressant
PVC	premature ventricular contraction	TD	tardive dyskinesia
PVD	peripheral vascular disease	TE	transesophageal
qd	every day	TEE	transesophageal echocardiography
RA	rheumatoid arthritis	TEF	tracheoesophageal fistula
RAAS	renin-angiotensin-aldosterone system	TENS	transcutaneous electrical nerve stimulation
RBBB	right bundle branch block		
RBC	red blood cell	TFT	thyroid function test
RCA	right coronary artery	TG	triglyceride
RCC	renal cell carcinoma	TIA	transient ischemic attack
RCT	randomized clinical trial	TIBC	total iron-binding capacity
RDS	respiratory distress syndrome	TIPS	transjugular intrahepatic portosystemic shunt
REM	rapid eye movement		
RF	rheumatoid factor, risk factor	TLC	therapeutic lifestyle changes, total lung capacity
RHF	right heart failure		
RLQ	right lower quadrant	TM	tympanic membrane
ROM	range of motion, rupture of membranes	TMP-SMX	trimethoprim-sulfamethoxazole
RPR	rapid plasma reagin	TOA	tubo-ovarian abscess
RR	relative risk, respiratory rate	TOEFL	Test of English as a Foreign Language
RSV	respiratory syncytial virus	tPA	tissue plasminogen activator
RTA	renal tubular acidosis	TPN	total parenteral nutrition
RUQ	right upper quadrant	TRH	thyrotropin-releasing hormone
RV	residual volume, right ventricle	TSH	thyroid-stimulating hormone
RVRR	renal vein renin ratio	TSS	toxic shock syndrome
SA	sinoatrial	TSST	toxic shock syndrome toxin
SAAG	serum ascites albumin gradient	TTP	thrombotic thrombocytopenic purpura
SAB	spontaneous abortion	TURP	transurethral resection of the prostate
SAH	subarachnoid hemorrhage	UA	urinalysis
SBO	small bowel obstruction	UMN	upper motor neuron
SBP	systolic blood pressure	UPEP	urinary protein electrophoresis
SCC	squamous cell carcinoma	URI	upper respiratory infection
SCD	sickle cell disease	U/S	ultrasound
SCID	severe combined immunodeficiency	USDA	U.S. Department of Agriculture
SCLC	small cell lung cancer	USIA	United States Information Agency
SD	standard deviation	USMLE	United States Medical Licensing Examination
SEM	systolic ejection murmur		
SIADH	syndrome of inappropriate antidiuretic hormone	UTI	urinary tract infection
		UV	ultraviolet
SIL	squamous intraepithelial lesion	VA	Veterans Administration
SIRS	systemic inflammatory response syndrome	VC	vital capacity
		VCUG	voiding cystourethrogram
SLE	systemic lupus erythematosus	VDRL	Venereal Disease Research Laboratory
SMA	superior mesenteric artery	VF	ventricular fibrillation
SOB	shortness of breath	VMA	vanillylmandelic acid
SP	standardized patient	VSD	ventricular septal defect
SPEP	serum protein electrophoresis	VT	ventricular tachycardia
SRP	sponsoring residency program	VZV	varicella-zoster virus
SS	single strength	WBC	white blood cell
SSRI	selective serotonin reuptake inhibitor	WPW	Wolff-Parkinson-White [syndrome]
STD	sexually transmitted disease		

Index

Pages followed by f indicate figure. Pages followed by t indicate table.

Human chorionic gonadotropin (hCG)
(*continued*)
   pelvic inflammatory disease, 359
   testicular cancer, 472
   uterine bleeding, abnormal,
      348
Humerus fracture, 266t
Hunter's syndrome, 373
Huntington's disease
   CAG triplet repeats on chromosome
      4p, 294
   differential, 294
   evaluation, 294
   history/pe, 294
   treatment, 294
Hurler's syndrome, 373
Hutchinson's triad, 221
Hydantoins, 103
Hydatidiform mole, 318, 333
Hydralazine, 71t, 73, 262
Hydrocephalus, 221
Hydrochloroquine, 98
Hydrochlorothiazide, 462t
Hydrocortisone, 102, 232
Hydronephrosis, 320t
Hydrops fetalis, 333
Hydrotherapy, 256
Hydroxychloroquine, 261, 263
11-hydroxylase, 122
17-hydroxylase, 122
21-hydroxylase, 121, 122
Hydroxyproline, 258
Hydroxyurea, 198, 204
Hymen, 349t
Hyperaldosteronism
   differential, 121
   evaluation, 121
   history/pe, 121
   hypokalemia, 458
   treatment, 121
Hyperbilirubinemia, 388, 391, 392
Hypercalcemia
   acute pancreatitis, 184t
   causes, common, 458
   evaluation, 458
   history/pe, 458
   hyperparathyroidism, 127
   multiple myeloma, 206
   sarcoidosis, 445
   treatment, 459
Hypercalciuria, 127, 445
Hypercapnea, 52
Hypercarotenemia, 410
Hypercholesterolemia
   cholesterol increase leads to coro-
      nary artery disease, 64
   etiologies, 65
   evaluation, 65
   history/pe, 65
   stroke, 302, 305
Hypercoagulable states
   causes, common, 202t
   deep venous thrombosis, 77
   nephrotic syndrome, 462
   overview, 201

pulmonary embolism, 443
   stroke, 303
Hypercortisolism, 119
Hyperemesis gravidarum, 326, 333
Hyperglycemia
   Cushing's syndrome, 119
   diabetic ketoacidosis, 116
   diuretics, 71t
   gestational diabetes mellitus, 326
Hyperkalemia
   ACE inhibitors, 71t
   adrenal insufficiency, 120
   angiotensin II receptor antagonists,
      71t
   evaluation, 457, 457f
   history/pe, 457
   treatment, 457–458
Hyperkeratosis, 96, 106
Hyperlipidemia, 462
Hypernatremia
   diabetes insipidus, 467
   evaluation, 456
   history/pe, 456
   hyperaldosteronism, 121
   treatment, 456
Hyperosmolar nonketotic coma, 124,
      125
Hyperosmolar states, 299
Hyperparathyroidism
   differential, 127
   evaluation, 127
   history/pe, 126–127
   hypercalcemia, 458
   multiple myeloma, 206
   stones, 465
   treatment, 127
Hyperpigmentation, 321t
Hyperprolactinemia, 349t, 417
Hypersensitivity. *See also* Contact der-
      matitis
   anaphylactic and atopic, 84
   Arthus reaction, 84
   cytotoxic, 84
   delayed, 84
   immune complex, 84
   serum sickness, 84
Hypersensitivity pneumonitis
   antigens of, 436t
   differential, 437
   evaluation, 437
   exam, physical, 436
   history, 436
   treatment, 437
Hypertension
   acromegaly, 127
   acute renal failure, 460
   angina pectoris, 66
   aorta, coarctation of the, 376
   aortic aneurysms, 75
   aortic dissection, 487
   congestive heart failure, 62
   Cushing's syndrome, 119
   defining terms, 69
   erectile dysfunction, 472
   gestational, 327–328

gestational trophoblastic disease, 333
   hyperaldosteronism, 121
   hypercholesterolemia, 65
   left bundle branch block, 56t
   monoamine oxidase inhibitors, 413
   nephritic syndrome, 461, 462
   neuroblastoma, 117, 395
   parenchymal hemorrhage, 291
   pheochromocytoma, 122
   polycystic kidney disease, 466
   polycystic ovarian syndrome, 364
   portal, 155, 180–182, 181t
   primary
      agents, major classes of antihyper-
         tensive, 71t
      complications, 72
      differential/evaluation, 69–70
      history/pe, 69
      measurements, classification/ in-
         terpretation of blood pressure,
         69, 70f
      treatment, 70, 70t–71t
   scleroderma, 262
   secondary, 72
   seizures, 299
   sleep apnea, 446
   stroke, 302, 305
   urgency/emergency, hypertensive
      defining terms, 72
      evaluation, 72
      treatment, 73
   vulvar cancer, 360
Hyperthermia, 116, 217, 299
Hyperthyroidism
   causes, common, 129
   differential, 130
   evaluation, 130
   exam, physical, 130, 130f
   gestational trophoblastic disease,
      333
   history, 129
   propylthiouracil, 118
   treatment, 130
Hypertrophic cardiomyopathy
   evaluation, 62
   history/pe, 61
   treatment, 62
Hypertrophy and systolic dysfunction,
      63
Hyperuricemia, 71t
Hypnosis, 405
Hypoalbuminemia, 462
Hypocalcemia
   acute pancreatitis, 184t
   etiologies, 459
   evaluation, 459
   history/pe, 459
   seizures, 299
   treatment, 459
Hypocarbia, 443
Hypochloremic-hypokalemic meta-
      bolic alkalosis, 381
Hypochondriasis, 421t
Hypoglycemia, 120, 299, 305
Hypogonadism, 182, 473

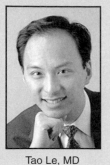
Tao Le, MD

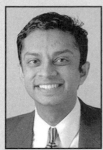
Vikas Bhushan, MD

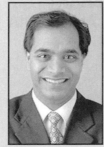
Chirag Amin, MD

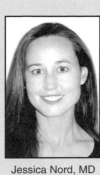
Jennifer LaFemina, MD

Jessica Nord, MD

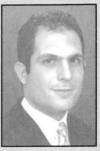
Nader Pouratian, MD

Tao Le, MD

Dr. Le has led multiple medical education projects over the past seven years. As a medical student, he was editor-in-chief of the University of California, San Francisco Synapse, a university newspaper with a weekly circulation of 9,000. Subsequently, he authored *First Aid for the Wards* and *First Aid for the Match* and led the most recent revision of *First Aid for the USMLE Step 2*. At Yale, he was a regular guest lecturer on the USMLE review courses and an adviser to the Yale University School of Medicine curriculum committee. Dr. Le earned his medical degree from the University of California, San Francisco in 1996 and completed his residency training and board certification in internal medicine at Yale-New Haven Hospital. Dr. Le subsequently went on to co-found Medsn and currently serves as its Chief Medical Officer.

Vikas Bhushan, MD

Dr. Bhushan is a world-renowned author, publisher, entrepreneur, and board-certified diagnostic radiologist who resides in Los Angeles, California. Dr. Bhushan conceived and authored the original *First Aid for the USMLE Step 1* in 1992, which, after ten consecutive editions, has become the most popular medical review book in the world. Following this, he co-authored and led three additional *First Aid* books as well as the development of the highly acclaimed 17-title *Underground Clinical Vignettes* series. He was an active researcher in medical informatics and digital radiology and completed his training in diagnostic radiology at the University of California, Los Angeles. Dr. Bhushan has more than 12 years of entrepreneurial experience and started two successful software and publishing companies prior to co-founding Medsn. Over the course of his career, he has worked directly with dozens of medical school faculty members, colleagues, and consultants and corresponded with well over a thousand medical students from around the world. Dr. Bhushan earned his bachelor's degree in biochemistry from the University of California, Berkeley, and his MD with thesis from the University of California, San Francisco.

Chirag Amin, MD

Dr. Amin has extensive experience in the field of medical education and has served as a co-author with Drs. Bhushan and Le on the entire *First Aid* series. He also led the completion of *The Insider's Guide to the MCAT,* published by Lippincott Williams & Wilkins. Dr. Amin has an extensive background in Internet-related enterprises; he actively follows a number of development-stage Internet companies. Dr. Amin earned his BS in biology at the University of Illinois in 1992. He then went on to get his MD with Research Distinction from the University of Miami School of Medicine in 1996 and completed three years of residency training in orthopedic surgery at Orlando Regional Medical Center.

Jennifer LaFemina, MD

Jennifer recently graduated from the University of California at Los Angeles School of Medicine and will be moving to the freezing winters of Boston to complete her surgical residency at Massachusetts General Hospital. She has a research interest in soft-tissue tumors and hopes to pursue a career in Surgical Oncology. She is originally from Thousand Oaks, CA and went to the University of California at Irvine, where she received her BS in Biological Sciences. She would like to thank her parents, Michael and Florence, as well as her siblings, Michael, Steven, and Maureen, not only for helping her move to Boston (just kidding!!), but also, for their support and love. She can be contacted at jlafemin@yahoo.com.

Jessica Nord, MD

Jessica graduated from the UCLA School of Medicine in 2002. After taking a year off to travel, do research, and enjoy life before internship, she is entering a Psychiatry residency at UCLA-NPI. A Northern California native, she attended Harvard University where she studied Psychology and developed an aversion to cold weather. She now lives happily near the beach in Santa Monica with her husband and two cats and plans to stay put. This is her second year working on the First Aid series.

Nader Pouratian, MD

Nader just completed medical school at the UCLA School of Medicine and is beginning his neurosurgical residency at the University of Virginia. Nader earned a BS in Neuroscience in 1996 from UCLA, where he started to develop an interest in brain mapping and linguistics. During medical school, he continued research in these areas, earning a Ph.D. in Neuroscience, with an emphasis in brain mapping. Nader has a keen interest in developing and implementing new brain mapping techniques and analysis methods to improve neurosurgical guidance and outcomes, especially with respect to understanding the organization of language in the human brain and preserving language in neurosurgical patients. Nader has also been extensively involved in teaching, at the high school, undergraduate, and medical school levels. To date, he has authored over 40 abstracts, 10 papers, and 3 book chapters. This is Nader's second book in the First Aid series.

About the Authors

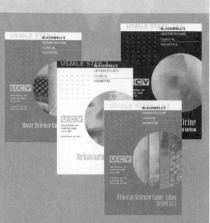
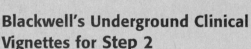